Essential
Life
Choices

HEALTH CONCEPTS AND STRATEGIES

Essential Life Choices

HEALTH CONCEPTS AND STRATEGIES

Eleanor Noss Whitney and **Frances Sienkiewicz Sizer**
with
Lori Waite Turner

West Publishing Company
St. Paul   New York   Los Angeles   San Francisco

Copyediting: Elaine Levin
Illustrations: Cyndie Clark-Huegel, Wayne Clark, John Waller, Judy Waller, Darwen Hennings, Vally Hennings, Carlisle Graphics, Rolin Graphics
Cartoons: Gary Carroll, Robert Celander, William Celander
Composition: Carlise Graphics
Cover Art: Edward Hopper. *Grand Swell*, 1939. Oil, 36½″ × 50¼″. The Corcoran Gallery of Art, Washington, D.C.

Library of Congress Cataloging-in-Publication Data

Whitney, Eleanor Noss.
   Essential life choices/Eleanor Noss Whitney, Frances Sienkiewicz Sizer.
      p.   cm.
   Includes index.
   ISBN 0–314–47686–5
   1. Health.   I. Sizer, Frances Sienkiewicz.   II. Title.
RA776.W563   1989
613—dc19   88-33327
                                                                              CIP

Acknowledgements and Photo Credit appear following the index.

Look to this day!
For it is life,
the very life of life.
In its brief course
lie all the verities
and realities of your existence . . .
For yesterday is already a dream,
and tomorrow is only a vision;
But today, well lived,
makes every yesterday
a dream of happiness,
and every tomorrow
a vision of hope.

From the Sanskrit

About the Authors

Eleanor Noss Whitney, PhD, RD received her BA in biology from Radcliffe College in 1960 and her PhD in biology with an emphasis on genetics from Washington University, St. Louis, in 1970. She has taught community classes and workshops in health, weight control, and addiction recovery and has served as a paraprofessional counselor in the treatment of people with alcoholism. Formerly an associate professor of nutrition at the Florida State University, she now devotes full time to research, writing, and consulting in nutrition and health. Her publications include articles in *Science,* the *Journal of Nutrition, Genetics,* and other journals, and the textbooks *Nutrition: Concepts and Controversies* and *Understanding Nutrition* among others. She is president of Nutrition and Health Associates and cofounder of the Coastal Plains Institute, a foundation that conducts environmental education projects in North Florida.

Frances Sienkiewicz Sizer, MS, RD attended Florida State University where, in 1980, she received her BS, and in 1982, her MS in nutrition. She has counseled clients in the University's stress-reduction clinic and served as nutrition consultant to schools and alcoholism programs in Florida. She coauthors the textbooks *Nutrition: Concepts and Controversies,* now in its fourth edition, and *Life Choices: Health Concepts and Strategies,* on which this book is based. She has published in *Shape* magazine, in the health newsletter *Healthline,* and in the *Journal of Chemical Senses.* She is a founding member of Nutrition and Health Associates, an information resource center in Tallahassee, Florida, and writes monographs for professionals on current topics in nutrition and health. She is a member of the American Public Health Association, the American Alliance for Health, Physical Education, Recreation, and Dance, and the Association for the Advancement of Health Education, and she is active in environmental groups in the Coastal Plains area.

Lori Waite Turner, MS, RD attended Florida State University where, in 1980, she received her BS in Food and Nutrition with a minor in physical education. In 1983 she completed her MS in Dietetics and Nutrition at Florida International University. She worked for Capitol Foods of Atlanta, Georgia where she marketed a computerized menu system to health care institutions. She served as a Therapeutic Dietitian at Kennestone Hospital in Marietta, Georgia, as Chief Clinical Dietitian for Doctors' Hospital in Coral Gables, Florida, and as a Nutrition Consultant for a Cardiac Rehabilitation program, also in Coral Gables. She has coauthored the *Instructor's Manual, Test Bank,* and *Student Activity Manual* that accompany this text, and she is a member of the American Dietetic Association. She is an active member of the Florida State University Synchronized Swim Club.

Contents in Brief

Contents

Chapter 14   Accident and Injury Prevention   280

Chapter 15   Infectious Diseases   298

Chapter 16   Heart and Artery Disease   320

Appendixes

Preface

Ten years ago, the U.S. Public Health Service completed a review of the health status of the population and established specific goals to be achieved by 1990. With 1990 just around the corner, progress has been made, but the goals still express our nation's foremost health needs:

Infants. Reduce the incidence of low birthweight and birth defects.
Children. Improve health and development patterns, reduce childhood deaths.
Young adults. Prevent accidents, prevent the misuse of alcohol and drugs, prevent unwanted pregnancies.
Adults. Reduce the incidence of stroke, heart attack, and cancer.
Older adults. Increase independence; reduce the incidence of flu and pneumonia.*

We therefore adopted these objectives as missions of this book. We describe health promotion for infants and children in the chapters on pregnancy and parenting. To address young adults' major health threats, we devote a chapter each to alcohol, other drugs, smoking, and accident and injury prevention. As for the problems of adults, the book addresses all of the educational objectives the Public Health Service identified.

This book is not intended for the public, however; it was written for the individual: you. Thus each chapter contains not only basic information (*concepts*), but also the other two elements of our title: the options that the information gives people (*choices*) and applications (*strategies*). We have set out in the margins the lists of **strategies** that accompany the text, and have gathered others into boxes throughout the chapters. Both are identifiable by the strategy logo. An objective for each chapter is not only to learn optimal health behavior, but also to learn the steps toward establishing that behavior as a routine.

Clear definitions of terms ease the mastery of information; we have made it a high priority to supply such definitions. To facilitate learning them, we have highlighted all key terms in the chapters in boldface type and defined them in end-of-chapter **glossaries. Miniglossaries,** presented at intervals throughout the chapters, contain groups of terms related to single concepts. The intent of the Miniglossaries is twofold: to ease study by presenting the information in small, manageable blocks; and to offer flexibility to the instructor who wants to assign some but not other sets of terms. The **index**

*This list was adapted from the Public Health Service implementation plans for attaining the objectives for the nation, *Public Health Reports Supplement*, September-October 1983.

serves as an alphabetical list of all glossary terms: page numbers where definitions appear are in the index in boldface type.

The book addresses the reader as a consumer, not only of health products and services, but also of health information. Strategies for evaluating health claims are offered in Chapter 1, and in **Consumer Cautions** throughout the rest of the book. Further, it is vital to distinguish between needs created by advertisers or quacks and real needs—and the **magic bullet** logo appears throughout the book to identify suspect claims. The book cites its references, modeling the characteristics of a reliable health information source. (To keep the pages uncluttered, though, the references are gathered together in Appendix D).

A theme of the book is that a person's state of health is, to a great extent, that person's own responsibility. At the same time, it is important to acknowledge that not all of life's outcomes are chosen. Each chapter makes clear what people can control (their lifestyle habits) and what they cannot (their heredity, some of the circumstances of their lives, and chance events, including some accidents). Guidelines are offered, wherever relevant, to suggest when to get help with states of mind and body that are the subjects of the chapters that follow.

Another thing we emphasize is that someone else's choices are not a person's responsibility. From teaching, we know that students often ask what they can do to persuade friends and relatives to change their behavior. No matter how much a person may want to persuade Aunt Sally to give up smoking, or a sister to quit using pills, or a spouse to go jogging, one person cannot make the choice for another. The best bet is often to keep quiet about the choices others are making. We offer suggestions in the chapters about facilitating versus enabling behavior.

The book is positive. Its emphasis is on what *to* do, not on what *not* to do, to enhance the quality of life. Therefore, the chapters on diseases make it clear how different (and how preferable) *prevention* is in comparison with *cure*. The chapters on nutrition encourage the reader, not to diet, but to eat well. The book does not suggest that people just give up destructive habits, but that they find adaptive habits to substitute for them.

The abundant thought we have put into the topics of this book has brought about changes in our own awareness and behavior. If reading the book has one-tenth of the impact on its users that writing it has had on us, it should be a successful book as we define success.

We hope it will be successful. As we define it, success is bringing about behavior change that will enhance the quality of our readers' lives.

Eleanor N. Whitney

Frances S. Sizer

January, 1989

Acknowledgments

We are grateful to our associates Linda DeBruyne and Sharon Rolfes for their support throughout the preparation of this book. We also thank Betty and Bob Geltz for the data from which Appendix E was generated. We thank our editors Kristen Weber and Peter Marshall for their many efforts in behalf of the book.

We also appreciate the efforts of our reviewers:

Judy Baker
East Carolina University

Sharon Garcia
Diablo Valley College

Mark Kittleson
Youngstown State University

Barbara Wilks
University of Georgia

Health Information and Behavior

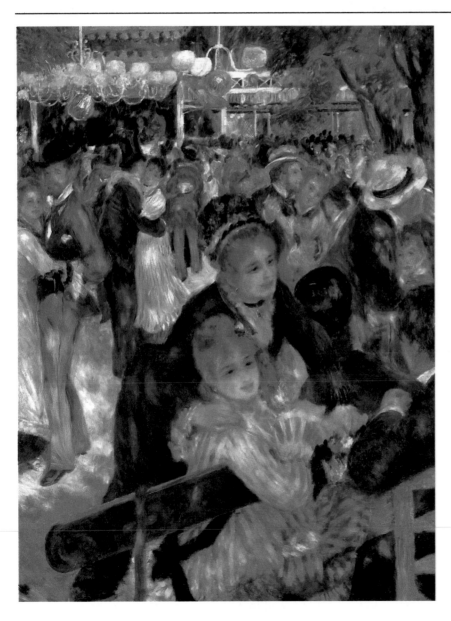

For Openers . . .

True or false? If false, say what is true.

1. Being well is best defined as being free from disease.
2. Adults catch the most prevalent diseases of today the same way as they caught malaria and smallpox in earlier times.
3. People can make themselves physiologically younger or older by the ways they choose to live.
4. Knowing how to relax can lengthen your life.
5. Women generally live longer than men do.
6. Accidents are among the major causes of death for middle-aged to older adults.
7. If a product label makes the claim "organic" or "natural," this means the product has unusual powers to promote health.
8. A person who wants to change a harmful health habit, and knows how, will do so.
9. Some people fail at making positive behavior changes because they undertake too many changes at one time.
10. You are responsible for changing the harmful health behaviors of the people you care about.

(Answers on page 16.)

health: a range of states; at a minimum, freedom from negative states such as physical disease, physical deterioration, social maladjustment, mental illness, and so on.

At a maximum, a state that some call **wellness**: the achievement of full potential mentally, emotionally, physically, interpersonally, socially, and spiritually.

Well people enjoy outdoor play.

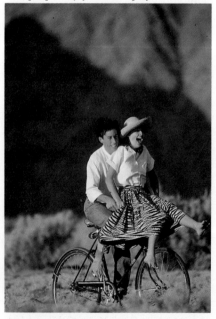

This book is about enjoying life. It challenges you to increase your knowledge, strengths, and skills in many areas—in self-awareness, consumerism, stress management, emotional health, intimate relationships, nutrition, fitness, accident and disease prevention, and many others. Its aim is to enhance your confidence and competence in all these areas.

This is a tall order—especially since everyone already possesses considerable experience and knowledge about all these things. Why read a book about them? Oddly, the experience and knowledge people pick up about life are always somewhat haphazard. Standard schooling, no matter where obtained, ensures that people learn the basics of language and mathematics, but the skills they need to manage their lives are taught only in bits and pieces. This book hopes to fill in some of the gaps for everyone who reads it.

How, then, can people maximally enjoy their lives? By feeling well, confident, and as far as possible, in control of their worlds. And what does it mean to be well? This book defines a well person as one who has not only physical but also mental, emotional, interpersonal, social, and even spiritual, strengths.

Imagine for a moment that you are a magnificently healthy person, with strengths in every one of these realms. The following paragraphs define **health**, using you as an example.

Ideally, then, as an emotionally healthy person, you have a strong sense of self. You are willing to attempt new learnings and behaviors, and are able to handle setbacks without loss of self-esteem. You have a realistic grasp of current information, and you are sufficiently assertive to resist being victimized by misinformation and fraud. You manage stress with skill and enjoyment, and don't let it become overwhelming. You keep tabs on your emotions, and you manage and express them appropriately. Finally, you know when to seek help. These strengths and how to cultivate them are described in Chapters 2 and 3.

A healthy person cultivates physical health, too. To be physically healthy does *not* mean to be without illness, of course, for illnesses sometimes attack us without our consent or control. But it does mean to manage your food intakes, body weight, physical fitness, and sleep needs so as to support your own health, and it also means to abstain from harmful drug use. Chapters 4, 5, and 6 are devoted to nutrition, weight control, fitness, and sleep; and Chapters 7, 8, and 9 discuss the appropriate uses of medical drugs and to the effects of harmful drugs and the importance of abstinence from them.

A healthy person also has social and spiritual strengths. It is important to be able to develop and maintain intimacy with others and to form successful long-term partnerships. It is important to understand and appreciate your own sexuality, and manage your sexual relationships in a way that enhances the quality of your life. If you are sexually active, you need to understand the principles of contraception, to be able to communicate about it, and to make informed decisions on its use. If you are a woman, then on choosing to bear a child, you need to learn to manage your pregnancy and childbirth with attention to the health of both yourself and your infant. When you become a mother or father, you need to understand human development sufficiently to be able to nurture children or younger people, even if your own parents were not nurturing parents. As you grow older, you will continue learning and facing new challenges; and finally, you will be willing to learn what is required in facing death (your own or someone

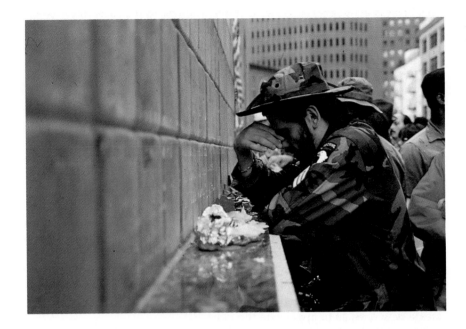

A well person expresses emotions appropriately.

else's). Chapters 10, 11, 12, and 13 take up these concerns of the human life cycle, and the Spotlight at the end of Chapter 13 is devoted to spiritual health, the part that inspires all the rest.

Since life's events are at times outside an individual's control, you also have to be aware that accidents and infectious diseases (including sexually transmitted diseases) are a real possibility, and take appropriate measures to prevent them. You also know your own familial risk factors for diseases such as heart disease, diabetes, or cancer, and adopt the behaviors that will minimize your risks. Prevention of accidents and diseases is the subject of Chapters 14, 15, 16, and 17. Because you cannot always prevent accidents and diseases, you need to know how to use the health care system to advantage and when to attend to your own medical needs (self-care). Pointers on these important subjects are given in Chapter 18.

Last, and encompassing all of these other health concerns, is your relationship to the larger environment—the earth. You carry your share of the responsibility for this realm. Its importance, and the roles that are rightfully yours in connection with it, are the subjects of Chapter 19.

This long description not only defines health but also implies actions to achieve it. It could be termed a list of **life management skills**. People who have already developed these skills to some extent, and who are actively moving forward toward health goals, are maximizing their chances for enjoyment of life.

life management skills: the skills that help a person realize his or her potential to be well and enjoy life; this book's strategies.

▓ HEALTH: YOUR CHOICE

You change your health by the choices you make every day, whether you mean to or not. The choices you make today will either improve or harm your health, and their effects are compounded by time. Today's choices, repeated for a week, will have seven times the impact. Repeated every day

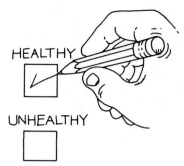

HEALTHY

UNHEALTHY

For most people, health through life is largely determined by the choices they make.

This book uses these terms interchangeably: Infectious disease = communicable disease. Lifestyle disease = degenerative disease. See the glossaries in and at the ends of chapters for all terms that appear in boldface type.

locus of control: the location of control inside or outside a person. Before a person will take responsibility and act to acquire health, that person must see that the locus of control of the situation is within. A simpler way to say this is that the person *owns* the responsibility.

FIGURE 1–1 Invest in Learning

For the majority of people it pays to learn about health and apply the knowledge.

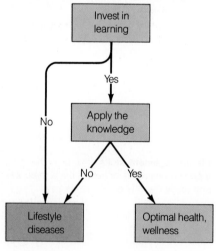

Your age as measured in years from the date of your birth is your **chronological age**. Your age as estimated from your body's health and probable life expectancy is your **physiological age**.

for a year, they will have 365 times the impact on your health. Over years, the effects accumulate still further.

With the information available today and presented in this book, you can make choices that will improve the quality of your life and even your statistical life expectancy.

This statement reflects a reality that differs from the reality of the past. People's health has always been influenced by the same factors—their heredity, their environment, and their personal lifestyle choices—but the weights of these factors have changed. Today, personal choices have a much greater influence on health than they had in the past. The reason is that the world we live in is different in many significant ways.

For one thing, far more information is available, thanks to scientific advances. We know more about psychology, physical health, and sexuality than ever before. We know more about the causes of **infectious diseases** and their prevention, and we are beginning to learn enough about the **lifestyle diseases** to have a grasp of what we need to do to prevent those, too. Perhaps only in the spiritual realm can it be said that we are no further advanced than our ancestors; for some age-old truths seem to hold as true today as they ever have, and our task in mastering them is not so much to create new ones as to appreciate the old.

Figure 1–1 shows the probable course of a person who invests in learning about health. The investment leads to improved quality of life.

That people have more control over their lives than before means that they have more responsibility. As psychology puts it, the **locus of control**, with respect to many health factors, is inside the individual; people are not the hapless victims of external chance. It is vital to know the difference, because only when people realize that they can change things do they take action. People do not helplessly "catch" the consequences of poor lifestyle choices as they once caught smallpox. A different word is used: they "contract" lifestyle diseases through their own choices.

Researchers have given a dramatic demonstration of how personal choices affect health. They studied nearly 7,000 adults in California and noticed that some people seemed young for their age; others, old for their age. To find out what made the difference, the researchers focused on health habits and identified six factors that had maximum impact on **physiological age**: regular, adequate sleep; regularity of meals; regular physical activity; abstinence from smoking; abstinence from, or moderation in, alcohol use; and weight control. The effects of these factors were cumulative. That is, those who followed all six positive practices were in better health, even if older in calendar years, than people who failed to do so. In fact, the physical health of those who reported all positive health practices was consistently about the same as that of people *30 years younger* who followed few or none.[1]* These findings demonstrated that although you cannot alter the year of your birth, you can alter the probable length of your life. In effect, you can make yourself younger or older by the way you choose to live. This chapter's Life Choice Inventory illustrates this point.

Middle-aged to older people served as subjects for the California study just described. For younger people, accidents are a seventh significant cause of loss of life and health. The Life Choice Inventory includes accident

*Reference notes are in Appendix D.

LIFE CHOICE INVENTORY: HOW LONG WILL YOU LIVE?

How long will you live? No one can answer this question for sure, of course. But you can increase or decrease your *probable* life expectancy by a good many years depending on what choices you make. That is, your statistical *chances* of dying younger or older are affected by how you live.

The Longevity Game illustrates this principle. To play the game, start on the top line (age 74, the average life expectancy for adults in the United States today). Then answer the 11 questions that follow. For each question, add or subtract years as instructed. If a question doesn't apply, go on to the next one. If you are not sure of the exact number to add or subtract, make a guess. Don't take the score too seriously, but do pay attention to those areas where you lose years: they could point to choices you might want to change.

Start with: ____74____
  1. Exercise   _____
  2. Relaxation   _____
  3. Driving   _____
  4. Blood pressure   _____
  5. 65 and working   _____
  6. Family history   _____
  7. Smoking   _____
  8. Drinking   _____
  9. Gender   _____
10. Weight   _____
11. Age   _____
Your final score   _____

1. **Exercise.** If your work requires regular, vigorous activity or you work out each day, add three years. If you don't get much exercise at home, work, or play, subtract three years.
2. **Relaxation.** If you have a relaxed approach to life (you roll with the punches), add three years. If you're aggressive, ambitious, or nervous (you have sleepless nights, you bite your nails), subtract three years. If you consider yourself unhappy, subtract another year.
3. **Driving.** Drivers under 30 who have had traffic tickets in the last year or have been involved in an accident, subtract four years. Other violations, minus one. If you always wear seatbelts, add one.

4. **Blood pressure.** High blood pressure is a major cause of the most common killers—heart attacks and strokes—but most victims don't know they have it. If you know you have it, you are likely to do something about it. If you *know* your blood pressure, add one year.
5. **Sixty-five and working.** If you are 65 or older and still working, add three.
6. **Family history.** If any grandparent has reached age 85, add two; if all grandparents have reached age 80, add six. If a parent died of a stroke or heart attack before age 50, minus four. If a parent or brother or sister has (or had) diabetes since childhood, minus three.
7. **Smoking.** Cigarette smokers who finish:
   More than two packs a day, minus eight.
   One or two packs a day, minus six.
   One-half to one pack, minus three.
8. **Drinking.** If you drink two cocktails (or beers or glasses of wine) a day, subtract one year. For each additional daily libation, subtract two.
9. **Gender.** Women live longer than men. Females add three years, males subtract three years.
10. **Weight.** If you avoid eating fatty foods and don't add salt to your meals, your heart will be healthier, and you're entitled to add two years.
    Now, weigh in:
    Overweight by 50 pounds or more, minus eight.
    30 to 40 pounds, minus four.
    10 to 29 pounds, minus two.
11. **Age.** How long you have already lived can help predict how much longer you'll live. If you're under 30, the jury is still out. But if your age is:
    30 to 39, plus two.
    40 to 49, plus three.
    50 to 69, plus four.
    70 or over, plus five.

SOURCE: From ''The Longevity Game'' by Northwestern Mutual Life Insurance Company, with permission.

prevention as one of the strategies most likely to promote physical health for adults.

This section of the chapter has offered the reasons why it makes sense to study health. The next two sections answer the questions of how to study it and how to apply the information.

THE SOURCES OF HEALTH INFORMATION

Many sources of information claim that their statements are facts. For example, claims made in advertisements often appear to do this. Actors dressed as scientists or physicians appear on the screen or on the magazine page and make solemn pronouncements to the effect that "research has shown this product to be effective. . . ." But when you look closely, where is the evidence? Not on the screen, and not on the magazine page.

How, then, can the consumer of health information decide whether to believe the claims made by the promoters of health products and services? This section's main purpose is to enhance your skill in distinguishing between valid health information and health **fraud**.

When you encounter a claim for a product or service, you can use a set of basic strategies to help you evaluate it. Ask and find answers to the following questions: Who is making the claim? What are that person's qualifications for making such statements? On what evidence is the claim based? Where was that evidence published? In what language style is it stated?

A simple rule governs the evaluation of claims on the basis of who is making them. If the person or organization making the claim stands to profit by selling you something you would not otherwise buy, discount the claim. It is as simple as that. To get honest, unbiased information on any product or service, find an outside expert who can make an assessment. An example familiar to most people is buying a used car. The salesperson's word alone isn't sufficient, nor is the word of someone who has another car to sell; an independent garage mechanic should be hired to assess the car. The mechanic is not personally involved in the sale and stands to gain most by telling the truth, because the satisfied customer will give a favorable report to other customers.

If the person making the claim does not appear to be motivated by personal gain, then there are some other questions to ask—notably, about the person's education, training, skill, and reputation. A person may be justly famed and admired for one specialty, but that does not indicate qualifications to speak in another specialty area. A noted poet is probably not as well qualified to speak on physical fitness as the trainer of Olympic athletes; a famed heart surgeon may not be knowledgeable about sex therapy; the governor of a state is not an authority on nutrition; and so forth. When an authority makes pronouncements on a given topic, ask yourself whether the person has the education and experience to speak on that topic.

We mentioned four characteristics to look for in sizing up a person's qualifications as an expert. Education is indispensable; there is no substitute for the hundreds of hours of book learning that provide the foundation for a person's expertise. Training is another, for all the book learning in the world is useless until the person has practiced using it in real-life situations. Skill is a third; it normally develops as the result of education and training, but some people do not become skilled even with the best of both. Finally comes reputation: a person earns that by developing the first three assets.

Another thing to notice about a claim is the information source. Health information purveyed by the mass communication media—newspapers, magazines, radio, television—is notoriously unreliable. Books on health written for the public are also so unreliable that most professional organizations maintain committees to combat the misinformation in them. A list of organizations that provide reliable scientific information appears in

✿ **STRATEGIES**
for Evaluating Health Claims

To evaluate a claim:

✿ **Ask who is making the claim. Does that person stand to gain from your believing it?**

✿ **Ask about the person's education, training, skill, and reputation.**

✿ **Ask where the claim is published: newspaper, magazine, book written for the public, textbook, journal?**

✿ **Consult the professional society concerned with the subject matter in question.**

||| Credentials of Physicians and Other Health Care Providers

This book uses the term **health care provider** to describe those people to whom you can safely turn for medical care: the physician (M.D., D.O.), the physician's assistant (P.A.), or the nurse practitioner (R.N., R.N.P.). These people can all provide care for ordinary medical problems; all can refer you to specialists for extraordinary problems. The term **client** in place of **patient** is also appropriate. A patient is, literally, a passive person, one who waits, who is dependent on someone else, the physician, for the solution to a medical problem. A client is an active person, one who is in charge of his or her own health and who pays the health care provider for services that person is trained to provide. Sometimes one term, sometimes the other, is used in the chapters that follow, depending on the attitude toward self of the person seeking medical assistance.

Appendix A, and any of them can serve as sources for your own inquiries about the authenticity of scientific information in their areas.*

One way you can gather clues about the validity of health information is to study the language in which a claim is stated. Many buzzwords and phrases can alert you to false or misleading information—among them, the following:

⊛ Write to the National Council Against Health Fraud.

⊛ Be alert to the language in which claims are made.

- *Organic, health, herbal, natural.* These terms have no legal meaning as used on labels, and although intended to imply unusual power to promote health, they do not.
- *Scientific breakthrough, medical miracle.* Seldom do popular reports prove true when they make statements in defiance of current scientific knowledge—new cure for cancer, a way to lose weight without cutting calories, a tiny pill with enormous power. In advertisements, such claims almost never prove true.
- *Doctors agree, authorities agree.* When the identity of the doctors is not revealed, or when no reference to an authoritative publication is provided, these statements are meaningless. They may mean only that the advertiser persuaded three doctors to agree.

Some false claims are recognizable if you can spot the confused thinking that underlies them. Examples:

- "Tiredness is a symptom of iron-poor blood." This is true. "Therefore, if you are tired, you have iron-poor blood, and you need iron supplements." This is not true because tiredness is also a symptom of other conditions. You need a diagnosis.

⊛ Don't guess at a diagnosis; be sure.

*If you have questions about a medical book, product, or service, write to the American Medical Association; about an anticancer book, product, or service, to the American Cancer Society; about a heart disease preventive, to the American Heart Association; about a diet or nutrient supplement, to the American Dietetic Association; and so forth. Many of the professional organizations have also banded together to form the National Council Against Health Fraud (NCAHF), which has branches in many states. The NCAHF monitors radio, television, and other advertising, investigates complaints, and maintains a bimonthly newsletter to keep consumers informed on the latest health misinformation. You can write to the NCAHF at P.O. Box 1276, Loma Linda, CA 92354.

✳ **Recognize that no food is essential.**

✳ **Recognize the child in yourself who frightens easily and delights in magic.**

■ "People need the essential nutrients or else they'll get sick." This is true. "Therefore, they need food X, which contains nutrients." This is not true, because no food is the unique possessor of any nutrient. Other foods can supply essential nutrients in the amounts needed.

Symptoms especially likely to be used to draw in the unsuspecting consumer are those everybody has—tiredness, aches and pains, occasional insomnia, colds. Another class of such symptoms includes those everyone can see because they involve external parts of the body: the skin, hands, face, hair, scalp, eyes, fingernails.

Some claims are outright tricks that work because we consumers can be like children who frighten easily and delight in magic. The tricks are simple, but they are still attractive. Who hasn't been tempted to buy a product or try a service because it sounds so easy ("no effort"), because it costs so little and produces such a big reward ("something for nothing"), because it will protect you from terrible things (scare tactics), because it will relieve you of some natural characteristic you are being taught to despise, or because it will restore your vitality or youth or beauty or all of these (magical thinking)? Remember: aging is inevitable; so is death. Don't be misled into thinking you can totally prevent them. Learn what is preventable about aging and what isn't. Promote your health in the ways that truly work—they involve your lifestyle choices. None of them is magic.

The first part of this chapter illustrated how health choices affect the quality of life. This middle section has shown how to sort health facts from fads and frauds. Following is information on how to put health facts to work in your own life.

▧ HEALTH BEHAVIOR AND BEHAVIOR CHANGE

Health knowledge is hardly beneficial if it merely enables people to make A's on tests. It is valuable only if people use it to make informed choices. These choices may require them to change their behavior. The next sections describe this process. They define motivation and itemize the steps to action, explain behavior modification, and, finally, discuss how expectations affect behavior change.

Motivation

In general, **motives** are forces that move people to act. They may be either instinctive or learned. Instinctive motives, or **drives**, are strongest: hunger and thirst impel you to meet your needs for food and water. Learned motives may also be powerful—consider the desire for possessions, recognition, or achievement. A powerful motive virtually impels a person to act.

A person's **motivation** is modified by three factors: the value of the reward (how big is the reward and what does it cost?), its **latency** (how soon will the reward come or how soon will the price have to be paid?), and its probability (how likely is the reward, how certain the price?).

Contrast these situations:

■ Eat ice cream now (immediate reward); notice your weight gain tomorrow (pay later).
■ Forgo ice cream now; expect weight loss next week.

- Enjoy a cigarette (a certainty) now; pay with lung disease (a probability) in the future.
- Give up smoking now; enjoy better health in the future.

No wonder it's difficult to motivate people to change their health habits! Nevertheless, if persuaded of the importance, they sometimes do.

The steps that lead to behavior change seem to be these:

- Awareness: "I could choose to change."
- Cognition: "I know how to change."
- Emotion: "I want to change."
- Decision: "I will change."
- Action: "I am changing."

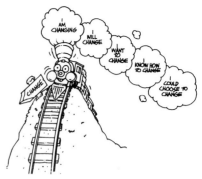

The elements of behavior change.

They don't always appear in the same order, but they always seem to appear.

Being overweight is a problem familiar to many people. (If you can't identify with this problem, substitute some other while reading this.) No doubt you know someone who wants to lose weight. He has taken the first two steps: he is aware of the need, and he knows how—at least, to some extent—yet he still takes no action. Eating fattening foods brings him great pleasure, for one thing. For another, without being aware of it, he may receive some benefits from being fat. (He doesn't have to cope with many sexual advances, for example.) He may *claim* he wants to lose weight, and he may be chronically upset with himself for not getting thinner, yet deep inside he may not really want to change. Many people get stuck at this point.

Wanting is emotional—and when the emotions become positively charged, a rush of energy enables the person to act. Still, even if the wanting is so strong that it brings tears of frustration or anger, emotion is not enough to change behavior. We all can name people who know how to diet and who desperately want to lose weight, and yet who still do nothing. The person has to make a decision—a step in which the **will** is engaged.

Even psychologists don't fully understand how people make decisions. But everyone knows how it feels to arrive at a decision point. One day, your friend who needs to lose weight says, "I'm going to eat wisely from now on," and from that point on, possibly for months, he may not deviate from an unbroken course of restricting calories and losing weight until he seems to have become a completely different person.

In a sense, he is a different person. He has had to let go of his old habits absolutely. He has had to go through a grief experience—the loss of a cherished habit with its rewards. His self-image has had to change. He *was* an overeater; he is now an *ex*-overeater, an abstainer. He *was* a person who avoided facing certain problems by overeating; he is now a person who owns those problems and deals with them constructively. He knows himself better, and he asserts himself more effectively.

The commitment that comes with a firm decision to make a significant life change is profound and transforming. It has been called "the moment of truth," "conversion," "submission," or "total surrender." And total it has to be, for a long road of effort lies ahead.

In case you are reflecting on your own behavior and possible changes, it is as important to know when you are *not* ready as to know when you are. Much needless time and anxiety is wasted struggling with "I should; I ought to; I must" and with shame and guilt over "I can't; I failed again." An important part of arriving at permanent desired behavior change is the awareness that success may require many practice runs. You don't have to succeed totally the first time.

Suppose a person has firmly decided to make a change and is now about to begin. Many changes in individual, small, daily behaviors are going to be necessary. It will help to understand the basic principles of **behavior modification**.

Behavior Modification

Some psychologists view human behavior as regulated by environmental factors. In simple terms, they see each behavior as sandwiched between two environmental conditions, those that precede it and those that follow it— the **antecedents** and the **consequences**:

$$A \text{ (antecedents)} \longrightarrow B \text{ (behavior)} \longleftrightarrow C \text{ (consequences)}$$

A behavior occurs in response to antecedents (cues or stimuli); the more intense the antecedents are, the more likely the behavior will occur. The behavior leads to consequences, and the more intense these are, the more or less likely the behavior will occur again. Behavior modification involves manipulating these environmental conditions so as to favor the repeated occurrence of a desired behavior and extinguish the occurrence of unwanted behaviors.

Figure 1–2 illustrates strategies to modify antecedents, behaviors, and consequences to cement a desired behavior in place: in this example, studying effectively. Strategies 1 and 2 eliminate or suppress the strength of cues to the unwanted behavior. Strategy 3 increases the strength of cues to the desired behavior. Strategy 4 repeats the wanted behavior itself: the more

FIGURE 1–2   Behavior Modification Used to Facilitate Effective Studying

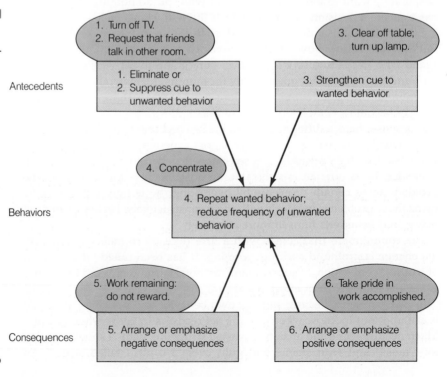

often the desired behavior is repeated, the weaker the tendency to repeat the unwanted behavior. Strategy 5 arranges or emphasizes negative consequences of the unwanted behavior, thus weakening it; and strategy 6 arranges or emphasizes positive consequences of the wanted behavior, thus strengthening it.

The example in the figure illustrates how behavior modification works. Kristin needs to write a paper but lacks enough motivation to get started on it. Conditions are unfavorable: the TV is blaring, two friends have dropped in and are conversing, and there is no inviting place to settle down and work. It is tempting to procrastinate (unwanted behavior). Knowing the principles of behavior modification, though, Kristin modifies the antecedents. Turning off the TV eliminates one cue to procrastination (strategy 1 of Figure 1–2). Requesting that the friends talk in another room suppresses another (strategy 2). Clearing off the table and turning up the lamp provide cues to studying (strategy 3). Once Kristin begins to concentrate, the tendency to procrastinate fades and the work begins to move forward (strategy 4). Self-congratulation is now in order (strategy 6).

A note about emphasizing negative consequences (strategy 5): if Kristin had chosen to procrastinate, the result would have been work left undone— a negative consequence. But to pay much attention to this would be to reward it. Punishment is a form of attention—and attention is a reward. That is why, sometimes, unruly children misbehave more when they are punished. The most effective way to use strategy 5 is to ignore the unwanted behavior, not to call attention to it, and not to punish it.

Behavior modification techniques equip people with a means of effectively changing their behavior if they want to. A particularly attractive feature of these strategies is that they don't involve blaming onself or putting oneself down. The person who understands these techniques can say, "I know how to change— when I'm ready."

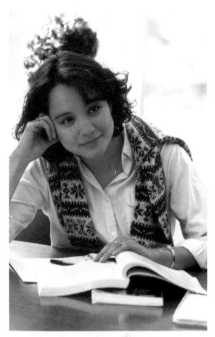

Once you have all your ducks in a row, congratulate yourself.

Expectations

Sometimes, even after what seems to be a firm commitment to changed behavior, a person slips back. Why? Once you have instituted a change in your life, you will persist in maintaining that change only if the benefits continue to outweigh the barriers.

Let's switch our attention to a woman who smokes, to examine the broader application of behavior-change principles. She has decided to give up smoking, but after a day without cigarettes, she is a nervous wreck. After two days, she is climbing the walls and driving her friends and lifemate crazy. At this time, the long-distant rewards of eventual respiratory health have receded far into the background in her thinking, and all that she is aware of is her desperate desire for a cigarette. This being the case, it is not surprising that she fails to give up smoking and returns to the habit within one or two days after making the initial effort.

To succeed, this person needs to have realistic expectations and a plan of action. She needs to know from the outset how hard it will be and especially how long it will take before the pain goes away and the rewards begin to come in. It helps, too, to be alert to the immediate rewards—immediate, that is, in terms of days, not years. After a week, she is free of thoughts about cigarettes for several hours at a time, and in climbing stairs, she does not become as winded as before. If she tunes in to these immediate rewards, she may make it through the hard part.

In contrast, the person who returns to the habit may have been unaware that the pain of withdrawal was about to diminish and that rewards were so soon to come. These awarenesses will help to cement the desired behavior change in place.

People need to know, too, that they can't undertake too large a change and expect to succeed. Suppose a person decides to give up cookies and cakes and candies and colas, in fact to avoid all sugar—and not only to do that, but to avoid all fatty foods too—and not only that, but also to give up all alcoholic beverages—and to switch from whole milk to nonfat milk and never to use cream—and to give up salt—and to start jogging a mile every morning and do situps every night—to go to church on Sundays—and to spend at least two added hours each day on homework . . . That person may be in for a rude surprise. All these changes can be made, but not all at once. After only a few days, such a person will be exhausted and will give it all up. We congratulate the person on having identified many worthy goals. Now it's time to plan realistically. New behaviors require energy. They need to be taken up a few at a time—in fact, probably one by one.

This section has not identified all the many steps you can take to ensure that your behavior change efforts will be successful, but it has outlined some of the more important ones. A plan of action that incorporates these steps and others might read like the one in this chapter's Strategies box.

Sometimes people act on a new behavior only for a short time. We don't understand exactly what happens when a person reverts to a negative health habit, but it is clear that at least two things are involved: magical thinking and forgetting. An ex-smoker's magical thinking might sound like this: "I'm a different person now. I can take just one cigarette; I won't get hooked." People sometimes have to make this kind of mistake several times before they finally learn they cannot afford it.

People who have long maintained a new way of life sometimes report episodes in which the old way springs back to consciousness, in dreams or unexpected memories. An ex-drug addict reports that she suddenly felt high again, and it scared her. A dieter dreams that he's been bingeing on chocolate. An ex-alcohol abuser awakens in a cold sweat from a nightmare in which she got drunk. No one seems to know why these episodes occur, but they do serve a useful purpose: they bring back a vivid memory of the old behavior—and its price. Alcohol counselors say, "If you can't remember the last drink, then it wasn't your last." The maintenance of a new behavior sometimes depends on not forgetting that a return to the old behavior would be worse.

Finally, people changing their behavior have to realize that their self-image must change as well. Sometimes the self-image is slow to change, and the behavior slips back. People have to do some psychological work with their physical work to change through and through. A person who gives up smoking has to learn to see herself as a confirmed ex-smoker. A person who takes up swimming every day has to own his new identity: "I am a swimmer."

In summary, the maintenance of changed health-promoting behavior is facilitated by:

■ Continued motivation (remembering vividly the price of the old behavior and remaining aware of the benefits of the new).
■ A changed self-image.

STRATEGIES: How to Change Your Behavior

If you want to change a behavior, try taking the following steps:

1. Identify the goal, the behaviors that will lead to it, and those that will prevent it. List the advantages and disadvantages of the desired behaviors. Learn what will be involved.

2. Commit to changing. Plan. Dedicate the necessary time and money. Face what you'll have to give up or displace to give high priority to making the change. Mobilize the support of family and friends.

3. Divide the behavior into manageable portions. Set small, achievable goals, and plan periodic rewards.

4. Envision your changed future self. Role-play the new you in your imagination. Buy the equipment you need (owning a pair of jogging shoes gives you a boost toward being a jogger).

5. Pick a time to start, and write it down. Tell others, if that will help reinforce your determination.

6. Plan stepwise progression if suitable. ("The next time, I'll take only one drink on each weekend day.")

7. Try out the plan.

8. Modify the plan in ways that will succeed.

9. Try the modified plan.

10. Evaluate your progress often.

11. Savor your results and value the benefits.

One additional factor helps immensely if behavior change is to succeed, a factor that may be more important than any of those named above:

■ Self-esteem.

The person who starts out feeling worthwhile, who cares enough to invest energy and effort in attaining optimal health, is a step ahead of the game from the beginning. The person who begins to succeed in changing behavior gains improved self-esteem from the effort and so wins an advantage for the efforts ahead.

OTHER PEOPLE'S HEALTH BEHAVIOR

Perhaps you are not resistant to change but are concerned about someone else's behavior: "How can I get my father (mother, friend, child) to change?" These people's choices are *not* your responsibility. You can care about them and you can help them, but you can't change their behavior. No matter how much you may want them to do what you think is best, you cannot make the choice for them. In fact, your best bet is usually to say nothing and let the awareness of what they need to do come upon them from inside. Most importantly, make no negative judgments; these reduce the other person's self-esteem and make change less, not more, likely.

You can, however, facilitate the dawning of awareness. These strategies are especially effective:

- Give straightforward feedback.
- Set an example with your own behavior.
- Offer authenticated information, or make sure it is available.

Here is an example of the first strategy. A student in a health course was earning money by evening babysitting for a young mother who went out to several parties a week. The student observed that the mother usually had two or three drinks before she left home and often came home dangerously drunk. All she dared to say to the woman was, "Gee, every time I see you, you have a drink in your hand."

As it turned out, this was all she needed to say. The woman chose to seek treatment for alcoholism and later thanked the student for her help. "What did I do to help?" the student wanted to know. "You made me aware that I had a problem," the woman replied. "I hadn't realized how far I had gone until I saw myself as you saw me." The student had delivered straightforward feedback, as a mirror does, with no judgment implied.

The second strategy, setting an example, is also effective because it is nonjudgmental. No one likes to be told, "You really ought to quit [behavior A]" or "You really ought to start [behavior B]." In fact, people often do not even like to be reminded of resolutions they themselves have made: "Aren't you going to work out today?" If you change a health habit yourself, however, the person you are concerned about will surely notice and may begin thinking about doing the same thing. When ready, this person may ask you how you did it or ask to join you.

The third strategy, to supply authenticated information, helps increase people's knowledge, so that when they become ready to make a change, they are equipped to do it. The information you offer may be statistics on the effects of a certain health behavior or "how-to" facts such as the meeting time and place for the next smoke-enders class. It is often better not to push such information at people, rather simply to make sure it is available in case they want it.

If you try to influence someone and think you've failed, take comfort in the fact that the "failure" may really be success waiting to happen. Your feedback and information may not tip the scale right now but together with other factors will weigh on the favorable side. It may take years before someone decides to make a lifestyle change for health's sake, but when the change happens, the person may well credit it to something someone said years earlier. Don't hesitate to care. Do what you can, then take satisfaction in having done your best, and let it go.

When someone does make the choice to change to a health-promoting behavior, you then have a further opportunity to help:

- Offer positive reinforcement and support.

Often it is best to keep the verbal praise moderate; some people don't like to have too much attention drawn to their first, tentative efforts. Also, make sure the reinforcement you give is positive, not negative: "I'm glad to see you doing that," not "It's about time you did that" (which takes the credit from your friend). Also: "You look wonderful," not "You look better" (which implies that your friend looked awful before).

Much more could be said about promoting positive choices, but these ideas are enough for a start. Whether it is your own life or other people's that you keep in mind as you read this book, we hope the following chapters will bring you the information you need to make informed health choices.

STUDY AIDS

1. Identify the areas of life to which the term *health* applies.
2. Itemize life management skills to promote health in the following areas: (a) emotional; (b) physical; (c) interpersonal, social, and spiritual; and (d) life events such as accidents and diseases.
3. Contrast the lifestyle diseases and the infectious diseases. Explain how the nature of the lifestyle diseases makes us responsible to some extent for our own health.
4. Explain the concept of locus of control and how it relates to disease prevention and health promotion.
5. Describe the difference between chronological and physiological age.
6. Identify six factors shown by research to have maximum impact on the physiological age of adults and an additional factor that affects life expectancy in younger adults.
7. List elements a person should consider when evaluating health claims and explain why they are important.
8. Describe ways to recognize false or inflated health claims.
9. List some factors that influence motivation.
10. List and describe the steps that lead to behavior change.
11. Describe six ways in which people can manipulate antecedents, behaviors, and consequences to facilitate behavior change.
12. Identify some requirements for maintaining a changed behavior.
13. Describe a plan of action for ensuring successful behavior change.
14. Describe effective strategies for facilitating desirable health behavior change in other people.

GLOSSARY

antecedents: see *behavior modification*.
behavior modification: the changing of behavior by the manipulation of *antecedents* (cues, or environmental factors that trigger behavior), the behavior itself, and *consequences* (the penalties or rewards attached to behavior).
chronological age: age as measured in years from date of birth. See also *physiological age*.
    chron = time
client: a person who pays another to perform a service. This term is gradually replacing the term *patient*, as *health care provider* is replacing *physician*. See *health care provider*.
communicable disease: see *infectious disease*.
consequences: see *behavior modification*.
degenerative disease: see *lifestyle disease*.
disease: a diagnosable disorder such as heart disease or tuberculosis. Two terms often used to describe disease conditions are *acute* and *chronic*. An acute condition is one that comes on suddenly and may be intense, such as attacks of influenza or heart attacks. A chronic condition is one

that progresses and does not go away, such as heart disease, arthritis, or tuberculosis. See also *infectious disease*, *lifestyle disease*.
drives: instincts that propel individuals into action, such as hunger, thirst, fear, and needs for sleep and sex. Drives may prompt an individual to act alone or to act in relation to others.
fraud: conscious deceit, practiced for profit.
health: a range of states with physical, mental, emotional, interpersonal, social, and spiritual components. At a minimum, health means freedom from negative states such as physical disease, physical deterioration, social maladjustment, mental illness, etc. At a maximum, it means the achievement of full potential physically, mentally, emotionally, interpersonally, socially, and spiritually—a state that some call *wellness*.
health care provider: a term used in this book to refer to people who are qualified and credentialed to provide safe, expert general medical care—physicians (M.D., D.O.), physician assistants (P.A.), or nurse practitioners (R.N., R.N.P., for registered nurse practitioner). The credentialing of

these people is described in Chapter 18.
infectious disease: a disease that can be passed from person to person and is caused by a specific disease-carrying agent. Also called *communicable disease*.
latency: the time lag between an action and its consequence. (With respect to behavior, latency modifies motivation; that is, the longer the time lag, the weaker the motivation.)
life management skills: the skills that help a person to realize his or her potential to be well and enjoy life; this book's strategies.
lifestyle disease: a disease characterized by degeneration of body organs due to misuse and neglect. Lifestyle diseases cannot be passed from person to person; they are often influenced by personal lifestyle choices such as eating habits, smoking, alcohol use, and level of physical activity; and they are usually chronic and irreversible. Lifestyle diseases are often called *degenerative diseases*. Examples are heart disease, cancer, and diabetes. See also *disease*.
locus of control: the place where responsibility lies. If the locus of control is within a person, then the person is

responsible; if it is outside, then the person may be helpless. When a person perceives correctly that the locus of control is within, then that person is said to *own* the responsibility.

motivation: the desire and impulse to act.

motives: forces that move people to act. Some motives are instinctive (*drives*); others are learned.

owning: being responsible. See *locus of control*.

patient: a person who is dependent on a physician or other medical care provider for medical help. See also *client*.

physiological age: age as estimated from the body's health and probable life expectancy. See also *chronological age*.

wellness: maximal health, the achievement of full potential mentally, emotionally, physically, interpersonally, socially, and spiritually.

will: a person's intent, which leads to action.

QUIZ ANSWERS

1. *False*. The definition of wellness is more ambitious than this. It includes a high level of physical well-being—and emotional, social, and spiritual well-being, too.

2. *False*. The major diseases of adults today are contracted largely as a result of people's lifestyle choices, rather than being "caught."

3. *True*. People can make themselves physiologically younger or older by the ways they choose to live.

4. *True*. Knowing how to relax can lengthen your life.

5. *True*. Women generally live longer than men do.

6. *False*. Accidents are among the major causes of death for younger adults.

7. *False*. "Organic" and "natural" have no legal meaning as used on labels, and although intended to imply unusual power to promote health, they do not.

8. *False*. Wanting and knowing how to change a harmful health habit are not enough; a person also must have the will to change.

9. *True*. Some people fail at making positive health behavior changes because they undertake too many changes at one time.

10. *False*. You are not responsible for the health choices of other people, and you can not change their behavior. You can assist by non-judgmentally enhancing their awareness and providing accurate information to facilitate change when they demonstrate the desire to change.

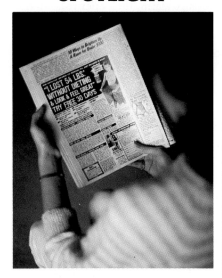

The Consumer and Health Fraud

A theme throughout this book is consumerism. Consumers face many problems in a free-enterprise market where competition for their dollars encourages advertisers to push their wares aggressively and not always honestly. Many advertisements twist the truth to create problems for us, exaggerate problems, or scare us with them, and then they twist the truth again to persuade us that they have the solutions we need. To give just one example, suppose you have a gray hair or two (or ten thousand). A television commercial might start there, and take these steps:

- You have gray hair (so far, that's true).
- It makes you look old (that may be true, too).
- That's unattractive (suddenly a problem has been created and projected onto you).
- You need Product X (now that you have this problem).

Consumers buy many "Product X's" they don't need because they have been led to follow such twisted reasoning. This book uses the term **magic bullets** to refer to unneeded products or products for which false claims are made.

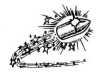

A common case of created problems is premenstrual syndrome (PMS), which has been said to "disable" women before their menstrual periods each month. PMS is not a fiction; it does seriously afflict some women (see Chapter 3). Advertisers, however, make it out to be more common than it is, and claim that it needs treatment when it does not. Women who have no unusual discomfort are led to think they do, and then to purchase remedies for it. These remedies are classic magic bullets, and the informed consumer sees through the claims made for them. Chapter 18 offers more help on recognizing the difference between a real need and a created one.

We do, however, need to buy products sold on the market. The question is, which ones do we really need? For what? When?

That's a good question. I sometimes wonder whether I really need the products I buy.

Let's go over the body head to toe and think it through. Shampoo is one of the first things to consider. If the question that comes to mind is "Which shampoo do I need?" then you haven't started at a basic enough level. The question is whether a shampoo is necessary at all—and the answer is no, at least not for the sake of a person's health. Hair gets dirty like the rest of the body, and dirt can harbor disease-causing organisms. Therefore, soap is necessary because it makes the organisms slippery enough to be washed away, but a person can use the same soap for the hair as for the body. Cleanliness is important to health, but glossiness, silkiness, manageability, and "body" are not. Nor do dandruff shampoos eliminate dandruff, despite the ads, so even for dandruff, a person still needs only soap.

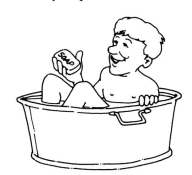

All you need is soap.

Are you recommending that I buy cheap soap?

Not necessarily. Just distinguish between what you need for health and what you may need for vanity or other reasons. If you're on a camping trip, cheap soap will do.

Clean water is also essential, baking soda makes an effective toothpaste, dental floss helps clean the teeth, and talcum powder is handy as an antibacterial measure. It can prevent chafing of the skin, which can lead to infection, and it keeps the body and the clothing dry. That's about all you need.

Wait a minute. You promised me a head-to-toe analysis. What about eyewash, facial cream, shaving cream, mouthwash, lip balm, deodorant, douche powders, vaginal deodorant sprays, nail buff, body lotion, and cologne?

No, clean water, soap, baking soda or toothpaste, dental floss, and powder are about all that a person needs for routine body maintenance. The rest of those products may do something for appearance and morale, but they aren't essential for health. Spotlight 18, "Your Body—An Owner's Manual," outlines a program of maintenance that includes daily, weekly, and annual routines, using these few basic supplies.

In addition to these health care products, people are wise to keep items on hand with which to meet common medical needs. A table in Appendix C makes suggestions for stocking a medicine chest.

That's funny. People buy a host of other products and devices, don't they?

People buy a multitude of products unnecessarily for supposed health or medical reasons. If you wish to restrict yourself to what you truly need, you will be astonished at the number of items and the amount of expense you can eliminate from your life. Health fraud (or **quackery**) encourages people to make some of these purchases. An example is medical devices. The Food and Drug Administration (FDA) has grouped quack medical devices into nine categories:

■ Figure enhancers (examples: bust developers, penis enlargers, fanny shapers, waist cinchers, muscle developers).
■ Arthritis and pain-relieving gadgets.
■ Sleep aids.
■ Hair and scalp devices (example: most baldness cures).
■ Youth prolongers (example: wrinkle removers, royal jelly).
■ Sex aids (example: cures for impotence).
■ Air and water purifiers.
■ Disease diagnosers.
■ Cure-alls (example: anemia preparations).[1]*

We would add a list of unnecessary medical products:

■ Mouthwashes (they don't eliminate the germs that cause bad breath; they only wash a few away for a very short time).
■ Cold medicines; arthritis medicines; sleeping pills and potions; headache remedies (see Chapter 7).
■ Cancer preventives and "cures" (see Chapter 17).
■ Health foods and nutrient supplements (see Chapter 4).
■ Fad diets and diet aids (see Chapter 5).
■ Colon treatments (examples: enemas for irritated colon, hemorrhoid ointments); laxatives (they create a dependency that can make the situation worse).
■ Vaginal deodorant sprays and douches (the natural odor is not offensive; a bad odor indicates a hygiene problem or a medical problem).
■ PMS medications.

How do promoters succeed in selling so many unnecessary things?

Most advertising of such products uses the basic magic bullet scheme

*Reference notes are in Appendix D.

already presented. Advertisements induce alarm, then offer reassurance or promise a benefit in the form of bottles, jars, tubes, or devices. Promotional advertisements use testimonials, opinions, exaggerations, and vague generalizations, without stating specific facts. Other techniques include the many kinds of claims familiar to every television-watcher today:

■ Our product is better than theirs (appeal to brand loyalty).
■ Everyone uses our product (bandwagon appeal).
■ Rich people use our product (snob appeal).
■ Famous people use our product (fame appeal).
■ We will give you bonuses and free merchandise if you buy our product (bribery).
■ Our product is new and improved. You can tell, because the packaging has changed (newness appeal).
■ Ordinary people use our product (just plain folks appeal).
■ Funny, happy people use our product (smile appeal).
■ Beautiful people use our product (vanity appeal).
■ Scientific people approve our product (science appeal).

Consumers who use their heads instead of the product wonder where the science is in all of this. Where are the statistics, surveys, professional health organization endorsements, or laboratory test results? Sometimes ads use these, too, but seldom with the serious expectation that the consumer will make a rational analysis of the results. The promotions may be sophisticated and hard to see through.

Quacks also offer special machines (technology appeal), secret formulas (chemistry appeal), and medical breakthroughs (miracle appeal). These appeals work; otherwise they would not be used.

I know they work. I'm sorry to say, I've had several experiences in which they were successful with me. With so many grasping fingers reaching for my wallet, how can I protect myself? Can I get any help from the government?

Yes, you can. Three major federal agencies are charged with aspects of consumer protection: the FDA (Food and Drug Administration), the FTC (Federal Trade Commission), and the U.S. Postal Service.

The FDA has jurisdiction over the ingredients of foods, drugs, medical devices, cosmetics, and labeling. Foods and cosmetics must by law be safe, and the FDA is empowered to test or order testing to see that they are. Drugs and medical devices must be both safe and effective, and the FDA can require proof and order them seized or withdrawn from the market if such proof is not presented. The FDA's efforts against quackery have been weakening, though. Originally founded in 1906 to fight unsafe and fraudulent foods and drugs, the FDA now spends only $1 of every $200 to do so. Since 1960, the FDA has directed much of its effort toward regulating the labeling of foods and drugs.[2]

FDA is ineffective against health fraud perpetrators for several reasons. For one thing, FDA is slow, and while it takes the time to fulfill federal regulations in pursuing a fraud, the fraud can easily make a quick move and go free. A former FDA commissioner confesses, "There are too many quacks, too skillful at the quick change of address and product name."[3] For another, the penalties are not stiff enough, and are not levied soon enough, to deter frauds who get away with millions before they are caught. A case in point is Dreamaway, a fraudulent product that was supposed to make people lose weight while they slept. By the time the district attorney in the California county where Dreamaway originated had instituted a suit against the company, it had already raked in a profit of over $1 million. It agreed not to market the product any more in California, and had to pay over $150,000 in court costs, but it walked away several hundred thousand dollars richer and free to defraud the public again in 49 other states.

Another reason why health fraud is flourishing is because lawsuits are time consuming, labor-intensive efforts. FDA cannot begin to prosecute all perpetrators; it has to go after the most medically dangerous. Those that are merely economic frauds go free.

The FTC's province is to fight the concentration of economic power and to investigate unfair or deceptive business practices, including deceptive advertising. The FTC has also been weakened, as its powers have been eroded by budget cuts and changed definitions of its mission.

The Postal Service deals with mail fraud cases, which amount to $500 million a year or more. Inspectors are available to investigate reports of such fraud, and when a case is uncovered, the Postal Service can take several actions. For example, it can refuse to deliver mail to the perpetrator of a fraud, thus shutting down the operation. It can sue, and demand a $1,000 fine for each individual mailing made in perpetration of a fraud, or impose a five-year imprisonment penalty per mailing.

Besides these and other federal agencies, private agencies also deal with consumer issues. The Better Business Bureau investigates consumer complaints and uses its influence to prevent unethical business practices in communities. Consumers Union systematically studies new products and services from the point of view of the consumer. *Consumer Reports* magazine, which it publishes, informs individuals about products and services judged to be safe, effective, and economical.

Also, the National Council Against Health Fraud (NCHAF) deserves a mention. Its members, vigilant against fraud wherever it occurs, feed information to central headquarters, and the newsletter passes the word on to consumers. However, agencies cannot predict or prevent fraud; they can pursue quacks only after they have *injured* many people. You may find yourself choosing a service or product that has been promoted by a health scam before you have heard anything from the authorities about its safety or effectiveness. It is up to you to beware. The rest of this book gives you pointers to help you on the way.

Chapter 2

Stress and Stress Management

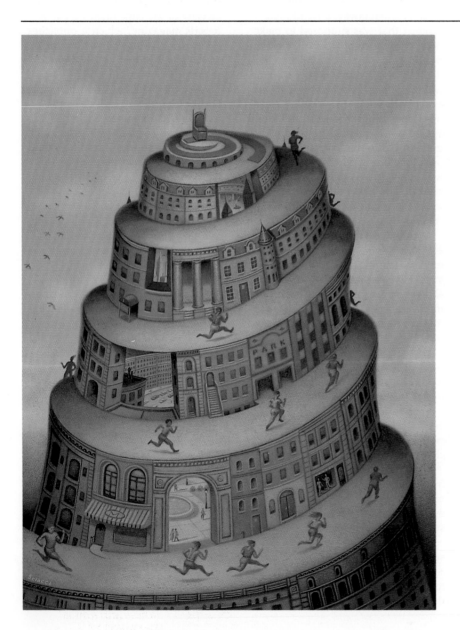

FOR OPENERS . . .

True or false? If false, say what is true.

1. The less stress a person experiences, the better for that person's health.
2. Having a skiing accident and getting married are more similar than different, as far as your body is concerned.
3. Whether an event is stressful depends more on the person experiencing it than on the event itself.
4. The feeling of helplessness makes people more likely to get sick.
5. There is a limit to how much stress a person can take; when the limit is reached, the person dies.
6. Being able to talk to close friends about personal matters helps people manage stress.
7. Once you are in a crisis you can do nothing to reduce its physical effect on you until it is over; then you can rest.
8. It's all right to refuse to face emotional injury as long as you do so only for a while.
9. Some people just can't relax, no matter what they do.
10. Meditation and self-hypnosis are similar relaxation techniques.

(Answers on page 37.)

The word **stress** is widely used today. The experience has been known since prehistoric times, but the term as applied to modern society was not used until Hans Selye examined stress scientifically earlier in this century.[1]* Now it is so widely used that it seems to apply to every life situation. When a person says, "I am under stress," he may mean that he is ill, that his love life has gone awry, that he is under financial pressure, or any of many other things.

In contrast, another person who says she is under stress may mean that she is thriving. Stress can be a threat to health, or it can be the fuel for progress and achievement. For some, it almost borders on inspiration. This chapter shows how people respond to stress and how you can deal with stress on a daily basis.

■■■ STRESSORS AND STRESS

To say that a person is under stress means that the person is responding to **stressors** in a characteristic way. A stressor is anything that requires you to cope with or adapt to a situation. Physical stressors include all environmental stimuli. Psychosocial stressors include life-changing events, both desirable and undesirable (see Tables 2–1 and 2–2).

To mobilize a healthy reaction to stress is to **cope**.

Among the most common kinds of stressors experienced by students are those that involve pressure to achieve. On top of the demands of school are needs for parental approval and students' own high standards. Meeting these demands can lead to the satisfaction of achievement, but sometimes these demands arouse anxiety that can cause mental and physical harm.

More about anxiety—Chapter 3.

Figure 2–1 (page 23) illustrates stressors. Through all stress situations runs a common thread: the hormonal and nervous systems respond in a characteristic way, producing an **adaptive** mobilization of resources to meet the need.

The stress response has three phases—alarm, resistance, and recovery or exhaustion. Figure 2–2 (page 24) shows the first sequence: alarm—resistance—recovery. Alarm is the initial reaction that occurs when you perceive that you are facing a new challenge. The second stage is resistance: a state

Three stages of stress:
alarm—resistance—recovery
or
alarm—resistance—exhaustion

*Reference notes are in Appendix D.

TABLE 2–1 **Physical Stressors**

The Greater the Intensity, the Greater the Stress
Light and changes in light
Heat/cold and changes in temperature
Sound and changes in sound level
Touch/pressure and changes in touch stimuli
Airborne chemical stimuli (odors, smoke, smog, air pollution)
Waterborne chemical stimuli
Drugs/medicines/alcohol
Foodborne chemicals and contaminants
Bacteria/viruses/other infective agents/allergens
Injury, including surgery
Exertion, work
X rays/radioactive rays/other forms of radiation

TABLE 2–2 Psychosocial Stressors

People ranked these events, according to how stressful they perceived them to be, on a scale from 1 to 100. Note that some "happy" events are included here. Individual people may score these events higher or lower than they are here. We have added in brackets events that might be comparable to these in the lives of students.

Life Event	Stress Points	Life Event	Stress Points
Death of spouse	100	Son or daughter leaving home	29
Divorce	73	Trouble with in-laws [trouble with parents]	29
Marital separation [breakup with boyfriend/girlfriend]	65	Outstanding personal achievement	28
Jail term	63	Spouse beginning or stopping work	26
Death of close family member (except spouse)	63	School beginning or ending [final exams]	26
Major personal injury or illness	53	Change in living conditions	25
Marriage	50	Revision of personal habits (self or family)	24
Being fired from a job [expulsion from school]	47	Trouble with boss [trouble with professor]	23
Marital reconciliation	45	Change in work [or school] hours or conditions	20
Retirement	45	Change in residence [moving to school, moving home]	20
Change in health of a family member (not self)	44	Change in schools	20
Pregnancy	40	Change in recreation	19
Sex difficulties	39	Change in church activities	19
Gain of new family member [change of roommate]	39	Change in social activities [joining new group]	18
Business readjustment	39	Taking on small mortgage or loan	17
Change in financial state	38	Change in sleeping habits	16
Death of close friend	37	Change in number of family get-togethers	15
Change to different line of work [change of major]	36	Change in eating habits	13
Change in number of arguments with spouse	35	Vacation	13
Taking on a large mortgage [financial aid]	31	Christmas	12
Foreclosure of mortgage or loan	30	Minor violations of the law	11
Change in responsibilities at work [change in course demands]	29		

Check the list and identify the events that have happened to you in the past year or that you expect within the next year. Use the number system to determine how many stress points you are experiencing in this period of your life. Then score yourself as follows: over 200—urgent need of intelligent stress management; 150–199—careful stress management indicated; 100–149—stressful life, keep tabs on your mental health; under 100—no present cause for concern about stress.

SOURCE: Adapted from Lifescore: Holmes scale, *Family Health*, January 1979, p. 32.

of speeded-up functioning in which your resources of strength, adaptability, and skill are mobilized. When normalcy returns, all systems slow down, and recovery readies them for the next round of excitement. If you have to stay in overdrive for too long, however, resistance finally breaks down. This is exhaustion (Figure 2–2).

You may have noticed these sequences in yourself. At first, when you are under stress, you perform at peak efficiency. Your energy is tremendous, you never get sick, and you amaze yourself with all you can accomplish. This is the high-resistance stage of stress. But you may have noticed, too, that if you push yourself too hard for too long, you get sick when the stress lets up. It is not uncommon for students to go through final exams getting too little sleep, only to find that at the end of the examination period, they become ill. This often coincides with their returning home, where they can afford to relax.

Your ability to withstand stress depends on several factors. Some have to do with you, others with the stress itself. With respect to you, one factor is inborn: some people simply have stronger resistance than others, both physically and psychologically. Another is the skill with which you have

How well you handle a stressor depends on:
  Inborn resistance.
  Coping skill.
  Total load of recent/current stressors.
  Earlier experience with this kind of stressor.
  Self-esteem.

FIGURE 2–1 **Stressors in the Lives of Students**

Social pressures

Parental conflict

Academic competition

Lack of privacy

College red tape

Illness and injury

Religious conflicts

Love/ marriage decisions

Choice of major/ future job

Social alienation, anonymity

The College Student

Sexual pressures and fears

Military obligations

Family responsibilities

Money troubles

Loneliness, depression, anxiety

learned to handle stress: your coping skill. A third factor is the amount of stress you have already experienced, especially recently. Repeated bouts, too close together, weaken you. Still another factor is your past experience with stressors of the kind you are facing: if you have handled them well in the past, you will experience them as less stressful today. Your self-esteem plays a part, too: if ''I can handle it'' is a stock phrase for you, then chances are, you *can* handle it.

Many factors also modify the impact of stress. One is the intensity of the stressor—whether mild or extreme. Another is its duration—whether short or long term. You may be able to withstand acute stress (intense but short) better than chronic stress (less intense but endless), because the latter may ultimately drain more of your resources. Acute stress is aroused by a sudden, time-limited event such as a bomb threat, a snarling dog, or wonderful news. Chronic stress occurs when you experience continuous or repeated exposure to a situation and cannot adapt to it. A frustrating job, unfairness at school, and an overstimulating social life represent chronic stress.

In a school setting, stressors likely to require adaptation include the following:

■ *Arrival*. The person has to adjust to new surroundings.
■ *Course demands*. Some new classes may be difficult or impossible; some may be badly taught, boring, or irrelevant.

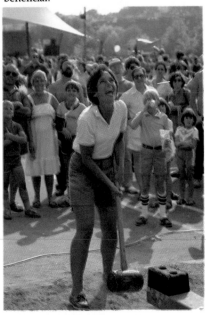

Physical challenges can be stressful—and beneficial.

FIGURE 2–2 Stress Ending in Recovery or Exhaustion

Alarm briefly lowers resistance but is followed by a high level of resistance. Recovery restores the normal level. If resistance is required for too long, exhaustion sets in, and resistance temporarily falls below the level normally maintained.

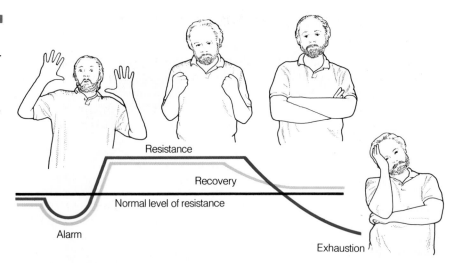

Resistance

Recovery

Normal level of resistance

Alarm

Exhaustion

- *Financial problems.* Students almost never have enough money.
- *Social life.* New students may need to learn new ways of speaking and behaving, and cope with new pressures (for example, the pressure to use drugs or alcohol).
- *Love life.* Developing intimate relationships can be stressful.
- *Sexual pressures and fears.* Students have to take responsibility for their own sexual behavior in the face of invitations and risks.
- *Family life.* Students have to balance family against school; some have to contend with attempted remote control from parents.
- *Self-definition.* Students have to choose and live by their own values: Do I have casual sex or don't I? Do I study or go out partying?
- *Self-continuity.* College can treat students as little more than Social Security numbers. The sense of self has to be strong to withstand this.

More important than either the person or the stressor alone is how the person perceives the stressor. If you know you can manage it skillfully, you may perceive it as beneficial. The kind of stress that challenges you to do your best, you experience as **eustress** (*eu*, pronounced "you," means good). When you feel that a stressor will require more resources than you have, it drains you. Stress that leads to exhaustion and defeat is termed **distress**. To feel that you can't cope with stress is to feel helpless. The brain's perception of inability to cope, called **learned helplessness**, is a major determinant of susceptibility to illness, and even of whether that illness will be fatal.[2]

An example will help to make this clear. Of two equally intelligent students in the same class, one feels inadequate and miserable, while the other feels challenged and enthusiastic. The first person experiences the class as a negative stressor; the second, as a positive one. This reveals that the person's reaction, not the situation, determines whether the stress is distress or eustress.

Your perception of yourself in the face of life's challenges is central to your state of health in every area—emotional, social, spiritual, and all the rest. It determines whether you function well or become ill. In a sense, you create your own reality.

The person's reaction, not the situation, determines whether the stress is distress or eustress.

BODY SYSTEMS: NERVOUS, HORMONAL, IMMUNE SYSTEMS

The stress response illustrates vividly how the whole person reacts to life's events. Whether stress at first seems to be "mental" or "physical," it always affects both mind and body. The reason is that the mind-body distinction is an illusion; the two are really one. To understand this fully, you need to become acquainted with the **anatomy** and **physiology** of the nervous and hormonal systems.

The Nervous System

Imagine for a moment that the body is a machine with millions of moving parts. The functioning of the whole depends on each part's doing its job exactly when needed and stopping when appropriate. The machine has an amazing central control system—a sort of computer—that can evaluate information about conditions, both within the machine and outside it. It can call into play whatever parts can best respond to any situation. It gets its information and transmits its instructions by way of a vast system of wiring. The system carries messages in two directions: signals about conditions from the parts to the center, and messages signaling work or rest from the center to the parts.

The system described here is, of course, the body's nervous system (see Figure 2-3). The control unit is the brain and spinal cord, called the **central nervous system**; and the wiring between the center and the parts is the **peripheral nervous system** (see Miniglossary of Nervous System Terms). The smooth functioning that results from the system's adjustments to changing conditions is **homeostasis**.

A second distinction is between the part of the nervous system that controls the voluntary muscles and the part that controls the internal organs. Your conscious mind wills the movement of your legs, but your pancreas operates automatically with no conscious demand from you. The unconscious nervous system, called the **autonomic nervous system**, has two parts, each of which opposes the other.

peripheral: puh-RIFF-er-ul

homeostasis: HO-me-oh-STAY- sis

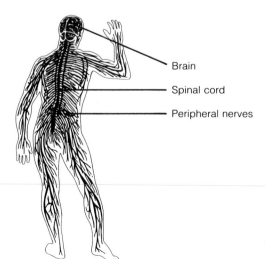

Brain

Spinal cord

Peripheral nerves

FIGURE 2-3   The Brain and Spinal Cord Comprise the Central Nervous System

An example will show how these parts work in balance to maintain homeostasis. When you go outside in cold weather, your skin's temperature receptors send "cold" messages to the spinal cord and brain. Your conscious mind may intervene at this point to tell you to wrap your sweater more closely around you, but let's say you have no sweater. Your autonomic nervous system reacts to the external stressor, the cold. It signals your skin-surface capillaries to shut down so your blood will circulate deeper in your tissues, where it will conserve heat. It also signals involuntary contractions of the small muscles just under the skin surface. A product of these muscle contractions is heat, and the visible result is goose bumps. If these measures do not raise your body temperature enough, then the nerves signal your large muscle groups to shiver; the contractions of these large muscles produce still more heat. All of this activity adds up to a set of adjustments that maintains your homeostasis (for temperature) under conditions of external extremes that would throw it off balance (cold). The cold was a stressor; the body's response was resistance.

Now let's say you come in and sit by a fire and drink hot cocoa. You are warm, and you no longer need all that heat-producing activity. At this point, the opposing set of autonomic nerves takes over; they signal your skin surface capillaries to dilate again, your goose bumps to subside, and your muscles to relax. Your body is back to normal. This is recovery.

Think about the autonomic nervous system this way: one part directs the body when homeostasis needs restoring and the other part controls it during normal times.

The Hormonal System

The body has yet another communication system—the hormonal system. Like the nervous system, it coordinates body functions by transmitting and receiving messages, but with several major differences. A nervous system message originates in a nerve and travels as electrical impulses along nerves from point to point within the body. A hormonal system message originates in a **gland** (see Miniglossary of Hormonal System Terms) and travels as a chemical compound (a **hormone**) in the bloodstream. The hormone flows everywhere in the body, but only its **target organs** respond to it, because only they possess the equipment to receive it. The point-to-point messages of the nervous system travel through a central switchboard (the spinal cord and brain), whereas the messages of the hormonal system are broadcast over the airways (the bloodstream), and any organ with the right receiver can pick them up.

Another difference between the two systems is that nerve impulses travel faster than hormonal messages do—although both are remarkably swift. Whereas your brain's command to wiggle your toes reaches the toes within a fraction of a second and stops as quickly, a gland's message to alter a body condition may take several seconds or minutes to get started and may fade away equally slowly.

Among the hormones familiar to everyone are:

■ Insulin, which helps regulate the blood sugar level.
■ Estrogen and testosterone, which help regulate the body's sexual development and functions.

■ Thyroid hormone, which regulates the body's metabolic rate.
■ **Epinephrine** and **norepinephrine**, the so-called **stress hormones**.

The hormonal system, together with the nervous system, integrates the whole body's functioning so that all parts act smoothly together.

The Immune System

You may think that you have not been exposed to any illnesses today, but the truth is that you are surrounded and constantly being attacked by health's enemies. If you are healthy now, thank your **immune system** (see Miniglossary of Immune System Terms), which has been serving as your personal bodyguard, successfully fighting off and destroying invaders every day.

It is hard to say just where the immune system is located, because parts of the system are everywhere. The bone marrow grows the white blood cells called **lymphocytes**. The **thymus gland** incubates some of the lymphocytes and releases them as **T cells** (T for thymus): they now possess the ability to recognize enemies. The liver and spleen make other lymphocytes into **B cells**,* which produce **antibodies**, large molecules that serve as ammunition against invaders.

The lymphocytes travel in the blood and lymph, reside in the tissues, and aggregate in the lymph nodes, which swell in response to infection. (Among the lymph nodes are the small, lima bean-shaped organs that you can feel swell up around your throat when you are getting a cold.) Some of the lymphocytes respond to invaders by producing a chemical called **histamine**, which inflames the site and attracts defenders to it.

When T cells have identified the enemy, and B cells have fired antibodies at it and killed it, still other lymphocytes (we'll call them scavenger cells) capture and devour it. In the background are still other cells (memory cells) that retain a memory of the invader so that the system can quickly destroy it at the next encounter.

The strike force of T and B cells works as a unit. If one of the T cells spots an enemy it recognizes, it sends out an alert (a chemical message). B cells respond by producing antibodies. The antibodies are proteins that recognize an **antigen**, attach to it, and package it up to be disposed of (see Figure 2–4). Other cells that respond to the T cells' chemical message are the T-killer cells. This group destroys body cells that have become infected with the invader.

As you might suspect, all of this death and destruction could be hazardous if it got out of hand, so the body has developed a shutoff system to control it. The immune response is shut down by T-suppressor cells, which become active as the battle comes to an end. When the action is over, all that remain are some antibodies and memory cells, which retain an imprint of what has happened.

Memory cells live for many years and remember the enemy. If it is ever spotted again, they act swiftly and prevent a major invasion. At this point, you have developed an **immunity** to that particular antigen and to the disease it produces. You have permanent protection against reinfection. That's why so many of the contagious diseases—measles, mumps, chicken pox—are once-only diseases. Today, you don't even have to get the disease once, in many

---

> ### MINIGLOSSARY
> ### of Immune System Terms
>
> **antibodies:** large protein molecules produced in response to the presence of antigens such as viruses; they immobilize the antigens so that scavenger cells can devour and digest them.
> **antigen:** a foreign body such as a virus, bacteria, or allergy-causing substance; any foreign substance that stimulates the production of antibodies.
> **B cells:** a class of lymphocytes that produces antibodies.
> **histamine** (HIST-uh-meen): a chemical of immunity that produces inflammation (swelling and irritation) of tissue.
> **immune system:** the cells, tissues, and organs that protect the body from disease, composed of the lymphocytes, bone marrow, thymus gland, spleen, and other parts.
> **immunity:** the body's capacity for identifying, destroying, and disposing of disease-causing agents.
> **interferon:** see *T cells*.
> **lymphocytes** (LIM-fo-sights): a class of white blood cells, involved in immunity.
> **T cells:** a class of lymphocytes that possesses the ability to recognize invaders dangerous to the body. T cells produce chemical messengers, such as *interferon*, that prompt the B cells to produce antibodies.
> **thymus gland:** an organ of the immune system.

The immune system resides in many body organs, including the bone marrow, the thymus gland, the liver and spleen, and the lymphatic system.

An example of a chemical message sent out by the T cells is **interferon**, which is used in medicine to step up the body's response to certain infections and is being used as an anticancer drug.

---

*B cells are named for the bursa, a part of the intestinal area of chickens, where they were first discovered.

FIGURE 2–4   Antigens and
Antibodies

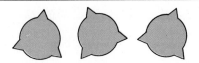

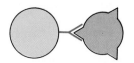

1. Body is challenged by foreign invaders
   (antigens).

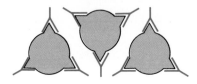

2. Immune system cells record shape of
   invaders.

Antibodies

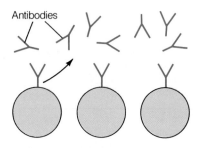

3. Cells use this memory record to make
   antibodies.

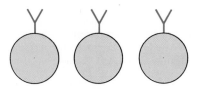

4. Later, antibodies inactivate foreign invaders.

5. Memory remains to make antibodies faster
   the next time this foreign invader attacks.

cases, because vaccinations introduce antigens in a form that doesn't cause disease but codes the memory cells to make you immune to it.

You may wonder why a person catches colds or flu over and over again. Actually, it is likely that the symptoms of sickness we call "a cold" represent a multitude of *different* colds, each caused by a different infectious agent. Also, some flu viruses can hide from the immune cells just well enough to keep the cells from remembering them from infection to infection. That is why a person who gets cold sores will have repeated outbreaks once the virus takes up residence in the body. The immune system doesn't fully recognize the old enemy.

■ THE STRESS RESPONSE

The **stress response** evolved as a reaction to immediate physical danger, the **fight-or-flight reaction**. The moment the brain perceives danger, a regulating center, the **hypothalamus**, initiates the response, and the nervous and hormonal systems go into an emergency alert.

Under stress, the nervous system works just as you would want it to, facilitating the most efficient possible response to physical danger. The pupils of the eyes widen so that you can see better; the muscles tense up so that you can jump, run, or struggle with maximum strength; breathing quickens to bring more oxygen into the lungs; circulation to the skin diminishes (to protect against blood loss from injury); circulation to the digestive system and internal organs (which can wait) also diminishes; while circulation to the muscles and brain (which are needed now) increases; the heart races and the blood pressure rises to rush oxygen to the muscles and brain so that they can burn the fuel they need for energy. The kidneys retain water, in case you should be injured and lose water by bleeding; the immune system shuts down, including the part of it that produces inflammation at a site of injury (the body can't afford to deal with irritation at a time when it needs to cope with external threats).

While the nerves bring about some of these effects, the hormones go to work, too. The hypothalamus initiates a hormone cascade that calls gland after gland into play, affecting every organ in the body. Among the compounds released in response are **endorphins**, the body's natural painkillers, to enable the person to continue functioning, even if injured.

The nerves and hormones of the stress response produce not only the effects you feel—tense muscles, sharp eyesight, speeded-up heartbeat and respiration—but also other deep, internal responses that make you ready for fight or flight in other ways. They alter the metabolism—the chemical changes affecting energy—of every cell.

When the stress response is called upon day after day and not discharged, harmful effects set in. Repeated shutdown of the immune system weakens the defenses against infection and cancer. Retention of fluid raises the blood pressure and can lead to heart attacks and strokes. Shutdown of the digestive system predisposes it to ulcers, constipation, diarrhea, and other disorders. Muscle tension strains the lower back and produces tension headaches. The skin is deprived of nourishment by way of the circulation, and of immune factors necessary to prevent infections, including acne. The hormonal system is upset, leading to menstrual irregularities, some forms of infertility, and growth failure in children. In short, prolonged stress damages many major body organs and systems.

The experience of chronic stress unrelieved by periods of recreation or relaxation takes a toll on the body that renders it less resilient and more susceptible to disease. Diseases themselves add further stresses. The toll, according to Selye, is ultimately paid in **adaptation energy**, a commodity that is limited. When you run out of adaptation energy, you die.

For a long time after Selye advanced this idea, it seemed vague. No physical basis for it had been identified. Now, researchers may be discovering what Selye's adaptation energy consists of: the ability of the brain cells to respond to stress. Each time they are hit with high doses of stress hormones, they age a little.[3] Laboratory experiments with animals show that brain aging is reflected in three measurable characteristics. First, higher stress hormone levels are required to elicit a response from the brain cells; second, the adaptation response is slower; and third, recovery is delayed.[4]

Failing recovery, exhaustion takes any of three forms. Physical illness is one. Mental illness is another, and social maladjustment is a third (see Chapter 3).

The length of the human lifespan appears to be primarily determined by the amount of available adaptation energy. Constant exposure to any stressor will use it up
—Hans Selye, *The Stress of Life*, 1956.

STRESS MANAGEMENT STRATEGIES

Managing stress well involves two sets of skills—one for sailing along, when moment-to-moment adjustments can keep you on course; the other for stormy times. The person who maintains a strong program of personal health during ordinary life is best able to withstand crises when they arrive. The foundation for that health is emotional stability; this chapter's Life Choice Inventory provides a checklist against which to measure yours.

Wise time management can help you to minimize stress. Time is similar to a regular income: you receive 24 hours of it each day. It is like money, too, in that you have three ways in which to spend it. You can save ahead (do tasks now so you won't have to do them later); you can spend as you go; or you can borrow from the future (have fun now and hope you will find the time later to do things you have to do). If you manage time wisely,

---

CONSUMER CAUTION

There are no quick-fix pills that will make you strong in a crisis.

LIFE CHOICE INVENTORY

Do you cultivate emotional well-being? Try answering these questions to get an idea. Don't take your score too seriously; this is just for fun.

1. I spend time doing work that I enjoy.
   (a) Almost always (b) Sometimes (c) Almost never
2. I find it easy to relax.
   (a) Almost always (b) Sometimes (c) Almost never
3. In my spare time, I participate in activities that I enjoy.
   (a) Almost always (b) Sometimes (c) Almost never
4. When I am about to be in a stressful situation, I realize it ahead of time, and I prepare for it.
   (a) Almost always (b) Sometimes (c) Almost never
5. I handle anger: (a) By expressing it in ways that hurt neither myself nor other people; (b) By bottling it up so that no one knows I'm angry (c) I never am angry, or I express anger aggressively.
6. I participate in group activities such as church and-community organizations.
   (a) Quite often (b) Very seldom (c) Never

7. I find it easy to express my feelings.
   (a) Almost always (b) Sometimes (c) Almost never
8. I can talk to close friends, relatives, or others about personal matters.
   (a) Almost always (b) Sometimes (c) Almost never
9. When I need help with personal matters, I seek it out.
   (a) Almost always (b) Sometimes (c) Almost never
10. When I am under stress, I make extra sure to exercise regularly, to work off my tension.
    (a) Almost always (b) Sometimes (c) Almost never

For each *a* answer, give yourself two points; for each *b* answer, give yourself one point; for each *c* answer, give yourself zero points. A score of 18 to 20 is excellent; 16 or 17 is very good; 14 or 15 is good; and 13 or below means that you need improvement.

SOURCE: Adapted from U.S. Department of Health and Human Services, "Health Style," HHS publication no. (PHS) 81- 50155, 1981 (a self-test, distributed by National Health Information Clearinghouse).

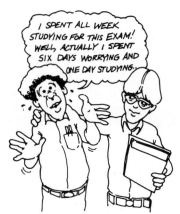

It only slows you down to worry about things you have to do.

you can gain the two advantages that wise money management also gives you—security for the future and enjoyment of the present. It takes skill to treat yourself to enough luxuries so that you enjoy your present life, while saving enough so that you will have time available when you need it. When your friends call on a Sunday to invite you out, you don't want to be caught with no money on hand, no clean clothes, and no studying done for the big exam on Monday. That is an avoidable stress, and planning ahead circumvents it. Make a time budget. Remember, you have to do it only once, and an hour of time spent organizing buys many hours of time doing what you choose.

Several planning techniques can help you get the most out of your day while keeping tabs on long-term time needs. One such technique is to make two records—one, a list of things to do, and the other, a weekly time schedule. To make the time schedule, set up a grid that lists the days of the week across the top and blocks of time (such as each hour from waking to bedtime) down the left-hand side. First, fill in your set obligations, such as class meetings, in the appropriate spaces. Then add study time, travel time, and mealtimes. Allot a space each day to exercise. In the time left, decide when to take care of your regular weekly obligations, such as laundry, bill paying, or grocery shopping. Part of your daily time should be allocated to maintaining yourself physically. Attend to your nutrition, your sleep needs, and your need for play and relaxation. When you have listed everything you can anticipate for the week, you are ready to make a daily schedule. Write out today's obligations and activities on a sheet to carry with you, and prepare to assign tasks from your list of things to do, to the empty spaces.

Study your list of things to do, and decide how urgent each one is ("This I can postpone; this I have to do today"). Enter the most urgent items into today's schedule, carry it with you, and check off each item when you have completed it. At the end of the day, return uncompleted tasks to the list of things to do.

To schedule a long-term assignment, such as a term paper, first identify every task you must do to complete the project. Then, working backward from the due date, schedule each task. For example, if it will take you six hours to type the paper, schedule those six hours on a grid that you have started for the due-date week. Back up and schedule time before that to write the final draft and time before that for the research. If you have been realistic about the time each step will take, you will not be caught short at the end.

These strategies strengthen your resistance between stressful times. Now, consider the times of stress themselves. You have to cope.

The means of handling pain and stress are behaviors known as **coping devices**, and some are more adaptive than others (see Miniglossary of Coping Devices). The less adaptive ones are ways of continuing to avoid the pain as much as possible, whereas the more adaptive ones are ways of dealing with it and working it through. The **maladaptive** coping behaviors are sometimes known as **defense mechanisms**, and they are listed in a Miniglossary of their own.

An intermediate type of coping behavior is **displacement**, the application of energy to another area altogether. Displacement is suitable for a time. Healthy people have a hierarchy of displacement behaviors with which they handle life's ups and downs. The behaviors need not be orthodox. It takes time to heal, and while the healing is taking place, it makes sense to do whatever works for you—as long as what you choose to do harms or endangers neither you nor anyone else. Many people elect to engage in familiar, even pointless, activity while sensation returns.

Ultimately, though, it becomes necessary to move on, and many people do so by way of **ventilation**, a truly adaptive coping behavior. Ventilating means letting off steam, by expressing feelings to another person.

Too many people believe they have to wait until the effects of stress are beginning to become severe before they take steps to relieve it. That's not true. At each step along the way, it's possible to intervene and obtain relief. The alarm step is the first at which you can intervene. Recognize your own alarm reaction. You can then seek to identify the source of the stress and begin to deal with it immediately.

We said earlier that the person's reaction, not the situation, determines the severity of stress. People can change the way they react to events so that the events aren't so stressful.

An example is public speaking. The stress response can help you get "up for it." Some excitement and anticipation ahead of the event, with the associated rapid heartbeat and breathing, will give you the physical energy to turn out a spectacular performance. You are at your most attractive when you are aroused and alert. But too much is debilitating. If you allow yourself to think about what a catastrophe it will be if you do less than a perfect job, you will be trembling visibly, your teeth will be chattering, and your knees will be knocking together. In such a state, you can hardly reach your audience at all, and you will be unduly exhausted afterward. It is to your advantage to learn to *perceive* the event as not-so-stressful.

MINIGLOSSARY
of Coping Devices

displacement: channeling the energy of suffering into something else—for example, using the emotional energy churned up by grief for work or recreation.
ventilation: the act of verbally venting one's feelings; letting off steam by talking, crying, swearing, or laughing.

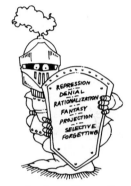

Defense mechanisms: Forms of mental avoidance.

"Do not distress yourself," a famous poem ("Desiderata") says. Doesn't this suggest that distress—the maladaptive response to stress—is a personal choice? You do it to yourself.

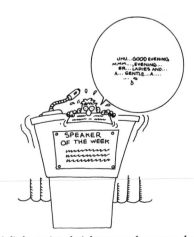

A little anxiety heightens performance, but too much anxiety can be debilitating.

To prevent harm from stress:

✳ Identify tensions when they first arise.

✳ Recognize stress and identify its source.

✳ Control responses.

✳ Identify inappropriate responses and change them.

✳ Focus your attention and energy right on the task you are facing.

✳ Recognize the warning signals of too much stress.

This example illustrates another strategy: use the stress response to your advantage. Direct and control the energy it gives you. Energy is a magnificent, adaptive response to challenges, after all. It's only when the energy is scattered and wasted that it drains you without giving you anything in return. (In other words, it's OK to have butterflies in your stomach as long as they're all flying in formation.)

It is helpful to monitor your body for the many warning signals of too much stress. If you are alert to their appearance, you can initiate preventive action before exhaustion sets in and does damage (see Table 2–3).

The length of the lists of signs of stress is impressive. Some people have some of the symptoms all the time. Everyone has some of them some of the time. The presence of a few symptoms is not cause for alarm, but there is a time to take them seriously. The thing to be concerned about is the appearance of these symptoms under conditions that you know are stressful

TABLE 2–3 Signs of Stress

Physical Signs	Psychological Signs
Pounding of the heart; rapid heart rate.	Irritability, tension, or depression.
Rapid, shallow breathing.	Impulsive behavior and emotional instability; the overpowering urge to cry or to run and hide.
Dryness of the throat and mouth.	Lowered self-esteem; thoughts related to failure.
Raised body temperature.	
Decreased sexual appetite or activity.	Excessive worry; insecurity; concern about other people's opinions; self-deprecation in conversation.
Feelings of weakness, light-headedness, dizziness, or faintness.	Reduced ability to communicate with others.
Trembling; nervous tics; twitches; shaking hands and fingers.	Increased awkwardness in social situations.
Tendency to be easily startled (by small sounds and the like).	Excessive boredom; unexplained dissatisfaction with job or other normal conditions.
High-pitched, nervous laughter.	Increased procrastination.
Stuttering and other speech difficulties.	Feelings of isolation.
Insomnia—that is, difficulty in getting to sleep, or a tendency to wake up during the night.	Avoidance of specific situations or activities.
Grinding of the teeth during sleep.	Irrational fears (phobias) about specific things.
Restlessness, an inability to keep still.	Irrational thoughts; forgetting things more often than usual; mental "blocks"; missing of planned events.
Sweating (not necessarily noticeably); clammy hands; cold hands and feet; cold chills.	Guilt about neglecting family or friends; inner confusion about duties and roles.
Blushing; hot face.	Excessive work; omission of play.
The need to urinate frequently.	Unresponsiveness and preoccupation.
Diarrhea; indigestion; upset stomach, nausea.	Inability to organize oneself; tendency to get distraught over minor matters.
Migraine or other headaches; frequent unexplained earaches or toothaches.	Inability to reach decisions; erratic, unpredictable judgement making.
Premenstrual tension or missed menstrual periods.	Decreased ability to perform different tasks.
More body aches and pains than usual, such as pain in the neck or lower back; or any localized muscle tension.	Inability to concentrate.
Loss of appetite; unintended weight loss; excessive appetite; sudden weight gain.	General ("floating") anxiety; feelings of unreality.
Sudden change in appearance.	A tendency to become fatigued; loss of energy; loss of spontaneous joy.
Increased use of substances (tobacco, legally prescribed drugs such as tranquilizers or amphetamines, alcohol, other drugs).	Nightmares.
Accident proneness.	Feelings of powerlessness; mistrust of others.
Frequent illnesses.	Neurotic behavior; psychosis.

for you and that have, in the past, proved to be the forerunners of serious illness or inability to cope.

The cumulative effects of stress create a situation in which even small details become overwhelming. The person under chronic stress may become unable to handle even small problems. Example: a student who is breaking up with his girlfriend, moving out of his home, and changing schools all at the same time is trying to get his personal effects packed. He picks up a paper clip and can't decide what packing box to put it in. He starts to sob; he can't cope.

At such a time, you need to reduce your stress. Ask yourself which elements of the situation you can control, and pay strict attention to only those. In the case of our friend, he needs to take a deep breath and calm down. Once the crying has relaxed him, he should ask himself what he can control right now and what he can't. The breakup, the move, and the change of schools are beyond his control right now. The packing is not. He can go on with it or stop. He may need to take a break—for food, sleep, or exercise. He may need to tap a friendship—get help moving boxes or just make plans for dinner. These are the tasks he has to handle right now. He can let go of the rest.

Finally, even in the midst of severe stress, you can learn to relax and indulge in moments of recovery.

⊛ Identify which stressors you can control. Put the others out of your mind. List priorities and start taking action.

⊛ Learn to release tension whenever appropriate, by exercising, laughing, or willing yourself to relax.

WILLED RELAXATION

The exact opposite of the stress response is the **relaxation response** (see Table 2–4). Relaxation occurs naturally whenever stressors stop acting on you, and it permits your body to recover from the effects of stress. But you can also will it to happen, even in the midst of a stressful situation.[5]

Many clinics use a **biofeedback** technique to teach people how to monitor their own physical condition. A machine (an electroencephalograph, or EEG) is wired to pads attached painlessly to the outside of the head. It displays patterns that reflect brainwave activity on a monitor. By watching the screen display, the subject notes that different brainwaves are associated with tension and relaxation and that different sensations occur along with them; she can then learn to bring on the states voluntarily.

Another way to achieve the same result is **progressive muscle relaxation**. The technique involves lying flat and relaxing the muscles all over the body,

MINIGLOSSARY
of Defense Mechanisms

denial: the refusal to admit that something unpleasant or painful has occurred: "No, I don't believe it."

fantasy: delusion, in the face of a painful or unpleasant situation, that something positive has happened instead: "He hasn't really left me. He's gone to buy me a present."

oral behavior: ingesting substances such as drugs, alcohol, or unneeded food.

projection: the conviction, in the face of an unpleasant or painful situation you have caused, that it is the other person's fault: "The teacher asked the wrong questions on the exam."

rationalization: the justification of an unreasonable action or attitude by manufacturing reasons for it: "I couldn't prevent the accident because I had to pay attention to something else."

regression: the reversion to inappropriate childish ways of dealing with painful realities, such as chronic crying or whining.

repression: the refusal to acknowledge an unpleasant or painful event or piece of news: not hearing it.

selective forgetting: memory lapse concerning an experience or piece of news too painful to bear: not remembering it.

withdrawal: disengaging from people and activities to avoid pain. Examples: engaging in extended periods of fantasy (daydreaming), refusing to talk with anyone, or sleeping excessively.

TABLE 2–4   The Stress Response and the Relaxation Response

Stress Response	Relaxation Response
Rapid metabolism	Normal metabolism
Fast heart rate	Normal heart rate
Raised blood pressure	Normal blood pressure
Rapid respiration	Normal respiration
Muscles tense	Muscles relaxed
Blood supply to digestive organs and skin diverted to muscles	Normal blood circulation restored
Water retained in body	Normal water balance restored
Immune resistance lowered	Immune resistance restored

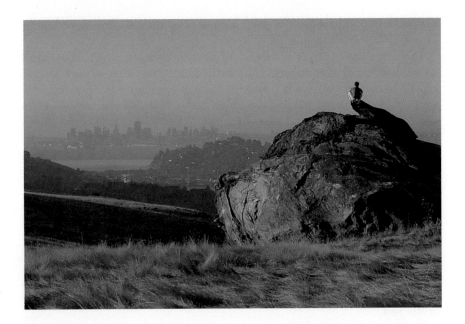

When you have symptoms of stress, they indicate that you are exhausting your ability to cope if:

■ You know you are under severe stress.
■ The same symptoms, in the past, appeared just before your resistance failed.

. . . but you can also learn to relax at will.

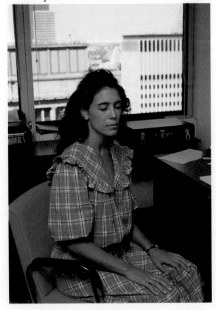

beginning with the toes. The goal is to locate and erase tension wherever it is occurring in the body. People who have never tried this are astonished to discover the number of different muscles used in creating tension, especially in the belly, the upper back and neck, and the face. A way to learn muscle relaxation is to use a machine (the electromyograph, or EMG) that can measure muscle tension. Harmless electronic sensors can be fastened to the forehead, neck, jaw, or anywhere muscles may be tense. A tone feeds back information to the person by changing pitch when the muscle tension changes. The pitch drops lower and lower as the person relaxes, and so the person learns what to do to become fully relaxed. Another biofeedback tool, the pulse monitor, can make the heartbeat audible, so that the subject can learn how to slow it down, thus achieving the same thing—relaxation.

You can practice muscle relaxation whenever you think of it—not only when you have time to lie down for 30 minutes. Professional mountain climbers train themselves to do it while climbing—the so-called mountain rest step. Any time you take a step, you have to tense one leg—but why tense the other one? At each step, relax the unused leg and let the tension go. That way, you're resting throughout the climb and don't have to be exhausted when you get to the top. Students don't have physical mountains to climb, but they do have intellectual ones. If your shoulders (for example) are tense while you are reading, what good does that do you? Relax them.

Two similar relaxation techniques are **meditation** and **self-hypnosis**. Both involve closing the eyes, breathing deeply, and relaxing the muscles. This chapter's Strategies box presents a summary of the steps used in a variety of relaxation techniques. A complete set of instructions would provide many more details. You can use the one given here once or twice daily, and after a while, the response will come with little effort. Practicing it before meals is better than after, since the digestive processes seem to interfere with the response.

To practice relaxation at intervals is to assume control of the body's responses, and it has a benefit beyond the simple pleasure it brings. Just as stress leads to disease, stress management helps prevent it.

STRATEGIES: Steps to Relaxation

To relax at will:
1. Assume a comfortable sitting position.
2. When you are ready, close your eyes.
3. Become aware of your breathing. Breathe in deeply, hold it, then breathe out. Each time you breathe out, say the word *one* silently to yourself.
4. Allow each of your muscles to relax deeply, one after another. Imagine that you are floating, drifting, or gliding.
5. Maintain a passive attitude and permit relaxation to occur at its own pace. (Any way that you are proceeding is correct.) Thoughts will pass through your mind; allow them to come and go without resistance.
6. Continue for 20 minutes. You may open your eyes to check the time, but do not use an alarm. When you finish, sit quietly for several minutes, and open your eyes when you are ready.

The joy of life is in meeting its challenges, developing new ways of dealing with them, engaging in experiences that will facilitate new learning. The next chapter delves further into factors that enhance emotional health and well-being.

STUDY AIDS

1. Define *stress*.
2. Distinguish between eustress and distress.
3. Show how the nervous and hormonal systems regulate the body's functioning during times of stress and between those times.
4. Identify the principal components of the immune system.
5. Describe how each of the immune system's components contributes to the body's defenses against disease.
6. Describe the harmful side effects of prolonged stress on the body's systems.
7. Describe an effective time management strategy.
8. Describe some ways of dealing with emotional pain (defense mechanisms and coping devices), together with the limits of their utility.
9. Enumerate some of the physical and psychological signs of stress.
10. Describe the relaxation response and several different means of achieving it.

GLOSSARY

For nervous system, hormonal system, and immune system terms, see separate Miniglossaries on pages 26 and 27.

adaptation energy: a term used to describe the limited capacity of the body to withstand stress.

adaptive: with respect to behavior, that which benefits the organism. Behavior that brings about results that are harmful to the organism is termed *maladaptive* behavior.
    mal = bad

alarm: see *stress response*.

anatomy: the study of the physical structures of the body.

biofeedback: a clinical technique used to help a person learn to bring about the relaxation response by providing mechanical feedback on brainwave activity, skin temperature, heart rate, muscle tension, or other measurable biological activities of the body.

cope: to mobilize a healthy, effective reaction to stress.

coping devices: behaviors, both adaptive and maladaptive, used to deal with the reality of an unpleasant or painful situation. See Miniglossary of Coping Devices (page 31).

defense mechanisms: automatic and often unconscious forms of emotional avoidance in reaction to emotional injury. See Miniglossary of Defense Mechanisms (page 33).

distress: see *stress*.

endorphin (en-DOR-fin): a natural painkiller manufactured in the brain in response to stress or injury. Endorphins are also known as *endogenous opiates*.
    endo = inside
    gen = produced

epinephrine (EP-uh-NEFF-rin), **norepinephrine**: two hormones of the adrenal gland, sometimes called the stress hormones, although they are not the only hormones modulating the stress response. (The *adrenal gland* is a gland that nestles in the surface of the kidney.)

> *ad* = on
> *renal* = kidney

eustress (YOU-stress): see *stress*.

exhaustion: see *stress response*.

fight-or-flight reaction: the response to immediate physical danger; the stress response.

homeostasis (HO-me-oh-STAY-sis): the maintenance of relatively constant internal conditions by corrective responses to forces that would otherwise cause life-threatening changes in those conditions. A homeostatic system is not static. It is constantly changing, but within tolerable limits.

> *homeo* = the same
> *stasis* = staying

hypothalamus (HIGH-poh-THAL-uh-mus): a regulating center within the brain that communicates with both the nervous system and the hormonal system.

> *hypo* = beneath, under

learned helplessness: the perception of inability to cope; a major factor in determining a person's susceptibility to stress-induced illness.

maladaptive: see *adaptive*.

meditation: a method of relaxing that involves closing the eyes, breathing deeply, and relaxing the muscles.

noradrenaline (NOR-uh-DREN-uh-lin): see *adrenaline*.

norepinephrine (NOR-ep-uh-NEFF-rin): see *epinephrine*.

physiology: the study of the functions of the body.

progressive muscle relaxation: a technique of achieving the relaxation response by systematically relaxing the body's muscle groups.

recovery: see *stress response*.

relaxation response: the opposite of the stress response; the normal state of the body.

resistance: the body's ability to withstand stress. See *stress response*.

self-hypnosis: a method of relaxing that involves closing the eyes, breathing deeply, and relaxing the muscles.

stress: the effect of stressors on a person. Stress that provides a welcome challenge is *eustress*; stress that is perceived as negative is *distress*. See *stress response*.

> *eu* = good, beneficial
> *dis* = bad, negative

stress hormones: epinephrine and norepinephrine, secreted as part of the reaction of the autonomic nervous system to stress.

stress response or **general adaptation syndrome:** the response to a demand or stressor, brought about by the nerves and hormones of the autonomic nervous system. It has three phases. In the *alarm* phase, the person perceives the demand or stressor; in the *resistance* phase, the body's systems are mobilized to deal with the demand. The third phase is either *recovery* (a return to the normal, relatively stress-free state) or *exhaustion* (breakdown of resistance with consequent harmful side effects).

stressor: a demand placed on the body to adapt.

QUIZ ANSWERS

1. *False*. Too little stress is as bad for health as too much.

2. *True*. Having a skiing accident and getting married are more similar than different, as far as your body is concerned.

3. *True*. Whether an event is stressful depends more on the person experiencing it than on the event itself.

4. *True*. The feeling of helplessness makes people more likely to get sick.

5. *True*. There is a limit to how much stress a person can take; when the limit is reached, the person dies.

6. *True*. Being able to talk to close friends about personal matters helps people manage stress.

7. *False*. You can intervene at several points during a crisis to minimize the negative effects it might have on you.

8. *True*. It's all right to refuse to face emotional injury as long as you do so only for a while.

9. *False*. People can learn to relax.

10. *True*. Meditation and self-hypnosis are similar relaxation techniques.

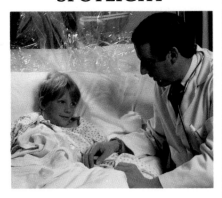

Faith and Healing

An extraordinary story about successful coping with stress is that of Norman Cousins's bout with a debilitating illness. Cousins, the editor of the famous *Saturday Review* magazine, took a stressful trip overseas and returned home exhausted. A week later, he found himself hardly able to stand up, and he had to go to the hospital.

Didn't he have some sort of miracle recovery?

Yes. At first, he was told that the diagnosis was a degenerative disease of the connective tissue of the spine, almost invariably fatal. His physicians predicted that he would remain an invalid for the rest of his life and that his spine would deteriorate until he was paralyzed. Stress and exhaustion had led to disease, the disease was expected to be totally disabling, the expectation caused further stress, and the end would be tragic.

Lying in his hospital bed, Cousins considered what he already knew about stress, diseases, and cures. It occurred to him that if negative emotional experiences could harm the body, then positive emotional experiences might restore health. To his way of thinking, the most positive emotional experiences would be "hope, faith, laughter, confidence, and the will to live." Finding the hospital an unpleasant environment, Cousins checked out and moved, with his physician's approval, into a hotel room, where he could be equally well taken care of without being surrounded by illness. There, he watched comedy films and had funny stories read to him. Having spent weeks with hardly any sleep and being now in acute pain, he made the wonderful discovery that after a hearty laugh, he could relax and sleep soundly for an hour or two at a time. (He also believed in the curative power of vitamin C for diseases of connective tissue and so employed large doses as part of his cure regimen.) The laughter, relaxation, and sleep (and, according to Cousins, the vitamin C) brought about a healing that no amount of medical attention could have achieved. The long of the story is in Cousins's article "Anatomy of an Illness," which was published in the *Saturday Review* and the *New England Journal of Medicine* as a landmark in medical history.[1]* The short of it is that Cousins recovered completely, and was able after some weeks to walk on the beach, to use all of his limbs, to return to work, and to lead a normal life.

Well, how do you suppose he did it? What accounts for his recovery?

There has been much speculation about that, but most people (including Cousins himself) agree that there was certainly an element of **placebo effect**. A **placebo** is an inert, or dummy, substance labeled "medicine," used for its psychological effect. The placebo effect is the healing that occurs in people given such medication.

How common is the placebo effect?

It is not unusual for experiments using placebos to record an effect in 30 to 60 percent of subjects. That is, people given only distilled water or sugar pills will recover about half the time, as completely as if they had received a curative medication.

Placebos, given with persuasive encouragement ("This will make you better"), are sometimes so effective that physicians have on occasion prescribed them when they didn't know what else to prescribe. The curious thing is that people will recover, given placebos, when they would not recover without them. In other words, the placebo effect is valuable; it is an important weapon against illness.

Are you telling me that my physician may give me fake medicine?

*Reference notes are in Appendix D.

No, that would be unethical. But the point is that your response, even to the real drug, may be aided by your faith in the treatment, whether you or your physician know it or not.

We want to warn you, though: quacks will sell you placebos every chance they get. Since 30 to 60 percent of people given anything will recover, there will be plenty of testimonials extolling the virtues of the quack's miracle cures.

How does the placebo effect work?

Recall how the nervous system works. The patient is anxious, wonders what might be wrong, feels helpless, and worries so much that symptoms become aggravated. Then the patient goes to a famous healer. The healer names the disease, and the patient feels reassured: the expert has the answer. The healer then prescribes a treatment, and the patient relaxes. Help has replaced helplessness. The stress response diminishes, and symptoms begin to disappear. The placebo actually brings about a measurable physiological response: blood pressure falls, pulse rate slows, and so forth.[2] With resistance restored, the patient proceeds to get well, whatever treatment has been prescribed.

So you think it works through the relaxation response?

That certainly must be part of it. Research has often illustrated the effect. For example, it had been thought, at various times, that ulcers were caused by poor circulation to the stomach or intestine, by hot foods, by cold foods, by coarse foods, by spices such as pepper, by alcohol, by caffeine. Patients were cautioned against all these things. One physician, however, attempted to treat ulcers simply by giving shots of distilled water with the guarantee that they would heal the ulcers. The patients recovered.[3] We now know that the common thread in all such ulcers is anxiety. In such cases, the placebo effect reliably works its magic. Faith heals.

I see what you mean. I suppose witch doctors, shamans, and all healers work their cures the same way.

Probably so. Don't forget, too, that the body will often heal itself, given time. Frequently, all that healers have to do is to wait out the duration of the malady. If they can offer reassurance and confidence, they will be providing support as important as any chemical or physical procedure might be. In fact, health care providers in training are taught not only to manage their clients' medical care but also to dole out liberal doses of TLC, tender loving care. Children given TLC recover far faster than those deprived of it. They even grow better.[4]

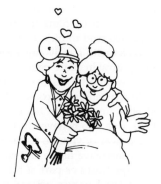

Love heals.

Does the placebo effect work for pain?

Yes. A physician describes a study in which people in pain had to go through some medical procedures. Some people were fully informed in advance; others were deprived of the comfort of knowing what to expect. The informed people needed only half as many pain-killing drugs and were discharged from the hospital an average of two and a half days earlier.[5] This suggests an effect specifically in those nerves that register pain.

Research on exactly how brain and body chemistry interact is only beginning, but some clues have already been collected. They point to natural brain chemicals (endorphins) that relieve stress and pain. People in pain, given placebos, often experience relief of their pain; those given placebos with naloxone, a chemical agent that blocks the brain's production of these natural painkillers, experience no such relief. This shows that placebos relieve pain by triggering endorphin production.

How powerful can the placebo effect be?

The endorphins are more powerful painkillers than morphine, which has been used for centuries to relieve extreme distress, such as that caused by wounds in war. The endorphins don't necessarily produce a cure—you still need a surgeon to operate on the wound—but mobilizing the body's natural resources speeds healing.

In this connection, some fascinating stories are told about healing in the hospital. Just physically touching people has been documented as hastening healing. Not only do researchers now know it works; they are beginning to find out how and why.[6]

So faith really heals. But I'm skeptical—to say the least—about those

faith-healing scenes we sometimes see on television.

Rightly so. Anything as dramatic as faith healing is bound to attract quacks in multitudes. Fraud is most successful when it mimics amazing true events. A viewer should always watch such scenes skeptically and judge each one on its own merits. Just remember, though: the fact that a shyster can try to rip off the public, faking "miracle cures," does not negate the value of the effect of confidence. Faith does heal—or at least it helps enormously—in any situation where stress has contributed to illness.

I see what you mean. I think you've partially explained the healing effect of love, too.

You may be right. Anything that makes people feel cared for helps them to produce their own internal tranquilizers and strengthens their immune systems. As Dr. Francis Weld Peabody of Harvard University put it, "The secret of the care of the patient is in caring for the patient."

"I have seen a paper with some writing on it, strung round the neck, heal such illness of the whole body, and in a single night. I have seen a fever banished by pronouncing a few ceremonial words."
—Plato, 500 B.C.

Chapter 3

Emotional Health

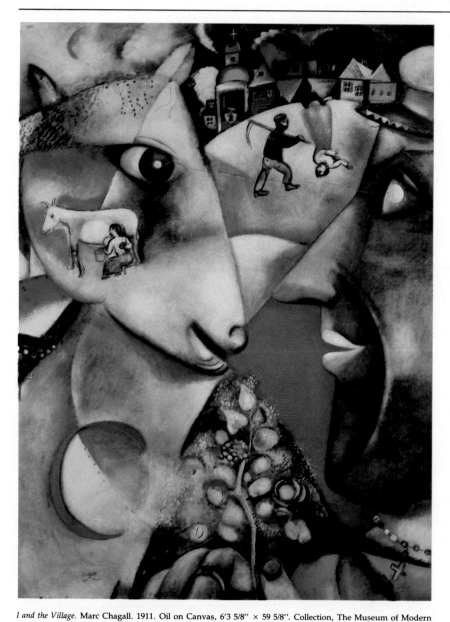

I and the Village. Marc Chagall. 1911. Oil on Canvas, 6'3 5/8" × 59 5/8". Collection, The Museum of Modern Art, New York. Mrs. Simon Guggenheim Fund.

FOR OPENERS . . .

True or false? If false, say what is true:

1. An emotionally healthy person is a person who has few or no emotional problems.
2. You can change what you think, but you cannot change how you feel.
3. A person's values are fixed from childhood on.
4. Talking to yourself can enhance your self-esteem.
5. An adult who sometimes still has childish feelings needs to grow up.
6. The primary problem shy people have is the fear of being rejected.
7. People are responsible for their own emotional problems. They should be able to pull themselves together.
8. The experience of loss always causes depression.
9. Anxiety can be beneficial.
10. Guilt is the appropriate response of a person who has gone against conscience.

(Answers on page 62.)

Self-knowledge is not given at birth. Human beings normally are conscious of only a small part of themselves, and to discover more takes learning and practice that, ideally, continue for a lifetime. This chapter offers some suggestions on knowing yourself.

To begin with, you have to be acquainted with, and able to manage, three aspects of your internal world: your thoughts, emotions (feelings), and values. Your **thought** processes take place in your cerebral cortex, the outermost layer of your brain. They are conscious; you are always aware of them. But much of the work of your brain goes on without your continuous awareness, and the **emotions** fall in this category. Brain centers deeper than the cortex integrate the emotions, and these centers do much of their work without your detection.

Your **values** are your set of rules for behavior. You learned the first ones from your family and society, and later you continued working them out for yourself. They are both conscious and unconscious; sometimes you can state them in words, but sometimes they influence your behavior without your awareness.

Thoughts are easy to get in touch with because you are aware of them. Emotions and values are not always so accessible, and the first task of this chapter is to make you more conscious of them.

■ EMOTIONS

An emotionally healthy person is not a person who has no problems; rather, such a person does have problems, but copes with them. To do so, you have to continuously monitor emotions, stay aware of them, own them, and use them wisely. The cortex is connected to the deeper brain centers, so your conscious mind has access to your emotions. When your mind has to make decisions, it can either ignore your emotions or take them into account. If it is necessary to ignore an emotion momentarily (for example, if fear would be incapacitating and action is needed), then it's fine to do so, but it's best to attend to the feeling as soon as possible. Unconscious emotion has a way of accumulating and ultimately making it difficult for a person to function either emotionally or physically.

An emotion is defined as a felt tendency to move toward something assessed as good or favorable or away from something assessed as bad or unfavorable. Emotions arise in response to events and experiences. The experience of hearing a twig crack in the woods may arouse the emotion of fear or joy or interest, depending on what you are expecting. The experience of being frustrated in your attempt to reach a goal may arouse a mixture of emotions including impatience, anger, and irritation. Losing a loved one (the experience of grief) evokes a series of emotions including both anger and sorrow.

A key word in the definition of emotion is *assessed*. Your emotional reaction to an event or experience depends not on what the event or experience is, but on your assessment of it, which is unique to you. Suppose you see a snake at your feet; your assessments and reactions may be any of the following:

- ■ "Snakes are poisonous"—fear.
- ■ "Snakes are beautiful"—happiness.
- ■ "Snakes do not belong in my garden"—anger.
- ■ "Snakes are my chosen subject of study"—interest.

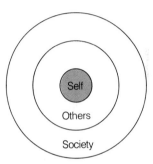

The emotionally healthy person functions well in three spheres—in relation to self, to others, and to society.

A sampling of emotions and their extremes:
Affection—love.
Anger—rage.
Desire—lust.
Dislike—revulsion.
Distress—anguish.
Excitement—frenzy.
Fear—terror.
Happiness—ecstasy.
Interest—fascination.
Possessiveness—jealousy.
Shame—humiliation.
Sorrow—agony.

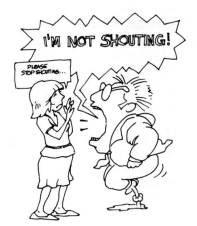

People deny anger because, in our society, it seems unacceptable or inappropriate.

Feelings are natural.
Feelings are OK—all of them.

(We're using OK here to mean acceptable and healthy.)*

Some of your emotional reactions to experiences may be instinctive—that is, programmed from birth. You instinctively feel fear when you are being physically hurt, for example. This emotion makes you tend to move away—an adaptive response. Other emotional reactions to experiences are learned: you learned that a certain experience was painful, so now you fear all such experiences.

Correct assessments, reinforced by emotional tendencies, lead to rational actions, or what we have called adaptive behavior. It is rational to avoid snakes in settings where most snakes are poisonous. But some emotions are based on incorrect assessments, and they lead to maladaptive behavior. In a setting where there are only harmless snakes, the fear of them is unreasonable.

Even when feelings are unreasonable, they are not "wrong"; they are as natural as the wind. It is acceptable to feel anything, although it may not be acceptable to act on all feelings. Some feelings can be destructive and need to be dealt with, but first, we have to be aware of them.

In the cartoon example in the margin, the person shouting is angry and won't admit it. Anger is not accepted in most social settings, so people often deny it. Other emotions people often deny are hurt, loneliness, and the like—feelings that reveal weakness and vulnerability.

Some people are closely in touch with their feelings and easily let them show. Others find it hard to show their feelings and even to know what they are. Generally, people who are aware of their feelings and who express them appropriately are more emotionally healthy than people who bottle them up.

*The term OK, with reference to one's feelings of self-esteem, originates with the transactional analysis system of therapy, discussed later. The term was popularized in T. A. Harris, I'm OK—You're Ok (New York: Avon, 1973)

Emotions are expressed physically.

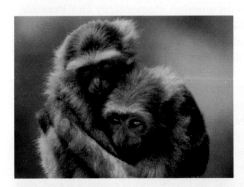

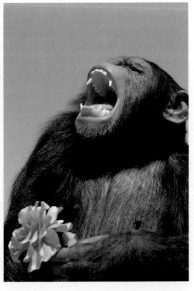

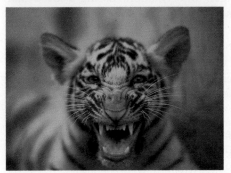

To express feelings means to do something physical—to speak, cry, shout, laugh, or otherwise act out emotions. Let's take the first alternative: speaking. How often in the last two or three weeks have you made any of the statements listed in the margin, either to yourself or to someone else? Knowing that you have these feelings is one step in dealing with them. Being able to verbalize them is another step, and acting them out (appropriately) is still another.

People often have a hard time accepting some of their feelings, because the actions they imply may be unacceptable. It helps to keep in mind the distinction between feelings and actions. Some actions are not OK, of course, but impulses toward them are OK. A young mother, listening to her baby crying, may have a sudden impulse to hit the baby; that is natural, and all mothers have such impulses. A person who feels sexual desire may imagine having sex with a stranger; the impulse is natural. A rejected lover, in a flood of self-pity, may feel like committing suicide; that feeling, too, is natural. It is at the borderline between feelings and action that the judging self steps in and prevents unacceptable behavior. When you can recognize, own, and express in acceptable ways even your negative feelings, you have gained some self-acceptance, a major factor in emotional health.

Communicating feelings is sometimes best done physically. Calmly saying, "I'm angry," for example, doesn't fully express the feeling. It releases more of the emotion to speak angrily, or even to beat on a punching bag. It is not acceptable to knock down another person with a blow to the jaw just to express your anger, but doing nothing at all is harmful to you. Once you have let off steam by yelling, crying, weight lifting, dancing, or whatever, then you can relax again and reassess the situation that triggered your emotion in the first place.

The expression of an emotion may be all you need to deal with it. But sometimes negative emotions come back over and over again. If they do, you have to make a choice: change the situation or change the feeling. The idea that people can change their feelings may be new and deserves some attention.

Emotions are instant, involuntary responses, and it isn't easy to change them. With persistence, however, people can "unlearn" emotional responses so that they are not trapped in behaviors that limit their enjoyment of life.

Someone we know was furious at a lifemate. In addition to recognizing the anger, owning it, and verbalizing it, this person expressed it physically in a socially acceptable way every day after work—by digging a hole in the back yard. After a year the hole was big enough for a swimming pool, and our friend was a superb physical specimen—but still an angry person. It was now necessary either to change the situation or the emotions involved. Three alternatives presented themselves: to seek marital counseling, to decide to separate, or to emotionally accept their differences and become peaceful about them.

We don't have to know which choice the person made. Any of the three would work. The first two alternatives (counseling or separation) would resolve the situation and so would lead to changed feelings in time. The third alternative (acceptance) may seem impossible at first, but acceptance is a genuine adjustment, and sometimes it is the preferred choice. Outwardly it may resemble the bottling up of feelings, but inwardly the person who truly accepts what cannot be changed is serene. Acceptance is absolutely necessary

✳ STRATEGIES
for Dealing with an Emotion

To deal with an emotion, you must:

✳ **Recognize it: What am I feeling?**
I'm angry.
I'm upset.
I'm hurt.
I'm excited.
I'm resentful.
I'm envious.
I'm frustrated.
I'm afraid.
I'm thrilled.
I'm stressed.
I'm touched.
I'm lonely.

✳ **Own it: Accept that you feel it.**

✳ **Verbalize it: Express it in words to yourself or someone else.**

✳ **Express it: Take physical action to relieve stress.**

✳ **If a negative emotion persists or returns, change the feeling or change the situation.**

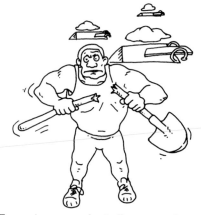

Expressing anger physically may produce fitness but no resolution. Either action or acceptance is needed.

43

at times—for example, when someone has died. The experience of grief includes a succession of feelings beginning with anger and (in the healthy person) leading ultimately to acceptance; Chapter 13 comes back to it.

Consider two other examples of changing feelings as a way of dealing with emotional distress: a woman who seethes with impatience at red lights and a man afraid of the new woman in his life. The woman at the traffic light assesses delays as "terrible," and so is impatient and angry. As a result, her blood pressure is high as she drives to and from work. She cannot change the traffic patterns (and we'll assume she cannot change her route or time of travel, either), but she can learn to change her reaction. She can learn to assess delays as "inconvenient" at worst and put up with them more calmly. If she is creative, she can even learn to assess them as opportunities (to organize her thoughts, plan or review her day, or even meditate) and enjoy them. It may strike you (and you are right) that in learning this new way of waiting at traffic lights, the woman is deactivating her stress response and practicing the relaxation response.

Similarly, the man may have learned, from a painful experience with a woman, to distrust and fear all women. (This is like saying "all snakes are poisonous.") The woman he is now encountering may be different, though, and he risks losing a rewarding relationship if he cannot revise his expectations. With patient work, he may learn to feel more pleasure than fear, so that when a trustworthy woman is available, he will allow himself to get to know her.

People cannot change their feelings directly but can change the assessments that lead to the feelings.

Notice that both these people do not change their feelings directly but change the assessments that lead to the feelings. The woman at the light changes her assessment from "It's terrible to be delayed" to "It's inconvenient" or even "It's an opportunity." Similarly, the man changes his assessment from "This woman is dangerous" to "This woman may be worth getting to know." The changing of assessments is a way of reducing extreme feelings to manageable ones.

■ PERSONAL VALUES

Your values are closely tied to your emotions. Values assign positive and negative weights to things and lead to decisions. You can tell how strong your values are by stating them as beliefs and then asking some questions about them. For each value that you state, ask the questions in the margin.[1*] Values change and one of the skills in moving through life is to learn when it is time to change a value.

To discover your values, ask:
■ How strongly do I cherish this value?
■ Would I be willing to affirm it publicly?
■ How faithfully will I stand by this value in the face of negative consequences?
■ Do I act consistently and repeatedly in line with this value?[2]

Sometimes values conflict with emotions or with each other, so that it may be difficult to act. It takes self-study to discover your feelings and values, and it may take effort to get them all pulling one way. "I know what I think, I know how I feel, and I know where I stand on this issue"—so say people who are well acquainted with themselves. Such self-knowledge supports self-esteem.

■ SELF-ESTEEM: SELF-IMAGE AND BODY IMAGE

Self-esteem underlies emotional health. People with real self-esteem do not think they are perfect; in fact, they know they are not, but they like them-

*Reference notes are in Appendix D.

LIFE CHOICE INVENTORY

How high is your self-esteem? In whatever areas you answer *yes* or *usually*, your self-esteem is strong. In the areas you answer *no*, you may want to work on increasing your strength. This test is not for passing or failing, but for enlightening.

1. Do you believe strongly in certain values and principles, so that you are willing to defend them?
2. Do you act on your own best judgment, without regretting your actions if others disapprove?
3. Do you manage your life so as not to waste time worrying about what is coming tomorrow or what happened yesterday?
4. Do you have confidence in your ability to deal with problems, even in the face of failures and setbacks?
5. Do you feel equal—neither inferior nor superior—to others?

6. Do you take it more or less for granted that other people are interested in you and value you?
7. Do you accept praise without pretense of false modesty?
8. Do you resist the efforts of your peers to dominate you?
9. Do you own a wide range of feelings, whether or not you act on them?
10. Do you genuinely enjoy yourself in a wide range of activities, including work, play, creative self-expression, companionship, and just plain loafing?
11. Do you sense and consider the needs of others?

SOURCE: Adapted from D. E. Hamachek, *Encounters with the Self* (New York: Holt, Rinehart, and Winston, 1971), pp. 248–251.

selves anyway. (In contrast, a person who claims to be perfect probably has low self-esteem; that's why the person can't own imperfections.) This chapter's Life Choice Inventory shows you how to measure your own self-esteem.

High self-esteem facilitates personal growth. If you know you are a worthwhile person, then you will take care of your health in all ways—education, spiritual development, personal relationships, nutrition, fitness, and all the rest. You might think that so much attention to self is selfish, but as it happens, these efforts to support yourself usually also benefit your family, friends, and society. You can enhance your self-esteem in two ways: one, by fostering a positive view of your inner self; the other, by developing a healthy relationship with your outer self, your body.

A technique for viewing your inner self positively is to practice making affirmative statements about yourself. This is called **positive self-talk**. These statements can be ones you perceive as true now or statements you plan to make true by means of practice. They should all be "I" statements, phrased positively: "I am learning to relax when under stress"; "I can be alone without being lonely"; "I am a sensitive listener"; "When I laugh, other people laugh with me." A similarly helpful technique is **positive imaging**: visualizing yourself succeeding at whatever task you choose. Positive imaging has helped people battle disease, win athletic contests, and overcome social awkwardness. Other steps you can take to improve your self-esteem are to pursue activities (occupational and recreational) that reflect your skills and interests, to appreciate what you do have, to continue your efforts even when discouraged, to compliment yourself when you do well, and to relax.[3]

Also, accept what cannot be changed. Someone who had made many mistakes in life is said to have spoken a prayer, which became famous. This person could not go back to change the past but wisely chose to invest energy in the present:

Grant me the serenity to accept the things I cannot change,
The courage to change the things I can,
And the wisdom to know the difference.

The second part of self-esteem is developing a positive body image. Each year, millions of people try to change the way they look. Half a milion undergo cosmetic surgery; 40 million go on diets; and multitudes try contact lenses, facials, and new cosmetics in hopes of becoming more attractive.[4] Our society intensely values what it defines as physical attractiveness, and the pressure to compete, especially among the young, is extreme. People feel that they must be sexually attractive—meaning that women must have flat bellies, firm round breasts, smooth slim thighs, and so forth; and that men must have broad flat chests rippling with muscles, bulging biceps, slim firm hips, hard flat bellies, full heads of hair, and so on. As you might guess, the intense desire for a sexier appearance makes us sitting ducks for quacks (see Consumer Caution).

Improving your body appearance by means of exercise and good nutrition is appropriate and can benefit your physical health as well as your self-esteem. Once you've attained a healthy body, though, it's important to accept your physical structure. In dealing with body image, it is appropriate to work at a realistic strategy that emphasizes both physical and emotional health, rather than mere looks.

THE EVOLVING SELF

Self-concept is a person's answer to the question "Who am I?" Many people begin answering this question by saying their names: "I am Leslie Owens." When pressed to say more, people may go on to describe their observable traits, such as sex, height, weight, age, occupation, and race. Beneath the surface, though, who are they, really? What are their intimate, secret thoughts about themselves? For each person, they are different. Self-concept is strongly influenced by impressions made by parents and other significant people in childhood. The next sections present views of how the self-concept develops in childhood and continues to evolve in adulthood.

Erikson's Developmental Stages—Childhood

The psychoanalyst Erik Erikson has been influential in shaping other theorists' thoughts about emotional health. His theory of personality development sees human life as a sequence of eight periods, in each of which the individual has a new learning task.[5] To the extent that individuals master each task successfully, they develop a strong foundation from which to proceed to the next. To the extent that they fail, they are handicapped in mastering the task at the next level. The stages in life and their respective learning tasks, as identified by Erikson, are as follows:

Infant	**trust** vs distrust
Toddler	**autonomy** vs shame and doubt
Preschooler	**initiative** vs guilt
School child	**industry** vs inferiority
Adolescent	**identity** vs role confusion
Young adult	**intimacy** vs isolation
Adult	**generativity** vs stagnation
Older adult	**ego integrity** vs despair

Erikson's theory has the potential to be destructive if it is oversimplified or applied too heavy-handedly. Keep in mind that the positive side of each pair of opposites represents an ideal to strive for, not a judgment from which anyone falls short. Neither the authors of this book, nor your instructors in school, nor your parents, nor anyone else has had a "perfect childhood." One of the services a theory like Erikson's can perform is to provide insight into the building blocks of personality so that people can work in later life on developing those they most need.

The Three Selves of Transactional Analysis

Erikson's theory focuses on poles within the self, whereas a school of thought that originated a type of therapy known as **transactional analysis (TA)** looks at personality as a cluster of selves that develop during the early years. If you ask yourself, "Who am I, *really*?" different people may come to mind—some of them remembered from your childhood and one being the child you once were.

It is as if each person carries three people inside: the Child, the Parent, and the Adult—which we can think of as personifications of the emotions, thoughts, and values described earlier.[6] The Child is the little person of the past. The Parent is composed of all the people who wielded parental authority in the past. The Adult is the reasoning person who collects information, weighs facts, and makes meaning of them. Table 3–1 lists the traits of the Parent, Adult, and Child; corresponding examples are in the margin.

TABLE 3–1 Traits of the Parent, Adult, and Child in Transactional Analysis

Parent	Adult	Child
Nuturing	Information giving	Loving
Tender	Fact finding	Impulsive
Helpful	Reality testing	Curious
Judgment making	Intelligent	Playful
Value conveying	Objective	Exuberant
Tradition transmitting	Able to estimate probabilities	Spontaneous
Critical	Able to compute dispassionately	Irresponsible
		Selfish
		Manipulative

MINOGLOSSARY of Erikson's Life Tasks

autonomy: the perception that one is a separate person with a will of one's own.
ego integrity: a mature person's perception of fulfillment, of having accomplished goals, values, and personal relationships well; a sense of personal worth.
generativity: the inclination of a mature person to encourage the development of others, especially persons in earlier stages of development.
identity: one's sense of self, goals, and values and of roles in family, social group, and job or career.
industry: the characteristic of working with vigor at selfchosen goals, whether personal, career, or social.
initiative: the characteristic of being self-propelled, as opposed to waiting for directions from others.
intimacy: emotional closeness to another, associated with honesty, vulnerability, tenderness, and love.
trust: the feeling or belief that one's needs will be met without fail.

Examples of T.A. personalities:

On seeing an older child wildly pushing a baby in a park swing;

Parent: Oh, dear, she'd better stop that before someone gets hurt.
Adult: The baby seems to be enjoying the ride, the swing is sturdy, and it looks as though he's buckled in pretty well.
Child: Whee! That looks like fun! Me next!

On seeing a row of tulips in early spring:

Parent: Mustn't touch!
Adult: I wonder how a person goes about growing such lovely flowers.
Child: I want to pick them all for myself!

On waking up in the morning feeling extra sleepy:

Parent: Stay in bed, honey; you need your rest.
Adult: If I stay in bed, I could catch up on rest, but I stand a chance of missing something important today.
Child: Zzzzzz . . .

No one of these personality states is "better" than the others, but a balance is needed between them. For example, a person with an overbearing Parent state would probably impress others as critical, judgmental, perhaps prejudiced, perhaps overly concerned for others' welfare. A person with an overactive Child state might be impulsive, irresponsible, or selfish. A person whose Adult state was overly active would seem like the character Mr. Spock from the science fiction adventures of "Star Trek"—emotionless, dull, measured, and factual. (Of course, these descriptions are exaggerated.)

According to the theorists, the figures we carry within us, and especially the Parent figure, have a major influence on our self-esteem. Parents (simply stated) are of two kinds: critical and nurturing. The critical Parent reacts to the child in a predominantly negative, judgmental way, and adults who have internalized this type of Parent may have a predominantly negative self-concept. Having heard messages throughout childhood to the effect that he was no good, sloppy, and lazy, and having adopted this critical Parent as part of his own personality, he continues to hear negative judgments from within. In contrast, the nurturing Parent reacts to the child positively as being cute, funny, industrious, achieving, and the like. This child carries a more self-approving Parent inside as an adult, and the positive messages, repeated throughout adult life, are confirming.

Maslow's Hierarchy of Needs

According to the psychologist Abraham Maslow, people have certain basic needs that they will struggle to meet before they even begin to think about "higher" things.[7] For example, a person who is hungry may not be interested in listening to music. Once that basic need is met, however, other needs naturally arise. In other words, the needs form a hierarchy, and when you have met the basic ones, you become more aware of the "higher" ones.

Most primitive are needs related to physical survival—needs for food, clothing, and shelter (physiological). Next is the need to feel physically safe and secure (safety needs). If safe and secure, people are free to notice their need to be loved, to feel emotionally secure (love needs). If that need is met, they can be in touch with the need for other people's esteem; and given that, they can seek to achieve the ultimate—**self-actualization**, or the realization of their full potential. Only a few people, perhaps 1 to 2 percent, ever evolve that far.

Maslow's theory offers hopeful perspectives both for people who feel good about where they are and for people who do not. For those who are dissatisfied, it suggests that life will not always be this way: it will get better. For those who are satisfied, it offers inspiration: there is still more to aspire to.

The Stages of Adult Life

Several theorists have studied the changes that take place during adult life. According to Erikson, the first two decades of adult life are spent resolving the issue of intimacy versus isolation. In this stage, the individual works out the details of relationships with others and society. Sometime after age 30 the so called midlife crisis may strike. People may painfully come to fear that their dreams may not be fully realized. With full adulthood (often around age 40), the person is established and self-accepting. At 60 or so,

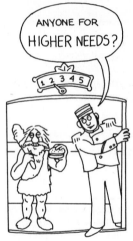

Once basic needs are met, a person can aspire to meet higher needs.

the shift into old age begins. The challenge is to maintain the sense of personal worth (ego integrity) during retirement, when the self may begin to seem less important.

Journalist Gail Sheehy has taken Erikson's work on adult life a step further. She collected 115 life stories of men and women and wrote about them in her book *Passages: Predictable Crises of Adult Life*.[8] Sheehy's important contribution is her insights into the differences between men's and women's patterns of development and into the transitions that occur in the lives of couples. Table 3–2 lists and describes the predictable crises of adult life according to Sheehy.

It hardly does justice to any of the authorities mentioned here to present their life story theories so briefly. One thing is clear, though: the theories display patterns with which people can identify. When people see the patterns of their lives, they can assume some control and make conscious choices that would not be possible otherwise.

◾ SELF AND OTHERS

We have said that the emotionally healthy person functions well in three spheres—in relation to self, to others, and to society. So far, this chapter has been devoted primarily to the most important relationship in anyone's life—the relationship with self. Now, what about relationships with others?

Developing Personal Relationships

People who value themselves cultivate a strong **support system** in case of need, which may consist of family; neighbors; friends; people at work, school, or church; **mentor** or adviser; and a therapy or self-help group. Of course, the person participating in such friendships and social groups stands ready to give, as well as to receive, and so does not need to be embarrassed about asking for support sometimes.

People also cultivate friendships—though many fear to do so at first. *Why Am I Afraid to Tell You Who I Am?* is the title of a book written to help shy

The emotionally healthy person maintains strong relationships with others.

TABLE 3–2 Predictable Crises of Adult Life According to Sheehy

Age	Crisis
18–22	"Pulling up roots"—breaking free from family.
22–29	"Trying Twenties"—getting started on life, locating peer group, gender role, occupation, philosophy of living.
30–34	"Catch 30"—making new choices, developing more realistic goals.
35–45	"Deadline Decade"—reevaluating of accomplishment, discovering of autonomy.
mid-40's	"Renewal or Resignation"—developing a hardened, stale attitude or revitalizing warmth and mellowing.

A support group lends security to its members.

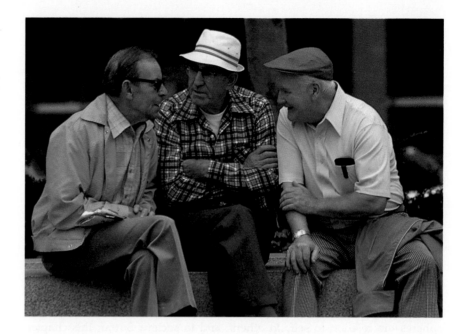

people overcome their fears about relationships.[9] Its title reveals the primary problem shy people have: fear—specifically, fear of being rejected.

Reaching out to other people usually does not lead to rejection, but to get started, you have to be willing to risk rejection and to handle it if it occurs. It helps to keep two things in mind: first, "If I'm rejected, I won't be any worse off than I am now"; second, "If it doesn't work out, it's no reflection on me; I tried. The other person had other needs." What more often happens when you reach out is that the other person is pleased to be approached. At least you have the benefit of some contact; at best, a rewarding relationship has a chance to form.

Multitudes of people who know this can't act on it, though, because they don't know how. A few specific suggestions can help. Each can be practiced in isolation, in front of a mirror, or with one close friend you already trust. One authority recommends remembering these suggestions by thinking of the word "soften" (see margin).[10] To these, we'd add:

- Disclose your own feelings (people always find feelings interesting).
- Ask questions about the other person's feelings (people like you to be interested in them).
- Listen attentively (people love to be listened to).

Personal relationships may not meet both persons' needs adequately. Sometimes they should end, but at other times they end for the wrong reasons. For example, a person's needs may not be met because they are expressed inappropriately. To form successful relationships, you must know how to express wants and needs without forcing them on the other person.

To find the happy compromise between the extremes of mousiness and assault is to be **assertive** rather than **nonassertive** or **aggressive**. There is always a gap, sometimes large, sometimes small, between what you want or need and what you are receiving in every setting—school, job, home, friendships, dealings with storekeepers or creditors, and more. To help close the gap, you need to have some appropriate and effective way to express

S Smile.
O Open posture.
F Forward lean.
T Touch.
E Eye contact.
N Nod.

your wants and needs. At the same time, you need to remain mindful of other people's feelings and not wound them unnecessarily.

To be assertive is to say what you mean, not to tiptoe around dropping hints, and not to attack the other person. This does not come naturally to many people and has to be learned and practiced. In each of the following situations, a person is behaving nonassertively; see if you can decide what the person really means (assertive responses are given in the accompanying box):

Situation	Nonassertive Behavior
A person steps in front of Ms. A, who has been standing in line for an hour.	Ms. A: "Well, excuse *me!*"
	or
	Ms. A: Says nothing aloud; mutters, "Some people. . . ."
Mr. B comes home, gets a drink, sits down, and starts reading the paper.	Ms. B (from kitchen): "I sure wish I could rest like that at the end of the day. But no, I have to cook dinner, bathe the baby, wash up . . . I'm tired, too."
Mr. C notices that Child C hasn't cleaned up her room even though he told her to do so earlier:	Mr. C: "Child, I told you to clean up your room. What's the matter with you? You're the laziest child I ever saw."

▌▌▌ Assertive Behaviors for Ms. A, Ms. B, and Mr. C

> *Ms. A:* "Excuse me. I was here first. The end of the line is back there." (points)
>
> *Ms. B:* "Would you please cook dinner while I bathe the baby?"
>
> *Mr. C:* "I told you to clean up your room. Now do it." (and sees that she does)

In the first example, Ms. A is not assertive at all; she simply does not speak up for herself. In the second, Ms. B makes it clear to her husband that she feels overworked, tired, and grumpy, but she doesn't tell him what she wants him to do about it. In the third example, Mr. C tells his child what to do, which is assertive, but then goes on to insult the child, which is aggressive.

Ms. B and Mr. C share a problem common to people who have trouble being assertive. They have let their resentments build up for so long that when they do speak, they express not a simple wish of the moment but an age-old gripe. Ms. B does it slow-burn style; Mr. C does it by way of a loud explosion. Both are painful to express and painful to witness. By contrast, notice how the appropriate responses differ in tone and content: they each express a single, specific, concrete request of the moment. Assertive statements are like that: "Please wash the dishes." "Please pay me the five dollars you owe me." Also, they speak of the action they want, not of the person. The responder knows exactly what to do and does not have to feel attacked. To make your wishes known assertively but not aggressively:

■ Isolate the incident. Don't discuss everything that has been bothering you for months.
■ Be specific. Identify the behavior you want.

A way to choose what to mention is to ask yourself, "Does this bother me every time it happens, or is it an isolated incident?" If it happens often, mention it. If not, handle it yourself by walking it off or waiting it out.

If a major grievance has built up, then don't just casually mention it the next time the occasion arises. Here are pointers for expressing major grievances:

■ Pick a time to express them; don't just burst forth with them.

- Pair a resentment with an appreciation: "I appreciate [this], but resent [that]."
- Make feeling statements about yourself ("It hurts my feelings when you . . ."), not judgment statements about the other person ("You are insensitive").

Assertiveness is the key to obtaining cooperation: it makes you easier, not harder, to get along with. It is worth practicing for the person who wants to achieve harmonious relationships with others. Chapter 10 develops this theme further with respect to intimate relationships.

Finding a Place in Society

Self and others relate to a larger circle—society. Societies have sets of values of their own and sets of expectations that they impose on their members. Sometimes the fit is easy, sometimes not.

Our society is dominated by the middle class, which confers on it many of its prevailing characteristics. The middle class tends to value the future more than the present, putting off enjoying today so that tomorrow there will be money or prestige or time to have fun. It also values the doers, those devoted to action and achievement. In another culture, a mother may enjoy her child because he is sitting in her lap and laughing in her face, but in our culture, a mother is more likely to be preoccupied with how well the child is preparing for tomorrow. Not all societies uphold the same values for their members, and no law says people must abide by the values of their own society. However, they pay a price if they don't, because they lose approval and support.

Take society's view of progress and achievement, for example. If you share these values, they will give you incentive to work hard. If you don't, you may experience feelings of **alienation**; you will be unable to relate to the values that make life meaningful for the people around you. This also creates a problem for your society: if you don't fit in, you are a **nonconformist**. The consequence is some degree of **ostracism**— disapproval and shunning by others.

In any case, each person has to establish some relationship with the larger world. One person may choose to live a relatively isolated life, pursuing goals of personal value. Another may choose to associate with a subgroup in society whose values differ from the majority's values. Society is really a mosaic of many small societies, each a group of like-minded people.

An increasingly important component for many people in establishing a place in society is finding a job or career. A book written for people trying to find their place in the world of work is *What Color Is Your Parachute?*[11] The title implies that the leap into a job is somewhat like jumping from an airplane. You have no guarantee of success; all you have is what you came with—yourself. The better you know yourself, the better you can choose, and succeed at, a job or career.

To be satisfying, a job ideally meets several of a person's needs including security, feeling of competence, autonomy, creativity, variety, and feeling of performing worthwhile work.[12] Your work may be school or homemaking right now; it is still a job, in a sense. Ask yourself how many of your needs are met by your work.

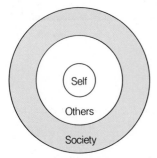

The emotionally healthy person has a strong relationship with society.

Three levels of work:
- Job—meets basic needs for survival and physical security.
- Career—can help meet needs for other people's esteem and respect, for a position in life.
- Life's work—helps meet needs for self-actualization.

Some authorities believe that to be engaged in rewarding work is the single most important determinant of well-being in the adult.[13] Those who are lucky enough to have satisfying jobs, then, have a built-in life advantage. Those who are not so lucky may be well-advised to invest their energy preparing to seek future work that will be satisfying. No job can meet all needs, of course. Even people who love their work can obtain further satisfaction through activities such as hobbies or volunteer work.

The relationship with self, others, and society requires periodic checking and adjustments. People who experience difficulty in making needed adjustments or who fail to establish a working relationship with self, others, or society may have an emotional problem that is blocking the way to emotional health. Problems serious enough to require professional help affect 1 in every 15 children and a larger number of adults. In Canada, it is estimated that disorders such as anxiety are a factor affecting *half* of all the people who visit physicians in general medical practice.[14] U.S. statistics are similar. In a typical city of 400,000 people, about 1,000 may be in the hospital for emotional problems at any one time.

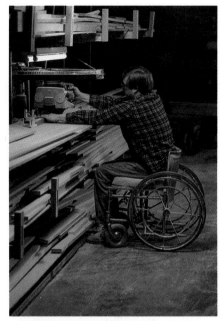

A satisfying job meets a person's need for a feeling of competence.

Three areas in which inability to function indicates mental illness:
1. Social or family relations.
2. Occupation (including school).
3. Use of leisure time.

A MATTER OF DEFINITION: WHAT IS EMOTIONAL/MENTAL ILLNESS?

Some people refer to *mental* illness, some to *emotional* illness. We use both terms, in the hope of conveying that, by whatever name they are called, such problems are problems of both the emotions and the mind. They are also often problems of the body. In many instances we don't know *yet* (but we will know, in the future) what physical abnormalities are associated with these illnesses.[15] Even tuberculosis (TB) was once classed as a mental disorder; people with TB were thought to experience things too intensely. We know now, of course, that it is a bacterial infection.

Despite much study, knowledge about **mental disorders** is limited. For example, it is not known whether mild and severe depressions differ from each other in kind or only in degree. A lesson for nonprofessionals is that we are not experts and we had better remain humble about our qualifications to make judgments in the field of mental health. Especially, we are not qualified to diagnose our friends' or family members' problems.

CAUSES OF EMOTIONAL PROBLEMS

Some people may be genetically predisposed to certain mental illnesses. Others may develop disorders by way of learned thought patterns or behaviors that do not work—maladaptive habits. Still others remain emotionally healthy even under severely stressful environmental circumstances, as if they were born with exceptional mental resilience. We do not know why people exhibit these differences.

We can define several classes of mental disorders. First, a person who fails to adjust to stress at a reasonable pace suffers prolonged and severe disturbance—major depression, disabling anxiety, inappropriate behavior, withdrawal, or some combination of these. Such a person has an **adjustment disorder**.

The second cause of mental disorders rests more in society than in its members. Sometimes a person simply cannot adjust to some requirement that society sets up. For example, suppose that a man is expected to enlist

Times of transition can be lonely times.

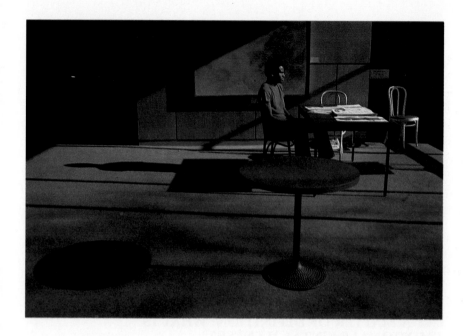

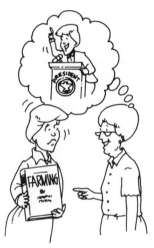

Society's ideals don't always fit the individual.

in the armed forces and go to war—but cannot or will not do so, and so is called a coward. Or suppose that a woman feels pressure to keep a tidy house and garden—but does not and becomes the talk of the neighborhood because her home is messy and dirty. Such a person has an adjustment problem, and society may define this, somewhat unfairly, as a mental disorder. Psychologists disagree in some cases: "When the disturbance is *limited* to a conflict between an individual and society, this may represent social deviance, which may or may not be commendable, but is not by itself a mental disorder."[16]

The third class of mental illness is that arising from known chemical causes. Some mental illnesses run in families. This suggests one of two possible causes. They may be inherited or learned, but in several cases, researchers have shown that major mental disorders are inherited, and in fact have discovered the exact location of the responsible gene within the genetic material.

A mental disorder suspected to be caused by biochemical changes in the brain is major depression. Among symptoms of major depression are loss of appetite, lack of energy, and lack of interest in sex. It is difficult to distinguish major depression from mild depression, but people with major depression produce much less of a certain hormone in response to a chemical stimulus than do people with mild or no depression. A blood test is becoming increasingly useful in diagnosis of this mental disorder.[17]

A condition not yet known, but suspected, to have a chemical cause is **premenstrual syndrome (PMS)**. The two hormones that regulate the menstrual cycle ebb and flow with a monthly rhythm, and when one hormone is high and the other is low, some women experience a range of symptoms including both physical and emotional pain. Perhaps in this case the causes are both chemical and emotional. The woman who has trouble with PMS is advised to tend sensibly to all aspects of her health, sleep, exercise, and nutrition, and to avoid drugs, alcohol, and tobacco—as well as quack remedies.

If you have any questions about your own state of well-being, you are not alone. Whatever you fear, others have feared it, too—and have conquered it or come to terms with it. Isolation prevents personal growth and blocks escape from problems. Whatever you least dare share is what most needs sharing. When you have expressed it, you almost invariably find that others have experienced it, too; that it is not as bad as you thought; and that there is a way to deal with it. If you have any questions about your own mental health, ask someone. Ask an expert, and not just a self-advertised expert, but a proved expert. The end of this chapter lists many sources of information and help on personal problems.

▨ COMMON EMOTIONAL PROBLEMS

With these thoughts as introduction, let us turn to the more common kinds of emotional problems. Foremost among them are **depression** and **anxiety**—the most common of all mental disorders. Because so many people experience these conditions in greater or lesser degrss, the emphasis of the following sections is practical: how to recognize them, how to decide whether they are serious, how to counteract them, and how to get help if necessary.

Depression

If you have never felt "down," you are a most unusual person. More likely, you know exactly what it is like to be depressed, because you have been there: taking no joy in life, not looking forward to anything, wanting to withdraw from people and activities. Being extremely tired can make you feel this way, but in the case of depression, it doesn't go away, even after a night's sleep.

Depression can be mild and short-lived or severe and long-lasting. Sometimes it goes away by itself, but often you can hasten its departure. Over the course of a lifetime, most people learn what kinds of things characteristically cause them to become depressed, at what times of the day or year they typically become depressed, how to recognize the signs of an impending depression, and how best to prevent or relieve it.

Sometimes the reason for being depressed is obvious. People always become depressed, for example, when they have experienced a loss—whether of a loved one, a pet, a job, a possession, money, a belief, a habit, or anything they cherish. Adverse external circumstances can cause depressions, too: a prolonged drought on the farm, a long spell of rain during a vacation, the threat and fear of war, or widespread financial disaster. Note that the name for an economic slump—depression—is the same as for the emotional disorder.

Abundant evidence gathered before 1984 supported the view that people who exercised regularly experienced less depression and anxiety than people who did not.[18] A further study showed that running could be used in place of psychotherapy to treat mild depression.[19] A spate of studies have followed since then, showing that exercise alters mood and attitude for the better in numerous disease states, including heart disease and alcoholism.[20] More recently still, both running and weight-lifting routines have been demonstrated to improve mood in depressed women compared with others who did neither.[21] Other ways of combating mild depression are listed in this chapter's Strategies Box, page 56.

⊛ **STRATEGIES: Relieving Mild Depression and Anxiety**

To ease the passing of mild depression:

1. Recognize the cause.

2. Take productive action to benefit the situation.

3. Avoid unpleasant tasks, if possible.

4. Take a nap.

5. Exercise.

6. Plan a pick-me-up snack.

7. Do something fun.

8. Find reasons to laugh.

9. Go outdoors (the green color of living plants in the sun has a known therapeutic effect on the viewer).

10. If necessary, get outside help.

To reduce anxiety:

1. Identify the cause. What do you fear? State it in words.

2. Deal with it. Can you change it? How? Do it.

3. If you can't change it, let it go. Worry is not helpful, and it wastes energy. Substitute concentration, where useful. Discard the worry.

4. Visualize a positive outcome, and work toward that. Live in the solution, not in the problem.

5. Use any accumulated energy in some physical way: exercise. People who exercise regularly experience less anxiety than people who don't. Lack of exercise aggravates and can even cause anxiety.

6. Practice the relaxation techniques already described in Chapter 2.

A person in a prolonged depression needs outside help.

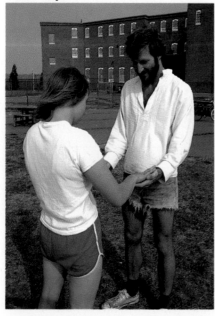

Persistent depression, whatever the cause, can be terrifying. Some people who have experienced it say that they would rather have any kind of physical pain than the mental anguish of total hopelessness and helplessness. A person in a prolonged depression needs outside help. The signs are:

■ Withdrawal from friends; cessation of hobbies and activities.
■ Slackening interest in schoolwork and decline in grades.
■ Not caring what happens, good or bad; passive behaviors.
■ Feeling bad about oneself, pessimistic, and helpless.
■ Ceasing to groom oneself or care for one's room, possessions, or clothes.
■ Ceasing to meet responsibilities (pay bills, return calls, or answer the phone).
■ Changes in eating habits, alcohol or drug use, or sleeping habits.
■ Abrupt changes in personality; acting out: aggressive, hostile behavior; impulsiveness; sudden mood swings.
■ Anxiety at times of separation.

- Inability to concentrate.
- Refusal to leave the room or the bed.
- Making a will; obsession with death; a death wish.

Depressed people, by their very behavior, repel others as if they were saying, "Leave me alone." Too often, they get what they seem to be asking for. It takes a discerning friend or family member to recognize such unattractive behavior as a call for help. Depressed people may consider suicide. Those who do usually believe they are not loved or accepted. A suicide attempt is actually a cry for help. Most people who commit suicide suffer from deep despair, loneliness, and hopelessness. Suicide is a possibility, and therefore it is important to take seriously the warning signs of depression. If you suspect an oncoming suicide, get involved. Don't wait; ask outright if the person is planning suicide. Talking about it can help. If the person seems on the verge of making a suicide attempt, phone a suicide hotline or crisis intervention center immediately. Dial 911, the operator, or the police, and stay with the person until help arrives.

This may sound strange to you now, but there may come a time when you feel like ending your own life. Almost everyone feels that way at one time or another. Things can seem very bad, but they always get better, given time. You can talk to someone during the bad times without the person knowing who you are by calling the helping hotline in your area. Or you can ask someone you trust to listen to your thoughts; you'll both be glad you did.

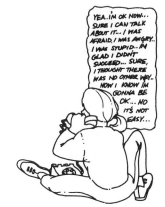

Ask someone to listen to you; you'll be glad you did.

Anxiety

Like depression, anxiety is familiar to everyone. And like depression, anxiety is a normal state, some of the time. Whereas depression is a low-energy state, however, anxiety is characterized by high energy and therefore can be beneficial on occasion. A small dose of anxiety can spur a student to tackle a test with intense concentration, but excessive test anxiety can also freeze the test-taker's mind. Too much anxiety is disabling.

Anxiety can also hit people who have been through stressful experiences such as bombings, rape, floods, torture, kidnapping, or hurricanes. After such an experience a person may have disturbed sleep and an impaired memory (especially of the stressful time) and is said to have a **post-traumatic stress disorder**. The person may repeatedly relive the experience and may be unable to concentrate or focus on present responsibilities, sometimes acting unresponsive to other people and sometimes overreacting to minor disturbances.

Sometimes post-traumatic stress disorders last long after the stressful periods have ended. Many of the veterans who fought in Vietnam during the 1960s, for example, still had symptoms 15 to 20 years later and were just beginning to come to terms with their experiences in the 1980s. Also, many women after being raped show signs of distress months or years after the actual incident.

The body's reaction to anxiety is the stress response: rapid heartbeat and respiration, extreme alertness, and the other aspects of readiness needed for fight or flight. You can take steps to alleviate anxiety, such as those listed in this chapter's Strategies box.

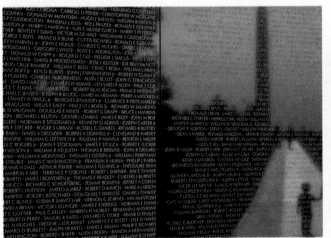
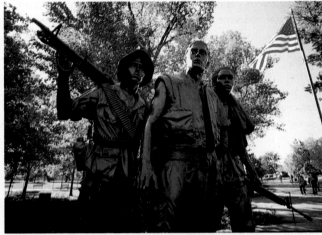

The experience of Vietnam was so traumatic that even the memorial could not be built until twenty years later.

Prolonged or intense anxiety out of proportion to any real danger or threat is a signal that the situation is getting out of hand. Signs of extreme anxiety are the same as those of extreme stress (see Table 2-3 in Chapter 2). If these symptoms persist, it is time to get help.

Guilt and Resentment

Ordinary guilt, like anxiety, is desirable up to a point. A guilty feeling says that you have crossed a line your values dictate you should not cross; it is a reminder from your conscience to act consistently with your own values. But guilt in the extreme can handicap a person's functioning, especially in relationships. The person whose conscience is too controlling is likely to suffer from too much guilt at small transgressions, whereas the healthy person could let them go.

An example may help to show the difference between appropriate and inappropriate guilt. Let's say you have agreed to take care of your neighbor's dog. You miss a day, and on your return, you find that the water is gone. You feel guilty, and you resolve not to take responsibility for the dog again unless you are sure you won't have to miss a day. The guilt is appropriate, and your reaction is appropriate; you won't let it happen again.

By contrast, we read the story of a 12-year-old who shot and killed a bird in a meadow and who felt so guilty about it that he hanged himself. "I killed myself on account of me shooting a redbird," he wrote in his suicide note. Clearly, the child's guilt was irrational and extreme.[22]

On occasion, a person who feels anger and is afraid to express it may choose to feel guilt instead. "Guilt is resentment turned inward," it has been said, and it is healthier to own and express the resentment in appropriate and assertive ways than to be consumed by guilt.

Suppose your roommate entertains friends in your crowded quarters when you would rather be alone. Instead of expressing your resentment, you burn inwardly. Later, when your roommate makes a simple request, you snap irritably. Now you have only two choices—feel resentful or to feel guilty. Guilt is less explosive, so that is what you choose. You pay a price, though: your relationship with your roommate will be impaired until the resentment is expressed and dealt with by both of you.

To handle situations like this without hurting yourself or others, it is important to remember that even unkind feelings are acceptable. In flashing momentarily on an angry thought, you have not transgressed. You have simply expressed your feelings to yourself, giving them an outlet. It was adaptive to do so; it made them easier to bear. Resentments need expression.

ABOUT GETTING AND GIVING HELP

The choice to get help is a choice that the emotionally healthy person can make. You don't have to be sick, and you certainly don't have to be very sick, to ask for help. The exact moment when a person decides to get help is often the moment when that person starts to get better.

If you have concluded that you might benefit from having psychological help, be selective. Not all "therapists" are well qualified. Try the following possibilities:

- If you are reading this book as the text for a course, check with the instructor, who is likely to be well informed about local helping agencies.
- Look in your telephone book for a telephone counseling service; call; ask what to do. You don't have to identify yourself.
- Look up "Mental health," "Health," "Social services," "Drugs," "Alcohol," "Family services," "Suicide prevention," or "Counseling" in the telephone book; call; ask what to do.
- Call a hospital or any physician and ask for advice.
- Ask your mentor whom to see. Call or ask around for a member of the clergy who is known to be helpful.

Persist. The first source you try may not work out well, but there *is* someone out there for you to talk to. Often several referrals will take place before a problem is resolved. You might start by seeing a counselor for anxiety but end up getting help from someone in your bank who will teach you to balance your checkbook—and that might solve the anxiety problem. Often

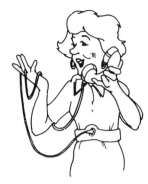

It's normal for people to talk to themselves.

Talking to Yourself

A person who has a serious mental disorder and is having hallucinations sometimes talks out loud. As a result, people who talk to themselves sometimes are afraid that they are "crazy." This is not true. Talking to oneself indicates an emotional problem only when the conversation shows that the speaker is out of touch with reality. Otherwise self-talk can be useful. It is easier, if you think out loud, to hear what you are thinking. Advice from a mental health worker is: "Just relax and start listening. You may have something important to say." Source: Problems? Have a chat with yourself, *Family Health*, May 1981, p. 58.

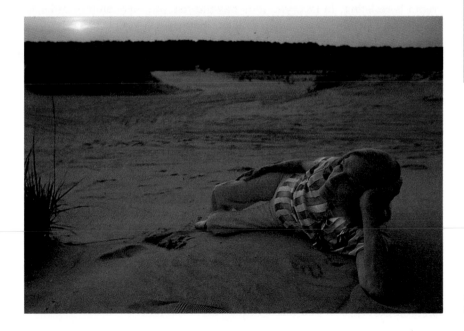

Any activity that has a healing effect is therapy.

a single clearheaded discussion will lead to a simple solution. People often hesitate to consult professional helpers for fear of what they may be forced to discover about themselves. Yet the most earthshaking discovery people are likely to make is that they are not alone—that other people have the same problem, and that, with help, they can deal with it.

It is sometimes possible to deliver significant help to another person who has an emotional problem. Simply caring and offering support is often beneficial. Listening is therapeutic, too. Often a person can work out problems with sufficient opportunity to discuss them.

Not many people, however, are born with the skills necessary to help others. The untrained person can do more harm than good by saying or suggesting the wrong things. Sometimes, too, a person who intends to help may do harm by allowing a troubled person evade feelings that should be confronted and dealt with. This misguided attempt to help is termed **enabling**, because it supports maladaptive behavior. Enablers, with the best intentions in the world, actually prolong drinking, gambling, or other self-destructive behaviors, by helping people avoid facing the consequences of their own actions (see Chapter 8).

Another way in which the "helper" may actually do harm is by paying attention only when the other person is in trouble rather than when the person is functioning in a positive manner. This reinforcement encourages people to become embroiled in problems so that they can get attention. Some therapists and self-help groups also make this mistake.

Still another caution: a person may help another for the wrong reasons. Helping others may be a way of avoiding facing one's own problems. It can provide an excuse: "I couldn't go to class because I was helping Jane." It takes a mature sense of proportion to know when to get involved and when to suggest professional help. Life offers many opportunities to make this choice.

Helping people in crisis requires a special set of strategies. You sometimes have to break out of ordinary social norms. If a person is clearly irrational and in danger, you may have to insist on action, to take charge when your friend is resisting. In fact, you may have to risk the friendship in order to benefit the person. To tell when to take this risk, ask yourself:

■ Do I perceive that the person's life or health is in serious danger?
■ Is the person threatening someone else's life or health?
■ If I fail to intervene, will the situation get worse?

If the answer to any of these questions is yes, then intervene. It is a risk, but the risk of not intervening is worse. Your judgment may not be perfect, but it is the best you have available, so use it.

When a crisis requires professional help, the person who needs help should be the one to actually make the contact. Mental health agencies will not step in on your say-so. If your friend resists, place the telephone call yourself and then persuade your friend to talk to a helping person on the other end of the line. Failing that, or in the case of a very sick, weak, or debilitated friend, call the police or an ambulance. If the need is imperative, the awkwardness of the situation is outweighed by its urgency.

When you are unsure what to do in a crisis, call the telephone hotline, the hospital, or the police. Keep on until you are satisfied that you have done all you can. Then let go. Should the outcome disappoint you, remember, you did the best you knew how to do at the time.

MINIGLOSSARY
of Therapists

counselor: term for a helping person, not particularly definitive; people with a number of different qualifications can practice under this description. A graduate degree in counseling (M.S. or Ph.D.) from an accredited university is the degree to look for. Many states require licensing for counselors to practice.

psychiatrist: a physician (M.D.) who, after completing medical school, received additional special training to treat emotional problems and is licensed to prescribe drugs.

   psych = mind, soul
   iatros = doctor

psychoanalyst: a psychiatrist who specializes in analysis, seeking the root psychological causes of emotional problems.

psychologist: a person with a graduate degree (M.S. or Ph.D.) in psychology from a university. This person, although called "Doctor," is not licensed to write prescriptions; a desirable credential for a psychologist is certification by the American Psychology Association (APA). Many states require licensing for psychologists to practice.

social worker: a person with a graduate degree in social work (M.S.W.); a respected degree that includes training in counseling.

Other practitioners may call themselves by many titles. Some may be truly helpful individuals, but unless they have the appropriate credentials, you can't be sure of their qualifications to practice therapy.

Be sure to protect yourself. For your emotional well-being, it is important to be aware of the limits of your ability to give support. A depressed person can be a sort of emotional sink into which you pour your energy without getting anything back. Such a relationship drains you, to no useful purpose, yet you may not want or dare to turn your back on a person in time of need.

The person who constantly appeals to your sympathy and desire to be helpful is engaging in **manipulative behavior**. (To manipulate is to manage, in an underhanded way—often unconsciously.) By involving you in their problems, such people are managing in a roundabout fashion to get your attention, love, and support. But allowing them to depend on you is not healthy for them. A dependency relationship inflates the giver and diminishes the receiver so that neither is appreciated, loved, or supported on their own merits.

If such a situation drags on for very long, wisdom dictates that it is best for you and the other person if you extricate yourself from it. Your continued listening may be postponing a solution. Put the person in touch with expert help and bow out. Make it clear that you are taking this action to obtain truly effective help for your friend and peace of mind for yourself.

Your friend may have an emotional problem that needs some form of **psychotherapy** (which means, literally, therapy for the spirit). Any activity that has a healing or health-promoting effect is **therapy**. Psychotherapy is offered in many different places, such as those listed in the margin. You can take relief in knowing that your friend will probably end up in good hands because these centers are linked by a system of referrals, so that wherever people get into the system, they will—at least in theory—be able to find their way to the part of it that will best meet their needs.

Additional help might be found at one of the "anonymous" groups: Alcholics Anonymous (AA), Overeaters Anonymous (OA), Narcotics Anonymous (NA), Gamblers Anonymous (GA), and others like them.

The mind and body are really one, but Chapters 2 and 3 have emphasized the mind, with the body's continuous, though quiet, involvement an implicit theme. The next chapters reverse this emphasis, exploring the body's contributions to this partnership, while the involvement of the mind remains implicit.

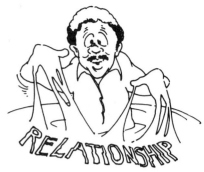

If you are mired in a dependency relationship, you may need help getting out of it.

Therapy can be obtained at:
- The community mental health center.
- The offices of psychiatrists, psycho-analysts, and psychiatric nurses.[23]
- Private counseling centers and psychological clinics.
- Counseling centers at schools or colleges.
- Employee assistance programs.
- Crisis centers (drug crisis, spouse abuse, and others).
- Alcohol and drug abuse programs.
- Self-help groups.
- Telephone counseling.

▩ STUDY AIDS

1. Define and distinguish among the terms *thoughts*, *emotions*, and *values*.
2. Explain why it is important to be aware of, express, and deal with emotions.
3. Explain what is meant by the *assessment* that leads to an emotion.
4. Outline the steps to take in changing one's feelings.
5. Explain how people can discover their values.
6. Explain what self-esteem has to do with being perfect.
7. Identify the stages of emotional growth throughout life (according to Erikson).
8. Identify and characterize the different selves according to trans-actional analysis.
9. Describe the order in which people's needs must be met (according to Maslow).
10. List some examples of support systems.
11. Describe some ways of reaching out to others.
12. Distinguish among nonassertive, assertive, and aggressive behaviors.
13. Describe the role a job or career plays in supporting a person's well-being.
14. Define emotional/mental illness, distinguishing it from normal, everyday problems.
15. Identify and contrast several causes of emotional problems.
16. Identify some strategies for dealing with depression.
17. List signs indicating that a depressed person needs help.
18. Describe how to go about getting help for emotional problems.

GLOSSARY

adjustment disorder: a maladaptive reaction to a life change—one that sets in within three months of the change and significantly impairs the person's functioning socially or on the job or causes symptoms in excess of the expected reaction to such a stress.

aggressive: insulting another person or otherwise invading the other person's territory; an inappropriate and ineffective way of expressing wants and needs.

alienation: withdrawal of personal involvement; being unable to relate to the values others live by.

anxiety: an emotional state characterized by high energy; the body's reaction to it is the stress response.

assertive: a term describing the appropriate expression of wants and needs; this mode of expression is effective and direct, without needless words or actions.

depression: an emotional condition of varying duration and severity in which the person feels apathetic, hopeless, and withdrawn from others. A *major depression* is an emotionally crippling depressed state; at the extreme, a suicidal state.

emotion: a felt tendency to move toward something assessed as good or favorable or away from something assessed as bad or unfavorable.

enabling: a term for misguided "helping." An enabler is a person who actually does harm by supporting a troubled person's continued indulgence in a self-destructive attitude or behavior.

manipulative behavior: behavior employed by a person in the hope of appealing to the helping impulses of others; managing others in a kind of underhanded way to obtain attention, love, and support.

mental disorder: a clinically significant behavioral or psychological syndrome that is typically associated with either a painful symptom (distress) or impairment in one or more important areas of functioning (disability).

mentor: a role model or spiritual adviser.

nonassertive: failing to express wants and needs at all.

nonconformist: a person who does not share society's values orbehave according to them and who therefore does not fit in.

ostracism (OS-tra- sizm): exclusion from society, often due to refusal to conform to its values.

positive imaging: a technique of imagining oneself achieving positive outcomes to experiences. Also called *guided imaging*.

positive self-talk: the practice of making affirmative statements to oneself about oneself, helpful in building self-esteem.

post-traumatic stress disorder: severe anxiety in reaction to psychological stress such as wartime trauma or rape, arising after the event is over.

　trauma = wound

premenstrual syndrome (PMS): a cluster of symptoms, including both physical and emotional pain, that occurs in some women just before menstruation.

psychotherapy: therapy directed toward the solution of emotional problems. See Miniglossary of Therapies.

self-actualization: the realization of one's full potential; the highest state in Maslow's hierarchy of needs, never completely realized.

support system: a network of individuals or groups with which one identifies and exchanges support.

therapy: any activity that has a healing or health-promoting effect. See also *psychotherapy*.

thought: a conscious mental process that takes place in the cortex of the brain.

transactional analysis (TA): a type of therapy that recognizes three components in people's personalities—the Child, Parent, and Adult—and studies the ways in which they interact.

values: set of rules for behavior, based on beliefs.

QUIZ ANSWERS

1. *False.* An emotionally healthy person is distinguished by owning and working on problems, not by not having them.

2. *False.* Feelings can be changed by changing the assessments that lead to them.

3. *False.* A person's values change as life goes on, and in fact can be changed intentionally.

4. *True.* Talking to yourself can enhance your self-esteem.

5. *False.* It is natural and desirable to stay in touch with childish feelings throughout life.

6. *True.* The primary problem shy people have is the fear of being rejected.

7. *False*, at least some of the time. Some emotional problems are beyond the scope of self-help and require professional treatment.

8. *True.* The experience of loss always causes depression.

9. *True.* Anxiety can be beneficial.

10. *True.* Guilt is the appropriate response of a person who has gone against conscience.

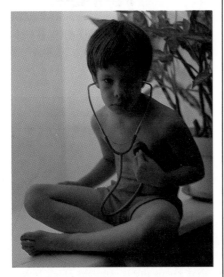

Signals from Within

Part of personal health is keeping in touch with your body. People often wonder just how much you can tell by simply "listening to your body."

I've wondered about that. Sometimes I feel as if I have a need to eat some particular food. Is there any scientific explanation for such cravings?

Nutritionists have wondered for years whether cravings are adaptive—that is, whether they reflect any physical need for the foods you crave. We know they do in some instances. Hunger and thirst, of course, reflect the body's needs for food and water. We don't even know exactly how these mechanisms work, though, and we know still less about other cravings.

Do you know what other cravings might be adaptive?

The craving for salt is a candidate. Pasture animals can easily become depleted of sodium, because grass and grain are naturally low in the mineral. To obtain it, they will travel miles to a salt lick. It isn't known whether human beings' apparent salt hunger signifies a real need for sodium. Usually it does not; we normally get much more sodium in our diets than we need.

An annual phenomenon related to cravings is that people tend to eat heavier foods—foods richer in fat—in the fall and winter than they do in the summertime. As a result, they ingest more calories, which can support the increased metabolic rate necessary to maintain their body temperatures in the cold. It may be no accident that the traditional Thanksgiving and Christmas feasts involve heavy eating. While winter feasting benefits people who face long periods of exposure to cold, it only puts unwanted fat on people who live and work in heated buildings. This is an example of a natural tendency whose adaptive advantage is lost to modern human beings.

As for other cravings, women commonly report craving carbohydrate foods right after they ovulate, and they eat 500 calories more per day, on the average, during the ten days before their menstrual periods than during the ten days after.[1]* The extra calories probably support the extra work of making the uterus ready for pregnancy. The woman who knows herself well will expect this tendency and not fight it. If she wants to restrict calories, she'll do well to cut down after her period, when it's easier to do so.

I wonder why women single out carbohydrate, particularly?

That is a question to which we may have a partial answer. Carbohydrate, in the form of blood glucose, enables a substance that may alter the way you feel to get into the brain. This substance contributes to the formation of a **neurotransmitter**, called **serotonin**, which conveys messages from nerve to nerve. The right amount of serotonin reduces pain to a minimum, eases sleep, and diminishes depression. Researchers studying serotonin have suggested that when its level in the brain is low, you may actually develop a "carbohydrate hunger." If you obey the urge and eat carbohydrate, it will lead to the raising of your brain's serotonin level; that makes you feel better and so reinforces the eating behavior.[2] (You don't have to eat candy to benefit from this effect, though. Read Chapter 4 on nutrition before jumping to any conclusions about the best ways to eat.)

Tell me something else. Is it true that during pregnancy, women crave the foods that are good for them?

You mean "pickles and ice cream"? There is certainly no evidence that pregnant women crave such strange combinations for the specific

*Reference notes are in Appendix D.

nutrients they contain, but yes, it
may be true in general. Pregnant
women have reported in interviews
that their tastes do change. They
drink less coffee and alcohol; they actually like them less. They like and
eat more sweets, milk, chocolate,
fruit, and fish; and they eat less meat
and poultry. It is not clear what
makes them do this.[3]

**That's interesting. It sounds like a
kind of natural rhythm.**

People have recognized natural
rhythms since the dawn of history.
Every living creature senses and responds to them. We human beings
have cycles corresponding to those of
the moon, the day-night cycle, and
the seasons, to name only a few. For
example, several human cycles seem
related to the lunar cycle. The best
known doubtless is the menstrual
cycle (*menses* refers to month and
moon), but men also respond to the
moon's cycles: their beards grow
faster near the full moon. People's
moods are thought to be influenced
by the lunar cycle, too. In fact, the
word *lunatic* originally referred to the
strange ways people behaved at the
time of the full moon. It is not just
that people cannot sleep because of
the light; they actually are more emotionally aroused at the time of the
full moon than at other times.

**Are you saying that people are not
responsible for their own behavior
at certain times of the month?**

To be truthful, it's not clear just what
is and is not true in this realm, but
people's moods tend to go in cycles,
even if we don't know the reason.
The information is useful: it helps us
to know ourselves. "I always feel lo-
neliest just before the dawn," says
one woman. "I tend to get depressed
in the springtime," says a man. We
may not know just what to do about
our cyclic rhythms, but being aware
of them helps us cope. At least we
can say, "I know that this will pass."

**Tell me more about the "time of
day" rhythms. I think I have a peak
time around ten in the morning. Is
that likely to be true?**

Yes, it could very well be. The day-
night cycle coincides with rhythms
known as **circadian rhythms**—from
root words meaning "about a day."
The body seems to have several biological clocks, which keep running
on a 24- to 25-hour cycle even when
the person is kept from seeing sunrise and sunset. Many body functions seem to operate on such cycles:
blood pressure, hormone levels,
heart rate, body temperature, mood,
and memory. Such cycles even affect
people's ability to perform mathematics problems, error rate,[4] and sensitivity to the effects of alcohol.[5] So it
may be best for us to do certain
things at certain times of day. In
your case, for example, you'd better
balance your checkbook in the
morning.

**Why should my temperature fluc-
tuate on a 24-hour cycle?**

Your body temperature helps determine how easily you can sleep. It is
lowest (for most people) in the middle of the night. It rises toward
morning, and at a certain critical
point, you wake up. It continues to
rise throughout the day and falls in
the evening. As it declines, you begin to feel sleepy, and you go to
sleep. People who "listen to their
bodies" and don't try to fight this
natural rhythm probably have the
easiest time sleeping and waking.

Can you reset your clock?

We're not certain, but it seems possible that habit can to some extent override the clock settings you were
born with. When a late sleeper has a
baby who wakes her early every
morning, for example, she may go to
sleep and awaken earlier of necessity,
and in time, her body-temperature
cycle may shift to accommodate the
change.

**I always fade right after lunch. Does
that mean my biological clock lowers my temperature at that time?**

No, the temperature does not fall at
that time, but you are describing a
universal human experience. Researchers have wondered why people get sleepy after lunch. For years,
people believed that eating a big
meal caused the sleepiness. They
thought the blood was routed away
from the brain to the digestive system. Research has shown, though,
that noontime sleepiness has nothing
to do with the food eaten for lunch.
People often eat larger evening meals
than lunches, but they tend to drop
off after lunch more predictably than
after dinner. The early afternoon low
is thought to be programmed into us
as a response to the heat of the day
in the tropics, where the human species evolved. In hot climates, it's best
to sleep at midday and save activity
for morning and later afternoon,
when moving about is easier.[6]

**It occurs to me that "jet lag" has
something to do with these biological clocks.**

It certainly does. People who fly long
distances around the world have to
adjust very quickly to radical changes
in the day-night cycle, and that can
be seriously upsetting to the system.

There are some tricks that can help, though. The body's clocks can apparently be reset (although they resist resetting) by changes in the times of sunrise and sunset and also by changes in mealtimes. A man who must fly from New York to California can function better on California time if he forces himself to start eating and sleeping on California time a few days before the trip. If he sleeps, wakes, and eats late by New York standards, then by the time he makes the trip, he'll be adjusted. Of course, he still goes through disruption, but the preplanned change makes the trip more pleasant.

What about the timing of exercise in relation to meals?

It's best not to exercise right after meals, because the body's hormones are set one way to digest food and another way to exercise muscles. The two needs conflict. Circulation can be routed to pick up absorbed nutrients from the digestive tract or to carry oxygen to exercising muscles, but not both at once—at least not with maximum efficiency. But more subtly, it seems that exercise within two or three hours after eating burns off more calories than the same amount of exercise beyond that time. And the day after you *over*eat, exercise will burn off more calories than the day after you eat a normal or small amount of food.[7]

I sometimes feel as if I have to get outdoors. Is there any physical basis for that?

There probably is a physical basis. Light, particularly sunlight, affects the brain, and the brain affects the body in such a way as to relieve depression. The color green may be most effective in this respect. Also, people need space. Depression is twice as frequent in the city as in rural areas.[8] There is a real possibility that we human beings are born with a need for natural environments—or at least with the capacity to be pleased and uplifted by them. We like vistas, the sound of running water, the songs of birds, the sound of rain and wind in the trees, scenes with a certain amount of variety in them, certain kinds of spaces. Successful architects build accordingly, meeting people's natural needs. Biologists are now attempting to discover just what it is about natural environments that human beings need for their survival and well-being.[9]

What does all this mean in terms of my behavior? How can I put into practice the skill of "listening to my body"?

Keep on learning, and start listening. It would be a mistake to impulsively do whatever you feel like doing; the impulse to eat two pounds of chocolate is not one to obey. But do pay attention to the impulses you are feeling. Give them credit for being signals from within. Try to guess what needs they may reflect. Experiment with meeting those needs in different ways, and see if you can tell which ways are right on target. Your first guess may not be correct, for many responses to internal stirrings are inappropriate.

It sounds simple-minded, but you'd be amazed how many people, even after years of living with themselves, fail to hear the messages their bodies are trying to send them. One person needs to learn, when he is lonely, to call a friend rather than to overeat or drink. Another needs to learn, when she is exhausted, to sleep rather than to drink coffee. Still another has found out, at the age of 45, that he should exercise when he is nervous, rather than biting his fingernails. And so forth. If you will keep on learning about the subject—yourself, that is—the results will mean a healthier, happier life.

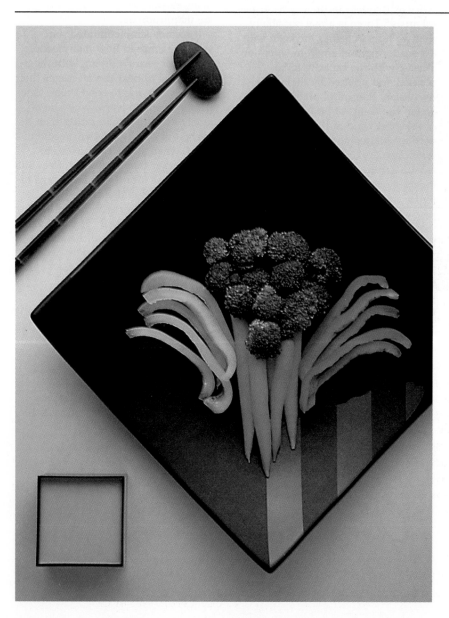

Chapter 4

Nutrition

FOR OPENERS . . .

True or false? If false, say what is true.

1. Malnutrition occurs in people in the United States and Canada.

2. It is possible to have an appetite without being hungry.

3. As far as nutrients are concerned, the more, the better.

4. Carbohydrate should contribute more than half of all the calories a person consumes in a day.

5. Honey and sugar are the same, as far as the body is concerned.

6. Of all the dietary factors related to diseases prevalent in developed countries, fiber is probably the most significant.

7. Low-carbohydrate diets cause the body to lose muscle tissue.

8. Adults need milk, just as children do.

9. In large amounts, all vitamins can be harmful.

10. Fast foods can be nutritious.

(Answers on page 83.)

You choose to eat a meal about 1,000 times a year. Eating is so habitual that often people give it hardly any thought, yet it is a voluntary activity. You can choose when to eat, what to eat, and how much to eat—70,000 times in a lifetime.

Not all selections of foods supply the nutrients needed for health. Some people in the United States and Canada, especially those with low incomes, suffer from **undernutrition**. Some pregnant women suffer nutrient deficiencies that retard their infants' growth. Among migratory workers and certain rural populations, more than 1 in every 10 children suffers stunted growth caused by a poor diet.[1]* Iron deficiencies occur in all people regardless of income, affecting 1 to 5 percent of people severely enough to cause the deficiency disease **anemia**. Many more are affected in subtly damaging ways.

At the same time, **overnutrition** also threatens people's health. About 15 percent of men and 25 percent of women are obese. People's average daily intakes of sodium are too high for the health of their hearts. People are choosing to eat foods higher in fat, cholesterol, and sugar than recommended, and high incidences of several degenerative diseases are attributed to these habits.[2]

Your accumulated choices profoundly influence your health, right now, today, and also in the years of tomorrow. The well-nourished person resists disease and other stresses better, enjoys greater energy, and can be physiologically years younger than the poorly nourished person. Your body derives its energy from foods and is made of materials obtained from them. You are, as the old saying goes, what you eat. It is worth questioning why you eat when you do, why you choose the foods you do—and, most important, whether they supply the nutrients you need.

To the question of what prompts you to eat, you may reply that it is **hunger**. That is often true, but hunger, the physiological need for food, is not the only stimulus that triggers eating behavior. Another cue is **appetite**, the psychological desire for food, which may arise in response to the sight, smell, or thought of food even when you don't need to eat. You may have an appetite when you are not hungry—or the reverse.

You choose particular foods for several reasons including personal preference, habit, social pressure, availability, convenience, economy, and nutritional value. The task of this chapter is to increase your understanding of nutrition and to provide strategies that may improve your nutrition status.

Food supplies **nutrients, fiber**, and other materials. There are six classes of nutrients: **carbohydrate, fat** (technically known as **lipid**), **protein, vitamins, minerals**, and **water**. Three of the classes of nutrients supply **energy**: carbohydrate, lipid, and protein. Carbohydrate supplies the body with the sugar **glucose**, the main energy fuel for the brain and nervous system. Lipid supplies the main energy fuel **fatty acids**, for muscles, including the heart muscle. Protein's building blocks, **amino acids**, are the major structural material of cells, but they can be broken down for energy if the body has run out of available glucose and fatty acids. They can also be transformed into glucose to feed the brain if carbohydrate is not available.

The energy from these nutrients is used by the body to do work or generate heat. The units of measure of energy are **calories**. The other nutrients, vitamins and minerals, do not offer energy but regulate its release and other

*Reference notes are in Appendix D.

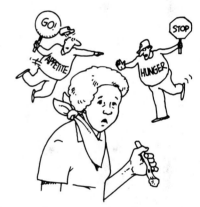

You may have an appetite when you are not hungry—or the reverse.

Nutrients:
    Carbohydrate—provides energy as glucose.
    Lipid—provides energy as fatty acids.
    Protein—provides structural material but can be transformed into glucose or fatty acids under some conditions.
Vitamins—play regulatory roles.
Minerals—play regulatory roles.
Water—provides the medium for life processes.

Water is the most vital nutrient of all.

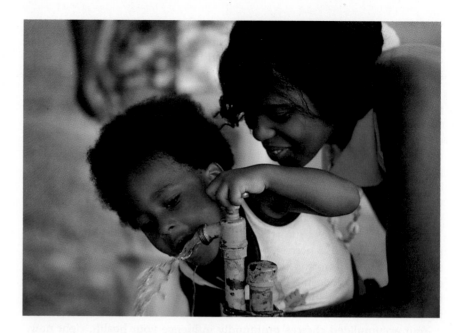

Calories are units in which energy is measured.*

Alcohol is not a nutrient but provides energy. For more information see Chapter 8.

processes. As for water, it is the medium in which all the body's processes take place. Probably about 60 percent of your body's weight is water. Since you lose water from your body daily, you must replace it daily. Second only to oxygen, water is the most vital substance you require; you could live only a few days without it.

ENERGY FROM FOOD

As mentioned, the body derives its energy chiefly from two fuels: glucose and fatty acids. The supply of glucose is temporary, and you have to eat to maintain it. The brain's hypothalamus sends out a hunger signal when blood glucose gets too low. If you refuse to eat, the body turns to its four or so hours' worth of **glycogen** (a concentrated storage form of glucose) in your liver that can be broken down to generate glucose. And if you still don't eat after the glycogen has been used, then your muscles and other lean body tissues begin to break down, releasing protein fragments, which your liver converts to glucose. But the wise eater turns to food before incurring tissue protein losses. Why dismantle your house for firewood, when the woodpile is nearby?

It has been advised by many—nutritionists, health professionals, and most likely, your parents—to eat a **balanced meal**. This is a meal that contains several different kinds of food, offering protein, fat, and carbohydrate (see Figure 4–1).

Carbohydrate

The terms *simple carbohydrate* and *complex carbohydrate* refer to one important distinction among carbohydrates. Another is that the simple carbohydrates come in both natural (dilute) and processed (concentrated) form.

*Food energy can also be measured in joules, or kilojoules. A joule is a measure or work energy (force), whereas a calorie is a measure of heat energy. Both are metric measures.

The **complex carbohydrates** are composed of long chains of glucose units. One of them, glycogen, has already been mentioned as the form in which glucose is stored in the human liver and muscle cells. The complex carbohydrate **starch** is the principal complex carbohydrate in grains and vegetables and the chief energy source for human beings. Other complex carbohydrates in foods are indigestible by human beings and so yield no calories but serve as fiber, or **roughage**, helping to maintain the health of the digestive tract.

The fibers in foods are not digestible. They move through the digestive tract essentially unchanged. They hold water and so provide bulk inside the intestines, enabling the muscles of the digestive tract walls to push their contents along. The more fiber in the foods you eat, the more water they hold, and the softer the stools they form. The subject may seem unglamorous, but it intensely interests anyone who suffers from the consequences of a lack of fiber: constipation, hemorrhoids, or a host of other intestinal ills.

Fiber is credited with many virtues. It helps prevent constipation. It helps prevent and relieve hemorrhoids. It may also, by keeping the intestinal contents moving, help prevent infection of the appendix (appendicitis) and may reduce the time of exposure of the intestinal walls to cancer-causing compounds. Fiber may also help prevent obesity. The person who eats fiber-rich foods chews longer and fills up sooner on fewer calories.

However, there is such a thing as too much fiber. Some years ago, many college students overdid the high-fiber diet, much to their intestinal distress. The consequence was diarrhea prolonged and severe enough to cause dangerous dehydration in some instances. Too much of anything, in nutrition as in all areas of life, is as harmful as too little.

Plant foods are high in fiber—particularly those with their skins and seeds intact. Fiber breaks down as the foods are refined or cooked. If you want to eat a diet high enough in fiber to benefit your health, choose whole grains, whole fruits, and whole vegetables most of the time. Cook sparingly those you cook, and eat some raw.

The **simple carbohydrates** are the **sugars**. All are chemically similar to glucose and can be converted into glucose in the body. Simple carbohydrates come mostly from fruits and milk, or in concentrated form, as sugar, honey, and other sweets relatively empty of nutrients. Nutritionists recommend that you consume abundant quantities of fruits and vegetables that contain sugars, but they urge you in the same breath to avoid consuming "too much sugar" (see Table 4–1). What's the difference?

Part of the answer lies in the phrase **empty calories**. A large apple and a 12-ounce cola beverage furnish similar amounts of calories. The apple, however, also contains vitamin A, thiamin, vitamin C, fiber, and potassium.

In contrast to claims stating that honey provides nutrients and is not empty calories, honey contains only traces of a few vitamins and minerals. Honey is a relatively empty calorie food. Honey is almost identical to sugar chemically, too.

Also, the bacteria that cause dental caries thrive on sugar. They can double their numbers when carbohydrate sticks to tooth surfaces for 20 minutes or more at a time—and sugar tends to stick. Caries form when three factors are present: a susceptible tooth, a carbohydrate supply, and bacteria to consume the carbohydrate and produce acid from it that decays the tooth enamel. A few people are born with decay-resistant teeth, but most need to protect their teeth to prevent decay. A prime mode of prevention is

Complex carbohydrates (long chains of glucose):
    Starch—people's main energy source.
    Glycogen—storage form of glucose.
    Fibers—indigestible carbohydrates.

RUFF-idge

FIGURE 4–1   A Balanced Meal

The meal supplies foods from every food group, as well as a recommended balance of energy sources: less than 30 percent of its calories are from fat, and about 60 percent are from carbohydrate. Note the moderate meat portion and the generous portions of vegetables and fruit. The bread is without butter, and the beverage is non-fat milk. Total calories: about 500.

A mistake people commonly make is to think that if fat should contribute 30 percent of the calories, then it should take up a third of the plate. On the contrary: Fat is much more calorie-dense than the other constituents of food, and much of it is invisible. In this 500-calorie meal, the only visible fat is in the chicken skin, and yet fat contributes almost 30 percent of the calories.

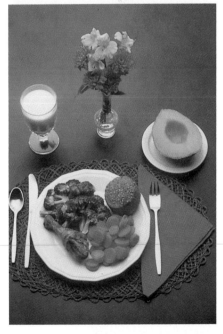

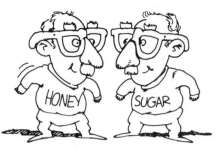

In terms of nutrition, there's no significant difference between honey and sugar.

Snacks dentists recommend:
  Milk, cheese, and yogurt (not fruit and flavored yogurts, though, which are as sugary as ice cream).
  Fresh fruits (not dried fruits, jams, and jellies).
  Unsweetened juice.
  Vegetables (but not candied or glazed).
  Grains (but not granola bars, which are as sticky as candy bars).

fluoridation of the water supply where natural fluoride levels are low, because fluoride combines with the crystals of tooth enamel to make teeth insoluble and resistant to decay. Another obvious preventive measure is to avoid exposing the teeth to carbohydrate for long periods and, after exposure, to brush and floss them promptly. If you drink a sugary soft drink, finish it quickly, and follow with a vigorous water rinse.

Fat

Nearly all the body's tissues (except the brain and nervous system) can use fat as an energy source. It is the major fuel for muscles, as long as they have enough oxygen to break it down.

Fat is stored in a layer of cells beneath the skin and also in many pads surrounding and underlying vital organs. It helps to insulate the body from heat, cold, and mechanical shock as well as providing an energy reserve. Whenever you eat, you store some fat, and within a few hours after a meal, you take it out of storage and use it for energy until the next meal.

Thus both glucose and fat are stored after meals, and both are released later when needed as fuel for the cells' work. But where excess carbohydrate and protein can be converted to fat, fat can serve only as an energy fuel for cells equipped to use it. The body has scanty reserves of carbohydrate and virtually no protein to spare, but it can store fat in practically unlimited amounts. A pound of body fat is worth 3,500 calories, and a person's body can easily carry 30 to 50 pounds of fat without looking fat at all. In fact, a man of normal weight might have about 15 percent, and a woman about 20 percent, of the body weight as fat.

Fat comes in different forms. In foods, most of it comes as **triglycerides**, and it is stored in the body's fat cells in the same form. Another form of fat is **cholesterol**. Cholesterol is made in the body and is necessary to health, but it also is associated with heart and artery disease. Cholesterol forms a major part of the deposits that accumulate along arteries and increase the risk of heart attacks and strokes. In reality, though, it is not the cholesterol you eat, but *cholesterol made by the body from the triglycerides you eat*, that forms these deposits. When you eat less fat, your body makes less cholesterol.

Reducing fat intake offers a fringe benefit to people who wish to cut calories. A spoon of fat contains more than twice as many calories as a spoon of sugar or pure protein. By removing the fat from a food, you can drastically reduce the calorie count (see Table 4–2).

Of all the dietary factors related to diseases prevalent in developed countries, high fat intakes are probably the most significant. Heart disease and many forms of cancer are linked to high fat intakes; probably many other diseases are, too, including arthritis, gallbladder disease, diabetes, and all diseases aggravated by obesity. The most important dietary steps that you can take to prevent these diseases are to control your fat intake and to control your weight.

Protein

Protein is famed as the body-building nutrient, the material of strong muscles, and rightly so. No new living tissue can be built without it, for protein is part of every cell, every bone, the blood, and every other tissue. Proteins constitute the cells' machinery—they do the cells' work, while carbohydrate and fat provide the energy to fuel that work.

Among the cells' working parts are a multitude of proteins called **enzymes**. Each enzyme performs a specific chemical step in the synthesis or breakdown of cellular materials. A single human cell may contain several thousand kinds of enzymes, each performing a different chemical reaction.

The instructions that tell cells how to make their proteins are inherited. When geneticists talk about hereditary differences among people, they are really talking about differences in the codes they have inherited for their proteins, most of which are enzymes.

Another set of proteins that confer individuality on people is the antibodies of the immune system, which facilitate resistance to disease. Antibodies participate in the rejection of foreign materials.

Proteins are made of amino acids—building blocks. There are 20 distinct amino acids that form proteins (much as letters form sentences), but your body can make only 11 of them. There are 9 essential amino acids, essential in that the body cannot make them and therefore they must be obtained from food.

Your body loses protein every day. Digestive tract cells wear out and are excreted in the feces. Skin cells flake off or are rubbed off. Hair and nails (made of protein) grow longer daily and are shed or cut away. An adult

Some forms of fat:
  Triglycerides.
    Saturated.
    Unsaturated (including polyunsaturated).
  Cholesterol.

Chapter 16 gives more details on heart and artery disease, saturated and unsaturated fats, and on the *lipoproteins*, LDL and HDL, which transport lipids in the body.

Nutrition-related factors known or strongly suspected to be partially responsible for heart disease:
  High blood pressure—high salt intake; obesity.
  High blood cholesterol—high fat and cholesterol intakes; obesity.
  Diabetes—high sugar and fat intakes; obesity.
For other factors, see Chapter 16.
Nutrition-related factors known or strongly suspected to be partially responsible for cancer:
  High fat intake.
  Low fiber intake.
  Low fruit and vegetable intakes.
For details, see Chapter 17's Spotlight.

TABLE 4–2 The Most Effective Way to Cut the Calories from a Food Is to Remove the Fat from It

Food	Calories
Pork chop with 1/2 inch of fat	275
Pork chop with fat trimmed off	165
Potato with 1 tbsp butter and 1 tbsp sour cream	260
Plain potato	130
Whole milk (1 cup)	150
Nonfat milk (1 cup)	90

loses about half a cup to a cup of pure protein a day. People need to eat protein-containing foods every day to replace the protein they lose.

You know you are eating protein when you eat foods that come from animals: meats, fish, poultry, eggs, cheese, and milk. It is easy to consume more than enough protein from these foods. An adult could obtain enough protein from one egg in the morning, two cups of milk during the day, and an assortment of grains and vegetables, without a single serving of meat. Yet many people eat two or three eggs for breakfast rather than one, hamburgers for lunch, and 12-ounce steaks for dinner.

Protein-rich foods from animal sources are almost invariably high in fat and calories, and all are low in fiber, so they pose a triple problem. It is beneficial to health for people to obtain at least half of their protein from plants, and it is possible to get enough protein from plant foods alone, as **vegetarians** do.

Animal proteins supply a balanced assortment of all the essential amino acids, but some plant proteins contain limited amounts of certain essential amino acids and so don't support the building of body protein by themselves. People who eat only plant foods have to eat them in combinations to receive the full range of needed amino acids. Alternatively, a vegetable meal that includes small amounts of animal proteins presents a balanced assortment of amino acids.

If people do not consume adequate protein or calories, they will become malnourished. The media have made **malnutrition** familiar to everyone as it occurs in faraway places, but it also occurs at home among neglected and homeless children, sick people in hospitals, substance abusers, and others.

A malnourished body may be deprived of protein or energy. Both deficiency states are marked by depletion of body protein. This is known as **protein-energy malnutrition (PEM),** which afflicts millions of people in the world and kills about a million children *a month.*[3]

People who starve themselves, even if they do it with the best of intentions, also incur malnutrition. A fat person attempting to lose weight by fasting may die of protein deficiency while still looking fat. A young person with anorexia nervosa also loses vital tissue and may die. Chapter 5 Spotlight offers information on anorexia nervosa.

Combinations of plant foods that deliver complete protein:
Beans and rice.
Peanut butter and bread.
Tofu and rice.
Any grain and any legume (bean).

CONSUMER CAUTION

The cautious consumer of diet information distinguishes between loss of fat and loss of weight.

When a person diets or starves, body fat is not the only tissue lost. Body protein is always sacrificed to meet the brain's glucose need when the carbohydrate supply runs short. Millions of dollars are made by the unscrupulous promoters of low-carbohydrate diets, high-protein diets, and fasts, because they bring about quick weight loss. Unwitting victims fail to realize that much of the weight being lost is from muscle and other vital tissue and that health is being lost along with it.

Thus far, this chapter has dealt with the energy-bearing nutrients—carbohydrate, fat, and protein. It remains to discuss the nutrients everyone thinks of when they think about nutrition—the vitamins and minerals.

THE VITAMINS AND MINERALS

The vitamins and minerals occur in foods in much smaller quantities than do the energy nutrients, and they make no contribution of energy themselves. Nor do they contribute building material, except for the minerals of bone. Instead they serve mostly as helpers, or facilitators, of body processes. They are nonetheless a powerful group of substances, as their absence attests. Vitamin A deficiency can cause blindness; a lack of niacin causes mental illness; a lack of vitamin D causes growth retardation. The consequences of deficiencies are so dire and the effects of restoring the needed nutrients so dramatic that they make wonderful stories for faddists to tell. Are you bald? Impotent? Do you have pimples? Are you nearsighted? The right vitamin will cure whatever ails you. Vitamin supplementation is discussed in this chapter's spotlight.

Actually, a vitamin or mineral can cure only the disease caused by a deficiency of that vitamin or mineral. Also, an overdose of any vitamin or mineral can make people as sick as a deficiency. It is remarkable, and lucky for people who haven't studied nutrition, that a balanced diet of ordinary foods supplies enough, but not too much, of each of the vitamins and minerals.

The vitamins and minerals are listed and some of their more important roles in the body shown in Table 4–3. To convince you of the urgency of meeting your body's needs for them, this section discusses two vitamins that deficient in large numbers of people in the United States—that is, those that you might most easily lack if you didn't take the needed precautions—thiamin and vitamin B_6.

Thiamin is a typical vitamin in that its presence is not felt, but its absence makes itself known all over the body. A severe thiamin deficiency causes a paralysis that begins at the fingers and toes and works its way inward toward the spine, extreme wasting and loss of muscle tissue, swelling all over the body, and enlargement of the heart and irregular heartbeat. Ultimately the victim dies from heart failure. You probably have never witnessed such an extreme deficiency, but consider how a mild lack manifests its presence: stomachaches, headaches, fatigue, restlessness, disturbances of sleep, chest pains, fevers, personality changes (aggressiveness and hostility), and a whole string of symptoms often classed as neurosis. Mild thiamin deficiencies are likely to be seen in consumers of "junk" diets—those built on foods low in nutrients and high in calories, sugar, fat, and salt.

Proof that thiamin was deficient in some people who snacked heavily on empty-calorie foods came from research that showed below-normal activity of a thiamin-containing enzyme in their blood. They also had symptoms of neurosis. When they took thiamin supplements for a month or more, the symptoms disappeared as the blood enzyme activity returned to normal.[4]

On hearing stories like this, people tend to want to rush out to the drugstore and buy bottles of vitamin pills. There's a problem, though: although you might get the amount of thiamin you need this way, there are some 40-odd other essential nutrients, and all are equally vital to your well-being. Foods are far more effective than pills in supplying the assortment of nutrients you need, because they contain such rich mixtures of nutrients in forms the body is adapted to use.

What foods in particular supply thiamin, then? Almost no one food you eat will supply your daily need in a single serving. In fact, thiamin is deliv-

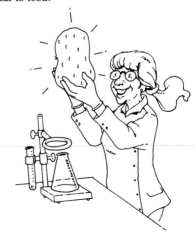

When science concocts the ideal supplement, it will probably turn out to be identical to food.

TABLE 4–3 Major Roles of the Vitamins and Minerals

Fat-Soluble Vitamins[a]

Vitamin A	A pigment of the eye important in vision, especially night vision. Participates in the modeling of bones during growth and in the mending of breaks. Helps maintain the body's many surfaces (skin and linings of lungs, digestive tract, urinary tract, vagina, eyelids). A participant in the repair of genetic damage that could otherwise lead to cancer. A factor in production of sperm and maintenance of pregnancy.
Vitamin D	A regulator of the calcium concentration in the blood.
Vitamin E	A protector of compounds that are susceptible to destruction by oxidation. Important in protecting red blood cells from bursting as they pass through the lungs.
Vitamin K	A factor necessary for the clotting of blood.

Water-Soluble Vitamins[a]

Thiamin **Riboflavin** **Niacin**	Factors that help enzymes to facilitate the release of energy from nutrients needed in every cell of the body.
Vitamin B_6	A factor necessary for the metabolism of protein.
Vitamin B_{12} **Folacin**	Factors that help cells to divide, especially blood cells and cells of the intestinal lining.
Biotin **Pantothenic acid**	Other B vitamins; seldom found deficient in human beings but known to be needed in the diets of experimental animals.
Vitamin C	A factor that maintains the body's connective tissue. Important to the healing of wounds. Part of the "glue" that holds cells together.

Major Minerals

Calcium **Phosphorus**	The principal minerals of bones and teeth. Calcium is involved with muscle contraction, nerve transmission, immune function, and blood clotting. Phosphorus is important in the genetic material and in energy transfer.

NOTE: The vitamin names given here are the official names as of 1979. Other names still commonly used and seen on labels are *alpha-tocopherol* for vitamin E, *vitamin B_1* for thiamin, *vitamin B_2* for riboflavin, *pyridoxine* for vitamin B_6, *folic acid* for folacin, and *ascorbic acid* for vitamin C.

[a]The fat-soluble and water-soluble vitamins were originally separated on the basis of their solubility. The fat-soluble vitamins tend to be stored in the body and so can be eaten in large quantities at intervals, whereas the water-soluble vitamins tend to be excreted daily in urine and not to accumulate, and so must be eaten daily.

TABLE 4–3 Continued

Major Minerals Continued	
Magnesium	Another factor involved in bone mineralization, protein synthesis, muscular contraction, and transmission of nerve impulses.
Sodium Chlorine Potassium	Electrolytes (see page 78) that maintain fluid balance and the balance of acids and bases inside and outside cells. Chlorine is also part of the hydrochloric acid of the stomach, necessary for digestion. Potassium also facilitates protein synthesis and the maintenance of nerves and muscles.
Sulfur	A component of certain amino acids. Part of the vitamins biotin and thiamin and the hormone insulin.

Trace Minerals	
Iodine	A component of thyroid hormone, which helps to regulate growth, development, and metabolic rate in the body.
Fluoride	An element involved in the formation of bones and teeth; helps to make them resistant to loss of their minerals.
Selenium	A factor that, with vitamin E, protects body compounds from oxidation.
Iron	Part of the red blood cell protein hemoglobin, which carries oxygen from place to place in the body, and of the muscle protein myoglobin, which makes oxygen available for muscle work. A factor necessary for the use of energy in every cell.
Zinc	A working part of many enzymes and of the hormone insulin. A factor involved in the making of genetic material and proteins, immune reactions, transport of vitamin A, taste perception, wound healing, the making of sperm, and the development of the fetus.
Copper	A factor necessary for the absorption and use of iron in the formation of hemoglobin. Part of several enzymes. A factor that helps to form the protective covering of nerves.
Cobalt	Part of vitamin B_{12} and therefore involved in cell division.
Chromium	A factor associated with insulin and required for the use of glucose.
Molybdenum Manganese	Facilitators, with enzymes, of many cell processes.
Vanadium, tin, nickel, silicon, others	Factors necessary for many biological functions in animals[b]

[b]Specific human requirements remain undetermined.

ered in adequate amounts only to people who eat *ten or more servings nutritious foods each day*, as the Four Food Group Plan advises (see Table 4–5, page 79).

As for vitamin B_6, it, too, is an indispensable cog in the body's machinery, and the price of a deficiency is a multitude of symptoms. Vitamin B_6 illustrates another nutrition principle— that excesses are also toxic. Whenever people start overusing a nutrient, no matter how nontoxic the nutrient may seem to be at first, it is only a matter of time before toxic effects appear. This happened in the 1970s with vitamin C after the publication of the popular book *Vitamin C and the Common Cold*.[5] In the 1980s, it is happening with vitamin B_6. People have been "diagnosing" vitamin B_6 deficiencies on grossly inadequate evidence and "prescribing" megadoses.

The first major report of toxic effects of vitamin B_6 appeared in 1983.[6] The physicians reporting them told the stories of seven different individuals who had been taking more than 2 grams a day of vitamin B_6 for two months or more (the recommended daily intake is 2 *milligrams*). Most of them were attempting to cure the symptoms of premenstrual syndrome (PMS; see Chapter 3). All seven cases were similar. The symptoms started with numb feet; the individuals then lost sensation in their hands, then became unable to work. Later, in some cases, their mouths became numb. In all but two cases they had started with low doses and progressed to higher and higher doses seeking an effect. They may have suffered irreversible nerve damage; at the last report, the symptoms still had not completely disappeared. Since then, other reports have followed, showing nervous system damage from more moderate doses of vitamin B_6.[7]

Not everyone is likely to suffer toxicity symptoms with a vitamin B_6 megadose. Because it is easily excreted in the urine, vitamin B_6 is a relatively nontoxic nutrient, but individual tolerances vary, and we cannot say that supplements are "safe" for anyone. The same fact holds for every vitamin.

Scientific studies have revealed true vitamin B_6 deficiencies in some people, notably those who eat inadequate diets and whose nutrient needs are higher than usual owing to pregnancy, alcohol abuse, or other unusual circumstances. However, doses of about ten times the requirement (25 milligrams a day) for a few weeks are sufficient to remedy these deficiencies.

Like the vitamins, the minerals occur in small amounts in the body, and you need only small amounts in foods daily. Minerals are vital to life, though. Two examples illustrate the importance of the 20-odd minerals that serve as nutrients for human beings—calcium and iron.

Calcium is well known as the major mineral of bones and teeth, and everyone is aware that children therefore need milk daily to support their growth. But abundant evidence now supports the contention that adults, too, and especially women, need calcium in their later years, just as they did when they were younger. A deficit of calcium during childhood and adulthood incurs a gradual bone loss, **osteoporosis**, that can totally cripple a person in later life.

Many people, even as young as 20, are gradually losing calcium, but the body sends no detectable signals saying that the bones are growing weak. The deficiency becomes apparent only when an older person breaks a hip or pelvic bone or suffers collapse of a spinal vertebra. It strikes at least one out of every three people over age 65.

Adult bone loss is eight times more prevalent in women than in men after age 50, for several reasons. Women generally have less bone mass to begin

A **megadose** is a dose ten times or more higher than the amount normally recommended (see RDA, Appendix B). An **overdose** is an amount high enough to cause toxicity symptoms. Megadoses taken long enough are usually overdoses.

The three major contributors to osteoporosis:
Lack of calcium in the younger years.
Lack of exercise.
Diminished hormone (estrogen) secretion after menopause in women.

with because of their smaller size; they more often use weight-reducing diets low in calcium; and they are less active, on the average, than men. Pregnancy and lactation tap the calcium reserves in bones whenever calcium intake is inadequate. Bone loss begins earlier in women owing to their different hormonal endowment, and the loss is accelerated at menopause; and finally, women live longer than men.

Figure 4–2 shows the effect of the loss of spinal bone on a woman's height and posture. It is not inevitable that people "grow shorter" as they age, but it does happen if they experience bone loss. Recommended for prevention are regular exercise, adequate calcium intakes throughout life, adequate fluoride and vitamin D intakes, abstinence from alcohol and other drugs, moderation in caffeine use, minimal prescription drug use, control of stress, and finally, estrogen replacement after menopause.

For most people, the obvious way to meet calcium needs is to include milk and milk products in the diet daily, because they are almost the only foods that contain significant quantities. Table 4–4 shows the amounts of milk recommended for children and adults. People who cannot tolerate fresh milk can use cheese or fermented dairy products as substitutes for fluid milk, but they need to use large quantities to obtain enough calcium. Calcium supplements may be of some value.

Another important mineral is iron. Iron is one of the **trace minerals**, so called because only tiny amounts are needed in the diet. Iron is the body's oxygen carrier, the protein **hemoglobin**. Bound into hemoglobin in the red

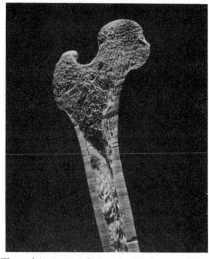

The calcium crystals inside this human hip bone give it its strength.

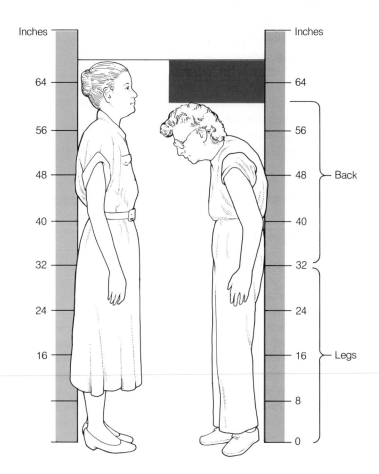

FIGURE 4–2   The Effect of Adult Bone Loss on the Height of an Older Woman

On the left is a woman at menopause (age 50); on the right *the same woman* 30 years later. Notice that collapse of her vertebrae has shortened her back; the length of her legs has not changed.

CHAPTER 4 ■ NUTRITION

TABLE 4–4   Recommended Fluid
             Milk Intakes

Children under 9	2 to 3 cups
Children 9 to 12	3+ cups
Teenagers	4+ cups
Adults	2 cups
Pregnant women	3+ cups
Lactating women	4+ cups
Older women	3 to 5 cups

Fluid replacement for sweat losses in heavy exercise or work is discussed in Chapter 6.

Excess sodium, or table **salt** can contribute to high blood pressure (**hypertension**) in those who are genetically susceptible. For more information, see Chapter 16.

blood cells, it enables them to ferry oxygen from lungs to tissues and so permit the release of energy from fuels to do the cells' work. Iron-deficiency anemia is characterized by weakness, tiredness, apathy, headaches, and a paleness that reflects a reduction in number and size of red blood cells. (In dark-skinned people this can be seen in the pink tissue, such as the corner of the eye.) A person with this anemia can do very little muscular work without disabling fatigue but will feel more energetic after a few weeks of eating the needed iron-rich foods.

Women often may be told that their blood iron level is normal, and yet they may need more iron because their body stores may be depleted. This condition is not detected by standard tests. Because most women are less active than men and therefore can eat less food, their iron intakes are lower. And because women menstruate, their iron losses are greater. These two factors predispose women to iron deficiencies.

Iron deficiency occurs in as many as half of all persons in some settings, even in developed countries—most predictably in inner-city and rural poor. People begin to lose energy long before iron deficiency is diagnosed. They have no obvious disease, they appear unmotivated and apathetic, they work and play less, and they are less physically fit. Incidence rates for iron deficiency anemia in developed countries range from 10 to 20 percent; rates are higher in the developing countries, and therefore the incidence of iron deficiency not severe enough to cause anemia must be higher still.[8] If this one worldwide malnutrition problem could be alleviated, millions of people's lives would brighten.

The cause of iron deficiency is usually poor nutrition—that is, inadequate intake, either from sheer lack of food or from high consumption of empty-calorie foods. Among non-nutritional causes, blood loss is the primary one, caused by infection. Meats, fish, poultry, and legumes are iron-rich, and an easy way to obtain the needed iron is to eat them regularly. But foods that are rich in iron are poor in calcium and vice versa. Thus it is important to use enough, but not too much, of each.

Some minerals serve as **electrolytes**, dissolved substances in blood and body fluid that carry electric charges. Electrolytes provide the environment in which the cells' work takes place—work such as nerve-to-nerve communication, heartbeats, contraction of muscles, and so forth. When people lose fluid—whether it be sweat, blood, or urine—they also lose electrolytes. When too-large amounts of body fluid are lost, as in heat stroke, infant diarrhea, or injury, their replacement is a task for a medical team.

▆ PERSONAL NUTRITION STRATEGY

About 40 vitamins and minerals are needed altogether. How can you meet your needs for all of these nutrients?

Each nutrient has its own unique pattern of distribution in foods. To get enough of every one of them from food is a balancing act that requires extensive practice. (People who manage this balancing act without conscious thought learned their eating habits from parents or grandparents who were taught with care how to do it.) Many people, whether they know it or not, use the Four Food Group Plan for planning adequate, balanced diets.

Table 4–5 shows the Four Food Group Plan. The number of servings recommended daily from each group (milk/milk products, meats/meat alternates, vegetables/fruits, and breads/cereals) for an adult is two, two, four,

TABLE 4–5 The Four Food Group Plan

Milk/Milk Products (2 servings a day for adults[a])

Major source of: Calcium, riboflavin, protein, vitamin B_{12}, magnesium

Sample serving sizes:

A. Nonfat or lowfat milk, buttermilk, plain yogurt
B. Whole milk, cheese, flavored yogurt, cottage cheese
C. Custard, milk shake, pudding, ice cream

Milk, pudding, yogurt—1 c
Cottage cheese—1 ½ c
Ice cream—2 c
Cheese—1 to 2 oz

Meat/Meat Alternates (2 servings a day)

Major source of: Protein, iron, niacin, thiamin, vitamins B_6 and B_{12}, folacin, magnesium, zinc

Sample serving sizes:

A. Poultry, fish, lean meat dried beans or peas, eggs
B. Beef, lamb, pork, lunch meat, refried beans
C. Hot dogs, peanut butter, nuts

Cooked meat, fish or poultry—2 to 3 oz
Tuna fish—¼ c
Peanut butter—4 tbsp
Beans or peas—1 c
Nuts—½ c

Vegetables/Fruits (4 servings a day[b])

Major source of: Vitamins A and C, folacin, fiber

Sample serving sizes:

A. Broccoli, cabbage, carrots, cauliflower, cucumber, grapefruit, green beans or peas, leafy greens, lettuce, melons, mushrooms, oranges, orange juice, tomatoes
B. Apples, bananas, canned fruit, corn, pears, potatoes
C. Avocados, dried fruit, sweet potatoes

Fruit, vegetable, or juice—½ c
Whole fruit (apple, banana)—1 fruit

Breads/Cereals (4 servings a day[c])

Major source of: Thiamin, iron, niacin, zinc, fiber

Sample serving sizes:

A. Whole-grain and enriched breads, rolls, tortillas
B. Rice, cereals, pastas (macaroni, spaghetti), bagels
C. Pancakes, muffins, cornbread, biscuits, sweetened cereal

Bread—1 slice
Cooked cereal—½ c
Cold cereal—1 c or 1 oz
Bun or bagel—½
Rice, grits, or pasta—½ c

Extra Foods (Extra Foods tend to be high in sugar, fat, salt, or alcohol and, in most cases, calories. Use only as calories permit after all servings of nutritious foods have been selected.)

Sugar	Fat	Salt (sodium)	Alcohol	Other
Cake, pie, cookies, doughnuts, sweet rolls, candy	Margarine, salad dressing, oils, mayonnaise	Potato chips, corn chips, pretzels	Wine	Spices, herbs
Soft drinks, fruit drinks	Cream, cream cheese, butter	Pickles, olives, bouillon	Beer	Coffee, tea
Jelly, syrup, gelatin desserts	Gravy, sauces	Mustard, soy sauce, steak sauce	Liquor	Diet soft drinks
Sugar, honey		Salt, seasoned salt		

NOTE: Foods labeled *A* are highest in nutrients for the calories, and generally cost the least. Foods labeled *B* are intermediate. Foods labeled *C* are highest in calories, and generally cost the most.
[a]For a pregnant or nursing woman, 3 servings; for a pregnant or nursing teen, 4 servings.
[b]One should be rich in vitamin C; at least one every other day should be rich in vitamin A.
[c]Enriched or whole-grain products only.
SOURCE: Dairy Council of California, 1983.

LIFE CHOICE INVENTORY

How well do you support your nutritional health?

This nutrition assessment questionnaire enables you to evaluate your own eating habits. The more points you get, the better your nutritional health is likely to be.

Part 1—Milk/Milk Products

1. I have two or more cups of milk or the equivalent in milk products every day.   Yes/No
2. I drink low-fat (2 percent or less butter-fat) or nonfat milk rather than whole milk.   Yes/No
3. I eat ice cream or ice milk twice a week at the most.   Yes/No
4. I seldom have more than about three teaspoons of margarine or butter per day.   Yes/No

Total yes answers   _____

Part 2—Meats/Meat Alternates

5. I usually limit my meat, fish, poultry, or egg servings to one or two a day.   Yes/No
6. I eat red meats (beef, ham, lamb, or pork) not more than about three times a week.   Yes/No
7. I remove fat or ask that fat be trimmed from meat before cooking.   Yes/No
8. I eat about three or four eggs per week, including those cooked with other foods.   Yes/No
9. I sometimes have meatless days and eat such protein-rich foods as legumes and nuts.   Yes/No
10. I usually broil, boil, bake, or roast meat, fish, or poultry; I usually don't fry it.   Yes/No

Total yes answers   _____

Part 3—Vegetables/Fruits

11. I usually have one serving (1/2 cup) of citrus fruit or juice (oranges, grapefruit, etc.) each day.   Yes/No
12. I have at least one serving of dark green or deep orange vegetables each day   Yes/No
13. I eat fresh fruits and vegetables when I can get them.   Yes/No
14. I cook vegetables without fat (if I use margarine, I add it after cooking).   Yes/No
15. I eat fresh fruit at the end of a meal more often than desserts.   Yes/No

Total yes answers   _____

Part 4—Breads/Cereals

16. I generally eat whole-grain breads and cereals.   Yes/No
17. Most of the breads and cereals I use are high in fiber.   Yes/No
18. The breads and cereals I use have little or no sugar added.   Yes/No
19. I generally use brown rice in preference to white rice.   Yes/No
20. I generally have at least four servings of bread or cereal grains each day.   Yes/No

Total yes answers   _____

Part 5—Extra Foods and Calories

21. I am usually within 5 to 10 pounds of the weight considered appropriate for my height.   Yes/No
22. I drink no more than two drinks of alcoholic beverages a day (see Chapter 8 for the definition of "a drink").   Yes/No
23. I do not add salt to food after preparation and generally use foods salted lightly or not salted at all.   Yes/No
24. I try to avoid foods high in sugar and use sugar sparingly.   Yes/No
25. I usually eat a breakfast of at least cereal and milk, egg and toast, or other protein-carbohydrate combination with fruit or fruit juice.   Yes/No

Total yes answers   _____

For each yes answer, give yourself one point. Place points earned in the appropriate box.

Your Nutrition Rating

	Excellent	Good	Fair	Poor	Your Score
Part 1	4	3	2	1	_____
Part 2	5 to 6	4	3	2	_____
Part 3	5	4	3	2	_____
Part 4	5	4	3	2	_____
Part 5	5	4	3	2	_____

Total Points Earned

Excellent	24 to 25
Good	19 to 23
Fair	14 to 18
Poor	9 to 13

Is your diet excellent, good, fair, or poor?

SOURCE: Adapted with permission from Roger Sargent, *Have a Good Life* series (Greenville, S.C.: Liberty Life).

✹ STRATEGIES: How to Select Nutritious Foods

To help you choose nutritious foods:

1. Given the choice between whole foods and refined, processed foods, choose the former (apples rather than apple pie; potatoes rather than potato chips). Fewer nutrients have been refined out of the whole foods; less fat, salt, and sugar have been added.

2. When choosing meats, choose the lean ones. Select fish or poultry often, beef seldom. Ask for broiled, not fried, to control your fat intake.

3. Use both raw and cooked vegetables and fruits. Raw foods offer more fiber and vitamins such as folacin and thiamin that are destroyed by cooking. Cooking foods frees other vitamins and minerals for absorption.

4. Include milk or milk products daily—2 cups or more—for the calcium you need. Use low-fat or nonfat items to reduce fat and calories.

5. Learn to use margarine, butter, and oils sparingly; only a little gives flavor; a lot overloads you with fat and calories.

6. Vary your choices. Eat broccoli today, carrots tomorrow, and corn the next day. Eat Chinese today, Italian tomorrow, and hot dogs and beans on Saturday.

7. Load your plate with vegetables and unrefined starchy foods. A small portion of meat or cheese is all you need for protein.

8. When choosing breads and cereals, choose the whole-grain varieties.

To select nutritious fast foods:

9. Choose the broiled hamburger with lettuce, tomatoes, and other goodies—and hold the mayo—rather than the fish or chicken patties coated with breadcrumbs and cooked in fat.

10. Select the salad bar—and use more plain raw vegetables than those mixed with oily or mayonnaise-based dressings.

11. Order chili with more beans than meat.

12. Drink milk rather than a cola beverage.

When eating out of a vending machine:

13. Choose cracker sandwiches over chips and pork rinds (virtually pure fat), and choose peanuts, pretzels, and popcorn over cookies and candy.

14. Choose milk and juices over cola beverages, or choose diet beverages over sugary ones to avoid empty calories.

and four from the food groups, respectively. The table shows some of the major nutrients each food group supplies and examples of foods in each group. This helps the planner design an adequate and balanced diet.

The plan also helps with calorie control, economy, and moderation. The foods labeled *A* are lowest in calories within the group; those labeled *B* are intermediate; and those labeled *C* are highest in calories. The foods labeled *A* are also lowest in cost per unit of nutrients, generally, and those labeled *C* are most expensive. Those labeled *C* are also highest in fat and sugar.

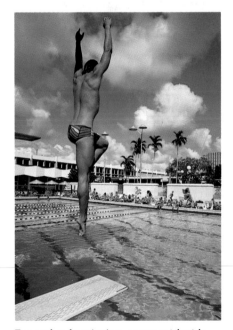

For perfect functioning, every nutrient is needed.

81

Diet planning principles:
  Adequacy—enough of each type of food.
  Balance—not too much of any type of food.
  Calorie control—not too many calories.
  Economy—not too expensive.
  Moderation—not too much fat or sugar.
  Variety—as many different foods as possible.

The Four Food Group Plan is flexible. For example, it permits you to substitute cheese for milk, because both supply the same nutrients in about the same amounts. You can choose legumes and nuts as alternatives for meats. You can also adapt the plan to casseroles and other mixed dishes and to different national and cultural cuisines. A study of the plan should provide the information you need to obtain a virtual guarantee of diet adequacy.

This chapter's Life Choice Inventory can help you determine your diet adequacy and the Strategies box can help you choose nutritious foods. No doubt you can create other ideas from the facts presented in this chapter. Apply them. And keep on learning about nutrition; it is worth a lot to your health.

STUDY AIDS

1. Describe what is meant by a *balanced meal*.
2. Explain why regular, balanced meals are important to a person's feeling of well-being throughout the day.
3. Explain why, although starch and sugar are both carbohydrates, starchy foods confer greater benefits on the body.
4. Describe what happens to the body's lean protein tissue when a person does not consume enough carbohydrate to meet the brain's and nervous system's energy needs.
5. Identify some symptoms of a vitamin or mineral deficiency.

GLOSSARY

amino acid: a building block from which proteins are made.

anemia: reduced size or number or altered shape of the red blood cells, a symptom of any of a number of different disease conditions, including several nutrient deficiencies.

appetite: the desire to eat, which normally accompanies hunger.

balanced meal: a meal containing sufficient but not excessive amounts of foods from each food group and therefore sufficient but not excessive carbohydrate, fat, protein, vitamins, and minerals.

calorie: a unit used to measure energy, determined by the heat the food releases when burned. Calories reflect the extent to which a food's energy can be stored in body fat.

  calor = heat

carbohydrate: one of a class of nutrients, most of which yield energy the human body can use. The *complex carbohydrates* include starch (energy yielding) and some fibers (primarily not energy yielding); the *simple carbohydrates* are the sugars.

cholesterol: a type of fat both made by the body and found in food; it is essential to health, but also forms the deposits that accumulate along arteries in heart and artery disease.

complex carbohydrate: see *carbohydrate*.

electrolyte: a mineral that carries an electric charge when dissolved in fluid.

empty calories: energy without nutrients, as in pure fat, an empty-calorie food.

energy: the capacity to do work, such as moving things or heating things.

enzyme: one of the working parts of a cell, a protein that performs a specific chemical step in building up or breaking down cellular materials.

fat (technically, *lipid*): a class of energy-yielding nutrients that includes triglycerides, cholesterol, and other compounds.

fatty acid: a simple form of fat that supplies fuel for most of the body's cells.

fiber: indigestible carbohydrates and other compounds in food that provide bulk in the digestive tract.

glucose: a simple carbohydrate, the principal sugar found in the blood, which supplies fuel for the brain's activities.

glycogen (GLIGH-coh-gen): the form in which the body stores glucose.

hemoglobin: a protein in the red blood cells, the body's oxygen carrier.

  hemo = blood

  globin = spherical protein

hunger: the physiological need for food.

hypertension: high blood pressure (Chapter 16 provides details).

lipid: see *fat*.

malnutrition: underconsumption, overconsumption, or unbalanced consumption of food energy or nutrients severe enough to cause disease or susceptibility to disease.

megadoses: doses of a nutrient that exceed the body's requirements by ten times or more—sometimes by up to 100 times. Megadoses are usually *overdoses*—that is, they cause symptoms of toxicity.

minerals: essential inorganic nutrients.

nutrient: a substance found in foods that the body requires for the maintenance of health and the growth and repair of tissues. The *essential nutrients* are not made in the body and must be obtained from food.

osteoporosis: adult bone loss, a crippling disease of later life caused partly by calcium deficiency.

  osteo = bone

  por = porous

overdoses: see *megadoses*.

overnutrition: overconsumption of food energy or nutrients sufficient to cause disease or susceptibility to disease, a form of malnutrition.

protein: a substance composed of amino acids that serves as structural components of cells, enzymes, and other cellular machinery or that can be broken down for energy.

protein-energy malnutrition (PEM): malnutrition involving protein deficiency (kwashiorkor), energy deficiency (marasmus), or both.

roughage (RUFF-idge): see *fiber*.

salt: a compound that, in water, dissociates into electrolytes.

simple carbohydrate: see *carbohydrate*.

starch: a complex carbohydrate, the predominant energy source for human beings.

sugar: simple carbohydrate. Examples are glucose, lactose, fructose, and sucrose.

trace minerals: minerals essential in nutrition, needed in small quantities (traces) daily. Iron and zinc are examples.

triglyceride (try-GLISS-uh-ride): the principal form of fat in foods and in the body.

undernutrition: underconsumption of food energy or nutrients severe enough to cause disease or increased susceptibility to disease, a form of malnutrition.

vegetarian: a person who omits meat, fish, and poultry from the diet. A *lacto-ovo vegetarian* uses milk and milk products and eggs as well as plant foods; a *strict vegetarian* uses only plant foods.

    lacto = milk

    ovo = egg

vitamins: essential organic nutrients.

water: an inorganic compound, necessary for life; it provides the medium for, participates in, and results as a waste product from, life processes.

QUIZ ANSWERS

1. *True.* Malnutrition occurs in people in the United States and Canada.

2. *True.* It is possible to have an appetite without being hungry.

3. *False.* Too much or too little of a nutrient is equally harmful.

4. *True.* Carbohydrate should contribute more than half of all the calories a person consumes in a day.

5. *True.* Honey and sugar are the same, as far as the body is concerned.

6. *False.* Of all dietary factors related to disease, fat is probably the most significant.

7. *True.* Low-carbohydrate diets cause the body to lose muscle tissue.

8. *True.* Adults need milk, just as children do.

9. *True.* In large amounts, all vitamins can be harmful.

10. *True.* Fast foods can be nutritious.

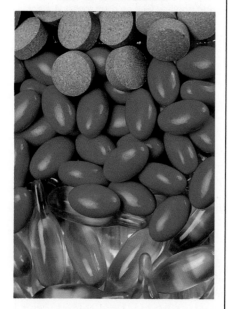

Vitamin Supplements

Billions of dollars are spent on vitamin pills in the United States each year. Two-thirds of our citizens use them. You may be one of these users. Perhaps, after studying nutrition, you are wondering if you should be. This discussion is intended to help you make that decision.

A lot of people have the impression that they can't get the nutrients they need from food alone.

People who haven't learned enough about nutrition think they need supplements as insurance against their own poor food choices. Indeed, their food choices may be poor, but taking supplements is no guarantee that they will get the particular nutrients they need. It's just as likely that they'll get a duplication of the nutrients their food is supplying and still lack the ones they need. The only way to be sure to get the needed assortment of nutrients is to construct a balanced diet from a variety of foods.

Are you saying that no supplement supplies all the nutrients you can get from food?

Yes, that's right. There is no way you can package in a pill the bulk nutrients you need—protein, fiber, carbohydrate, calcium, and others—because you need such large amounts that you couldn't swallow them in pill form. No one supplement can match a balanced diet, and no combination of supplements can, either. No one knows enough, yet, to construct a synthetic substitute for food. Even in the hospital, where the most advanced technology provides "complete" synthetic formulas for clients for months, the most these formulas can do is to enable clients to survive. They won't thrive until they are back on food.[1]*

Nutrient supplements are useful at times. A person may need a specific

*Reference notes are in Appendix D.

nutrient to counteract a specific deficiency—iron for iron-deficiency anemia, for example. But it takes medical training and tests to make a correct diagnosis; people can't diagnose themselves, and they would be foolish to try.

Do people ever have unusually high nutrient needs that justify their taking supplements?

No two people have exactly the same nutrient needs, but people's requirements differ, at the most, only twofold or threefold. An ordinary diet of mixed foods can easily meet the highest of those needs. And the argument still holds that you can't tell just by guessing which nutrients you need more of. One shouldn't self-prescribe nutrients based on speculations about having unusually high nutrient needs.

In rare instances, genetic defects may alter nutrient needs considerably, but only one person in 10,000 has such a defect. That person needs a diagnosis and treatment by a qualified health care provider.

What about high nutrient needs induced by different lifestyles? I've seen vitamins advertised for people under stress, alcohol users, cigarette smokers, athletes—things like that.

Yes, the purveyors of supplements like to make the claim that ordinary people need their products—of course, because they can sell more products that way. The claim works; lots of people buy nutrient supplements because they identify with the ads. Stresses, including smoking and moderate alcohol use, do deplete people's nutrient stores somewhat, but the composition of the supplements for those people is just guesswork on the part of the manufacturer. The way to counteract nutrient losses is still to eat well, not to take supplements.

People who drink to excess have major nutrition problems and need to stop drinking, of course, not to take supplements. As for athletes, they need supplements *less* than other people, because they are able to eat more food. Later chapters offer more nutrition information for these people.

Are there any times when I should be taking a vitamin pill?

Yes, when a health care provider recommends it, and yes, in at least two other instances:

- When your energy intake is below about 1,500 calories, so that you can't eat enough food to meet your vitamin needs. (People who can't exercise have this problem.)
- When you know that, for whatever reason, you are going to be eating irregularly for a limited time.

Remember that if vitamins are needed, minerals are needed, too, and a vitamin pill is not enough. A vitamin-mineral supplement is called for.

When I do need a vitamin-mineral supplement, what kind should I take? I've heard the organic, natural ones are preferable to the synthetic ones.

Organic and *natural* are terms that have no meaning in relation to the contents of vitamin-mineral supplements. All vitamins are organic, no matter where they come from. *Natural* has no legal meaning at all. These terms mean only that the product will be expensive. Don't let them fool you. Read the ingredient lists, and buy the product that contains the nutrients you are looking for, at the lowest price.

Whenever a health care provider recommends a supplement, carefully follow directions as to the type and dose to take. When you are selecting one yourself, a single, balanced vitamin-mineral supplement should suffice. Look for one in which the nutrient levels are at or slightly be-low the RDA. (The RDA, or Recommended Dietary Allowances, are shown in Appendix B.) Avoid preparations that exceed the RDA. Remember, you will still be getting some nutrients from foods.

What about taking supplements as a preventive measure? I've heard that certain vitamins prevent cancer.

Good nutrition certainly helps protect you. Diets that are *deficient* in nutrients render you defenseless against cancer and many other ills. But to say that a pill containing certain specific nutrients will protect you is to drastically oversimplify the case. You need foods, with all the multitude of nutrients and related compounds they contain, if you really want protection.

Suppose I just want to take a vitamin-mineral supplement as insurance against slight deficiencies. There's no harm in that, is there?

Perhaps not—if you keep the dose low. But it is a myth that the vitamins are nontoxic. All of them, not only the well-known vitamins A and D, but also the B vitamins and vitamin C, have been shown to have toxic effects, at least in some people, when taken in large doses.[2] Takers of self-prescribed pills need a warning about the risks of overdosing with vitamins, and they need a more urgent warning about minerals. Excess minerals can be toxic—often in quantities not far above normal intakes.

A good friend of mine routinely takes a pile of nutrient supplements. I am worried that some of her practices are dangerous. What should I tell her?

What supplements does she take?

Before breakfast, she takes 500 milligrams of vitamin C, 1,000 units of vitamin E, several tablespoons of nutritional yeast, some kelp tablets, a capsule of vitamins A and D, a spirulina tablet, some green pills, and other pills containing trace minerals. Then she sprinkles desiccated liver, powdered bone, bone meal, and wheat germ on her granola, and pours on some reconstituted powdered nonfat milk. Then for lunch . . .

Never mind what she takes for lunch. You have good reason to worry about her using such a huge stockpile of nutrient preparations. The potent supplements of vitamins A and D and the minerals are dangerous. Not all her choices are dangerous, though. The wheat germ and powdered skim milk are nutritious and reasonable in cost. The other choices have drawbacks. Powdered bone and bone meal may contain the toxic mineral lead and kelp has been found to contain arsenic, a poison and possible cancer-causing agent. As for dessicated liver and green pills, the foods that these pills imitate are more nutritious and economical. One green pill contains the nutrients in one small forkful of fresh vegetables—minus the losses incurred in processing, and sixty pills costing over $15 deliver vegetable matter worth about $1.50.

Your best bet in advising your friend (if she wants your advice) is to suggest she consult a qualified professional such as a registered dietitian (R.D.) for nutrition advice. Congratulate her, because she cares about her health. Reinforce her use of the nutrient-dense foods, the nonfat milk and wheat germ. Then single out for attention her most dangerous practices, the overdoses of toxic vitamins and minerals. As for the others, keep your own counsel about them unless you are asked. That way you probably won't lose a friend, and you may provide a substantial boost to exactly what she treasures most— her good health.

Weight Control

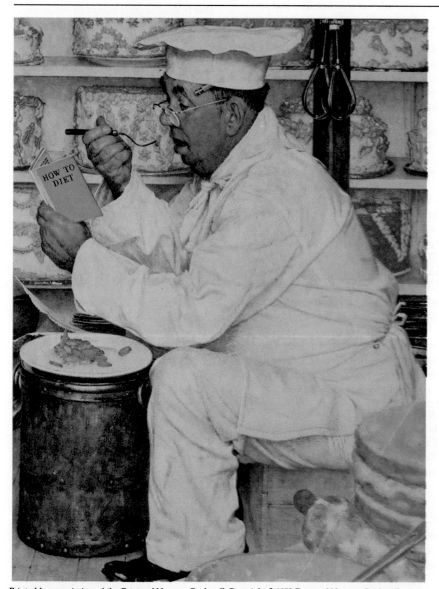

Printed by permission of the Estate of Norman Rockwell Copyright © 1953 Estate of Norman Rockwell.

FOR OPENERS . . .

True or false? If false, say what is true.

1. Being underweight presents a risk to health.

2. Excess fat around the abdomen presents a greater risk to health than excess fat elsewhere on the body.

3. The dieter who sees a large weight loss on the scale can take this as a sign of success.

4. An advertisement broadcast on nationwide television is likely to present the truth.

5. To succeed in losing weight, you have to stop eating carbohydrate.

6. The way to lose body fat most rapidly is to stop eating altogether.

7. The healthiest state for a person's body is to have less than 10 percent of the body weight as fat.

8. If an inactive person takes up a daily hour of exercise, the person will end up spending more calories all day, even during sleep.

9. You can eat any food on a weight-loss diet, as long as you don't eat too much of it.

10. It is harder to lose a pound than to gain one.

(Answers on page 101.)

Are you pleased with your body weight? If you answered yes, you are a rare individual. Nearly all people in our society think they should weigh more or less (mostly less) than they do. Usually, their primary reason is that they want to look acceptable by society's standards, but they often perceive, correctly, that weight is also somehow related to physical health.

People also think they should control their weight. A pair of misconceptions makes their task difficult. The first is to focus on *weight*; the second is to focus on *controlling* weight. To put it simply, it isn't your weight you need to control; it's the amount of fat in your body in proportion to the lean. And it isn't possible to control either one, directly; it is possible only to control your *behavior*.

THE PROBLEMS OF DEFICIENT AND EXCESSIVE BODY FATNESS

Both deficient and excessive body fat carry health risks. It has long been known that thin people will die first during a siege, in a famine, or in a concentration camp. A fact not always recognized, even by health care providers, is that overly thin people are also at a disadvantage in the hospital, where they may have to go for days without food so that they can undergo tests or surgery. Women need a certain minimum amount of body fat to menstruate normally; if they become underweight, their cycles are disrupted. Underweight also increases the risk for any person fighting a wasting disease. In fact, people with cancer die as often from starvation as from the cancer itself. Thus underweight people are urged to learn how to nourish themselves optimally—to gain body fat as an energy reserve and to acquire protective amounts of all the nutrients that can be stored.

As for overfatness: for one thing, it makes hypertension worse. Often weight loss alone can normalize the blood pressure of an overfat person. Some people with hypertension can tell you exactly at what weight their blood pressure begins to rise. Weight gain can also precipitate diabetes in genetically susceptible people. If hypertension or diabetes runs in your family, you urgently need a sensible program to keep from getting too fat.

Excess body fatness also increases the risk of heart disease. Excess fat pads crowd the heart muscle within the body cavity, and excess fat demands to be fed by miles of extra capillaries, increasing the heart's work load to the point of damaging it. Other conditions brought on or made worse by overfatness include abdominal hernias, breast cancer, varicose veins, gout, gallbladder disease, arthritis, respiratory problems, complications in pregnancy, and even a high accident rate. The health risks of overfatness are so many that it has been declared a disease: **obesity**. If you are obese, you are urged to reduce. You can expect your health risks to diminish as you do.[1]*

Some obese people can escape these health problems, but no one who is fat in our society quite escapes the social and economic handicaps. Fat people are less sought after for romance, they pay higher insurance premiums, they pay more for clothes, and they suffer job discrimination. Psychologically, too, a body size that embarrasses a person diminishes self-esteem. How thin, then, is too thin—and how fat is too fat? The next section attempts to draw the lines.

*Reference notes are in Appendix D.

fatfold test: a clinical test of body fatness in which the thickness of a fold of skin on the back of the arm (triceps), below the shoulder blade (subscapular), or in other places is measured with an instrument called a caliper. The older, less preferred, term for this is **skinfold test**.

Quick Ways to Access Body Fatness

These ways to answer the question "What is an appropriate weight for you?" are just for fun:

■ A crude measure of body fatness is the **pinch test** (this is a fatfold measure without the equipment to make it accurate). Pick up the skin and fat at the back of either arm with the thumb and forefinger of the other hand. Keep your fingers still, so as not to lose the "measurement" when you pull them away from your arm. Measure the thickness on a ruler. A fatfold over an inch thick reflects obesity.

■ Another shortcut method is to measure your waist compared with your chest (not bust). Every inch by which your waist measurement exceeds your chest measurement is said to take two years off your life.

■ Another crude measure: lie down, relax, and place a ruler across your abdomen from one hipbone to the other. If it doesn't easily touch both bones while you're relaxing, you're too fat.

DEFINITION OF APPROPRIATE WEIGHT

It is true that to have either too little or too much body *fat* presents a health risk. Body *weight* roughly corresponds to body fatness, so weight on the scale is used as an indicator of body fatness. A more accurate indicator would be a direct measure of body fatness, but this is hard to obtain.

The traditional way of assigning desirable weights to people is to use one of the insurance-company tables of weights for height, which used to be called the "ideal weight tables" (see inside back cover). You find your height in the table; decide whether you have a small, medium, or large frame (see Frame Size Table on inside back cover); and then find your weight range. That weight range is consistent with good health for most people, and you can narrow it down further, based on your own personal preferences. Traditionally, a weight 20 percent or more above the table weight defines obesity—that is, too much body fat for health; a weight 10 percent or more below the table weight defines **underweight** (too little body fat).

The use of body weight as an indicator of overfatness is unsatisfactory for some purposes. For one thing, weight and fatness do not always coincide: a healthy person with dense bones and muscles may seem overweight on the scale, while a person whose scale weight seems reasonable may have too much body fat for health. For another thing, frame size measures are not valid, and it is frustrating to have to use them.[2]

Health care professionals would prefer to have some direct measure of body fatness, but it is hard to measure. Most resort to the use of a fatfold caliper—a pinching device that measures the thickness of a fold of fat on the back of the arm, below the shoulder blade, on the side of the waist, or elsewhere. About 50 percent of the body's fat lies beneath the skin, and its thickness reflects total body fat. However, not everyone's body fat is distributed in the same way, and to complicate matters still further, the distribution itself turns out to have health implications. Excess fat around the abdomen represents a greater risk to health than excess fat elsewhere on the body; it correlates with an increased incidence of diabetes and heart disease.[3] The methods in the margin provide approximate measurements.

In any case, most people have access only to height measures and scale weights, and have to make do with them. Since the definition of appropriate weight is only approximate anyway, the scales are fine for most purposes. This chapter's Life Choice Inventory guides you to a tentative answer to the question, "What should I weigh?"

ENERGY BALANCE

Suppose you decide that you are too fat or too thin. How did you get that way? By having an unbalanced energy budget—that is, by eating either more or less food energy than you spent. In other words, your body fat is similar to a savings account, the only difference from money being that more is not better; there is an optimum. A day's energy balance can be stated like this:

Change in fat stores (calories) = Food energy taken in (calories) − Energy spent on metabolic and other activities (calories).

More simply:

Change in fat stores (calories) = Energy in (calories) − Energy out (calories).

LIFE CHOICE INVENTORY

How much should you weigh? When physical health alone is considered, a wide range of weights is acceptable for a person of a given height. Within the safe range, the definition of appropriate weight is up to the individual, depending on factors such as family history, occupation, physical and recreational activities, and personal preferences.

1. Determine the safe range for a person of your height and sex:

   ■ Record your height: _____ feet, _____ inches. Note that the Height-Weight Table (see inside back cover) assumes you measured your height in shoes with 1-inch heels. If you measured your barefoot height, add an inch; if you wore shoes with heels higher or lower than an inch, adjust accordingly.
   ■ Determine your frame size, using Frame Size Table (see inside back cover). Record whether you have a small, medium, or large frame: _____ frame.
   ■ Look up the appropriate weight for a person your height, sex, and frame size in the Height-Weight Table. Record the entire range: _____ to _____ pounds.
   EXAMPLE: For a man 5 feet 7 inches tall (in shoes) with a small frame, the range of weights is 138 to 145 pounds.
   ■ Determine the bottom end of the safe range. A person who is more than 10 percent below the lowest indicated weight for height is considered underweight to a degree that might compromise health. Take 10 percent off the bottom end of your range: _____ pounds.
   EXAMPLE: Ten percent of 138 pounds is 13.8 pounds (rounded off to 14 pounds). Bottom end of range is 138 minus 14, or 124 pounds.
   ■ Determine the top end of the safe range. A person who is more than 20 percent above the highest indicated weight for height is considered obese. Add 20 percent to the top end of your range: _____ pounds.
   EXAMPLE: Twenty percent of 145 pounds is 29 pounds. Top end of range is 145 plus 29, or 174 pounds.

   ■ Record your safe range here: _____ to _____ pounds.
   EXAMPLE: 124 to 174 pounds.

   If your weight is below the bottom end of this safe range, you need to gain weight; if above the top end, you need to lose weight for your health's sake.

2. Check your health history for further confirmation. A family or personal medical history of diabetes (non-insulin-dependent type), hypertension, or high blood cholesterol indicates the need for weight loss.

3. Choose a goal weight within the safe range. Answering the following questions should help you to determine where, within the safe range, your personal appropriate weight may be:

   ■ Does your occupation demand that you have a certain body shape? Record the weight, within the safe range, that would most nearly approximate this body shape: _____ pounds.
   ■ Do you engage in a sport or other physical activity that requires a particular body weight for optimal performance? Consult your instructor or other expert in that sport or activity, and record the weight recommended on that basis: _____ pounds.
   ■ Do you hope to start a pregnancy soon? If so, consult your health care provider as to the ideal weight with which to begin a pregnancy: _____ pounds.
   ■ Undress and stand before a mirror. Do you think you need to gain or lose weight? Add or subtract pounds from your current weight to arrive at a personal goal weight (but be sure to stay within the safe range): _____ pounds.

Now choose a goal weight, giving consideration to each of the weights you just listed above. No formula exists for this estimate: you decide, but don't choose a weight outside the safe range.

YOUR GOAL WEIGHT: _____ POUNDS

Rule-of-Thumb Method of Estimating "Ideal" Weight

To estimate a female's ideal weight by a quick method, give the height of 5 feet (barefooted) an ideal weight of 100 pounds. For every inch above 5 feet, add 5 pounds. Thus a woman who is 5 feet 4 inches tall would add 20 pounds (4 inches times 5 pounds per inch) to 100 pounds, making her ideal weight 120 pounds.

For a male, start with 110 pounds at 5 feet, and add 5 pounds per inch above 5 feet. Thus a 6-foot man would have an ideal weight of 170 pounds: 110 + (12 multiplied by 5).

You know about the "energy in" side of this equation. An apple brings you 100 calories; a candy bar, 425 calories. (Calorie amounts for several hundred foods are listed in Appendix E.) You probably also know that for each 3,500 calories you eat in excess of expenditures, you store one pound of body fat.*

As for the "energy out" side, the body spends energy in two major ways: to fuel its **basal metabolism** and to fuel its voluntary activities. You can change both of these to spend more or less energy in a day.

The basal metabolism supports the work that goes on all the time, without conscious awareness. The beating of the heart, the inhaling and exhaling of air, the maintenance of body temperature, and the sending of nerve and hormonal messages to direct these activities are the basal processes that maintain life. Basal metabolic needs are surprisingly large. A person whose total energy needs are 2,000 calories a day spends 1,200 to 1,400 of them to support basal metabolism.

The number of calories spent on voluntary activities depends on three factors. The larger the muscle mass required, the heavier the weight of the body part being moved, and the longer the activity takes, the more calories are spent.

A typical breakdown of the total energy spent by a moderately active person (for example, a student who walks from class to class) might look like this:

a. Energy for basal metabolism: 1,400 calories
b. Energy for voluntary activities: <u>500 calories</u>
          Total energy needs: 1,900 calories

The first is the larger component, and you can't change it much, today. You can, however, change the second component—voluntary activities—and so spend more calories today. If you want to increase your basal metabolic output, make exercise a daily habit. Your body composition will change, and your basal energy output will pick up the pace as well.* The end of this chapter shows how to alter both—with diet and exercise—to regulate body weight.

WEIGHT GAIN AND LOSS

When you step on the scale and note that you weigh a pound more or less than you did the last time you weighed, this doesn't mean you have gained or lost body fat. Changes in body weight reflect shifts in many different materials—not only fat, but fluid, bone minerals, and lean tissues such as muscles. It is important for people concerned with weight control to realize this.

A healthy man or woman about 5 feet 10 inches tall who weighs 150 pounds carries about 90 of those pounds as water and 30 as fat. The other 30 pounds are the so-called lean tissues: muscles; organs such as the heart, brain, and liver; and the bones of the skeleton. Stripped of water and fat,

For a healthy woman or man, 5 ft tall, who weighs 100 lb, the comparable figures would be 60 lb of water, 20 lb of fat, 20 lb of lean.

---

*Pure fat is worth 9 cal/g. A pound of it (450 g), then, would store 4,150 cal. A pound of body fat is not pure fat, though; it contains water, protein, and other materials (hence the lower calorie value).
*A third component of energy expenditure: The presence of food stimulates the general metabolism. This diet-induced thermogenesis, or the specific dynamic effect of food, is thought to represent about 6 to 10% of the total food energy taken in. For rough estimates, it can be ignored.

then, the person weighs only 30 pounds! This lean tissue is vital to health. When a person who is too fat seeks to lose weight, it should be fat, not this precious lean tissue, that is lost. And for someone who wants to gain weight, it is desirable to gain weight in proportion—lean *and* fat, not just fat.

The type of tissue gained or lost depends on how the person goes about it. To lose fluid, for example, one can take a "water pill" (diuretic), causing the kidneys to siphon extra water from the blood into the urine. Or one can exercise heavily in the heat, losing abundant fluid in sweat. (Both practices are dangerous, incidentally, and are not being recommended here.) To gain water weight, a person can overconsume salt and water; then for a few hours the body retains water until it can excrete the salt. (This, too, is not recommended.) Most quick-weight-loss diets promote large fluid losses that register temporary, dramatic changes on the scale but accomplish little loss of body fat. The rest of this chapter underscores this distinction, and a later section on strategy stresses exercise as a means of maintaining lean tissue during weight loss.

Weight Gain

When you eat more food than you need, where does it go in your body? This is illustrated in Figure 5–1. The energy nutrients—carbohydrate, fat, and protein—contribute to body stores as follows:

- Carbohydrate is broken down to small units (sugars) for absorption. Inside the body, these may be built up to glycogen or converted to fat and stored.
- Fat is broken down to its component parts (including fatty acids) for absorption. Inside the body, these may be built up to fat for storage.
- Protein, too, is broken down to its basic units (amino acids) for absorption. Inside the body, these may be used to replace lost body protein. Any extra amino acids lose their nitrogen and are converted to fat.

Notice that although three kinds of energy nutrients enter the body, they are stored there in only two forms: glycogen and fat. Also notice that when excess protein is converted to fat, it cannot be recovered later as protein. The amino acids lose their nitrogen—it is actually excreted in the urine. No matter whether you are eating steak, brownies, or baked beans, then, if you eat enough of them, the excess will be turned to fat within hours. And no matter how much protein you may eat today, you will still need some more tomorrow (hence the RDA, Recommended *Daily* Allowance, for protein).

Weight Loss and Fasting

When the tables are turned and you stop eating altogether, the body has to draw on its stored nutrients to keep going. Nothing is wrong with this; in fact, it is a great advantage to us that we can eat periodically, store fuel, and then use it up between meals. (Some animals, such as cattle, have to spend virtually all their waking hours eating—a necessity that leaves them little time for stargazing.) The between-meal interval is ideally about four to six hours—about the length of time it takes to use up most of the available liver glycogen—or 12 to 14 hours at night, when body systems are slowed down and the need is less. If a person doesn't eat for, say, three whole days or a week, then the body makes one adjustment after another.

FIGURE 5–1   Feasting and Fasting

Excess energy nutrients from food are mainly stored as fat; a little carbohydrate is stored as glycogen.

In times of little food, the body draws on its stored fat and glycogen for the fuel it needs; note that body stores cannot supply needed protein, even though food protein contributes to body fat.

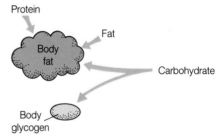

Excess energy nutrients from food are mainly stored as fat; a little carbohydrate is stored as glycogen.

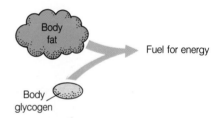

In times of little food, the body draws on its stored fat and glycogen for the fuel it needs; note that body stores cannot supply needed protein, even though food protein contributes to body fat.

RDA stands for Recommended Dietary Allowances, but they are amounts of nutrients recommended for *daily* consumption and so are often called daily allowances. See Appendix B.

Any food can make you fat. The total amount of calories is what makes the difference, and protein foods have calories, too.

Protein is not present in a storage form in the body; it is present only as working tissue. Working protein tissue is lost each day and can be replaced only by protein eaten that day.

After about a day, the liver's glycogen is essentially exhausted. Where, then, can the body obtain glucose to keep its nervous system going? Not from the muscles' glycogen, because that is reserved for the muscles' own use.

An alternative source of energy might be the abundant fat stores most people carry, but at first these are of no use to the nervous system. The muscles and other organs use fat as fuel, but the nervous system ordinarily cannot; nor can the body's fat be converted to glucose, because the body possesses no enzymes to perform this chemical reaction. It does, however, possess enzymes to convert protein to glucose.

As the fast continues, the body turns to this last resort, its own lean tissues, to keep up the supply of glucose. The reason why people who fast lose weight so dramatically within the first three days is that they are devouring their own protein tissues as fuel; since protein contains only half as many calories per pound as fat, it disappears twice as fast; and with each pound of body protein, three or four pounds of associated water are also lost.

If the body were to continue to consume itself at this rate, death would ensue within about ten days. After all, the liver, the heart muscle, the lung tissue, the blood—all vital tissues— are being burned as fuel. (In fact, fasting or starving people remain alive only until their body fat is gone or until half their lean tissue is gone, whichever comes first.) But now the body plays its last ace: it begins converting fat stores into a form it can use to help feed the nervous system and so forestall the end. This is **ketosis**.

In ketosis, the body combines partially broken-down fat fragments into ketone bodies (compounds that are normally rare in the blood), and lets them circulate in the bloodstream. About half of the brain's cells can use these compounds for energy. Thus, indirectly, the nervous system begins to feed on the body's fat stores. This reduces the need for glucose, spares lean tissue from being devoured so quickly, and prolongs the starving person's life. Thanks to ketosis, an initially healthy person deprived of food can live for as long as six to eight weeks.

Fasting has been practiced as a periodic discipline by respected, wise people in many cultures. However, ketosis may be harmful to the body. Some ketone bodies are acids, and when they are circulating in the blood they cause a dangerous imbalance. For the person who merely wants to lose weight, then, fasting is usually not the best way. For one thing, even in ketosis, the body's lean tissue continues to be lost at a rapid rate to supply glucose to those nervous system cells that cannot use ketones as fuel. For another, the body slows its metabolism during a fast to conserve energy. A low-calorie diet has actually been observed to promote the same rate of *weight* loss, and a faster rate of *fat* loss, than a total fast.[4] Just how to design a low-calorie diet is the subject of a later section, but first the low-carbohydrate diets deserve a moment's attention. They are examples of how *not* to design a diet.

Low-carbohydrate diets, by design, produce ketosis. The sales pitch is that ''you'll never feel hungry'' and that ''you'll lose weight fast—faster than

The nervous system cannot use fat as fuel, only glucose.
Body fat cannot be converted to glucose.*
Body protein can be converted to glucose.

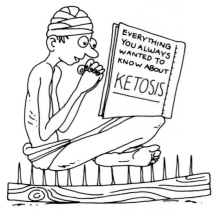

Fasting is an example of how *not* to design a weight-loss diet.

Names of low-carbohydrate diets:
Air Force Diet.
Atkins Diet.
Calories Don't Count Diet.
Drinking Man's Diet.
Herbalife Diet.
Mayo Diet.
Protein-Sparing Fast.
Scarsdale Diet.
Simeons HCG Diet.
Ski Team Diet.
Stillman Diet.
You Name It Diet.

*Glycerol, 5% of fat, can yield glucose but is a negligible source.

CHAPTER 5 ▬ WEIGHT CONTROL

you would on any ordinary diet." Both claims are true, but both are misleading. Loss of appetite accompanies any low-calorie diet. Fast weight loss means lean tissue loss.

The body responds to a low-carbohydrate diet as it does to a fast. It is receiving protein and fat (on a fast it draws on its own protein and fat), but it has used up its stored glycogen. It therefore turns to protein to make the needed glucose. On being converted to glucose, protein loses its nitrogen, which has to be excreted. This puts a burden on the kidneys. The low-carbohydrate dieter who fails to drink abundant water is risking kidney damage from nitrogen wastes and ketone bodies. Other physiological hazards of low-carbohydrate diets are high blood cholesterol, mineral imbalances, and many other metabolic abnormalities. Some low-carbohydrate diets, particularly the protein-sparing fast type, have caused deaths due to heart failure. The heart muscle disintegrates without sufficient nutrients to maintain it. These diets are never recommended by legitimate practitioners.

Low-carbohydrate diets appear every year under new names. Bringing out new diet books and products is a profitable business, and it will continue to be successful as long as people are deceived by the initial rapid weight loss into thinking that the diets work. To identify fraudulent, low-carbohydrate diets for what they are, learn to add up the carbohydrate grams they supply; less than 100 grams is too little. Appendix E shows the carbohydrate in foods.

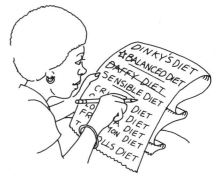

The cautious consumer distinguishes between loss of fat and loss of weight.

Wrong Ways to Lose Weight

The most valid criterion of a good weight-loss diet is not the speed or the magnitude of weight loss, but its maintenance, once achieved. By this standard, fasting and low-carbohydrate diets are not the way to lose weight. Other ways *not* to choose are water pills, diet pills, health spa regimens, muscle stimulators, hormones, and surgery. Water pills (diuretics) do nothing to solve a fat problem, although they may bring about the loss of a few pounds on the scale for half a day and cause dehydration. Diet pills (amphetamines, or "speed,") reduce appetite temporarily by triggering the stress response but leave the dieter with another problem: how to get off them without gaining more weight. Health spas may be a nice place to exercise, but you cannot "jiggle" or "melt" pounds away on their special machines. Muscle stimulators reduce body measurements by making muscles tighter, not by reducing their fat content—and only for an hour or so. Hormones are powerful body chemicals, and many affect fat metabolism, but all have proved ineffective and often hazardous as weight-loss aids.

Surgery for obesity has dangerous side effects. Bypass surgery, which involves disconnecting or removing a portion of the small intestine to reduce absorption, is seldom performed anymore, because results have been so disappointing. Stapling the stomach to reduce its capacity is preferred, but not perfect: stomach tissue is damaged, scars are formed, and staples pull loose.

At intervals, medical personnel develop new approaches to limit the stomach's capacity. One is slipping a balloon into the stomach and inflating it; another is confining the stomach within a web that keeps it from expanding. Risks of these procedures are unknown, but success, as measured by long-term weight maintenance, is seldom achieved by these methods.

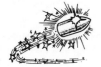

If it sounds too good to be true, it probably is.

One survey of 29,000 weight-loss strategies found fewer than 6 percent of them effective—and 13 percent dangerous.[5] People may respond to this fact with the question, "Can't the government do something about that?" The government is active in pursuing and cracking down on health swindles, but most agencies have insufficient staff and resources to handle the massive number of reported cases. They can eliminate only the most dangerous schemes at best. This results in a free market for other promoters who can rake in billions of dollars on products that are only slightly less dangerous than the worst ones. It is easy for a swindler to get a product on the market and hard for the government or other groups to get it off. That puts the burden of distinguishing frauds from reality on you, the consumer. To keep from getting taken in, remember: If it sounds too good to be true, it probably is.

WEIGHT LOSS STRATEGIES

Given that so many weight-loss approaches are guaranteed to fail, what works? How can a person lose weight safely and permanently? The secret is a sensible approach (we didn't say *easy*) that uses diet, exercise, and behavior modification. It takes tremendous dedication, especially at first, for a person whose habits have all promoted obesity to adopt as habits the hundred or so new behaviors that promote thinness. When people succeed, they do so because they have employed many of the techniques described in this chapter.[6]

To emphasize the personal nature of weight-loss plans, the following sections are written as advice to "you." This is intended to give you the illusion of listening in on a conversation in which an obese person is being competently counseled by someone familiar with the techniques known to be effective.

Diet Planning

No particular diet is magical, and no particular food must be either included or avoided. You are the one who will have to live with the diet, so you had better be involved in its planning. Don't think of it as a diet you are going "on"—because then you may be tempted to go "off." Think of it as an eating plan that you will adopt for life. It must consist of foods that you like or can learn to like, that are available to you, and that are within your means.

Choose a calorie level you can live with. A deficit of 500 calories a day for seven days is a 3,500-calorie deficit—enough to lose a pound of body fat. There is no point in hurrying, because you will never go off the diet—and adequate nutrient intakes can't be achieved on too few calories.

Make your diet adequate. This is a way of putting yourself first. "I like me, and I'm going to take good care of me" is the attitude to adopt. A good pattern to follow is the Four Food Group Plan of Table 4–5 (page 79). A plan that uses the minimum servings without frills and allows a teaspoon of fat at each meal provides less than 1,200 calories; most people could lose weight at a satisfactory rate following such a plan and meet their nutrient needs, too. Within each food group, learn what foods you like, and use them often. If you plan

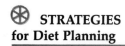

STRATEGIES
for Diet Planning

To control weight successfully:

❋ **Get involved personally.**

❋ **Adopt a realistic plan.**

❋ **Make the diet adequate.**

❋ **Emphasize high nutrient density.**

❋ **Individualize. Use foods you like.**

❋ **Stress dos, not don'ts.**

resolutely to include a certain number of servings of food from each group each day, you may be so busy making sure you get what you need that you will have little time or appetite left for high-calorie or empty-calorie foods. Foods such as vegetables and whole grains take a lot more eating, too—crunchy, wholesome foods offer bulk and satiety for far fewer calories than smooth, refined foods. Limit your meats: an ounce of ham contains more calories than an ounce of bread, and many of them are from fat.

Three meals a day is standard for our society, but no law says you shouldn't have four or five meals—only be sure they are smaller, of course. What is important is to eat regularly and, if at all possible, to eat before you are very hungry. When you do decide to eat, eat the entire meal you have planned for yourself. Then don't eat again until the next meal. Save "free" or favorite foods or beverages for a planned snack at the end of the day, if you need insurance against late-evening hunger.

⊛ Eat regular meals with no skipping—at least three a day.

At first it may seem as if you have to spend all your waking hours thinking about and planning your meals. Such a massive effort is always required when a new skill is being learned. (You spent hours practicing writing the alphabet when you were in the first grade.) But after about three weeks, it will be much easier. Use positive imaging: see yourself as a person who "eats thin." Your new eating pattern will become a habit.

⊛ Visualize a changed future self.

Do not weigh yourself more than every week or two. Gains or losses of a pound or more in a matter of days reverse themselves quickly; the smoothed-out average is what is real. Don't expect to lose continuously as fast as you did at first. A sizable water loss is common in the first week, but it will not happen again. If you have been working out lately, occasional weighings may show no loss or even a gain. This may reflect a welcome development: the gain of lean body mass—just what you want, if you want to be healthy.

⊛ Take well-spaced weighings to avoid discouragement.

If you slip, don't punish yourself. Positive reinforcement is effective at changing behavior, but punishment seldom works. If you ate an extra 1,000 calories yesterday, don't try to eat 1,000 fewer calories today. Just go back to your plan. On the other hand, you can plan ahead and budget for special occasions. If you want to celebrate your birthday with cake and ice cream, cut the necessary calories from your bread and milk allowance for several days *beforehand*. Your weight loss will be as smooth as if you had stayed with the daily plan.

⊛ Use positive reinforcement. Never blame, never punish.

You may have to get tough with yourself if you stop losing weight or start gaining unexpectedly. Ask yourself honestly (no one is listening in), "What am I doing wrong?" Seldom does an unpredicted weight plateau of any duration have no explanation in the dieter's own choices.

⊛ Be honest with yourself.

Finally, if you stop losing weight or begin to gain, be aware that you may be choosing that course. Your weight is under your control. Rather than feeling guilty or like a failure, hold your head high and take the attitude, "This is me, and this is the way I am choosing to be right now."

⊛ Stress personal responsibility.

⊛ Maintain self-esteem.

Exercise

Some people who want to lose weight hate the very idea of exercise. A word to reassure them: weight loss, at least to a point, is possible without exercise. But even if you choose not to alter your habits at first, let your mind be open to the possibility that you will want to take up some activity later on. As the pounds come off, moving your body becomes a pleasure.

The physical contributions exercise makes to a weight-control program are twofold: exercise alters body composition in favor of lean tissue, and it

Thinness is not the same as fitness.

FIGURE 5–2 The Ratchet Effect of Dieting

Each round of dieting, without exercise, is followed by a rebound of weight to a higher level than before.

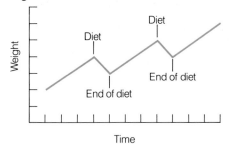

Benefits of exercise:
  Increased expenditure of energy.
  Long-term increase in resting metabolic rate.
  Appetite control.
  Stress reduction.
  Control of stress-induced eating.
  Increased self-esteem.
  Psychological and physical well-being.

raises the metabolic rate. It also offers the psychological benefits of looking and feeling healthy and the increased self-esteem that accompanies these benefits. Increased self-esteem tends to support a person's resolve to persist in a weight-control effort—rounding out a beneficial cycle.

Weight loss without exercise can have a negative effect on body composition. A person who diets without exercising loses both lean and fat tissue, as described earlier. If the person then gains weight without exercising, the gain is mostly fat. Compared with lean tissue, fat tissue burns fewer calories to maintain itself, so if the person eats the same amount as before, the person's weight will zoom higher than before, the so-called **ratchet effect**, or **yoyo effect**, of dieting (Figure 5–2).

On the other hand, the more lean tissue you develop, the more calories you spend, and the more you can afford to eat. This brings you both pleasure and nutrients. It must be clear by now that exercise speeds up your metabolism *permanently*—that is, for as long as you keep your body conditioned.

Exercise also, of course, spends energy while you are doing it. Table 5–1 lists energy costs of activities. The more intense the exercise, the more energy it requires, but much of the excess comes from glycogen, not fat. In any one person, the amount of fat burned during moderate and heavy exercise is about the same per minute.

People sometimes ask about "spot reducing." Can you lose fat in particular locations? Unfortunately, muscles do not "own" the fat that surrounds them. Fat cells release fat not into the underlying muscles, but into the blood, and the fat is shared by all the muscles. Spot-reducing exercises therefore do not work. A balanced exercise program will tighten muscles in trouble spots.

TABLE 5–1 Energy Demands of Activities

Activity	Intensity	Spent Energy (cal/lb/min)
Swimming (crawl)	20 yds/min	.032
	45 yds/min	.058
	50 yds/min	.070
Bicycling	13 mph	.045
	15 mph	.049
	17 mph	.057
	19 mph	.076
	21 mph	.090
	23 mph	.109
	25 mph	.139
Running	A mile in 11½ min (5.2 mph)	.061
	A mile in 9 min (6.7 mph)	.088
	A mile in 8 min (7.5 mph)	.094
	A mile in 7 min (9.0 mph)	.103
	A mile in 6 min (10.0 mph)	.114
	A mile in 5½ min (11.0 mph)	.131
Studying		.011

NOTE: Skiing, squash, and handball require about the same energy as biking at 13 mph.

SOURCE: All data except that for studying from G. P. Town and K. B. Wheeler, Nutritional concerns for the endurance athlete, *Dietetic Currents*, 1986, available from Ross Laboratories, Columbus, OH 43216.

The next chapter gives you many pointers about developing fitness, but a few strategies are in order here. For one thing, you must keep in mind that if exercise is to help with weight loss, it must be active exercise. Being moved passively, as by a machine or a massage, does not work. The more muscles you move, the more calories you spend. On the other hand, workouts do not have to be fast. If you choose to walk the distance instead of run, you will use up about the same energy; it will just take you longer. Weight loss is not the only reason to work out—if you incorporate regular aerobic exercise into your schedule (as described in the next chapter), your heart and lungs, as well as your muscles, will be fit.

Another strategy is to incorporate more exercise into your daily schedule in many simple, small-scale ways. Park the car at the far end of the parking lot; use the stairs instead of the elevator; do a deep knee bend each time you get up from your chair. These activities add up to only a few calories each, but over a year's time they become significant.

Behavior Modification

Behavior modification works to change the behaviors of overeating and underexercising that lead to and perpetuate obesity. Figure 1–2 in Chapter 1 showed six strategies you could use to modify your behavior. The discussion that follows and this chapter's Strategies box apply behavior modification principles to weight loss.

First, behavior modification experts say, you should establish a baseline, a record of your present eating behaviors against which to measure future progress. Keep a diary, in order to learn what your particular eating stimuli, or cues, are.

Second, set about eliminating or suppressing the cues that prompt you to eat inappropriately. There may be many such cues: watching television, talking on the telephone, passing a convenience store or a vending machine, being offered food, and many more. Resolve to respond no longer to these cues by eating, but to respond only to one set of cues designed by you: one particular place in one particular room.

Third, try to strengthen the cues to appropriate eating and exercise. For example, keep good foods in the front of the refrigerator and make exercise equipment easily available. Fourth, alter the activity itself. Eating more slowly is one way to do this (overeaters eat faster than others).

Fifth, arrange as far as possible to have negative consequences follow inappropriate eating behavior and activity. Scolding is *not* a negative consequence (it is a form of attention-giving, which is positive), so don't ask to be scolded. Sixth and finally, make sure that positive consequences, including material rewards, follow your display of the desired behaviors.

You may find it helpful to join a group such as TOPS (Take Off Pounds Sensibly), Weight Watchers, or Overeaters Anonymous. A modest expenditure for your own health is worthwhile (but avoid ripoffs, of course). Many dieters find it helpful to form their own self-help groups. If you are especially sensitive to social situations where you feel you have to eat, it will also help to have some assertiveness training. Learning to say "No, thank you" might be one of your first objectives. Learning not to "clean your plate" might be another.

From all the behavior changes available to you, you can choose the ones to begin with. Don't try to master them all at once. No one who attempts

STRATEGIES: Behavior Modifications for Weight Loss

To eliminate inappropriate eating cues:

1. Eat only in one place, in one room.

2. Don't buy problem foods (shop when you aren't hungry).

3. Don't serve rich sauces and toppings.

4. Let spouse and children buy, store, and serve their own sweets.

5. Clear plates directly into the garbage.

6. Create obstacles to the eating of problem foods (for example, make it necessary to unwrap, cook, and serve each one separately, allowing time for resistance to develop).

7. Minimize contact with excessive food (serve individual plates, don't put serving dishes on the table, leave the table when finished).

8. Make small portions of food look large (spread food out, serve on small plates). Garnish empty spaces with lettuce.

9. Control states of deprivation (eat regular meals, don't skip meals, avoid getting tired, avoid boredom by keeping cues to fun activities in sight).

10. Watch television that doesn't show food commercials.

To strengthen the cues to appropriate eating and exercise:

1. Encourage others to eat appropriate foods with you.

2. Keep a variety of appropriate foods available.

3. Learn appropriate portion sizes.

4. Save permitted foods from meals for snacks (and make these your only snacks).

5. Prepare permitted foods attractively.

6. Keep your ski poles (hiking boots, tennis racket) by the door.

7. Move more (shake a leg, pace, fidget, flex your muscles).

To alter the eating response itself:

1. Slow down (pause for two to three minutes, put down utensils, swallow before reloading the fork, always use utensils).

To arrange negative consequences of inappropriate eating:

1. Have others nearby when you eat.

2. Ask that others respond neutrally to your deviations (make no comment). This is a negative consequence because it withholds attention.

To arrange positive consequences of appropriate behaviors:

1. Update records of food intake, exercise, and weight change regularly.

2. Arrange for rewards for each unit of behavior change or weight loss.

3. Provide social reinforcement (ask to be encouraged).

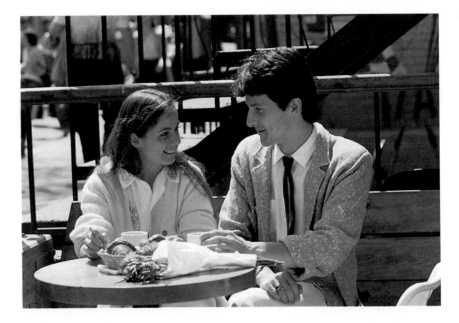

To control weight successfully, arrange to enjoy eating.

too many changes at one time is successful. Set your own priorities. Pick one trouble area that you think you can handle, start with that, and practice your strategy until it is automatic. Then select another trouble area to work on.

Enjoy your new, emerging self. Inside every fat person is a thin person, struggling to be freed. Get in touch with—reach out your hand to—your thin self, and help that self to feel welcome in the light of day.

Finally, be aware that it can be harder to maintain weight loss than to lose weight. On arriving at the goal weight after months of self-discipline and new habit formation, the victorious weight loser must at all costs avoid "celebrating" by resuming old eating habits. They are gone forever—remember? Membership in an ongoing weight-control organization and regular, continued physical activity with others can give indispensable support for the formerly fat person who wants to remain trim.

▨ WEIGHT GAIN STRATEGIES

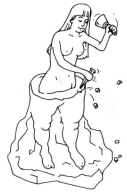

Make your thin self feel welcome in the light of day.

It is as hard for a person who tends to be underweight to gain a pound as it is for a person who tends to be overweight to lose one. Like the weight-loser, the person who wants to gain must learn new habits and learn to like new foods.

Although physical activity costs calories, it is essential for health, unless an underweight condition has become life-threatening. The healthy way to gain weight is to build up by patient and consistent training and, at the same time, to eat enough calories to support the weight gain. If you are not dangerously underweight:

■ Adopt an exercise program designed to increase lean body tissue (for more details, see Chapter 6).

In addition to exercising appropriately, you must eat enough calories to support weight gain. If you add 700 to 800 extra calories of nutritious foods a day, you can achieve a healthful weight gain of l to 1-1/2 pounds per week.

A person who wants to gain weight often has to learn to eat different foods. No matter how many helpings of boiled carrots you consume, you won't gain weight very fast, because carrots simply don't offer enough calories. The person who can't eat much volume is encouraged to use calorie-dense foods in meals (the very ones the dieter is trying to stay away from). Dietary modifications for the person trying to gain weight are:

■ Eat an additional 700-800 calories per day.
■ Use more calorie-dense foods; those items labeled C in Table 4–5 (page 79).

The underweight individual must be aware that a low-fat diet plan is recommended for the general U.S. population because the general population is overweight. Ignore most dietary recommendations designed for overweight individuals, including low-fat diet plans. Consumption of high-fat foods is essential for most underweight individuals trying to gain weight. Therefore:

■ Consume milk shakes instead of milk, peanut butter instead of lean meat, avocados instead of cucumbers, whole-wheat muffins instead of whole-wheat bread.
■ Eat butter on cooked vegetables, add cream and sugar to coffee, use creamy dressings on salads, whipped cream on fruit, sour cream on potatoes, and so forth. (Because fat contains twice as many calories per teaspoon as sugar, it adds calories without adding much bulk.)

Since you need substantially more calories per day, in addition to eating more calories per meal, you will need to:

■ Eat more frequently. Make three sandwiches in the morning and eat them between classes in addition to the day's three regular meals.

Most people who are underweight have simply been too busy (sometimes for months) to eat enough to gain or maintain weight. Therefore:

■ Preplan your meals.
■ Spend more time eating each meal; if you fill up fast, eat the highest-calorie items first. Don't start with soup or salad; eat meaty appetizers or the main course first.

Expect to feel full, sometimes even uncomfortably so. Most underweight individuals are accustomed to small quantities of food. When they begin eating significantly more food, they complain of uncomfortable fullness. This is normal and it passes over time.

When a person decides to gain or lose weight, that person would do well to examine the motives behind the decision. Is over- or underweight truly a problem? Much precious effort is wasted when people chase a wild goose by dieting to attain a "perfect" body as seen in a magazine or on television. That effort would be much better spent on things that actually need attention, perhaps stopping smoking, or gaining physical fitness, or developing spiritual perspectives. The Spotlight to come describes the harshest consequences of unrealistic weight-loss goals—the loss of self-esteem, loss of health, and sometimes, loss of life itself.

STUDY AIDS

1. Identify the major health risks associated with being overweight or underweight.
2. Explain, in terms of body composition, the various possible ways in which weight may be gained or lost.
3. Describe how the body maintains itself when a person eats:
   a. Too much food.
   b. Just enough food.
   c. Not enough food.
   d. No food.
4. Outline the principles of sound diet planning as they relate to weight loss, weight gain, and weight maintenance.
5. Show how diet, exercise, and behavior modification each can contribute to weight control.

GLOSSARY

basal metabolism: the sum total of all the chemical activities of the cells, necessary to sustain life, exclusive of voluntary activities. Basal metabolism, sometimes called *basal metabolic rate* (*BMR*), is the largest component of a person's daily energy expenditure.

fatfold test: a clinical test of body fatness in which the thickness of a fold of skin on the back of the arm (triceps), below the shoulder blade (subscapular), or in other places is measured with an instrument called a caliper. The older term for this is *skinfold test*. An informal means of doing the same thing is to perform the *pinch test*: simply lift a fold on the back of the arm with the fingers, and estimate its thickness (if it's over an inch thick, the person is said to be obese; if less than half an inch, underweight).

ketosis (kee-TOE-sis): an adaptation of the body to prolonged (several days') fasting or carbohydrate restriction: body fat is converted to ketone bodies, which can be used as fuel for some brain cells.

obesity: overfatness defined as weight 20 percent or more above the appropriate weight for height defined by body mass index; greater than 27.2 in men or 26.9 in women.

pinch test: see *fatfold test*.

ratchet effect, or yoyo effect (of dieting): the effect of repeated rounds of dieting without exercise; the person rebounds to a higher weight (and higher body fat content) at the end of each round.

skinfold test: see *fatfold test*.

underweight: weight too low for health. Traditionally defined as weight 10 percent or more below the appropriate weight for height.

yoyo effect: see *ratchet effect*.

QUIZ ANSWERS

1. *True.* Being underweight presents a risk to health.

2. *True.* Excess fat around the abdomen presents a greater risk to health than excess fat elsewhere on the body.

3. *False.* A weight loss may reflect loss of water or lean tissue rather than loss of fat.

4. *False.* Fraudulent advertisements are common on television.

5. *False.* Carbohydrate is a necessary part of a balanced weight-loss diet.

6. *False.* Fasting promotes rapid *weight* loss, but a balanced low-calorie diet can promote more rapid *fat* loss.

7. *False.* It is probably more nearly ideal for a woman to have 20 percent or more of her body weight as fat and for a man, 15 percent.

8. *True.* If an inactive person takes up a daily hour of exercise, the person will end up spending more calories all day, even during sleep.

9. *True.* You can eat any food on a weight-loss diet, as long as you don't eat too much of it.

10. *False.* It is as hard for a person who tends to be thin to gain a pound as it is for a person who tends to be fat to lose one.

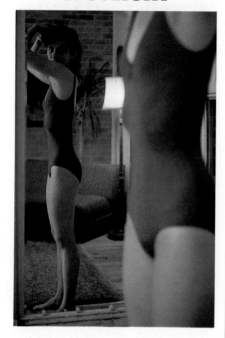

An Obsession with Thinness

"Right now I weigh 58 lbs., which isn't too bad for 5'2", though I want to lose a few more pounds—my hips are still fat. Lately I've got it down to no breakfast, a can of mushrooms for lunch, and a can of wax beans for dinner with lots of iced tea. I reward myself with a big, green apple at the end of the day, if I've stuck to The Plan.
"—A. Ciseaux

In developed nations such as the United States, society favors thinness in women. Magazines, newspapers, and television display camera-ready women, flaws concealed, unreasonably thin. The message is clear—the way you are isn't good enough. You are worthy only so long as you are lovely to look at. You should become like the cover girl who doesn't sweat; doesn't grow hair on her slender legs; has firm, small breasts, a flat stomach, a perfect face, small feet; and is always perfectly happy. If *you*, young woman, are not perfectly happy, it is because your body is not beautiful enough. Acceptance of such unreasonable expectations has driven nearly everyone in our society to be engaged in the "pursuit of thinness."

I thought being thin was healthy. Isn't it OK to pursue thinness?

Pursuing an appropriate body weight in a safe manner is healthy. An obsession with excessive thinness, however, can be dangerous. In fact, two eating disorders, **anorexia nervosa** and **bulimia** focus on an obsession with and extreme pursuit of thinness.

What happens to someone who has anorexia nervosa?

The story of Julie illustrates a typical case of anorexia nervosa. Julie is 18 years old. She is attractive, she is a superachiever in school, and she prides herself on her fine figure. She watches her diet with great care, and she exercises daily, maintaining a heroic schedule of self-discipline. She is thin, but she is not satisfied with her

weight and is determined to lose more. She is 5 feet 6 inches tall and weighs 85 pounds, but she's still trying to get thinner.

How could she possibly think she's too fat measuring 5 feet 6 inches tall and weighing 85 pounds?

Her self-image is distorted. Her constant complaints of being fat and her obsessive behavior are strong indicators of abnormal mental processes. Against her will, Julie's family insisted that she see a psychiatrist who tested her. She was given a visual self-image test and drew a picture of herself that was grossly distorted. When asked to draw her best friend, Julie rendered an accurate image.

Can't she see that she's hurting her body by being too thin?

Julie is unaware that she is undernourished, and she sees no need to obtain treatment. She stopped menstruating several months ago and has become very moody. Although her eyes lie in deep hollows in her face, and she is obviously close to physical exhaustion, she denies that she is ever tired.

How can someone get so thin and continue to diet?

Julie controls her food intake with tremendous discipline. If she feels that she has slipped and eaten more than intended, she runs or jumps rope until she is sure she has exercised it off, or she takes laxatives to hasten the exit of the food from her system. (She is unaware that this doesn't work to reduce the calories.) It is her fierce determination to achieve self-control, not lack of hunger, that prevents her from eating.

What could have caused her to behave this way?

A characteristic cluster of family and social circumstances often, though not always, surrounds the person with anorexia. Such a family is described as being dominated by the mother, with the father absent or distant, and it values achievement and outward appearances more than an inner sense of self-worth and self-actualization. The young person values her parents' opinion and works hard to attain perfection for them.

Young women look to their male parents or parent substitutes for important feedback on their self-worth, and when they don't receive it, tend to be oversensitive to negative cultural influences such as the drive for thinness and the view of emaciation as beautiful.[1*] Julie's father has alcoholism, and her mother left him a year ago. Anorexia, being obsessive-compulsive behavior, resembles an addiction, and often there are other addictions in the family.

As a child, when Julie cried with hunger, her parents didn't respond by feeding her. Rather, they fed her on a rigid schedule. They forced food on her at times when she didn't want it, and they withheld it when she was hungry. Julie lost the ability to detect her own hunger signals. Now, she feels she has to control her eating from outside, as her parents did.

*Reference notes are in Appendix D.

It sounds as though this could be dangerous. What is happening to her physically?

Julie is suffering the physical effects of starvation, in which hormone secretions become abnormal and blood pressure drops. The heart pumps less efficiently; its muscle becomes weak and thin, its chambers diminish in size, and its rhythms may change, with a characteristic abnormality appearing on the heart monitor. Sudden stopping of the heart, due to lean tissue loss or mineral deficiencies, accounts for many cases of sudden death among severely emaciated subjects.

Can a person with anorexia be cured?

In many cases, the hospitalized patient will describe herself as proud of her achievements in dieting, eager to achieve more, and resentful of her confinement in the hosptial. She has, after all, made significant progress toward achieving society's goal for her—to be thin.

Treatment outcomes are better than they used to be. Residential treatment centers specializing in eating disorders are often especially successful. Three-quarters of those in treatment may regain weight up to within 25 percent of the desired weight. Half to three-quarters may resume normal menstrual cycles. About two-thirds fail to eat normally on follow-up, but they may eat better than they did before. About 6 percent die, 1 percent by suicide.*

*This is from a review of 19 studies of about 1,000 clients over a five-year period. Other deaths are from infection, heart disease, lung disease, and treatment-related causes including aspiration, electrolyte imbalance from intravenous therapy, and vitamin D poisoning. M.A. Balaa and D. A. Drossman, *Anorexia Nervosa and Bulimia: The Eating Disorders, Disease-a-Month* (Chicago: Year Book Medical Publishers, June 1985), p. 34.

You previously mentioned bulimia. What happens to someone who has this disease?

The case of Sophie illustrates the plight of the person with bulimia. Like the "typical" person with bulimia, Sophie is single, Caucasian, in her early 20s, is well educated, and close to her ideal body weight. Sophie is a charming, intelligent woman who thinks constantly about food. She alternatively starves herself and binges, and when she has eaten too much, she vomits.

Her periodic binges take place in secret, usually at night, and they last an hour or more. She seldom lets bingeing interfere with her work or social activities, although a third of all bingers do. She is like most people with bulimia in that she starts the binge after having gone through a period of rigid dieting, so that her eating is accelerated by her hunger. Each time, she consumes thousands of calories of easy-to-eat, high-calorie food. Typically, she chooses cookies, cake, ice cream, or bread, although sometimes she binges on atypical foods—such as vegetables—when she is dieting. The binge is not like normal eating. It is a compulsion and usually occurs in several stages: "anticipation and planning, anxiety, urgency to begin, rapid and uncontrollable consumption of food, relief and relaxation, disappointment, and finally shame or disgust."[2]

What are the physical effects of bulimia?

Immediately following a binge, Sophie pays the price of having swollen hands and feet, bloating, fatigue, headache, nausea, and pain. Repetition of this behavior causes more serious consequences. Fluid and electrolyte imbalance caused by vomiting can lead to abnormal heart rhythms and injury to the kidneys. Vomiting causes irritation and infection of the pharynx, esophagus, and salivary glands; erosion of the teeth;

103

and dental caries. The esophagus may rupture or tear, as may the stomach. Sometimes the eyes become red from pressure on vomiting. The hands may be bruised and lacerated from scraping on the teeth while inducing vomiting.

Some people use **cathartics**—laxatives that can injure the lower intestinal tract. Others use **emetics** to induce vomiting; it was overuse of emetics that caused the death of popular singer Karen Carpenter in 1983.

What makes a person become bulimic?

We don't know, but the family dynamics suggest some clues. Much like Julie, who has anorexia nervosa, Sophie has been a high achiever, with a strong feeling of dependence on her parents. Her mother is a bright, well-educated woman who chose to stay home with the children; her father is a powerful and respected, but distant, figure.

Her family often combined hearty eating with much socializing around the dinner table. Food was always involved in celebrations and used to console the family during periods of mourning. She felt it would be disrespectful to not celebrate or mourn by not eating; equally strong was the demand to be thin.

Sophie experiences considerable social anxiety and has difficulty in establishing personal relationships. She is sometimes depressed and often behaves impulsively. Some people with bulimia engage in antisocial behavior, including drug abuse, compulsive stealing, and sexual promiscuity. Sophie feels inadequate, because she is unable to control her eating, and so she tends to be passive and to look to men for confirmation of her sense of worth. When she is rejected, either in reality or in her imagination, her bulimia becomes worse; in fact, many women point to male rejection as the event that led to the first binge.[3]

How common are anorexia nervosa and bulimia?

Both anorexia nervosa and bulimia occur only in developed nations and become more prevalent as wealth increases. The incidence of anorexia in our country and in other industrially advanced countries is steadily increasing. The disease afflicts women mostly (although men are not immune), and it now occurs in almost 1 of every 100 women.[4]

Bulimia occurs more frequently than anorexia nervosa. Although bulimia predominately afflicts women, bulimia is more common among men than anorexia. More people are claiming to have bulimia than ever before. In a survey of 300 suburban women shoppers in Boston, over 10 percent reported a history of bulimia, and almost 5 percent were currently practicing it.[5] Among college women, the incidence may range anywhere from 5 to 20 percent.

What can be done about this situation?

The causes of both bulimia and anorexia nervosa are unknown, but one school of thought labels them social problems. Perhaps they began when privileged young women internalized a message of their own low worth and adopted the ideal of some unachievable, "perfect" image.

Slowly, society is changing. Recognition of the success and desirability of a growing number of outstanding women in such traditionally male-dominated fields as athletics, science, law and politics has raised women's collective self-esteem. Perhaps anorexia nervosa and bulimia will disappear as feminine roles and ideals change. Prevention may be most effective if begun early in the children's lives. Warnings to children that the Madison Avenue female figure is simply an advertising gimmick designed to sell products, and not an ideal with which to compare one's own living body, may help. The simple concept—to respect and value your own uniqueness—may be lifesaving for a future generation.

Chapter 6

Fitness

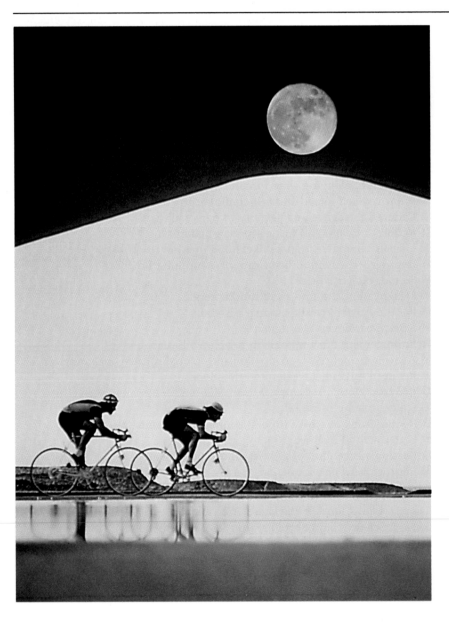

FOR OPENERS . . .

True or false? If false, say what is true.

1. You should never overload your body, because overload can cause damage.

2. Stroke volume is the amount of water moved by one stroke of an oar in a rowing competition.

3. The person who wishes to gain strength must use weights to provide resistance for the muscles to work against.

4. If you feel pain in your feet or legs while running, it is best to keep going and try to work through it.

5. On a hot day, if you perspire freely when you exercise, you should take a salt tablet.

6. Water is the beverage of choice to replace body fluids lost during exercise.

7. When you exercise a muscle until it is exhausted, you increase its strength.

8. A vigorous 20-minute aerobic workout every other day is all a person needs to stay fit.

9. To deal with the stress of conditioning, you need one or more vitamin-mineral supplements every day.

10. If you drink more than a swallow of fluid before you run, or certainly if you stop running and satisfy your thirst, you risk stomach cramps.

(Answers on page 122.)

Throughout history, human beings have used their wiles to invent machines that replace human exertion. The power of such machines spares us from having to climb stairs, take long walks, or even open cans of prepared food by hand. We now take our sports by way of TV, watching others perform. The sticker price of these inventions may be high, but it would be much higher if it included the health costs of the sedentary life they permit.

WHY EXERCISE?

Heredity gave Stone Age men and women bodies that needed exercise. Yours does, too. The human body is designed to fight enemies; push, pull, and carry heavy objects; and run long distances. Modern people still need to develop the same physical equipment, but modern life usually doesn't require as much physical exertion as we need to remain healthy. We therefore have to use our brains—the same ones that designed modern conveniences for us—to develop our **fitness**. Some of the information presented here is for people who are just learning that exercise is important; other information is intended to help the seasoned athlete. No matter at what level of fitness you find yourself, you can apply these basics to your own life.

The benefits of regular exercise make an impressive list, which is growing longer as new discoveries are made:

- More enjoyable, perhaps even longer, life.[1,2*]
- Improved mental capacity.
- Feeling of vigor.
- Feeling of belonging—the fun and companionship of sports.
- Improved self-image and self-confidence.
- Reduced incidence and severity of personality disorders.[3]
- Reduced fatness and increased lean body tissue.[4]
- Greater bone density (less likelihood of adult bone loss).[5]
- Improved circulation, heart capacity, and lung function.[6]
- Sound, beneficial sleep.
- Healthy skin and improved muscle tone.
- Reduced risk of cardiovascular disease.[7]
- Slowed cardiovascular aging.[8]
- Improvement of symptoms in people with diabetes.[9]
- A lower incidence of constipation and colon disorders, including cancer.[10]
- Reduced fat and cholesterol in the blood.
- Reduced blood pressure.
- Slower resting pulse rate.[11]
- Reduced risk of stroke (in oral contraceptive users, too).
- Faster wound healing.
- Possible prevention of arthritis and rheumatism.
- Improvement or elimination of menstrual cramps.
- Improved resistance to colds and infections.[12]

Exercise is also one of the most effective strategies against stress-related disease. Science cannot promise you all of these benefits if you exercise, but almost everyone who exercises reaps some of them. If only half of these rewards were yours for the asking, wouldn't you step up to claim them?

Blood lipids, including HDL, LDL, and other risk factors for heart disease, are discussed in Chapter 16.

*Reference notes are in Appendix D.

Imagine that this list is associated not with regular exercise but with a newly discovered "miracle pill." A stampede of people would try to buy it. In fact, miracle products claim to offer many of these benefits, and people do spend money in hopes of obtaining them. Why is money so much easier to spend than effort?

Despite evidence of the benefits, not all of the population of the United States exercises regularly,[13] although the number may be increasing. Sadly, regular exercise requires more effort than pill taking, and more time. Sometimes it's inconvenient and hard to get started. But once an exercise routine is established, the felt benefits far outweigh the inconveniences, and excuses carry less power to interfere.

■ THE CHARACTERISTICS OF FITNESS

To be physically healthy, you don't have to be spectacular looking. You don't have to develop a Miss America or Mr. Universe body. Rather, what you need is a reasonable weight and enough fitness to meet the everyday demands life places on you, plus some to spare. Fitness is expressed by different body systems. For the joints, **flexibility** is important. For the muscles that move the limbs, muscle **strength** and **muscle endurance** are important. The heart and lungs also need **endurance**: this type of endurance is called **cardiovascular endurance**.

Some people think of fitness as fitness for a particular sport, and in fact describe it in terms of *performance*, rather than overall *health*. They describe the goals not in terms of flexibility, strength, and endurance but in terms of skill, balance, speed, and coordination. This chapter aims at overall health and recognizes sports (respectfully) as a way of making fitness fun and challenging.

Let us consider what each of the compounds of fitness does for the body and how it can be attained. Flexibility depends on the **elasticity** of muscles, tendons, and ligaments and on the condition of the joints. If flexibility is maintained, the body can move as it was designed to move and will bend instead of tearing or breaking in response to sudden stresses. In addition, the movements of a flexible body are graceful and youthful. Flexibility improves in response to stretching.

Strength is a familiar concept. It is the ability of the muscles to work against resistance: to pull weeds from the ground, to push a stalled car, or to open a jar of jam. Many of today's mechanical helpers invented to spare effort rob us of the opportunity to develop strength—for example, the strength we would gain from chopping firewood instead of turning up a thermostat.

Muscle endurance, the third component of fitness, is the power of a muscle to keep on going for long periods. You are probably familiar with tests of muscle endurance: how many sit-ups, pull-ups, or lifts you can do in a row. But there is another realm in which endurance is important: how long you can keep going with an elevated heart rate—that is, how long your heart can endure a given demand. This kind of endurance is cardiovascular endurance. The heart is a muscle, and it, like your other muscles, can respond to repeated demands by becoming larger and stronger. Exercise of the cardiovascular system, then, improves all muscles: not just those you can control, but also the heart muscle, the muscles of glands that eject their secretions, and the muscles in the walls of arteries and the digestive tract.

Components of fitness:
  Flexibility.
  Muscle strength.
  Muscle endurance.
  Cardiovascular endurance.

The muscles you can control consciously are the **voluntary muscles**. The muscles of the internal organs, including the heart, are the **involuntary muscles**.

Cardiovascular conditioning:

- Increased blood volume and oxygen delivery.
- Increased heart strength and **stroke volume**.
- Slowed resting pulse.
- Increased breathing efficiency.
- Improved circulation.
- Reduced blood pressure.
- Firming of muscles throughout the body.

Cardiovascular conditioning requires aerobic exercise, as described on page 115.

FIGURE 6–1   Delivery of Oxygen by the Heart and Lungs to the Muscles

The more fit a muscle is, the more oxygen it draws from the blood. That oxygen has to be drawn from the lungs, so the person with more fit muscles extracts from the inhaled air more oxygen than a person with less fit muscles. Researchers can measure cardiovascular fitness by measuring the maximum amount of oxygen a person can consume per minute while working out, a measure called the VO_2 max.

The improvements from workouts that call for cardiovascular endurance are called cardiovascular **conditioning**, part of the **training effect**. The total blood volume increases, so the blood can carry more oxygen. The heart muscle becomes stronger and larger, each beat pumps more blood, fewer beats are necessary, and the pulse rate falls. The muscles that work the lungs gain strength and endurance, and breathing becomes more efficient. Blood moves easily through the body's arteries and veins and the blood pressure falls. Muscles throughout the body become firmer. Figure 6–1 shows major relationships among the heart, circulatory system, and lungs. Cardiovascular endurance is the physical achievement that many people rightly prize the most highly, because it reflects a healthy heart and circulatory system and a generally healthy body.

To see if you have a heartbeat rate consistent with cardiovascular fitness, you may want to take your pulse right now. As a rule of thumb, the average resting pulse rate for adults is around 70 beats per minute, but the rate can be higher or lower. Active people can have resting pulse rates of 50 or even lower. Instructions for taking your pulse are given in Figure 6–2 on page 110.

You can get an estimate of your activity level by answering the questions in this chapter's Life Choice Inventory. Tests that require physical activity would reveal more about your body's condition, and if you were to have measurements taken by a professional, you would obtain an accurate estimate of your fitness.

STRATEGIES FOR IMPROVING FITNESS

This section is addressed to you, although it may not apply to you right now. Some people are already exercising, some are just now ready to start, and some may make the choice in the future. The information here is available whenever you are ready to use it.

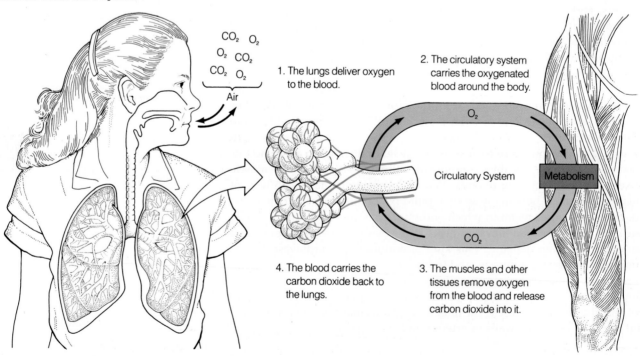

CO_2 O_2
O_2 CO_2
CO_2 O_2

Air

1. The lungs deliver oxygen to the blood.

2. The circulatory system carries the oxygenated blood around the body.

O_2

Circulatory System   Metabolism

CO_2

4. The blood carries the carbon dioxide back to the lungs.

3. The muscles and other tissues remove oxygen from the blood and release carbon dioxide into it.

LIFE CHOICE INVENTORY

How physically active are you? For each question answered yes, give yourself the number of points indicated. Then total your points to determine your score.

Occupation and Daily Activities

1. I usually walk to and from work or shopping (at least 1/2 mile each way).   1 point
2. I usually take the stairs rather than use elevators or escalators.   1 point
3. The type of physical activity involved in my job or daily household routine is best described by the following statement (select one):
   a. Most of my day is spent in office work, light physical activity, or household chores.   0 points
   b. Most of my work day is spent in farm activities, moderate physical activity, brisk walking, or comparable activities.   4 points
   c. My typical work day includes several hours of heavy physical activity (shoveling, lifting, etc.).   9 points

Leisure Activities

4. I do several hours of gardening or lawn work each week.   1 point
5. I fish or hunt once a week or more on the average. (Fishing must include active work, such as rowing a boat. Dock sitting doesn't count.)   1 point
6. At least once a week, I participate for an hour or more in vigorous dancing, such as square or folk dancing.   1 point
7. In season, I play golf at least once a week, and I do not use a power cart.   2 points

8. I often walk for exercise or recreation.   1 point
9. When I feel bothered by pressures at work or home, I use exercise as a way to relax.   1 point
10. Two or more times a week, I perform calisthenic exercises (sit-ups, push-ups) for at least ten minutes per session.   3 points
11. I regularly participate in yoga or perform stretching exercises.   2 points
12. I participate in active recreational sports such as tennis or handball:
    a. About once a week.   2 points
    b. About twice a week.   4 points
    c. Three times a week or more.   7 points
13. At least once a week, I participate in vigorous fitness activities like jogging or swimming (at least 20 continuous minutes per session):
    a. About once a week.   3 points
    b. About twice a week.   5 points
    c. Three times a week or more.   10 points

Total points earned _____

Scoring:

0 to 5 points—inactive. This amount of exercise leads to a steady deterioration in fitness. Improvement needed.

6 to 11 points—moderately active. This amount slows fitness loss but will not maintain fitness in most persons.

12 to 20 points—active. This amount will maintain an acceptable level of physical fitness.

21 points or over—very active. This amount of activity will maintain a high state of physical fitness.

SOURCE: Adapted with permission of Russell Pate (University of South Carolina, Human Performance Laboratory).

Whether you want to excel in a sport or simply achieve fitness, the goal in the physiologist's terms is to attain physical conditioning. Conditioning is the microscopic nuts and bolts of fitness, entailing a multitude of adaptations that cells make to promote the work that training demands of them. The sections that follow show both the training methods and the conditioning that results.

First, though, make sure it is safe to begin. If you have ever been told that you have a health problem of any kind, you would be wise to first consult an exercise physiologist or a health care provider trained in fitness. It is prudent to seek an **exercise stress test** before proceeding with a new

FIGURE 6–2 How to Take Your Pulse

Get a watch or clock with a second hand. Rest a few minutes for a resting pulse. Place your hand over your heart or your finger firmly over an artery in any pulse location that gives a clear rhythm. Start counting your pulse at a convenient second and continue counting for 10 seconds. If a heartbeat occurs exactly on the tenth second, count it as one-half beat. Multiply by 6 to obtain the beats per minute. To ensure a true count:

■ Use only fingers, not your thumb, on the pulse point (the thumb has a pulse of its own).

■ Press just firmly enough to feel the pulse. Too much pressure can interfere with the pulse rhythm.

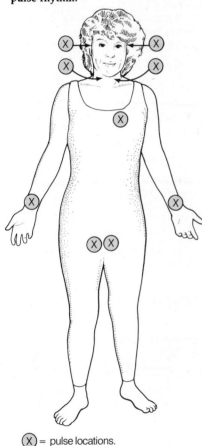

X = pulse locations.

high-PER-tro-fee

AT-ro-fee

Aerobic means "requiring oxygen." *Anaerobic* means "not requiring oxygen."

plan for exercise, particularly for those over 35 years of age and those who have been sedentary for several previous years. That way, you won't have to rely on symptoms that might not appear promptly enough to warn you of impending injury. If during exercise, you notice *any* change in comfort or experience pain, stop exercising and consult a health care provider before continuing.

The rest of this chapter assumes your exercise program will go well. Chapter 14 discusses preventing sports injuries and heat stroke.

First Facts

Every day your body works. The stronger and more fit you are, the less you must strain to do that work. If your body is weak, you can't trade it in as you might trade in a car too small to do its job, but fortunately, you don't need to. Unlike a small car, which will break down when consistently overloaded, your body responds to **overload** in a positive way—it gets itself into better shape to meet the demand next time.

Don't do too much too soon, though. It doesn't make sense to start a lifelong fitness program with activities so demanding that pain stops you within two days. Learn to enjoy the small steps along the way, because fitness builds slowly.

You have to overwork just a little. When you push yourself beyond the normal level of demand, you break down body tissue ever so slightly, so that immediately following exercise, your condition is actually at a slightly lower level than before. But not for long: in 24 to 48 hours, nature not only repairs the slight injuries but also builds extra tissue to a point that makes the body better conditioned than it was before the workout. This ensures that next time the muscles will meet a more vigorous challenge more easily.

You can apply overload in several different ways. You can do the activity more often—that is, increase its **frequency**; you can do the activity more strenuously—that is, increase its **intensity**; or you can do it for longer periods of time—that is, increase its **duration**. All three strategies work well, and you can pick one or a combination, depending on your preferences. For example, if you have little time, increase intensity. If you hate hard work, take it easy and go longer.

Fitness develops in response to demand and wanes when demand ceases—this is the **use-disuse principle**. When a muscle enlarges after being called on repeatedly to do a certain type of work, this is called muscle **hypertrophy**. When the activity is stopped for a few days, and the muscle group grows smaller and loses strength, this is called **atrophy**. Muscles also develop differently in response to different *kinds* of demands. They possess two different types of fibers—**slow-twitch muscle fibers** and **fast-twitch muscle fibers**. These are suited to two different kinds of work, **aerobic** and **anaerobic** and different ones develop, depending partly on what you ask your muscles to do.

The way your muscles develop also depends partly on your heredity. A person's athletic potential or talent is inborn, partly because every person is born with a set number of each type of fiber. In a sense, you are born to be either a sprinter or a long-distance runner. If you choose to develop your inborn capacity, you can excel at it. But even if you were not born with "the right stuff" to be a particular type of competitor, you can still choose to develop within your own limitations by choosing the right exercises. In any case, the way to begin is by understanding a few basic facts about muscle fibers and the work to which they are suited.

Metabolism during exercise requires that the muscles be supplied with three things: oxygen and the two muscle fuels, glucose and fatty acids. The lungs pass oxygen to the blood, which carries it to the muscles. The glucose used as muscle fuel comes chiefly from glycogen stored within the muscle itself, while the fatty acids come chiefly from fat stored elsewhere, delivered by the blood. Oxygen availability determines which of the two fuels will be burned. For the muscles to use the virtually unlimited supply of body fat to fuel their work, they must have ample oxygen, because the breakdown of fat is a strictly aerobic process.

The heart and lungs can provide only so much oxygen, only so fast. When the muscles' exertion is great enough that their energy demand outstrips their oxygen supply, they can no longer meet their fuel needs with fat. They must draw more on their limited supply of glucose, a fuel that can be metabolized either with or without oxygen.

During moderate exercise, your lungs and circulatory system have no trouble keeping up with the need for oxygen. You breathe deeply and easily, and your heart beats steadily. But some exercise is so demanding that you can't seem to breathe fast enough, and your heart is racing. This is when your body is building up an **oxygen debt**. You may even have to stop or at least slow down "to catch your breath" and replenish your oxygen supply. If you do, your body begins producing energy aerobically once more.

You may have heard the name of one of the waste products generated during oxygen debt: lactic acid. Its buildup causes burning pain in the muscles. A strategy for dealing with lactic acid buildup is to relax the muscles at every opportunity, so that the circulating blood can carry away the lactic acid and bring oxygen to support aerobic metabolism and reduce the oxygen debt. This is what mountaineers are doing when they relax their leg muscles at each step (the "mountain rest step").

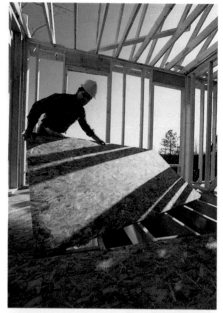

Work that requires physical activity helps build fitness.

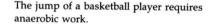

Muscles need oxygen to burn fat.
Muscles can use glucose as fuel either with or without oxygen.

The jump of a basketball player requires anaerobic work.

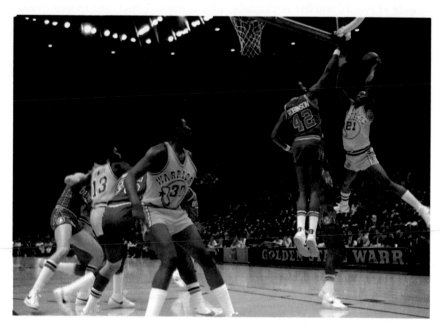

These go together:
    Muscle fibers—fast-twitch.*
    Fuel—glucose.
    Metabolism—anaerobic.
    Exercise—high-intensity, short-duration.
These go together:
    Muscle fibers—slow-twitch.*
    Fuel—fat.
    Metabolism—aerobic.
    Exercise—lower-intensity, longer-duration.

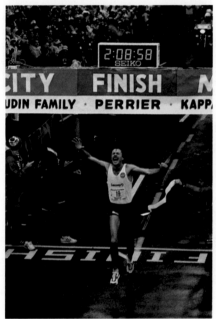

Running a marathon is mostly aerobic work.

High-intensity, short-duration activity depends mostly on fast-twitch muscle fibers and on glucose to provide energy anaerobically. Lower-intensity, longer-duration activity depends more on slow-twitch muscle fibers and on fat to provide energy aerobically.

Imagine a track meet. A sprinter bursts across the starting line in an explosion of energy. The burst lasts only a few seconds, followed by exhaustion at the finish line. Now envision a distance runner on an endless stretch of beach. The runner's steady stride has paced off miles of sand with only slight changes in speed, maximizing the distance covered.

The sprinter is engaging in mostly anaerobic activity. This activity is associated with strength, agility, and split-second surges of power. The jump of the basketball player, the slam of the tennis serve, the weight lifter's heave at the barbells, and the fullback's blast through the opposing line are all anaerobic work.

The distance runner is engaging in largely aerobic work. This work is associated with endurance. The ability to continue swimming until you reach the far bank, to continue hiking until you're at the camp, or to continue pedaling until you're home all reflect aerobic capacity. This capacity is also the crucial link to improving the health of the heart and circulatory system.

You can develop your body for different kinds of activities by choosing the right exercises. If you want to lift weights, you need to know that muscles develop anaerobic capacity best by working as hard as they can until they can go no further—that is, by working to exhaustion. Of course, you can't keep this kind of activity going for very long, but you don't have to. Just center your fitness program on weight work, progressively increasing the poundage. If you want to run, bike, or swim long distances, then aerobic capacity is your goal, and you should emphasize activities in which your breathing and heartbeat work steadily at an increased rate. This advice doesn't imply that you should concentrate solely on one type of exercise at the expense of the others, but only that you can tailor your program to achieve the results you want.

The overload principle applies equally to all aspects of fitness: flexibility, muscle strength, muscle endurance, and cardiovascular endurance. It also applies to other body systems. For example, to develop a strong, dense skeletal system, you must start by demanding that the bones bear slightly more stress (through weight-bearing exercises such as walking, running, or jumping) than they are used to. The bones respond by depositing more minerals. Eventually, a maximum is reached. People can develop their body systems to an amazing extent by increasing overload progressively. The elite athletes of today have done this.

When you are increasing your overload, remember to exercise to an intensity that only *slightly* injures tissues. It is better to progress too slowly than to risk serious injury by overexertion.[14] Allow enough, but not too much, time for recovery (at least, but not more than, 24 to 48 hours).

Other pointers:

■ Exercise regularly.
■ Train hard only once or twice a week, not every time you work out. Between times, do light workouts and plan for rest.

*Fast and slow twitch are the two best known of muscle fiber types. There are others.

■ Listen to your body and cooperate. If you feel energetic, work hard; but if you are tired or in pain, go lightly or stop, even if that wasn't in your plan.

Warm-up and Cool-down Activities

The body needs fair warning of exercise ahead. A warm-up activity increases blood flow to muscles and begins the hormonal changes that will liberate the needed fuels from storage. Heat produced by the activity warms the muscles and connective tissues, permitting them to stretch without tearing.

To warm up, some people use a brisk walk or light jog, followed by a stretching routine. Another strategy is to do a light version of what you plan to do intensively later. A runner may start out walking; break into a jog; and finally, when it feels right, pick up the pace to an outright run. A person who body builds may start with light weight repetitions; a tennis player, with a few lobs. Fitness experts think this strategy best prepares the main muscle groups required for the task ahead.

Cool-down activity eases the transition from exercising to normal functioning. A few minutes of light activity facilitates the relaxation of tight muscles and enhances the circulation of blood through them. It may also help prevent the dizziness that you may experience if you abruptly stop exercising.[15]

Gaining Flexibility

Flexibility is the easiest of all fitness components to improve and retain. Stretching exercises condition **muscles**, **tendons**, **cartilage**, and **ligaments** to greater tensile strength and elasticity (see Figure 6–3, page 114). A caution about stretching: your goal is to get limber, not to be a contortionist. (Observe a cat stretching, and notice the technique—the stretch is long and luxurious, a few moments of pure pleasure.) Do easy stretches, and only to the point of resistance.[16]

Do not bounce or push: overstretching may do permanent damage. A ligament may never regain its original elasticity once it is overstretched or torn; it can no longer support its joint, and the joint may become prone to injury. Nerves can overstretch painfully, too, if you are only slightly too enthusiastic. To get a full stretch, relax the muscles, allow the body part to move slowly through its full *range of motion*, and hold each stretch position for 10 seconds to begin with. Breathe normally; don't bounce. To improve, add 2 seconds to the time you hold each stretch until you can hold each for 30 seconds. Choose stretches that work all the major body regions: the neck, the shoulders, all back regions, pelvic regions, thighs (inner, front, and back), calf muscles, and ankles.

Developing Muscle Strength and Endurance

Two ways to gain muscle strength and endurance are **weight training** and **calisthenics**. Weight training is the most efficient way. Weight training strengthens muscles, tendons, ligaments, and bones so that they better protect the body's internal organs from injury. Appearance and muscle tone improve, and performance of practically all tasks becomes easier. Typically, weight training has been portrayed as a man's workout technique, but in

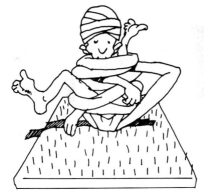

A stretch is long and luxurious, a few moments of pure pleasure.

CHAPTER 6 ■ FITNESS

113

FIGURE 6–3 Muscles, Tendons, Ligaments, and Cartilage

As a muscle contracts, it pulls the two bones to which it is attached closer together, creating movement. Joints can bend, and muscles, tendons, and ligaments can stretch, but each has its limits.

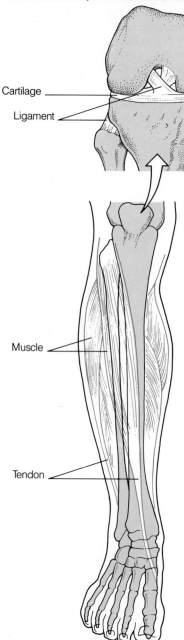

Cartilage

Ligament

Muscle

Tendon

reality it is ideal for both men and women. It need not produce big, bulky muscles, except in people who follow programs specifically designed to do just that. Nor does it produce muscle-bound inflexibility; that results from omission of flexibility training.

Do not hold your breath when you work with weights; it puts pressure on the heart and lungs and can damage them. Exhale as you raise or push the weight away (a way to remember is to "blow the weight away from you"), and inhale as you lower it. Also, raise and lower the weight smoothly. Jerking it up or letting gravity pull it down fails to improve strength and threatens to injure your joints. To develop maximum strength from the smallest number of repetitions, lower the weight especially slowly.[17] A complete group of ten repetitions of a particular exercise should take about a minute. Such a group of repetitions is called a **set**. Performing many sets with lighter weights mostly increases endurance, while doing fewer with heavier weights favors strength.

Small muscles fatigue quickly and can hinder your continuing the workout, so strengthen the larger muscle groups first, then the smaller ones. Make sure to distribute the weight work equally over the arms and legs, both sides—all the muscles. Overdeveloped muscles in one part of the body can stress other, weaker parts and cause damage. Weights can also be dangerous. Anyone who wishes to include weight training in a fitness program should seek guidance from a professional trainer; employees of spas and gyms may be unreliable sources.

Parts of your own body, working against gravity, can provide the same resistance as weights. Calisthenics are a series of exercises that use the body parts as weights to develop strength and endurance. Each repetition of a calisthenic exercise is easy, so improvement results from increasing the number of repetitions, the speed of performance, and the duration of the workout.

Gaining Cardiovascular Endurance

Professional athletes surround their endurance training with technical trappings like stopwatches and pulses. You don't have to get tangled up in all this. You can just go out and walk fast or run. A guideline for the fitness-minded who do not aspire to the Olympics is to do the exercise for 20 minutes at a rate at which you can talk but not sing; if you can sing, speed it up. The guidelines that follow are addressed to the athlete; you can modify them for your training.

To improve cardiovascular fitness, you must work up to a point where you can exercise aerobically for 20 minutes or more. This means you must elevate your heart rate (pulse) for 20 minutes or more. This heart rate must be considerably faster than the resting rate to "push" the heart, but not so fast as to strain it. Your **target heart rate** can be calculated from your age. The older you are, the lower your maximum heart rate. (But that's OK, because you can achieve improvement from working at a lower target heart rate.) As cardiovascular fitness improves, more intense exercise will be required to reach the same target rate. To calculate your target heart rate:

1. *Find your resting heart rate* (pulse) as described on page 110.
2. *Estimate your maximum heart rate*. Subtract your age from 220. This furnishes an estimate of the absolute maximum heart rate possible for a person your age. You should never exercise at this rate, of course.

3. *Locate your target heart rate.* Subtract your resting heart rate from your maximum heart rate. Multiply this figure by 60 percent, and add it to your resting heart rate.

When you can work out at the target heart rate for 20 to 30 minutes, you know that you have arrived at your fitness goal. In the building-up stage, you can make progress by using a pattern called **interval training**. A jogger might run at the target heart rate for 2 minutes before tiring, then rest by walking until ready to jog again, run another 2 minutes, then rest by walking, and so on for 20 minutes. At each session the jogger can make the running periods longer and the resting periods shorter. Eventually, in a few weeks or months, the rest periods will no longer be needed at all. Once you have worked up to that, you can maintain your level of fitness by repeating the workout about every other day. If you want to improve further, you can gradually raise your target heart rate, but seek professional advice before you do so.[18]

You will best develop cardiovascular fitness if you choose an activity that:

■ Is steady and constant.
■ Uses large muscle groups, such as legs, buttocks, and abdomen. If you move 50 percent of your muscle mass, the activity is aerobic.
■ Is uninterrupted and lasts for more than twenty minutes.

If you had to choose just one type of fitness to develop, you would do well to make it cardiovascular endurance, because it is the most basic to health and life. In fact, cardiovascular conditioning is all that some exercise specialists recommend. That has given some people the idea that 20 to 30 minutes of exercise every other day is all they need for fitness. It is not: it is all they need for the cardiovascular component of fitness.

Whether you spend 2 hours a day or 45 minutes every other day on fitness, you will want to allocate your efforts to the various components according to your goals. One ambitious person, whose goal is overall fitness, allocates 45 minutes several days a week as shown in the margin. Someone wanting more cardiovascular fitness might spend more time in activities at the target heart rate; if more muscle strength is the goal, then additional or more intense weight work is in order.

Occasionally, you may hear an expert state that 30 minutes *a week* or just a few minutes a day is plenty of exercise for the average adult. Indeed, there are a few individuals who have the genetic disposition to be healthy no matter what they do, and for these few, the advice is probably applicable. For most people, though, it is not. A well-conditioned body costs time and effort. It is true, though, that once a person builds fitness, less effort is required to maintain it, and at least some of the benefits persist for as long as six weeks during periods of inactivity.[19]

Special Circumstances

Sometimes circumstances make physical activity seem nearly impossible. Factors such as overweight, pregnancy, physical handicaps, arthritis, or the like can place the conventional get-up-and-run routines out of reach. But people in these circumstances need fitness *more* than other people, not less; a strong body and an active mind are essential to meet the challenges they face. People who have confronted limitations have developed excellent, if unconventional, activity programs to keep fit nevertheless.

Example: David Williams, age 25.
Resting heart rate = 62 beats per minute.
Maximum heart rate = 220 − 25 = 195.
Difference = 195 − 62 = 133.
60% of difference = 0.60 x 133 = 80 (rounded off).
Target heart rate = 62 + 80 = 142 beats per minute.

Some activities that will allow you to reach and sustain your target heart rate are:

Swimming.	Soccer.
Fast walking.	Hockey.
Jogging.	Basketball.
Bicycling.	Water polo.
Stair walking.	Lacrosse.
Rope jumping.	Rugby.
Aerobic dance.	

Sample fitness program, 45 minutes a day:
Monday, Friday:
10 minutes of stretching.
25 minutes of jogging.
10 minutes of calisthenics.
Tuesday, Thursday:
10 minutes of stretching.
25 minutes of weight training.
10 minutes of calisthenics.
Wednesday:
Rest.
Saturday:
Softball, walking, hiking, biking, or swimming.
Sunday:
Rest.

You can find out more about exercise during pregnancy in Chapter 12.

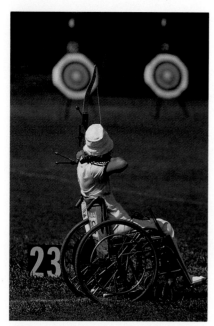
Circumstances need not deprive anyone of fitness.

Swimming is well suited to many people's needs. Joints that on land are stressed by the body's weight work well when weight is supported by water. For example, people who are overweight or pregnant can swim more safely than they can run, and they find it less exhausting, too.

People who are blind, deaf, or confined to wheelchairs climb mountains, swim, ski, play basketball, and engage in other activities tailored to their limitations. People who have had heart attacks can do special exercises and work up from one level to the next as they recover. Mentally handicapped people, too, can compete in sports at the community, state, national, and international levels through the Special Olympics. Fitness is important for everybody—don't let circumstances deprive you of it unnecessarily.

Dealing with Discouragement

The progress to fitness is not without setbacks. Today's workout may go well, but tomorrow's may be rocky. Irregular progress can discourage a person who doesn't expect it. Setbacks usually occur just before higher levels of fitness are achieved. A setback is not a time to give up; it is a time to celebrate impending success. If a workout goes badly, skip a day, or do a different workout.

Adopt appropriate expectations for your own performance. No one just starting out measures up to the standards of seasoned athletes. Standards are only a point of reference, usually somewhere in the middle of a range (there are as many people below them as above them). In the early stages of adopting an exercise habit, it helps to use your imagination to picture yourself performing well.

Other deterrents include bad weather, depression, loneliness, boredom, busy schedules, soreness, and lack of rewards. The following strategies may help:

- In bad weather, play racquetball or another indoor sport.
- If lonely or depressed, call a friend to go with you.
- If busy, remember that increased vigor will maximize your use of time.
- If sore, enjoy each ache as a badge of courage (and be gentler next time).
- If not encouraged by others, buy yourself a new sweatband or similar type of item to strengthen your identity as "one who does."

Other aids to overcoming discouragement: keep track of your progress to show where you started and how far you've come. Use positive self-talk: instead of "I'm too busy to exercise today," say, "I have to budget my time skillfully to plan for exercise today." The more positive thoughts you include, the better your chances of stamping out the negatives. Tell people about your exercise plan, and get them involved; or get involved with those who already exercise. Write a contract with yourself to accomplish specific goals. But don't hold yourself to a certain number of hours per week or a certain pace per mile; improvement over your previous level is enough. See this chapter's Strategies box for ways of including exercise in your day.

FOOD FOR FITNESS

Fitness and nutrition are tightly linked. People interested in fitness ask many questions about diet. They hear conflicting claims from different sources—popular books and magazines, athletes, health-food and supplement peddlers. Different people will recommend a high-protein diet, a high-carbohydrate diet, muscle-building powders or drinks, vitamin pills, and "energy-giving" foods. To distinguish fact from fiction, when you hear these claims, consider where the facts came from. Generally, you'll get the most valid information from an informant who has taken college or even graduate-school courses in the science of nutrition. Here, we attempt to sort the facts from the fantasies.[20]

Fuel for Muscles

Fit people have more muscle mass; exercise uses muscles; muscles are made largely of protein. It would seem, then, that to get fit, you might need more protein than normal. Muscular, active people do use more protein, both to build muscles and to fuel their activities, than others, but most people's diets contain about twice as much protein as they can possibly use, no matter how muscular or active they are. They are actually using about half the protein they eat, not to build body protein, but rather for energy.

That a claim has been made many times doesn't make it true.

Many athletes take protein powders because sellers and others say that extra protein will boost their muscle power. In reality, athletes usually lack nutrients found in vegetables, not protein. A head of broccoli would probably supply many more of the nutrients the athlete's muscles really need, but people—misguided or deceptive—continue to recommend protein powders, the more profitable product.

Even though the muscle-power claim for protein has been made many times, it is not true. Some health claims may appear to have been confirmed just because they have been repeated many times, but they have not been scientifically validated.

FIGURE 6–4 Fuels Used by the Muscles During Exercise

Exercise of high intensity requires more glycogen per minute than does exercise of lower intensity.

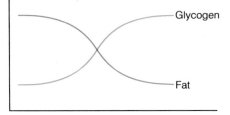

Increasing intensity of exercise

Even when muscles are adding protein to their mass, you can't force extra protein into them just by eating more of it. Cells don't respond to what is given to them by simply accepting it. They respond to the hormones that regulate them and to the demands put on them, and they select the nutrients they need from what is offered. The way to make muscles grow is to put a demand on them—that is, to make them work.

Men develop bulkier muscles in response to exercise than do women, because men produce larger amounts of certain **steroid hormones** in their bodies. Some people, both men and women, dose themselves with added steroid hormones in the attempt to grow bulkier muscles. This is a hazardous practice (see accompanying box).[21]

Exercising muscles do use a little extra protein for fuel (less than 10 percent of the total). Thus, the protein recommendation for athletes is slightly higher than the recommendation for sedentary people. Most people eat much more protein than even the amount recommended for athletes, so the wise athlete limits servings of protein-rich foods (which are also high in fat) and chooses more of the carbohydrate-rich foods to supply extra energy for exercise.

During times of intensive anaerobic work, such as sprinting or heavy weight lifting, muscles use mostly carbohydrate (glycogen) from stores saved during times of rest. When energy is needed to fuel long-term, low-intensity exercise, such as jogging, walking or swimming, the body wisely draws more on its most abundant fuel—fat. Figure 6–4 shows that muscles use more carbohydrate during high-intensity exercise and more fat during low-intensity exercise.

Competitors in long-distance endurance events need to have energy available to their muscles as long as possible. Unlimited energy is available from body fat stores, but glycogen energy is limited to the amount stored in the liver and muscles themselves, and glycogen is the limiting factor. Athletes' muscles use fat to the extent they are able to, but they need glycogen, too, especially for high-intensity sprints, especially at the end of the race. As Chapter 4 explained, glycogen has to be replenished periodically by eating carbohydrate. For the endurance athlete (and, in fact, for all athletes), a high-carbohydrate diet is therefore the best choice. Physical endurance is hampered by a high-fat, high-protein diet but enhanced by a high-carbohydrate diet, as Figure 6–5 demonstrates.[22]

A technique of tricking the muscles into storing extra glycogen is **glycogen loading**. When the technique was first introduced, it was found to produce side effects, including abnormal heartbeat; swollen, painful muscles (glycogen attracts and holds water); and weight gain immediately before com-

Steroid Drugs and Athletics

Some athletes self-administer steroid and other drugs in an attempt to gain extra muscle mass.* Indeed, some athletes reap improved strength, but others reap only health risks. Only a little more than half the research has found strength improvements attributable to the drugs, whereas the rest has shown no improvement beyond that attained with placebos. No extra aerobic capacity can be gained by drug use.

Steroid drug use produces a dilemma: athletes who are not superstar material genetically and who normally could not break into the elite ranks are, by using steroids, increasing the competition for the champions. Challenged by artifically endowed opponents, the champions may feel compelled to use the drugs themselves. Especially in professional athletics, where monetary rewards can be enormous, steroid use is common. In the 1980s, steroid use among national and world-class athletes was estimated at between 80 and 100 percent.

Steroid abuse is not safe. It brings a sharp change in blood lipids of the type associated with high risk of heart disease. Steroids also cause impaired liver function, permanent changes in the reproductive system, and altered facial appearance. Further, athletes who take human growth hormone develop symptoms of the disease **acromegaly**. Only a few users suffer the deadly effects but some of the side effects occur in all users. Testicular shrinkage in men and masculinization of women are inevitable. What may result from 20 years of abuse is unknown.

*The drugs most often taken by athletes are androgenic anabolic steroids (testosterone and its synthetic analogs), human growth hormone (and its synthetic analog), and human chorionic gonadotropin.

petition. The plan now recommended confers benefits but not hazards. To safely load glycogen, the athlete exercises intensely while eating a normal diet, then, the day before competetion, cuts back on exercise and eats a very high carbohydrate diet. Marathon racers who do this can keep going longer than their competitors. In the heat, extra glycogen confers an additional advantage, because as it breaks down, it releases water, which helps to meet the athlete's fluid needs.[23]

Active people need more food energy. By eating the extra calories they need from carbohydrate sources, they avoid having to use food protein for energy

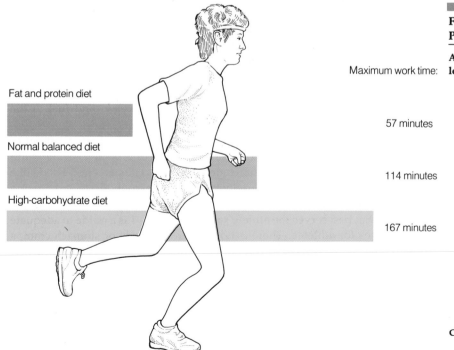

Fat and protein diet

Normal balanced diet

High-carbohydrate diet

Maximum work time:

57 minutes

114 minutes

167 minutes

FIGURE 6–5 The Effect of Diet on Physical Endurance

A high-carbohydrate diet can triple an athlete's endurance.

and can use it instead to replace lost muscle protein. With so much extra energy metabolism going on, they need adequate vitamins and minerals to make it all happen. To increase food energy intake, therefore, an active person shouldn't rely on just any high-calorie food, but should choose foods rich in nutrients as well—breads, cereals, fruits, vegetables, milk, and others.

Food and Fluid Needs

Before a competitive event, is there any special way that a person should eat? Many coaches and athletes believe intensely in special food rituals. Coach Casy's basketball team can't play without breakfasting first on T-bones. Coach David's swim team is forbidden milk at the meet because it "causes cotton mouth." Bicyclist Kara takes two tablespoons of honey before the race and savors the sweet on her tongue as she pedals away. Do these rituals work?

Scientifically, no particular food confers a special benefit before an athletic contest, but particular kinds of food make a difference. A meal of steak may boost morale, but it is high in fat and may take so long to digest that it hinders performance. The idea that milk causes cotton mouth is pure superstition. Honey demands water from the blood to dilute it, a handicap during exertion. Research on runners shows that a sugar drink taken directly before exercise can *reduce* athletic endurance by 25 percent.[24] In summary, some rituals have little effect, and some can impair performance. If a harmless but scientifically unproved practice gives a competitor a morale boost or extra confidence, it can make the difference between winning and losing and so should be respected. However, no foods have unusual power to promote performance.

Does it matter at all what the meal before an event consists of? Olympic training tables are laden with breads, pasta, rice, potatoes, and fruit juice. These are wise choices, for three reasons. They are high in carbohydrate—the fuel the athlete needs to store before the event. They are low in fat and protein, which would stay in the digestive tract too long. And they are low in fiber. Fiber is normally highly desirable, but not in the hours before physical exertion, because it remains in the digestive tract and attracts water out of the blood. Any meal or snack should be finished at least three or four hours before the event, because digestion requires routing the blood supply to the digestive tract to pick up nutrients. By the time the contest begins, the circulating blood should be available to carry oxygen and fuel to the muscles instead.

Fluid balance is crucial to successful performance. The first symptom of dehydration is fatigue. A rapid water loss equal to 5 percent of the body weight can reduce muscular work capacity by 20 to 30 percent.[25] Foods like gelatin, juices, and popsicles all deliver fluid with carbohydrate and are fine several hours before the event; after that time, plain, cold water is the beverage that best serves the athlete's needs. Table 6–1 is a guide to adequate fluid intakes for athletes. There is no danger of muscle or stomach cramps due to fluid intake before, during, or after an event, but salts are lost when fluid is lost through sweating. Salt replacement need not be immediate and should not be by way of salt tablets (even if they've been given the scientific-sounding name "electrolyte pills"). A person can sweat away as much as nine pounds of fluid and still perform well without salt supplements, provided he or she drinks enough water. A rule of thumb is to drink two cups

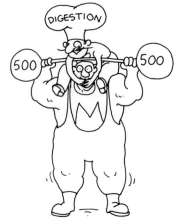

Digestion interferes with muscle work.

TABLE 6–1 Schedule of Hydration Before and During Exercise

When To Drink	Amount of Fluid
2 hours before exercise	About 3 c
10 or 15 minutes before exercise	About 2 c
Every 10 to 20 minutes during exercise	About 1/2 c or more
After exercise	Replace each pound of body weight lost with 2 c fluid

SOURCE: Adapted from J. B. Marcus, ed., *Sports Nutrition* (Chicago: American Dietetic Association, 1986), p. 57.

of water for every pound of body weight lost. When the event is over, eating regular food will reestablish salt balance.

Exercise works in harmony with all the other life management skills. It aids in stress management: the stress response readies the body for exercise, and exercise discharges the tension. It promotes emotional health physically, by improving the chemistry of the brain and circulation to it, and psychologically, by enhancing self-esteem. Hand in hand with nutrition, exercise renews and nourishes every body part. Spiritually, play contributes joy.

Your health is worth the time and energy it takes to include exercise in your day. Jog, play a game, ride a bike. Hike with friends. You work hard every day—you deserve a break every day, too. Go have fun.

▬ STUDY AIDS

1. List the benefits of keeping the body physically fit through regular exercise.
2. Describe the components of fitness.
3. List and describe the body improvements associated with cardiovascular conditioning.
4. Define the terms *overload* and *use-disuse* principle, and explain how they relate to physical fitness.
5. Describe the relationship of oxygen debt to lactic acid buildup.
6. Identify the types of exercises that would best develop each of the following: (a) flexibility, (b) muscle strength, (c) muscle endurance, and (d) cardiovascular endurance.
7. Describe fitness strategies suited to the special needs of people in atypical circumstances.
8. Describe how the availability of muscle fuels affects performance.
9. Describe the characteristics of the kind of diet that would best support athletic performance.

▬ GLOSSARY

acromegaly (ack-ro-MEG-a-lee): a disease caused by steroid hormone use, characterized by huge body size, widened jawline and nose, protruding brow and teeth, and an increased risk of death before age 50.

aerobic (air-ROE-bic): refers to processes using oxygen. Aerobic exercise is exercise performed at an intensity that places a sustained demand on the cardiovascular system; it speeds up breathing and heartbeat. Aerobic metabolism is that part of energy nutrient breakdown that requires oxygen for completion, such as the metabolism of fat.

 aero = air

anaerobic (AN-air-ROE-bic): refers to processes that do not use oxygen. Anaerobic exercise involves sudden, all-out exertions of muscles. Anaerobic metabolism is that part of energy nutrient metabolism that can take place without oxygen; for example, the first steps in the breakdown of glucose.

 an = without

atrophy (AT-ro-fee): a decrease in size due to lack of use.

calisthenics: exercise routines for muscular development that use the weight of the body as resistance.

 kallos = beautiful
 sthenos = strength

cardiovascular endurance: a component of fitness, the ability of the cardiovascular system to sustain effort over a long time.

cartilage: see Figure 6-3.

conditioning: the physical effects of training.

duration: length of time (for example, the length of time spent in each exercise session).

elasticity: the characteristic of being easily stretched or bent and able to return to original size and shape.

endurance: a component of fitness, the ability to sustain an effort for a long time.

exercise stress test: a test that monitors heart function during exercise to detect abnormalities that may not show up under ordinary conditions; exercise physiologists and trained health care professionals can administer the test.

fast-twitch muscle fibers: muscle fibers that use mostly glucose for fuel to perform high-intensity, short-duration work.

fitness: the body's ability to meet physical demands, composed of four components: flexibility, muscle strength, muscle endurance, and cardiovascular endurance.

flexibility: a component of fitness, the ability to bend without injury; it depends on the elasticity of muscles, tendons, and ligaments and on the condition of the joints.

frequency: the number of occurrences per unit of time (for example, the number of exercise sessions per week).

glycogen loading: a technique that forces muscles to store glycogen beyond their normal limits.

hypertrophy (high-PER-tro-fee): an increase in size in response to use.

intensity: degree (for example, degree of exertion while exercising).

interval training: a pattern for aerobic conditioning that involves exercising for longer and longer periods of time at the target heart rate with breaks between.

involuntary muscles: the muscles of the internal organs, not under conscious control; for example, those of the digestive tract or the arteries. These muscles are sometimes called the *smooth muscles*.

ligament: see Figure 6-3.

MOC (maximum oxygen consumption): see *VO₂ max*.

muscle: see Figure 6-3.

muscle endurance: the ability of a muscle to contract repeatedly within a given time without becoming exhausted.

overload: an extra physical demand placed on the body; an increase in the frequency, duration, or intensity of exercise. The *progressive overload principle* is the training principle that a body system, to improve, must be worked at frequencies, durations, or intensities that increase by increments over time.

oxygen debt: a deficit of oxygen built up by a body performing exercise so demanding that the circulation cannot bring oxygen to the muscles fast enough; it must be repaid by rapid breathing after the activity slows down or stops.

set: a specific number (for example, of times to repeat a weight-training exercise).

slow-twitch muscle fibers: muscle fibers that use mostly fat for fuel and require large amounts of oxygen to perform low-intensity, long-duration activities.

smooth muscles: see *involuntary muscles*.

steroid hormones: hormones of a certain chemical type (similar to the lipid cholesterol). In athletics, the sex hormones that build muscle bulkiness in response to exercise.

strength: a component of fitness; refers to the ability of muscles to work against resistance.

striated muscles: see *voluntary muscles*.

stroke volume: the amount of oxygenated blood ejected by the heart toward the tissues at each beat.

target heart rate: the heartbeat rate that will achieve cardiovascular conditioning for a person—fast enough to push the heart, but not so fast as to strain it.

tendon: see Figure 6-3.

training effect: the desired physiological changes that occur in the body in response to exercise.

use-disuse principle: the principle that fitness develops in response to demand and diminishes in response to the lack of demand.

VO₂ max: the maximum volume of oxygen that a person can consume during a minute of heavy work; a measure of cardiovascular and muscular fitness. Also called *MOC (maximum oxygen consumption)*.

voluntary muscles: the muscles under control of the conscious mind, such as the major muscles of the limbs. These muscles are called the *striated muscles*.

weight training: exercise routines for muscular development that employ mechanical devices or weights to provide resistance against which the muscles can work.

◼ QUIZ ANSWERS

1. *False.* Although an extreme and sudden exertion *can* damage the body, a gradual increase in overload will produce a strengthened body.

2. *False.* Stroke volume is the amount of blood pumped by one beat of the heart.

3. *False.* Weights do offer resistance, but so does gravity; calisthenics are designed to promote strength by using only the body's own weight against gravity.

4. *False.* You may aggravate an injury while running.

5. *False.* You need water, not salt. As for minerals, it is now believed that the best way to replenish those lost in sweat is by consuming ordinary foods and beverages that contain them naturally.

6. *True.* Water is the beverage of choice to replace body fluids lost during exercise.

7. *True.* When you exercise a muscle until it is exhausted, you increase its strength.

8. *False.* A 20-minute workout every other day will maintain cardiovascular fitness but won't maintain flexibility or overall body strength.

9. *False.* The best nutrition support for fitness is an adequate, balanced, and varied diet.

10. *False.* It's best to rehydrate as you go.

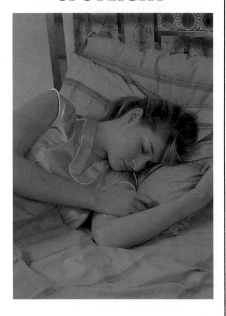

Sleep

Like fitness, sleep is indispensable to health. During sleep, people recover from physical and emotional stresses and injuries. People who regularly sleep about eight hours a night are physiologically younger than people who did not. This spotlight explores the importance of sleep and reveals what is known about its effects on health.

I've always wondered what goes on during sleep. What exactly does sleep do for me?

Oddly enough, this is the one question that may be the hardest to answer about sleep. Even though people spend a third of their lives sleeping, no one seems to know for sure what goes on during all that time. We know some of the things that happen physiologically, however: the blood pressure falls, breathing and heartbeat slow down, the muscles relax, and the body temperature falls. Perhaps most significantly, **growth hormone**, or **somatotropin**, is secreted during sleep almost exclusively—and growth hormone provides for growth and regeneration of body cells. Sleep is a time of renewal physically, as well as psychologically.

What happens to a person who doesn't get enough sleep?

No one has ever died from lack of sleep, but all systems work less and

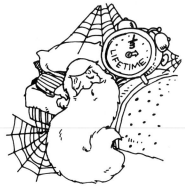

People spend a third of their lifetime sleeping.

less efficiently. People become irritable, can't concentrate, think slowly, and lose coordination. If sleep deprived long enough, people may start having hallucinations and feel that they are going insane—an observation that oppressive regimes have made use of in torturing people. Irregular sleep or chronic sleep deprivation over years can shorten life.

Does everybody need eight hours of sleep a night?

People's sleep needs vary. About 2 percent of adults habitually sleep 10 hours a night, and some even more. Children need more than 8 hours a night: babies sleep 16 hours or even more, 6-year-olds about 10 hours, most adults about 6 to 7 hours, and older adults about 6. These differences seem to reflect the rate of cell growth and replacement, which is fastest in the young and which slows throughout life. Amazingly, though, by the age of 60, you will have slept for about 20 years of your life.

Is there such a thing as beauty sleep? I've heard that an hour of sleep before midnight is worth two afterward.

There's nothing special about the hour of midnight, but it is true that early hours of sleep are "deeper" and more beneficial (more efficient, you might say) than others. You go through several predictable stages during sleep.

First, after you cross the threshold into sleep, your body temperature falls, and your brain goes into **alpha rhythm**. (The first four letters of the Greek alphabet are alpha, beta, gamma, and delta—*A*, *B*, *G*, and *D*. The brainwaves that occur during the four stages of sleep are named for them.) At this point, you may suddenly jerk half awake (the so-called **myoclonic jerk**)—the sign of a sudden burst of neural activity in your brain that heralds the beginning of stage 1 of sleep. In stage 1, your muscles relax, and your pulse slows down.

Minutes later, you enter stage 2. The brainwaves grow larger (**beta rhythm**), and your eyes roll from side to side, but if they were to open, they would not see. This lasts from about the tenth minute to about half an hour into sleep. Throughout this period, if you were awakened, you might feel that you had not had any sleep at all.

After 30 minutes, you enter stage 3 (**gamma**). Your brainwaves are large and slow, muscles are relaxed, and breathing is even. Then comes stage 4, or **delta** sleep. This is the deepest sleep of all. The longest delta periods occur early during the night's sleep.

Stage 4 sleep is interrupted, periodically, by **REM sleep** (REM stands for "rapid eye movements" and is pronounced as a single syllable, *rem*). The rapid eye movements seem to reflect dreaming, as if the person's eyes were following the actions of the dreams. During REM sleep, the heartbeat becomes irregular, the blood pressure fluctuates, and the brainwaves are characteristic of a person awake. The first REM pe-

riod lasts about ten minutes and is followed by stage 2 sleep. You cycle several times a night through REM, into stage 2, 3, and 4 sleep, and back into REM. Toward morning, stage 4 periods are shorter and REM periods longer.[1]*

That's amazing. I had no idea there was so much going on while I was asleep. What do you suppose it's all for?

We don't know, but we know that both delta and REM sleep seem to be essential to a person's well-being. People deprived of REM sleep become hostile, irritable, and anxious; people deprived of delta sleep become depressed and apathetic. When uninterrupted sleep is again possible, people who have been deprived of either type of sleep will experience longer periods of that type to "make up" for what they've missed. This is one reason why sleeping pills may actually harm people; many of them suppress these important phases of sleep.[2]

I often have difficulty sleeping. Are you saying that I shouldn't take sleeping pills?

Millions of people in the United States suffer from **insomnia** and spend tens of millions of dollars on medications to relieve it. But drugs may actually cause more sleeping problems than they solve, since they create a dependence in the user, as well as interfering with normal sleep patterns. The combination can leave a person exhausted and hooked, afraid to stop taking the pills and sleeping poorly because of them. A lot of sleep aids are quack devices, too: watch out for them.

Try, instead, to identify the cause of the insomnia, and then solve the problem—for example, try new bedding, a new schedule, get some exercise, or reduce your caffeine intake.

*Reference notes are in Appendix D.

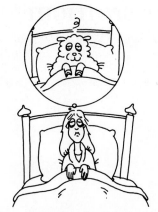

Millions of people suffer from insomnia.

Don't take an alcoholic "nightcap," though. Alcohol causes dangerous alterations in breathing during sleep.[3]

I've heard of a nutrient you can take to make yourself go to sleep—tryptophan. What do you know about it?

The amino acid **tryptophan**, when given in doses of 3 to 5 grams, can produce sedation and sleep in some wakeful people. The effect is thought to be the result of an increase in the neurotransmitter called serotonin (see Spotlight 3), which the brain makes from tryptophan. Serotonin is a natural sleep inducer. Neither tryptophan nor serotonin is addictive, nor does either alter sleep patterns.

Tryptophan is found in all proteins, so there may be more than just psychological comfort from a cup of warm milk at bedtime. The carbohydrate in the milk is important, too; it facilitates the brain's absorption of the tryptophan. Actually, any snack containing carbohydrate can ease your way to sleep, because enough tryptophan is already in your blood to produce the effect. Don't use tryptophan pills, though; they have not yet been proved safe.

My spouse always wants to stay up later than I do and then wakes me up by getting into bed. Which of us should change?

One of you could try, but larks and owls are born, not made.[4] You fall asleep when your body temperature falls to a certain degree, and that is governed by a preset cycle in your brain's hypothalamus. Neither one of you is wrong; you're just different.

Is it OK to sleep during the day?

Any combination of sleeping and wakefulness that serves to keep one refreshed and vigorous is acceptable. Some people choose to use some of the nighttime hours for working, and they find that an afternoon nap can allow them that privilege. Winston Churchill wrote that napping was essential for anyone who wanted to get the last scrap of energy out of the human structure. Many people famous for their personal energy have made similar statements. Some people accept sleep whenever it comes, but others take charge of their sleep and use it to great advantage.

Medicines, Other Drugs, and Drug Abuse

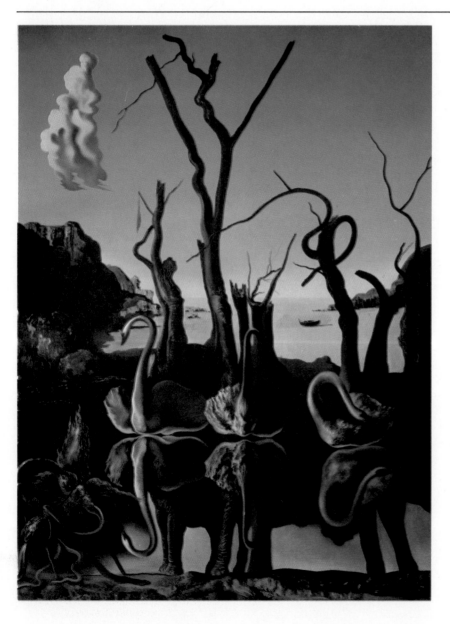

FOR OPENERS . . .

True or false? If false, say what is true.

1. Aspirin relieves pain, but insulin modifies the body's basic functioning.

2. People who take aspirin to relieve pain do not receive the same anticlotting effect as people who take it to prevent stroke.

3. A person who is not physically addicted to a drug may still crave it intensely.

4. The term *drug tolerant* describes a person who does not object to drug abuse.

5. Drugs sold over the counter are dangerous because people can buy them without consulting a physician.

6. Alcohol and marijuana impair driving ability, but medicines do not.

7. Alcohol is the most commonly abused drug in the United States and Canada.

8. When people become addicted to a drug, the primary reason they continue to use it is to experience pleasure.

9. The only way to get free of a drug habit is to quit "cold turkey."

10. Generic drugs, though less expensive, are chemically identical to brand name drugs and can be freely substituted for them.

(Answers on page 151.)

Some people think of drugs as **medicines** that help them get better when they are sick; some think of them as illegal, addictive substances. They are both. The general definition of a **drug** states that it is any substance taken into the living organism that modifies one or more of its functions.[1]* The medical definition acknowledges only medical drugs. Drugs can be separated into categories: nonprescription, or over-the-counter, drugs; prescription drugs; and illegal street drugs, but these categories of drugs are more similar than different. All drugs affect users physiologically, and their use carries risk. The next section is about all drugs, whether taken medically or otherwise. The end of this chapter discusses drug abuse, the Spotlight topic is caffeine, and Chapters 8 and 9 are devoted to alcohol and nicotine.

CHARACTERISTICS OF DRUGS

When people use medical or other drugs, they set in motion a series of actions in the body. Some of them are desirable; others may not be. Drugs work by setting in motion, or interfering with, the body's own processes. One drug is familiar to everyone; it is found in tiny, portable boxes or bottles, sometimes right next to the candy counter. It is cheap, ordinary, unglamorous. Consumers reach for a dose ten billion times a year, or once every three seconds.[2] It is aspirin, unsurpassed for the relief of certain kinds of pain.

Most people feel free to use aspirin. They think it is safe, because it is so familiar. If this is how you perceive aspirin, then you will probably be surprised by its far-reaching chemical effects on body systems.

Aspirin affects a set of powerful, hormonelike chemicals called **prostaglandins**. Prostaglandins are produced in all body tissues and released to do their work, after which they quickly break down and disappear. But during their brief existence, they help to produce fevers, they sensitize pain receptors, some cause contractions of the uterus, some stimulate digestive tract motion, some control nerve impulses, some regulate blood pressure, some promote blood clotting, and some cause inflammation. Aspirin retards the production of certain prostaglandins and so interferes with all these body responses. Thus, among other things, aspirin reduces fever and inflammation, relieves pain, and opposes blood clotting.

You cannot use aspirin for any one purpose without bringing on all its effects. A person who is prone to strokes and heart attacks might take aspirin to prevent blood clotting, but this same effect occurs also in people who take aspirin only for pain. For them, the anticlotting effect may be dangerous, since it can cause abnormal bleeding. A single two-tablet dose doubles the bleeding time of wounds, an effect that lasts from four to seven days. For this reason, it is important to refrain from taking aspirin before any kind of surgery.

These examples illustrate a general characteristic of all drugs: they have **side effects**, some of which are neutral, some of which are harmful. All drugs have many effects, and all of them occur when you take the drugs, whether you want them to or not.

Drugs that carry low risks to health are most desirable in the treatment of diseases. In fact, scientists use a risk/benefit ratio to assign safety ratings to drugs being considered for use as medicines. The ratio compares the **effective**

*Reference notes are in Appendix D.

FIGURE 7–1 The Therapeutic Index of a Drug

FIGURE 7–1 The Therapeutic Index of a Drug

The dose levels sufficient to kill members of two animal species of different sizes are used to determine the lethal dose for human beings by extrapolation. The therapeutic dose is determined by means of experiments with human beings. The ratio between the therapeutic dose and the lethal dose is the therapeutic index.

In one drug:

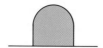

This is the therapeutic dose.

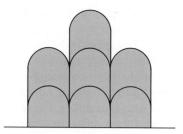

This is the lethal dose
(7 times the therapeutic dose).

The therapeutic index is 1/7.

In another drug:

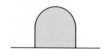

This is the therapeutic dose.

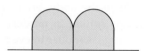

This is the lethal dose
(2 times the therapeutic dose).

The therapeutic index is 1/2. The margin of safety is too small; accidents are likely with this drug.

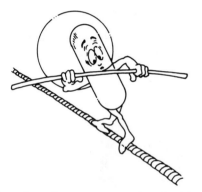

Some drugs have narrow margins of safety.

you-FORE-ee-uh

A way of remembering the factors that affect a drug's action:
   Substance.
   System (route of administration).
   Subject.
   Set (psychological set, or attitude).
   Setting.

or **therapeutic dose** with the **lethal dose**, asking the question, How much drug does it take to help a person, compared with the amount that will kill that person? The greater the difference, the greater the margin of safety. A drug's safety margin is called its **therapeutic index**, and Figure 7–1 illustrates it.

Some antibiotic drugs work against infection by stopping cell division. Bacteria divide rapidly, so the drugs halt their growth promptly. But some body cells are dividing, and the drugs halt their growth, too. Fortunately, bacteria divide faster than the body's own cells, and so succumb earlier to an antibiotic drug's effects. Once the drug is out of the system, the body's own cells soon recover. Thus, antibiotics have reasonable margins of safety.

Some drugs have narrower margins of safety. An example is the drug alcohol, which was used as an anesthetic during wartime, in surgery, and in childbirth before the development of safer anesthetics. A little alcohol produces feelings of drowsiness, dulls pain, and produces a characteristic feeling of exaggerated well-being known as **euphoria**, popularly called a **high**. More alcohol produces unconsciousness, and only a little more than that stops heartbeat and breathing. The amount of alcohol needed for an anesthetic effect is dangerously close to a lethal dose—making the margin of safety too narrow to tolerate. Other, better painkillers with wider safety margins are now used instead (see Figure 7–2).

When you take a drug, many factors work together to influence its effect on you. One is, of course, the drug itself—the substance. Another is its route of administration: a drug delivered into a vein will reach the brain faster, for example, than a drug injected into a muscle. Still another is you, the subject—both your physiology and your psychology. Still another is the setting in which you take the drug.

A person's drug-taking history also plays a role. A drug may produce one set of effects when used in the short term, but it may have an entirely

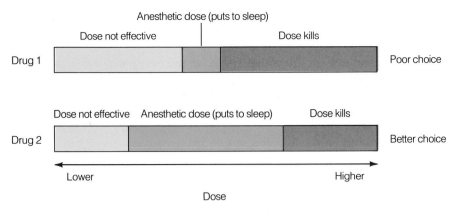

Drug 1 — Poor choice

Dose not effective | Anesthetic dose (puts to sleep) | Dose kills

Drug 2 — Better choice

Dose not effective | Anesthetic dose (puts to sleep) | Dose kills

Lower ← Dose → Higher

FIGURE 7–2   Anesthetics

An anesthetic has no effect at a low dose. As the dose increases, it puts the person to sleep. A still higher dose stops respiration and heartbeat, and so kills.

With a poor anesthetic (drug 1), the zone of doses within which the person is put to sleep is narrow. A slightly higher dose kills. Alcohol works this way and therefore has been abandoned (except in emergencies) as an anesthetic.

With a better anesthetic (drug 2), the zone within which sleep is induced without killing is wide, thus allowing for some variation in the dose without danger.

different set of effects when used over the long term. When increasing doses of a drug are needed to achieve a desired effect, it is because the body has developed **tolerance**. This is an adaptation: the more the body is exposed to the drug, the more enzymes it builds to break it down and the faster it disposes of it. Many organs may contribute: the liver dismantles the drug faster; the kidney excretes it faster; other tissues raise their resistance to its presence. Tolerance varies among individuals; some can come to tolerate certain drugs well; others can hardly adjust at all.

Another personal response to long-term drug use is **habituation**. Everyone knows what a habit is. Having done something once, we tend to do it again; the more often we do it, the more likely we are to repeat it. Finally a pattern is established. The automatic nature of the act reflects a physical adaptation: the nerve pathways involved in the action work easily, while the nerves that would interfere with the action are silenced.

A drug may be used initially to relieve a medical problem such as pain, to relieve a psychological problem such as anxiety, or to give pleasure. But the use of certain drugs progresses more or less rapidly to **addiction** or **physiological dependence**. Addiction is altogether different from habituation. In addiction, the body changes chemically so that it demands the presence of the drug to function normally. As the body begins to clear the drug from the system, the body chemistry becomes abnormal, and the symptoms of **withdrawal** ensue, creating a demand for another dose of the drug. Alternatively, the withdrawal symptoms can be managed medically.

Researchers identify addictive drugs using laboratory criteria. A drug is addictive if, on withdrawal, it alters brainwave patterns, affects mood, and elicits drug-seeking behavior (just as food deprivation elicits food-seeking behavior).[3] Addiction also includes tolerance, necessitating *increasing doses*.[4]

A person who is addicted to a drug always has a **psychological dependence** on it, too. The person craves the drug. But, depending on the nature of the drug, a person may develop psychological dependence without addiction. Euphoria-producing drugs can bring about changes in the brain that cause someone who is exposed to them to crave them. The distinction between physiological and psychological dependence is unclear, and this chapter uses the term *drug dependence* to refer to both.

Mind-altering drugs, including alcohol, marijuana, tranquilizers, and barbiturates, have been shown to change people's driving ability for the worse. Drugs influence people's judgment of speed and slow down their reactions. People fail simulator tests, crashing more frequently when under the influ-

CHAPTER 7 ■■ MEDICINES, OTHER DRUGS, AND DRUG ABUSE

MINIGLOSSARY
of Medicine Terms

For general terms relating to drugs, see Chapter Glossary on p. 150. Abusable drugs among the medicines are marked with an asterisk (*).

acetaminophen (ah-SEET-ah-MIN-o-fen): an *analgesic* drug.

*amphetamine (am-FET-uh-meen): a type of *stimulant* drug. Examples are Benzedrine, Dexedrine, and Ritalin.

analgesic (AN-ul-JEE-zick): a drug that relieves pain and fever, such as aspirin, ibuprofen, or acetaminophen.

  an = without
  alg = pain

anesthetic: a drug that produces loss of sensation, with or without loss of consciousness.

  esthes = sensation

antacid: a drug that neutralizes stomach acid.

antibiotic: a drug used to fight bacterial infection.

  biotic = life

anticoagulant (an-tee-coh-AG-you-lant): a drug used to prevent blood clotting.

antidiarrheal (an-tee-dye-uh-REE-ul): a drug used to relieve diarrhea.

antiemetic (an-tee-uh-MET-ick): a drug used to treat nausea and vomiting.

  emet = vomiting

antifungal: a drug used to treat fungus infections.

antihistamine: a drug that counteracts the effects of histamine, one of the chemicals involved in allergic reactions.

antipyretic (an-tee-pie-RET-ick): a drug that reduces fever.

  pyre = fire

aspirin: an *analgesic* drug.

*barbiturate (bar-BIH-chur-et): a type of *depressant* drug.

bronchodilator (BRONK-oh-DYE-lay-tor): a drug that opens the bronchial tubes within the lungs.

caffeine: a stimulant drug.

codeine: a narcotic drug.

cough suppressant: a drug that acts on the nervous system to suppress the cough reflex.

decongestant: a drug used to relieve nasal and sinus congestion.

*depressant: a drug that depresses the central nervous system. Types include sedatives, tranquilizers, barbiturates (such as Seconal), and alcohol.

continued

ence of drugs than otherwise.[5] In the case of alcohol and marijuana, the impairment of driving lasts for hours *after* the high from the drug has worn off.[6]

Amphetamines are drugs that speed up the nervous system. You might think they would improve people's driving, but accident studies show otherwise. Heavy amphetamine use allows fatigued people to override their feelings of exhaustion; driving ability decreases even though they think they are doing well.[7]

Nonprescription medications can endanger drivers, too. Cold preparations can cause drowsiness. If you have any question about a drug's effect on reaction time, a talk with a pharmacist or health care provider is in order.

DRUGS USED AS MEDICINES

Drugs selected as medicines must be proved both safe and effective before they are allowed on the market. The term **safe** means that an ingredient will not hurt you; **effective**, that it will do what the maker claims it will do. Drugs used as medicines produce six kinds of benefits:

- They can facilitate the *cure* of disease.
  Example: Penicillin kills the bacteria that cause pneumonia.
- They *lessen the severity* of disease.
  Example: Steroid hormones reinforce a bodily defense against arthritis.
- They *relieve symptoms*.
  Example: Aspirin relieves inflammation, aches, and pains.
- They help *diagnose* disease.
  Example: A dye is injected into a vein and its rate of travel is measured, to help locate obstructions in the circulatory system.
- They help *prevent* disease.
  Example: Vaccinations elicit the immune response, which strengthens the body's defenses against disease.
- They *produce a desired effect* not related to diseases.
  Example: Oral contraceptives prevent conception.

Medical drugs do not "cure" diseases by themselves. Only the body can fully accomplish that, but drugs can help.

The Food and Drug Administration (FDA), a watchdog agency of the federal government, divides medicines into two classes. **Over-the-counter (OTC) drugs** are sold without prescription, because they have these four characteristics:

- They are relatively safe with regard to accidental misuse.
- The dose is fairly universal.
- They can be used without professional guidance; instructions are not complex.
- They have a low abuse potential; they do not alone produce euphoria.

In contrast, **prescription drugs** can only be prescribed by physicians, because they have characteristics such as these:

- They may be dangerous if misused.
- The dose must be adjusted to body weight, age, or other drug use.
- They require following complex directions.
- They have higher abuse potential.

Some prescription drugs, notably the narcotics, are **controlled drugs**; their sales are registered, to track users.

People use two more terms in relation to medicines. First, **generic names** are the chemical names of drugs, and they never begin with a capital letter. Second, **brand names** are the names given to drugs by the companies that produce them, and they are always capitalized. (They also have a circled *R* by their names, indicating "registered trademark.") One generic drug may have several brand names (see margin). The Miniglossary of Medicine Terms defines classes of drugs used as medicines.

Nonprescription (Over-the-Counter) Medications

Imagine what would happen if you had to make an appointment to see a health care provider for every minor complaint. By the time you actually saw one, you would have suffered needlessly for many days and then had a medical fee tacked onto the price of relief. The quick availability of OTC medications gives you freedom—to listen to your body's messages, identify your own ailments, and try to gain relief from the ones that are minor. Figure 7–3, page 132 shows that self-care can benefit many conditions, and OTC drugs can contribute to that self-care.

How can you tell which medications to buy? You need to know how to read their labels. Drug companies are required to include only approved **active ingredients** in their products, and the FDA lists only a few hundred approved active ingredients. Yet 50,000 OTC drugs are on the market. How can there be so many, each claiming to be unique? The answer is that in addition to the active ingredients, each manufacturer adds others. Some are useful and necessary: carriers and fillers are examples. Others may be there simply because they have fancy chemical names that will lead buyers to believe the products are superior.

The FDA has suggested that producers of drugs list all **inactive (inert) ingredients** on labels, and most companies have voluntarily agreed to do so. Thus, by reading labels of OTC drugs, you can protect yourself against ingredients that may harm you. If you are allergic to the yellow dye tartrazine, for example, you can choose drugs not colored with it. The FDA also restricts medicine manufacturers to truth in labeling. A drug label must list approved uses for the drug—that is, conditions against which the drug is scientifically proved to be effective. If products have unsubstantiated claims on their labels, they can be removed from store shelves.

The drug label lists:

- Name and statement of identity of the product.
- What the product will do.
- Quantity of contents.
- Active ingredients and, usually, inactive ingredients.
- Name and address of the manufacturer, distributor, or packer.

It also lists directions:

- The correct amount of each dose.
- How frequently it should be taken.
- How to take it (by mouth, with water, and so on).
- How to store it and when to throw it away (the expiration date).

MINIGLOSSARY
continued

diuretic (DIE-you-RET-ick): a drug that increases the urine produced by the kidneys, used to rid the body of excess fluid.

expectorant: a drug that stimulates the flow of mucus and promotes coughing, used to eliminate phlegm from the respiratory tract.
   ex = out of
   pectus = the chest

ibuprofen (EYE-byoo-PRO-fen): an *analgesic* drug.

laxative: a drug that increases the frequency and ease of bowel movements.

muscle relaxant: a drug that relieves muscle spasms, used for disorders such as backache.

*narcotic: medically, a drug that slows down functioning of the central nervous system, including heroin, opium, morphine, methadone, codeine, paregoric, Demerol, and Darvon. Legally, the term includes any drug with potential for abuse.
   narko = to numb

sedative: a type of *depressant* drug.

*stimulant: any of a wide variety of drugs that speed up the central nervous system, including amphetamines, caffeine, and others.

thrombolytic (THROM-boh-LIT-ic): a drug that helps dissolve and disperse blood clots.
   thrombos = clot
   lysis = to loosen

tranquilizer: a drug that has a calming effect; *major tranquilizers* are used to control people with severe psychosis; *minor tranquilizers* (such as Valium and Librium) are mild versions.

Brand names of the three most common pain-killers: Advil, Motrin, Nuprin, Rufen (ibuprofen). Anacin-3, Datril, Panadol, Tylenol (acetaminophen). Bufferin (aspirin).

FIGURE 7–3 Ailments Benefiting
from Self-care

Of people visiting general health care providers, perhaps about 65 percent have minor ailments; another 25 percent have chronic ailments; and only 10 percent have acute conditions that demand dramatic medical treatment. Thus 90 percent of these people could appropriately select their own medicines and administer their own self-care.

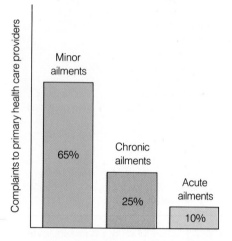

⊕ **STRATEGIES**
for Selecting OTC Drugs

To use OTC drugs to your best advantage:

⊕ **Identify the condition you are treating.**

Finally, it lists warnings:

■ A limit on the duration of use.

■ Side effects, if any (drowsiness, constipation, and the like); see Table 7–1.

■ Circumstances that may require a health care provider's advice before use.

■ A warning to the pregnant woman discouraging her use of the product without the advice of her health care provider.

Strategies: Over-the-Counter Medications

Understanding the condition you are trying to treat is essential to wise medicine selection. Say you have a cold. First, you might consult a home-reference medical guide.* According to most sources, a cold is a self-limiting respiratory infection, usually caused by a virus, which lasts from one to two weeks. The symptoms usually occur in progression, starting with a sore throat, sneezing, and a runny nose. In a few days the nose may be stuffed up and the eyes watery. Aches and pains may accompany these symptoms, along with tiredness and sometimes a fever. A cough usually develops

*Recommended references for your home library: the American Medical Association's *Family Medical Guide*; Better Homes and Gardens's *Family Medical Guide*; Consumer Guide's *Family Medical and Health Guide*; or Good Housekeeping's *Family Health and Medical Guide*. Look for the latest edition.

TABLE 7–1 Some Side Effects of OTC Drugs

Drug	Possible Hazard
Acetaminophen	Bloody urine, painful urination, skin rash, bleeding Liver damage from chronic low-level excesses
Antacids	Reduced mineral absorption from food Possible concealment of ulcer
Aspirin	Stomach upset and vomiting, stomach bleeding, worsening of ulcers Association with Reye's syndrome in children and teenagers[a]
Cold medications	Loss of consciousness (if taken with prescription tranquilizers)
Diet pills, decongestants, and caffeine[b]	Organ damage or death from cerebral hemorrhage
Ibuprofen	Liver damage similar to that from acetaminophen Enhancement of action of anticlotting medications
Laxatives	Reduced absorption of minerals from food
Toothache medications	Destruction of the still-healthy part of a damaged tooth (for medications that contain clove oil)

[a]Reye's (pronounced RISE) syndrome is a rare and potentially life-threatening condition linked to aspirin use associated with chicken pox or flu. Children and teenagers with chicken pox or flu should be treated with acetaminophen, not aspirin.

[b]These three OTC drugs are often combined in street varieties of abused drugs because they produce a high. They are sold in capsules called "look-alikes" that resemble prescription mind-altering drugs.

Sometimes, misleading information may remain on a label for a while after it has been reported, because the FDA hasn't had time to act. For example, a drug was sold for many years that claimed to benefit the liver; no such benefit was ever proved. The FDA took the company to court, and 14 years after proceedings began, the word *liver* was finally removed from the label. You can't depend on a label to conform to the law; the law may not have been enforced yet.

Even if the label conforms to the law, unscrupulous manufacturers may place "information" sheets or placards near the display shelf where the product is being sold. This trick is especially common in places that specialize in "health" or "natural" products, but such sheets can appear in regular drugstores and grocery stores, too. Be suspicious of claims of cures or benefits on any printed matter near products. Lies on labels are illegal, but placards can say anything and claim freedom of the press.

A similar trick is used in some magazines. You might read a magazine article written by Dr. Rip Off, M.D., which says, with absolute certainty, that zinc improves sexual performance. Already you have become uneasy—*the claim seems too good to be true.* As you scan the next page, an advertisement jumps out at you: "Full-Life zinc tablets—only $6.95 per bottle." The advertisement says only that the company sells zinc tablets, a legal claim. But chances are, the Full-Life Company sent the article on the previous page, as well as the advertisement, to be published. The article is a hoax, but its publication is legal. The FDA bars companies from printing lies in advertisements, but no law forbids lies in other writing. Your first clue to the hoax is the claims in the article; your second is the advertisement for the product in close proximity.

Lies on labels and in advertisements are against the law, but they still appear. Lies elsewhere in print may actually be protected by law.

A fever can help the body fight infection.

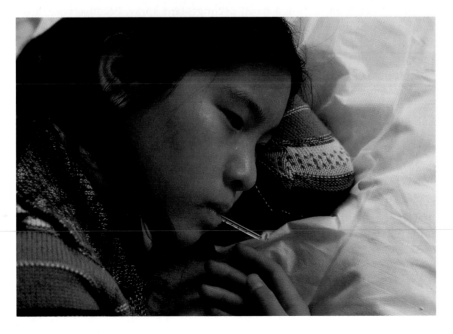

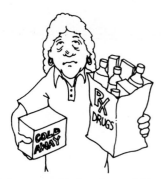

What *do* you need to buy for a cold?

⊛ **See a health care provider if symptoms persist.**

⊛ **Compare drugs by their chemical contents, not by their brand names.**

⊛ **Follow label directions about how to use drugs. Reread the label each time you rebuy.**

⊛ **Do not overbuy; throw away drugs whose expiration dates have passed.**

during the later stages. Health care providers suggest that the best medicine for a cold is bed rest, abundant fluids, plain aspirin (or acetaminophen or ibuprofen) if body aches are present, and a box of the softest facial tissues available. Since colds are, for the most part, caused by viruses, antibiotics are usually useless against them.

If you have a fever, you should know a few things about it before you reach for fever-relief medicine. People fear fever because it is associated with dangerous diseases, but the fever itself may actually assist the immune system (see Chapter 15).[8] Clearly, fever stresses the body—it raises the heart rate and increases the tissues' demand for oxygen. A weak heart could be damaged by such a strain. High temperatures (over 104° F or, in some cases, lower) can cause convulsions and should be treated by a health care provider, not only to control the fever but also to determine and treat the underlying condition. Generally, though, a mild fever should be allowed to do its job of assisting the immune system.[9] If the fever goes above about 100, you can lower it with aspirin, acetaminophen, or ibuprofen.

Now, suppose you decide to treat your cold yourself.[10] Knowing that no cold medicine will prevent, cure, or even shorten a cold, you seek OTC medicine only for relief of symptoms. You feel achy, so you study first the array of painkillers.

Being a shrewd consumer, you comparison-shop, ignoring the brand names and reading the labels to discover the contents of each. You overlook the claims of "extra strength," because you know you can adjust your dose yourself. (If you want an extra-strength dose, you can take two and a half pills of a regular-strength medicine; if you want a combination of pain relievers, you can take one and a quarter pills of each.) You also ignore the claims that "buffered" products protect your stomach, knowing that you can drink a full glass of water with any common pain reliever to achieve the same protection. (If aspirin irritates your stomach, though, switch pain relievers or use coated pills.) The prices of aspirins, acetaminophens, and ibuprofens vary threefold; you choose the cheapest, store-brand, regular-strength aspirin.

You refrain from buying a nasal decongestant spray, because your nose is not stopped up. Overuse of sprays can make nasal passages swell, necessitating medical treatment. You do not buy a spray for later, either, because the effectiveness of medicines have a time limit. You also refrain from buying "nighttime cold medicines." The labels list ingredients you do not need—antihistamines for relief of allergy (not cold) symptoms or cough suppressants (you are not coughing). The latter are loaded with alcohol, which can dehydrate you and disturb your sleep.

You have a sore throat, so you buy some anesthetizing spray. You plan to suck lozenges or gargle with warm salt water, just for comfort, but you need no costly mouthwashes. Most colds and sore throats are caused by viruses, and mouthwashes do not kill viruses. At the checkout counter, you ask whether your aspirin and spray interact; the pharmacist assures you that they do not.

On the way home, you buy some juices and soups to boost your liquid intake. One recent discovery in medical science is that the traditional home remedy of chicken soup actually does help relieve colds more than other hot drinks. Something in the broth promotes the flow of mucus, hastening recovery.[11]

Because drugs can mask symptoms, sick people who take them can be tempted to carry on with their regular routines, risking prolonged illness or relapse. You plan to rest in bed until you are well. You have made wise decisions based on hard facts, not on advertising. You have not spent money on wishful thinking, but only on the best relief for your particular cold.

Prescription Medications

Prescription drugs are true miracles of our time. One miracle: for a person whose cells do not absorb glucose from their blood, insulin is literally a life-saving treatment. Another miracle: a person whose heart lacks the ability to use calcium may take a calcium channel blocker, so that the life-giving heartbeat can go on.

Prescription medicines can be overused. Drug companies advertise them aggressively to physicians, who are led to overprescribe them. Also, the media hype new drugs and the public demand them from their physicians. The tranquilizer Valium is an example; in recent years it has been widely overprescribed, and has lead to addictions not unlike those of alcoholism. The risks of using prescription medicines may be as great as the benefits. In fact, as noted earlier, that is why they are available only by prescription: to administer them properly requires medical training. That does not mean you can leave the responsibility entirely to the physician, though. You have a part to play, too, and the next section describes it.

Strategies: Prescription Medications

To avoid most of the risks associated with prescription medicines, keep some basic rules in mind. Before you leave the physician's office, be sure you know:

- The diagnosis of your condition.
- That your physician is aware of all other drugs you are taking.

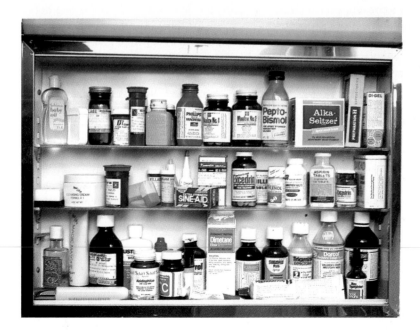

Medicines can be overused.

- The name of the medicine the physician has prescribed.
- How often, how long, and in what doses you should take it.
- When to take it in relation to meals.
- Whether side effects are likely to occur, and what they are.
- What to do if you forget to take a dose on time.

You can often save money by using a generic drug rather than the same drug sold with a brand name. Ask your physician first, though. The active ingredients are the same, but the inactive ingredients may change their absorption. If the exact timing of absorption is important, the physician may choose a particular brand name drug. To ensure that you receive the dose you need:

- Ask your physician to consider prescribing generic drugs, but don't ask the pharmacist to substitute them.
- Read and follow instructions on labels or on package inserts.
- Do not mix drugs (including OTC and other drugs) without checking first with your physician or pharmacist.
- Avoid alcohol when using medication.
- If the drug isn't doing what you expect it to, check with your physician.
- If you experience any side effects, report them to your physician at once.
- At night, turn on the light to be certain you take the correct medicine.
- Continue taking your prescription for the specified time, even if you feel better right away.
- Keep all medicines where young children can't get them.
- Discard any unused medication.
- Store drugs in a cool, dark place and in the original container.
- Do not share prescription medications with other people.

✳ **Do not mix drugs without checking with your health care provider or pharmacist.**

Chapter 14 gives more precautions on preventing child poisoning.

Chapter 14 gives more precautions on preventing child poisoning.

CONSUMER CAUTION

Today's prescription medications are products of sophisticated technology and regulatory procedures. They will act reliably and safely each time you use them, and you will get the same dose every time you take them. Some people, though, try to convince consumers that herbs and "natural" cures are safer than the products of technology.

Many drugs come from chemicals originally found in plants and animals, but technology has refined them into forms that are consistently helpful, predictable, and safe. The unrefined biological products do not have these qualities. In fact, they most often contain poisons along with the curing drugs. Sassafras, for example, contains the liver toxin safrole.[12] The overuse of ginseng produces high or low blood pressure, nervousness, sleeplessness, diarrhea, depression, and confusion.[13] Chamomile, often served as tea, can cause shock when overused.[14] Beware of "herbal cures"—doctoring yourself with them can be dangerous.

Natural cures are sometimes packaged with natural poisons.

ABUSE OF DRUGS

The terminology that describes abuse of drugs is controversial. Terms vary according to the people using them. The medical community and the FDA have created one set of formal definitions; society has created another set;

and individual people have created others that reflect their own drug histories and attitudes.

The FDA makes these distinctions: **drug use** is the taking of a drug for a medically intended purpose, and in the appropriate amount, frequency, strength, and manner. In contrast, **drug abuse** is the deliberate taking of a drug for other than a medical purpose and in a manner that can result in damage to a person's health or ability to function. For legally available drugs, the FDA also defines **drug misuse** as the taking of a drug for its medically intended purpose, but in an incorrect dose, timing, or manner. Recreational use of drugs is not defined by the FDA.[15] Medical terminology describes drug abuse simply as any nonmedical use or overuse of a drug.[16] These definitions classify any use of drugs for nonmedical reasons as drug abuse; there is no such thing as mere "use"—for example, to produce euphoria or hallucinations.

Society's view of drug use is reflected in its laws. Except for alcohol, no mind-altering (**psychoactive**) drug is freely available; most are available only by prescription or are outright illegal. By making these laws, society has defined the use of mind-altering drugs, except alcohol, as abuse.

Some individuals see drug use differently. Many people call themselves drug users, not abusers, when they take mind-altering drugs. They state that there is such a thing as **recreational drug use**, which produces no harmful health effects on the user and no deterioration of function in terms of job, family, or society. (People who call themselves *social drinkers* make the same distinction.)

It is not clear that such users of drugs are, themselves, well qualified to make the distinctions described here, because they are not impartial. Research is needed to measure the harm associated with various styles of drug taking, but research on illegal drugs is lacking. Even with alcohol, which is a legal drug, decades of research have been needed to show that social use produces significant physical harm with time (see Chapter 8). The question of whether any illegal drugs can be used without consequences remains unanswered.

Meanwhile, it is up to the individual to decide just how to handle mind-altering drugs. One thing is certain: these drugs are either available legally by prescription only or are altogether illegal, and punishment for their possession and sale can be harsh. This section is about some of the most commonly abused drugs, but keep in mind that the most abused drug in the United States and Canada is still alcohol. Chapter 8 is devoted entirely to it.

Why Do People Abuse Drugs?

Different factors may lead different people to abuse drugs. One factor is the nature of the individual. People's genetic makeup might dictate inborn tendencies toward drug abuse. Researchers are exploring the personalities of youngsters to identify traits that predict such tendencies.[17] These traits may well turn out to be hereditary, or they may result from the ways parents raise their children, or both.

Another factor is curiosity, which is a strong motivator. Many people try drugs to see what they are like, but most don't continue to use them; only a few do, and some become drug dependent.

A third factor is the individual's desire to fit in socially. Drugs are almost always, at least to begin with, part of a social event. People like to feel part of a group, and some groups have drug taking as their reason for being together. A person's self-perception may be a fourth influence on drug abuse. People may gravitate toward drugs because they pride themselves on their deviance from the rest of society. Drugs thus fit their image. Others may seek comfort from drugs because they have low self-esteem.

Still another factor is the nature of the drug itself. Some animal studies show clearly that drugs give pleasure. When animals are fitted with an apparatus to receive cocaine, they visit the device often. In fact, when they are offered either food or the drug, they consistently choose the drug until they eventually starve.[18] The feeling of pleasure the drug produces makes them forget to eat or sleep. Cocaine can have that effect on people, too.

Seeking pleasure is an inborn instinct, universal to all creatures on earth. In fact, it has been called the "primary biological steering mechanism for the whole animal world." In seeking pleasure and comfort, the species receives essential rewards such as warmth, food, and propagation.[19]

Abusable drugs produce pleasure directly in the brain, bypassing the necessity to work for it. Unfortunately, instead of being adaptive like the drive for normal pleasures, the artificially induced drive for drugs is maladaptive—it may lead to inability to function, and it brings no benefits, as do the natural drives. Furthermore, it may lead to addiction, as described earlier. In the case of some drugs, the pleasure may then dwindle while the pain of withdrawal intensifies, so that the person continues taking the drug no longer primarily for pleasure but for relief from pain.

The attachment to a drug can persist with astonishing strength. Curing drug dependence has been likened to trying to break a sexual bond, except that the drug attachment is stronger. Imagine to what lengths people may go to be with the object of their passion; the drug-dependent person will go much farther. Such people defend, cherish, and protect the drug habit as they would defend and protect a loved one. People need not be mentally disturbed to become drug dependent; they need only be exposed to the drug for a long enough time.[20] Even after the drug has been abandoned, a craving for it may persist, perhaps because of the memory of the pleasure it brought, and the forgetting of the pain.

Drug dependence is unexpected. Probably no one who starts out using a substance intends to get hooked, but it happens nevertheless. A person tries a drug for one reason but continues taking it for totally different reasons. For example, someone may begin to smoke cigarettes to look grown-up—but 30 years later, the person is still smoking. The original rewards are long gone; the addiction has taken over.

A person's choice to use a drug is influenced by the perception of how severely society punishes people for drug use. Research shows that tolerant drug policies spread drug addiction.* Research has also shown that education about drug hazards is not effective against drug abuse—physicians, despite their superior knowledge, have narcotic addiction rates at least 30 times higher than members of the general population.[21] The reason is unknown, but perhaps easy access to drugs combined with a false sense of security (they think they can handle it) overwhelm even superior knowledge.

Many complex factors work together to influence drug abuse:
1. The nature of the individual, including the tendency to become addicted, curiosity, sensitivity to peer pressure, self-image and self-esteem, and escapism.
2. The nature of the drug.
3. Perceived societal consequences.

*England and Sweden tried to combat addiction by making heroin legally available to addicts, with resulting epidemics of drug addiction. In both countries the policies were ultimately reversed. N. Bejerot, *Addiction, an Artificially Induced Drive* (Springfield, Ill.: Charles C. Thomas, 1972), pp. 46-59.

STRATEGIES: Drug-Free Highs

Pleasure is there for the taking, for those who know where to look. Go ahead and get high:

1. Run, walk, or skip across an open field or along a beach.

2. Ask one of your grandparents what life is about.

3. Play with a baby.

4. Give a friend a gift that you made with your own hands.

5. Work hard at something, and see it through to completion.

6. Have a good cry about that thing you have been hiding from for too long.

7. Learn to meditate.

8. Eat nourishing food.

9. Write some poetry for yourself (it doesn't have to rhyme).

10. Climb a mountain.

11. Visit a river.

12. Say "thank you" more often.

13. Beat the feathers out of a pillow next time you are very angry.

14. Stop biting your nails (or shed another bad habit).

15. Read a good book.

16. Give someone a long hug.

17. Call your parent and say, "I love you."

SOURCE: Adapted from S. J. Levy, *Managing the "Drugs" in Your Life* (New York: McGraw-Hill, 1983), p. 104.

People who experiment with drugs often want to believe that they won't become dependent, that only inferior people do. The truth is that no one is exempt—not people, not animals—no one. The only way to avoid drug dependence is to avoid experimenting with drugs that produce it. This chapter's Strategies box shows ways of enjoying life without using drugs.

Commonly Abused Drugs

People who take drugs often are unaware that drugs modify body functions. They do, though, just as medicines do, but in the case of illegally obtained drugs, no watchdog agency such as the FDA screens them for safety or purity. What a person ends up with may or may not be what the person expected to receive. Illegal drugs provide a profit at each level of sale, so sellers tend to mix them liberally with extenders at every turn. For example, "consumer-quality" cocaine is expected to contain some quantity of white powder other than pure cocaine, usually the powdered sugar lactose or talcum powder. Some sellers of cocaine, however, maximize profits by adding enormous quantities of sugar and then masking the weakened effect of the cocaine with cheaper drugs, such as amphetamines, caffeine, or anesthetics that mimic cocaine's effects.

This section discusses a few abusable drugs and compares the actual effects with the popular beliefs about them. Table 7–2 presents many more details. People considering taking any drug—even with a prescription—would do well to research its risks. But with street drugs, no amount of research ever guarantees that the risks can be fully calculated in advance.

TABLE 7–2 Abused Drugs

Class	Drug (with Selected Brand or Other Names)	Medical Use	Physical Dependence
Narcotics	Opium (Dover's Powder, paregoric, Parepectolin), Morphine (Pectoral Syrup), Codeine (Empirin with Codeine, Robitussin A-C), Others (Levo-Dromoran, Percodan, Tussionex, Fentanyl, Sublimaze, Darvon, Talwin, Lomotil)	Analgesic, antidiarrheal, antitussive	Yes
	Heroin (Diacetylmorphine, H, black tar, horse, smack)	Pain reliever	Yes
	Hydromorphone (Dilaudid), Meperidine (pethidine) hydrochloride (Demerol)	Analgesic	Yes
	Methadone hydrochloride (Dolophine, Methadone, Methadose)	Analgesic, heroin substitute	Yes
Depressants	Barbiturates (Phenobarbital, Alurate, Butisol, Nembutal, Secobarbital, Seconal, Tuinal), Chloral hydrate (Noctec)	Anesthetic, anticonvulsant, sedative, hypnotic	Yes
	Glutethimide (Doriden), Methaqualone (Quaalude, Sopor)	Sedative, hypnotic	Yes
	Benzodiazepines (Ativan, Clonopin, Dalmane, Diazepam, Librium, Serax, Tranxene, Valium), Others (Equanil, Miltown, Noludar Placidyl, Valmid)	Anxiety reliever, anticonvulsant, sedative, hypnotic	Yes
Stimulants	Cocaine (base, coke, crack, flake, rock, snow)	Local anesthetic	Possible
	Amphetamines (biphetamine, speed, uppers, black beauties, white crosses, Desoxyn, Dexedrine, Mediatric), Phenmetrazine hydrochloride (Preludin), Methylphenidate hydrochloride (Ritalin), Others (Adipex, Bacarate, Cylert, Didrex, Ionamin, Plegine, Sanorex, Tenuate, Tepanil)	Hyperkinesis, narcolepsy, weight control	Possible
Psychedelics (Hallucinogens)	Lysergic acid diethylamide, LSD (acid, microdot, lysergic acid diethylamide), Mescaline and peyote (mesc, buttons, cactus)	None	No
	Amphetamine variants (2,5-DMA, PMA, STP, MDA, MMDA, TMA, DOM, DOB)	None	Unknown
	Psilocybin and related mushroom species (mushrooms, shrooms)	None	Unknown
	Phencyclidine hydrochloride (PCP, angel dust, hog)	Veterinary anesthetic	Unknown
	Others (PCE, PCPy, TCP, DMT, DET, morning glory seeds)	None	No
Inhalants	Hydrocarbon vapors from many sources, such as plastic cement, gasoline, spray can vapors (glue, gas, poppers, locker room, rush, odor of man, Aspirols, Vaporal, amyl nitrite, butyl nitrite, nitrous oxide, laughing gas)	Amyl nitrite relieves angina pectoris (see Chapter 16); nitrous oxide relieves anxiety	Yes
Cannabis	Marijuana (pot, Acapulco gold, grass, weed, dope, reefer, sinsemilla, Thai sticks), Tetrahydrocannabinol (THC), Hashish (hash), Hashish oil (hash oil)	Relieves glaucoma, and cancer therapy side effects	Unknown
Other	Designer drugs (Ecstasy, Ex, MDMA)	None	Varies
	Clove cigarettes rolled from high-nicotine and high-tar tobacco, clove oil, cocoa, licorice, and other ingredients (Djarum, Kreteks)	None	Unknown

TABLE 7–2 Continued

Psychological Dependence	Tolerance	Usual Method of Administration	Possible Effect	Effect of Overdose	Withdrawal Syndrome
Yes	Yes	Oral, smoked, injected			
Yes	Yes	Injected, sniffed, smoked	Euphoria, drowsiness, respiratory depression, constricted pupils, nausea	Slow and shallow breathing, clammy skin, convulsions, coma, possible death	Watery eyes, runny nose, yawning, loss of appetite, irritability, tremors, panic, chills and sweating, cramps, nausea
Yes	Yes	Oral, injected			
Yes	Yes	Oral, injected			
Yes	Yes	Oral, injected		Shallow respiration, cold and clammy skin, dilated pupils, weak and rapid pulse, coma, possible death	Anxiety, insomnia, tremors, delirium, convulsions, possible death
Yes	Yes	Oral, injected	Slurred speech, disorientation, drunken behavior without odor of alcohol		
Yes	Yes	Oral, injected			
Yes	Possible	Sniffed, injected, smoked	Increased alertness, excitation, euphoria, increased pulse rate and blood pressure, insomnia, loss of appetite, skin lesions	Agitation, increase in body temperature, hallucinations, convulsions, possible death	Apathy, long periods of sleep, irritability, depression, disorientation
Yes	Yes	Oral, injected			
Unknown	Yes	Oral, injected			
Unknown	Yes	Oral, injected	Illusions and hallucinations, poor perception of time and distance, nausea, vomiting	Longer, more intense "trip" episodes; psychosis; death by accident or suicide	None reported
Yes, rarely	Yes	Oral			
Yes	Yes	Smoked, oral, injected			
Unknown	Yes	Smoked, oral, injected, sniffed			
Yes	Yes	Sniffed, vapors concentrated and inhaled	Altered time sense, brief euphoria, nausea, vomiting, dizziness, headache; liver, brain, and kidney cancer	Loss of consciousness, death by suffocation, cerebral hemorrhage	None reported
Yes	Yes	Smoked, oral	Euphoria, relaxed inhibitions, increased appetite, disoriented behavior	Fatigue, paranoia, possible psychosis	Insomnia, hyperactivity, decreased appetite
Varies	Varies	Varies	Varies	Varies	Varies
Unknown	Unknown	Unknown	Nausea, vomiting, respiratory dysfunctions and bleeding, allergic reaction	Possible death from severe lung infection	None reported

SOURCE: Adaptetd from R. D. Thompkins, *Before It's Too Late: The Prevention Manual on Drug Abuse for People Who Care* (Englewood, N.J.: Family Information Services, 1981), pp. 16–17.

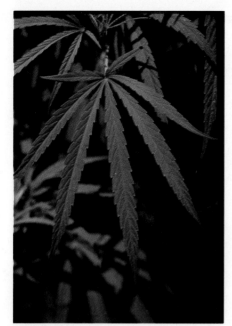

Drug dependence is unexpected. Plants like marijuana look innocent.

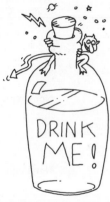

Many people who use drugs to chase away unpleasant feelings are unaware that the unpleasant feelings are the aftereffects of the drugs themselves.

MARIJUANA. Most people who use marijuana have the idea that since it has been around for thousands of years, it has proved itself: it gives the user a harmless high. Many people smoke it with no apparent ill effects, but scientific information is not all in yet. The situation is similar to the time when science knew little of the dangers of tobacco. People of the present generation are voluntarily "testing" the safety of marijuana as smokers tested tobacco in an earlier time.

Marijuana plants are harvested and dried, and then the leaves, flowers, and small stems are crushed and rolled into cigarettes (joints) or smoked in pipes. The ingredients are rapidly and completely (90 percent) absorbed from the lungs and then travel in the blood to the various body tissues that process them. They linger for several days in body fat and are excreted over a week or so thereafter.

The ingredient in marijuana that produces euphoria is delta-9-tetrahydrocannabinol, or THC for short. THC circulates to all the tissues, affecting hearing, touch, taste, and smell, as well as perceptions of time, of space, and of the body; it also produces changes in mental sensations and sleep patterns. Among the taste changes apparently induced is a great enjoyment of eating, especially of sweets ("the munchies"), but it is not known how this effect occurs.

The subjective experience of the high is influenced by people's expectations of how they will feel, how much of the drug they take, its potency, and other constituents of the particular batch. Scientists have identified at least 400 different chemicals in marijuana, and their ratios differ by genetic strain and even within the same strain from season to season. Marijuana's effects range from a mild euphoria to hallucinations. Users' inhibitions loosen, they may feel graceful (but act clumsy), they may feel brilliant (but make no sense), they may lose concentration and time sense. Lore has it that marijuana intensifies whatever feeling people are having at the moment: if they feel good, it will make them feel wonderful; if they feel bad, it will make them feel even worse; if they expect to enjoy sex, it will intensify that pleasure. Generally speaking, people's expectations are realized, but in the case of sex, marijuana dulls sexual pleasure for some and is more likely to make people feel sleepy than sexy. The morning after an evening of smoking is, for many, a morning of tiredness and irritability, and for many, time to roll another joint to get rid of unpleasant feelings. Many people who use drugs to chase away morning-after misery are unaware that the misery is the aftereffect of the drugs themselves.

THC is sometimes used as a medicine to treat nausea in people with cancer or to reduce eye swelling from the disease glaucoma. When THC is used this way, the high is the drug's side effect. A dangerous side effect, mentioned earlier, is marijuana's interference with driving ability. Even in doses that people use socially, the drug impairs driving performance, and the effect persists long after the high is gone. Another effect is an alteration in heart action, including rapid and sometimes irregular heartbeat. Marijuana may also reduce the body's immune response and, in young men, may reduce the sex hormone level and sperm count. Like other drugs, marijuana presents the greatest potential hazard to those who use it most heavily and frequently.

Users looking for a "better high" sometimes shift to hashish, a concentrated marijuana resin collected from the flowering top of the plant. With hashish, the risks probably increase dramatically, because the user receives a stronger THC dose.

Marijuana smoking, to a greater degree than cigarette smoking, sets the stage for lung damage, including lung cancer. Other hazards are significant: marijuana may be contaminated with pesticides, poisonous molds, or herbicides, or it may contain dangerous drugs. An example is the animal tranquilizer phencyclidine hydrochloride (PCP or "angel dust"), added to marijuana by sellers to deceive buyers into believing that its potency is high.

Marijuana is not thought to be physically addictive but is strongly habit-forming in some people. It could be that some people respond to long-term use by losing ambition and drive, the so-called **amotivational syndrome**.[22] Equally likely, though, lack of motivation and marijuana use simply appear together because of some other factor, such as boredom.[23] Some people find giving up the drug extremely difficult and require therapy to succeed.

AMPHETAMINES. In this high-speed society, a drug that reportedly provides some extra get-up-and-go might tempt even the most cautious. Amphetamines are said to be just such drugs; they are stimulants—drugs that stimulate the central nervous system, increasing activity, suppressing fatigue and hunger, and producing euphoria. They are available by prescription to treat diseases such as intractable obesity, uncontrollable sleeping, or, in children, hyperactivity.*

People may start using amphetamines to lose weight, to combat fatigue so they can work at night or study for exams; to party all night; or to offset the sleepiness brought on by alcohol, marijuana, or sedatives. Sometimes a daily cycle develops in which people use depressants such as barbiturates to relieve amphetamine overstimulation and then more amphetamines to pick themselves up again. (This cycle is especially common among physicians and nurses.) Physical tolerance to amphetamines builds up in just a few weeks, and soon, the user may be taking several hundred times the normally prescribed dose to achieve the desired effect. At this point, drug dependence is extreme.

When used as medicine, amphetamines are taken by mouth; the usual route for euphoria seekers is injection into a vein. The risks of using any drug increase dramatically when the drug is injected. Overdoses are likely. Needles may not be sterile, or the skin may not be properly cleansed; the needle puncture may introduce life-threatening microbes directly into the bloodstream, or a fatal air bubble may be injected. People may share needles and, at the same time, share infections such as AIDS or hepatitis (a dangerous, often incurable liver condition).

More about AIDS in Chapter 15.

A person injecting amphetamines experiences an intense short-lived euphoria likened to a sexual orgasm. The drug-taker may feel unusually strong; this, coupled with drug-induced hyperactivity and paranoid delusions, can lead to behavior dangerous to self and others. The user may repeat the injection ten times daily for several days consecutively, while not sleeping and taking very little food.

The euphoria wears off much more quickly than the drug's other effects. Accidents are likely because the user is unaware of fatigue until suddenly

---

*In the case of hyperactivity, the amphetamine acts not to stimulate the child but to stimulate a brain center that filters out distractions, so that the child can concentrate.

overwhelmed by it, perhaps while driving or crossing the street. When fatigue or confusion becomes so great that injection is no longer possible, the binge is over and the person sleeps for days, awakening with voracious hunger. Severe discomfort and psychological depression follow, and the person may turn again to the drug for relief. Injected amphetamines' side effects include acute anxiety, psychosis, malnutrition, and in high doses, brain hemorrhage resulting from high blood pressure, dangerously elevated temperature, convulsions, lack of oxygen, loss of consciousness, and death.

Amphetamines lead people to think they have desirable traits when they are under the influence. The undrugged self pales by comparison. They continue to take the drug to maintain their illusions, and in doing so, abandon real life, where they could become genuinely more sensitive, more fun, more intelligent, better lovers, or whatever else might improve the quality of their lives.

SEDATIVES AND BARBITURATES. These agents exert a depressant effect on many body systems, by a number of different means. Some sedatives slow the heart; some, the brain and nervous system; some, both. They may be used to calm agitation, dull sensation, or put to sleep—useful effects as tools of the medical professional, but potentially dangerous when self-administered. Some are more dangerous than others, but none are safe.

Barbiturates are a group of chemically related compounds that all have similar effects. They depress the nervous system, the heart rate, the respiration rate, the blood pressure, and the body temperature. They have legitimate medical uses, but they are easily abused. Long-term use can cause depression, forgetfulness, reduced sex drive, and many other adverse effects, including addiction; overdoses kill.

COCAINE. Cocaine's wonders have been extolled since Freud first wrote of it (although he later cursed it when he became intractably addicted). In contemporary life, cocaine has had an aura of sophistication, and until recently, its use was a badge of economic status. Mystique aside, cocaine's effects, when subjected to scientific examination, are found to be similar to those of two groups of medical drugs: the local anesthetics and the stimulants. In fact, experienced cocaine users cannot distinguish injected amphetamine from injected cocaine.[24]

The leaves of the coca bush are processed to yield the isolated drug cocaine. In coca-growing cultures, people chew the leaves to receive small doses of the stimulant to help them work longer. In other cultures, the isolated chemical is usually mixed with other white powders—some inert, some not—before it is sold. If an unwary consumer happens on pure cocaine and uses it in the same quantity as the diluted product, the reactions are severe or fatal.

People may use any of a number of methods to self-administer cocaine. One route is snorting—that is, taking the powder into the nose, usually by arranging it ceremoniously into neat lines on a mirror and inhaling it through a tube rolled from a currency bill that denotes status. Others may inhale from a gold "coke spoon," and still others may inject the drug. Many a person who starts by snorting a little escalates by increasing the doses, goes on binges, and moves to the more direct administration routes—injection or smoking. Such people have been known to rip through thousands of dollars worth of cocaine *each week*.

People also smoke cocaine products, "crack", or "rock," and "base." Smokable cocaine now rivals marijuana in frequency of use in some areas of the country. Crack opened whole new drug markets because of its low price, and deaths from the drug followed suit. As of this writing, still cheaper and even more dangerous forms are on the horizon.

Although not confirmed scientifically, hallucinations are reported to occur in regular users of cocaine. Some users describe flickering lights, called snow lights; or they perceive the presence of vermin on and about their bodies. Others may experience fears of persecution associated with paranoia.

The short-lived burst of exhilaration produced by cocaine is laced with a feeling of being out of control, and is followed by intense irritability. The intensity of the high and the low depends partly on the drug dose, partly on the route of administration, and partly on the user's expectations. Repeated use of the drug shuts off all drives, including the sex drive, and replaces them with the drug-seeking drive.

Cocaine causes constriction of blood vessels (and thus elevation of the blood pressure), dilation of the pupils of the eyes, and increased body temperature. It also banishes fatigue and hunger. Cocaine levels in brain tissues remain high long after euphoria has faded, and the stored drug is released slowly as blood levels start to fall.

By constricting the blood vessels, cocaine erodes nasal tissues in habitual snorters. At first, this causes such symptoms as sinus infection, runny nose, and nosebleeds. With increasing use, nasal tissues die, leaving a hole between the nostrils. Just over half of chronic users report nasal problems.

More commonly, people report chronic fatigue (yet they claim coke peps them up), poor sexual performance (but they claim coke is good for sex), and severe headaches. In one study, over a third of chronic cocaine users reported having considered suicide, and about a tenth had made suicide attempts.[25] Its use in pregnancy is linked to birth defects and infant death.

Cocaine occasionally causes death—usually by heart attack, stroke, or seizure in an already damaged body system. In other cases, the cocaine has been injected together with a drug having a narrow margin of safety, such as heroin.

A person who is cocaine dependent loses the ability to work, to keep a job, to play, or to stop using the drug. Between 60 and 80 percent of users questioned believe themselves to be addicted, unable to turn the drug down if offered and unable to limit cocaine use.[26] Recovery from addiction is described on page 147–148.

INHALANTS. Three categories of chemicals are sometimes inhaled to produce a high. The first type, solvents, consists of organic liquids that vaporize at room temperature; fumes from gasoline, glue, lighter fluid, cleaning fluid, and paint thinner are concentrated and inhaled. A second type, propellants, is added by manufacturers to products that are sprayed, such as paint, deodorant, hairspray, and oil. All these products bear labels that warn against inhaling their fumes because of the hazards they present. A person who experiments with them, even once, risks permanent disability or death from heart failure or suffocation.

A third group is manufactured as drugs; examples are chloroform, ether, nitrous oxide (laughing gas), and others. Amyl nitrite, a heart pain medicine, is sometimes abused this way, and so is butyl nitrite, sold legally as a "room odorizer." It has been claimed that sniffing the nitrites is a sexual stimulant; research shows that these chemicals interfere with erection and bring on headache, dizziness, accelerated heart rate, nausea, nasal irritation, or cough. They may, however, cause the user to think that sexual orgasm has been prolonged, because they interfere with time perception.

Inhalants' effects on brain cells are unpredictable and depend on the chemicals present and on the dose (although it is impossible to measure the quantity taken). In general, even short-term abuse brings on vision disturbances, impaired judgment, and reduced muscle and reflex control that may be difficult to reverse. Sniffing has caused many cases of permanent brain and nerve damage as well as damage to the kidneys, blood, liver, and bone marrow. Suffocation occurs when the lungs fill with gases that contain no oxygen or when the product coats the lungs' absorptive surfaces and thus blocks oxygen transfer to the blood.

LOOK-ALIKES. Another group of easily accessible drugs is the so-called **look-alikes**. Drug pushers, masquerading as companies, produce pills and powders that look like the prescription medications and illegal drugs that abusers seek. The pills are made from OTC drugs and other legal substances. For example, magazines publish ads for "legal stimulants" ("mail-order speed") that mimic the prescription drugs' appearance almost exactly, with one important difference: the capsules or tablets contain a combination of OTC stimulants, decongestants, antihistamines, and other drugs instead of amphetamines.

People who buy these bogus drugs may turn around and sell them to others as real, high-priced amphetamines. Because the look-alikes are weaker, users tend to take a lot of them. As a result, users may experience sleep disturbances, heartbeat irregularities, and sudden rises in blood pressure. The most dangerous situation occurs when a user can't tell the difference between the look-alikes and the real thing; when such a person gets some of the high-powered amphetamines and takes the same number of pills, a fatal overdose results.

The look-alikes are legal, so there are no limits on their sale and distribution. Those who sell them make huge profits at the expense of the consumer's health. It's the same with all street drugs—no one is looking out for the consumer.

DESIGNER DRUGS. Designer drugs are laboratory-synthesized compounds that closely resemble illegal drugs in chemical structure. The chemical definition of a substance determines its legality, and designer drugs are just dissimilar enough from the real thing to be legal, yet similar enough to produce like effects in the body—at least, that is the maker's plan.

A story of what actually can happen with designer drugs was told in an episode of the public television series "Nova."[27] A fumbling amateur chemist, using a crude basement laboratory in California, tried to produce a batch of designer heroin. His inept chemistry produced, instead, a substance so toxic to brain cells that when the heroin addicts who purchased it injected the stuff, they were immediately and permanently paralyzed.* The substance left them with Parkinson's disease—destruction of the parts of the brain that control motor activity. The police found and arrested the "designer"; he too had developed Parkinsonism from his creation, because the chemical had entered his body through his skin and lungs. Now, the same chemical is showing up in other chemists' drugs, under the names of designer heroin and designer cocaine.

This story accentuates the problem all users of street drugs face: lack of standardization. California is now taking steps to outlaw designer drugs, but new ones can be developed and sold faster than they can be classified and controlled. People who use them, or even simply handle them, are risking exposure to highly toxic chemicals.

STRATEGIES: FREEDOM FROM DRUGS

How can you tell whether someone close to you is abusing drugs? Here are some behavioral signs:

- Pallor and perspiration.
- Dilated pupils.
- Runny nose and nosebleeds.
- Jitters and hyperactivity.
- Ability to go without food or sleep for long periods of time.
- Lack of interest in sex and occasional inability to perform.
- Paranoia, anxiety, suspiciousness.
- Loss of memory.
- Increase in energy and talkativeness, followed by lethargy and depression.
- Sudden carelessness about personal appearance.
- Broken appointments, broken promises, lying.
- Inability to explain what happened to the paycheck or other money.[28]

Extreme caution should be used in attributing any of these signs to drug abuse; they may be caused by a hundred other things as well. Probably the best way to find out if a person is abusing drugs is to express concern and ask questions. If you care, this is a way to show it.

If a drug is causing chronic difficulty, that indicates a drug problem. A way to recognize such a problem is to give up the drug for a month. (Of course, if the drug is a medicine, the physician should decide whether it is safe to do without it.) Coffee, colas, cigarettes, OTC drugs, prescriptions, and alcohol all qualify for this test. Try doing without one, and write down your responses to this chapter's Life Choice Inventory (page 148).

Kicking the Habit

When people realize they have a drug problem, they have taken one important step: admitting it. Now comes a hard choice: suffer on and on, or quit. To quit involves suffering, too, but the suffering ends.

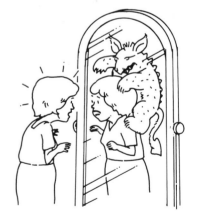

A person who faces up to a drug problem has taken the first important step.

*The substance is MPTP, a side product that usually arises in small amounts during chemical transformations to produce designer heroin. This particular batch was 90 percent MPTP. One of the early symptoms of MPTP exposure is an uncharacteristic burning at the site of entry, such as at the injection site or in the nasal passages.

LIFE CHOICE INVENTORY

Do you have a drug problem? For whatever drug comes to mind, this exercise is an informal way to find out. Give up the drug for a month, and answer these questions:

1. Do you miss the drug?
2. Are you experiencing withdrawal effects?
3. Does life seem less full or less fun without the drug?
4. Are you suddenly aware of problems in your life that you had been ignoring?
5. Are you feeling more tense or anxious than usual?
6. Are you feeling depressed?
7. Do you feel better without the drug?
8. Do you have more problems concentrating or meeting goals and deadlines than usual?

9. Do you find that you spend a lot of time thinking about the drug?
10. Did you ensure quick access to some of the drug just in case you missed it too much?

If you were unable to give up the drug for a month, you have a drug problem. If you answered yes to many of these questions, you may have a drug problem. If you gave up the drug for a month, you may want to kick the habit permanently. You need not figure it out alone; you may want to get someone to help you to do so.

SOURCE: Adapted from S. J. Levy, *Managing the "Drugs" in Your Life* (New York: McGraw-Hill, 1983), p. 41.

For those who face the problem and choose to quit, the next step is to get help. Rarely do people recover from drugs on their own. Help comes in many forms—hospital help, counseling, therapy, drug-quitting groups, and drug therapy. Forms of help for alcohol addiction are especially well worked out and are described in the next chapter.

An example of drug therapy is methadone as treatment for heroin addiction. Methadone is an addictive drug, as heroin is, but it is cheaper, and its effects are milder and longer-lasting. Taking a "maintenance" drug such as methadone or one of its relatives allows people addicted to heroin to recover

Some people make it.

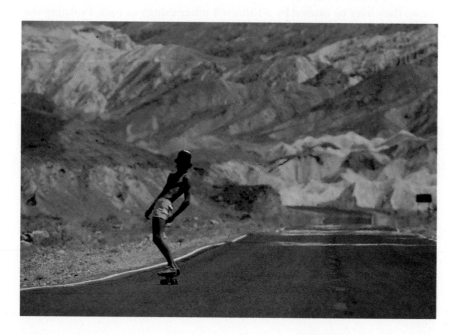

socially—that is, they no longer must struggle to purchase expensive, illegal drugs to hold off withdrawal. Another useful drug treatment employs drugs called narcotic **antagonists**, which block the effects of the addicting agent. The same drugs are used to treat overdoses. Each administration of the antagonist represents a renewed commitment by the taker not to use the addictive drug.

Few people who attempt recovery make a clean getaway. Instead of the normal life that awaits those few who make it, most people get caught in something like a revolving door: undergoing treatment, giving up the drug, getting out of treatment, taking the drug again, going back into treatment—and so on indefinitely. Many factors contribute to this pattern, a main one being the dependent person's failure to make necessary lifestyle changes. When the person first becomes free of the drug, problems are not only as numerous as ever, but now must be handled without the escape that drugs once provided. The person who develops a support system to facilitate confronting the problems has the best chance of staying free of drug abuse.

Another factor is the decrease in reinforcement once the person has become free of the drug. Drug-dependent people get negative attention while they are on the drug and positive reinforcement when they go for treatment. When they leave treatment, though, all forms of attention disappear, and they still crave the drug. Thus they fall back into drug use.

Still, some people make it. The first part is the hardest, for life seems empty without the drug; but later, looking back, the recovered person finds that the rewards of sanity and health outweigh whatever the drug seemed to offer. A great reinforcer of recovery is to turn and offer a helping hand to others.

Helping Someone Kick the Habit

If you care about a person with a drug problem, you will be willing to make the effort to help, even if this means being tough. You may have to risk confrontation, standing against your peers, and maybe even loss of a friend in the effort to save the person's health or life. Things you can do include:

- Making sure the person knows you won't endorse the drug habit.
- Making available all the information you can gather on the health effects.
- Making sure the person knows where to go for help on choosing to seek it.

Drug dependence does not mean a person is inferior. Blame is a useless concept; it can make people feel guilty, but it can't help them get better. Drug-dependent people pay heavily enough for past choices. If you want to help, you won't judge, and you won't blame.

No amount of effort on your part, however, can supply the crucial ingredient in someone else's choice to give up drugs: the will to quit. In fact, the toughest job for many people whose lives are affected by drug abusers is to learn how to manage their own lives without being dragged down. Often they have to learn simply to accept the other person's choice, painful as that may be. Beyond caring, you have to let go. To watch a person self-destruct with drugs is to witness a tragedy—but once you have done all you can, your best choice is to live your own life as fully as possible while it is yours to live.

STUDY AIDS

1. Define *drug*.
2. List the roles drugs play as medicines.
3. Explain why all drugs have risks and benefits.
4. Describe the proper uses of OTC and prescription medications.
5. List some considerations in selecting OTC medications.
6. List the factors that affect a drug's actions in the body.
7. Identify events that lead to drug tolerance and drug dependence.
8. Tell how generic and brand name drugs are similar and how they differ.
9. Give the medical definitions of *drug use*, *drug misuse*, and *drug abuse*.
10. Describe some of the hazards of abusing drugs (for example, marijuana, amphetamines, sedatives and barbiturates, cocaine, inhalants, look-alikes, and designer drugs).
11. Describe some signs that indicate that a person might have a drug problem.
12. State ways a person can help someone give up drugs.

GLOSSARY

(For names of medicines, see the Miniglossary of Medicine Terms on pages 130–131.)

active ingredients: the ingredients of a medical drug that bring about the desired effect. See also *inactive*, or *inert ingredients*.

addiction: the state of being physically dependent on a drug so that the drug must be administered periodically to prevent withdrawal symptoms.

amotivational syndrome: loss of ambition and drive; a characteristic of long-term users of marijuana.

antagonist (an-TAG-uh-nist): a drug that opposes the action of another drug.
  anti = against
  agon = struggle

brand name: the name a company gives to a drug; the name by which it is sold.

controlled drug: a drug placed on a schedule or in a special category to prevent, curtail, or limit its distribution and manufacture. A synonym for legal purposes is *narcotic*.

dependence: the state of reliance on (including addiction to) a drug. Dependence can be physiological or psychological.

drug: any substance taken into the living organism that modifies one or more of its functions. See also *medicine*.

drug abuse: the deliberate taking of a drug for other than a medical purpose and in a manner that can result in damage to a person's health or ability to function.

drug misuse: the taking of a drug for its medically intended purpose, but not in the appropriate amount, frequency, strength, or manner.

drug use: the taking of a drug for its medically intended purpose, and in the appropriate amount, frequency, strength, and manner. *Recreational drug use* is not defined by the FDA.

effective: having the medically intended effect, part of the legal requirement for a drug.

effective dose: see *therapeutic dose*.

euphoria (you-FORE-ee-uh): an inflated sense of well-being and pleasure brought on by some drugs, popularly called a *high*.

generic (jeh-NEHR-ick) **name:** the chemical name for a drug, as opposed to the brand name.
  genus = kind, type

habituation (ha-BIH-chu-AY-shun): the process of becoming accustomed to something by frequent repetition.

high: see *euphoria*.

inactive, or **inert, ingredients:** inactive, nontherapeutic ingredients in a medical drug, such as carriers, coloring agents, preservatives, or capsules.
  iners = idleness

lethal dose: the amount of a drug necessary to produce death.

look-alikes: combinations of OTC drugs and other chemicals packaged to look like prescription medications.

medicine: a drug used to facilitate cure of disease, lessen disease severity, relieve symptoms, prevent disease, facilitate diagnosis, or produce other desired effects.

overdose: see *therapeutic dose*.

over-the-counter (OTC) drug: a drug legally available without a prescription.

physiological dependence: see *addiction*, *dependence*.

prescription drug: a drug available only with a physician's order.

prostaglandins (PROST-uh-GLAND-ins): a group of hormonelike biological substances that affect a wide variety of body systems.

psychoactive: mind altering; a term used to describe drugs that produce euphoria or hallucinations.

psychological dependence: see *dependence*.

recreational drug use: a term not defined by authorities, but used by people who claim their drug taking produces no harmful social or health effects.

safe: causing no unacceptable harm, part of the legal requirement for a drug.

side effect: an effect of a drug other than the intended medical effect.

therapeutic dose: the amount of a drug required to bring about the desired therapeutic effect—the *effective dose*. Any dose above this is an *overdose*; or an *abusive dose*; a dose high enough to threaten health or life is a *toxic dose*.

therapeutic index: the margin of safety of a drug; the therapeutic dose compared with the lethal dose.

tolerance: a state that develops in users of certain drugs that requires them to take larger and larger amounts of the drug to produce the same effect. Tolerance underlies physical dependence.

withdrawal: the process of ceasing to use a particular drug, with accompanying psychological and sometimes physiological effects.

QUIZ ANSWERS

1. *False.* Both aspirin and insulin modify one or more body functions; all drugs do.

2. *False.* Everyone who takes aspirin receives all of its effects, whether or not they seek them.

3. *True.* A person who is not physically addicted to a drug may still crave it intensely.

4. *False.* A person who has developed a drug tolerance has physically adapted to the presence of a drug in the body.

5. *False.* Drugs that are sold over the counter are effective, relatively safe drugs that can be used, with appropriate caution, without the advice of a physician.

6. *False.* Medicines such as tranquilizers, amphetamines, and cold medications make driving hazardous to self and others.

7. *True.* Alcohol is the most commonly abused drug in the United States and Canada.

8. *False.* People keep taking addictive drugs to avoid withdrawal.

9. *False.* Substitutions may be helpful, such as methadone for heroin.

10. *False.* Generic and brand name drugs contain the same *active* ingredients but their other ingredients may differ, so decision to substitute should be made by a physician.

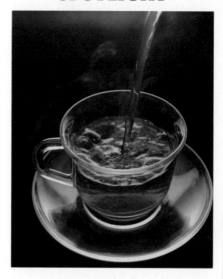

Caffeine

Most people have been consuming caffeine since their first cola drink, cup of tea, or chocolate bar. People are exposed to caffeine in coffee, wake-up pills, and other medications. Lately, though, some people have been cutting back on caffeine because they fear it may cause harm.

What effects does caffeine have?

Caffeine is a stimulant believed to work by interacting with the central nervous system. The familiar "pick-me-up" effects are reduced drowsiness and fatigue and a sharper focus on tasks at hand.

Does caffeine have side effects?

Yes, it does, but which ones you experience depends on how much you take in and how much you're used to, as well as your individual makeup. Most people, if they take the equivalent of two to five cups of brewed coffee, experience an accelerated heart rate, skeletal muscle tension, and a diuretic effect (frequent urination). Caffeine stimulates stomach acid secretion and so will irritate the stomach of a person prone to ulcer. (Decaffeinated coffee does the same thing because it contains caffeine relatives, and so people with ulcers are advised to drink no coffee, whether decaffeinated or regular.)

How can I tell if I'm getting too much caffeine?

If you take more caffeine than the amount in about five cups of coffee, you may experience irregular heartbeats, you may have trouble sleeping, or you may experience headaches, trembling, nervousness, and other symptoms of anxiety. It takes an astute medical professional to uncover the true cause of these symptoms, because they resemble the symptoms of anxiety neurosis.

All of caffeine's symptoms seem to hit children the hardest. If a child is cranky or unable to sleep, try to determine how many caffeine-containing foods and beverages that child consumed during the day.

I've heard people say, as a joke, "I'm addicted to cola!" Is caffeine addictive?

People who take large amounts of caffeine daily build up a tolerance to it; thus caffeine produces dependency. If they suddenly stop, they are likely to experience uncomfortable withdrawal symptoms: anxiety, muscle tension, and headache that no painkiller can relieve. A dose or two of caffeine makes them feel better and they soon learn that they can avoid withdrawal by taking the drug.

Does caffeine harm the body?

Caffeine is unlikely to be abused to extremes, because it does not produce feelings of pleasure. Researchers have been exploring possible links between caffeine and such disorders as birth defects, heart disease, adult bone loss, cancer, and a painful breast condition called fibrocystic breast disease. Most of these are still under investigation, but at present the researchers think that caffeine does not *cause* any of them. It may, however, *worsen* heart disease by raising the blood pressure and triggering the release of stress hormones, which in turn raise the concentration of the risk-posing blood lipids.[1]* Caffeine may worsen adult bone loss by causing increased calcium excretion, and it may worsen fibrocystic breast disease. Research does not support a connection with birth defects or cancer.

Do you think we should all do without caffeine?

Most likely not. To take in the equivalent of one or two cups of coffee a day is probably safe. Pregnant women would be especially wise not to exceed this limit, and parents should monitor their children's intakes—just because the research is

*Reference notes are in Appendix D.

TABLE S7–1 Caffeine Content of Beverages, Foods, and OTC Drugs

Item	Caffeine (mg)	
Drinks and Foods	Average	Range
Coffee (5-oz cup)		
Brewed, drip method	130	110–150
Brewed, percolator	94	64–124
Instant	74	40–108
Decaffeinated, brewed or instant	3	1–5
Tea (5-oz cup)		
Brewed, major U.S. brands	40	20–90
Brewed, imported brands	60	25–110
Instant	30	25–50
Iced (12-oz glass)	70	67–76
Soft drinks (12-oz can)		
Dr. Pepper		40
Colas and cherry colas: regular		30–46
diet		2–58
caffeine-free		0–trace
Jolt		72
Mountain Dew, Mello Yello		52
Big Red		38
Fresca, Hires Root Beer, 7-Up, Sprite, Squirt, Sunkist Orange		0
Cocoa beverage (5 oz cup)	4	2–20
Chocolate milk beverage (8 oz)	5	2–7
Milk chocolate (1 oz)	6	1–15
Dark chocolate, semisweet (1 oz)	20	5–35
Chocolate-flavored syrup (1 oz)	4	4
Drugs[a]		
Cold remedies (standard dose)		
Dristan		0
Coryban-D, Triaminicin		30
Diuretics (standard dose)		
Aqua-ban, Permathene H₂Off		200
Pre-Mens Forte		100
Pain relievers (standard dose)		
Excedrin		130
Midol, Anacin		65
Aspirin, plain (any brand)		0
Stimulants		
Caffedrin, NoDoz, Vivarin		200
Weight-control aids (daily dose)		
Prolamine		280
Dexatrim, Dietac		200

[a]Because products change in formulation, contact the manufacturer for an update.

SOURCES: C. Lecos, The latest caffeine scoreboard, *FDA Consumer,* March 1984, p. 14; Measuring your life with coffee spoons, *Tufts University Diet and Nutrition Letter,* April 1984, pp. 3–6; Expert Panel on Food Safety and Nutrition, Institute of Food Technologists, *Evaluation of Caffeine Safety,* a publication available from the Institute of Food Technologists, 221 N. LaSalle Street, Chicago, IL 60601, 1986.

unclear. People at risk for adult bone loss and heart disease should also be moderate in their use of caffeine. Consult Table S7–1 for the amounts of caffeine in beverages, foods, and drugs, if you want to monitor your intake.

Can you suggest some alternatives to beverages that contain caffeine?

No doubt you are aware that some cola products contain no caffeine, and of course, decaffeinated coffee is an old standby. (By the way, there is no truth in the popular belief that processing chemicals remain in decaffeinated coffee in dangerous amounts. They evaporate from the beans long before they could be ground into the coffee.) Other beverages include decaffeinated tea or teas made from mint or other herbs. Be careful when selecting herbal teas, though—many herbs contain toxic chemicals or chemicals that act as drugs. Use only herbal teas produced by major companies, whose reputations rest on the safety and purity of their products, and use even those in moderation. Don't forget that refreshment can be found in a glass of ice cold water, juice, or milk—the "natural" drinks with a health bonus.

Chapter 8

Alcohol: Use and Abuse

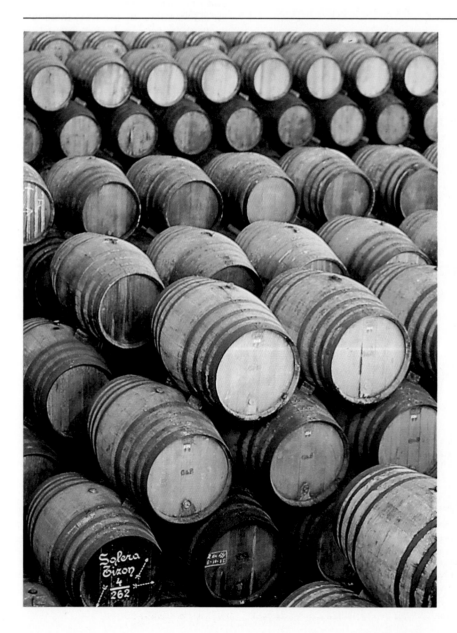

FOR OPENERS . . .

True or false? If false, say what is true.

1. Alcohol is a drug.
2. A person who drinks two drinks every day may be a moderate drinker.
3. Drinking can help a shy, inhibited person become outgoing, carefree, and bold.
4. Alcohol is a depressant drug; it slows people down.
5. In the body, alcohol is digested just as food is.
6. Impaired driving performance occurs when the blood alcohol level is 0.10 percent or higher.
7. Drinking alcohol kills brain cells.
8. Alcohol in any quantity will permanently damage organs in the human body.
9. A person who has had too much to drink should walk around so the muscles will metabolize the alcohol more quickly.
10. Drinking black coffee can help a drunk sober up.

(Answers on page 169.)

The term **alcohol** refers to a class of chemical compounds. One of these is the active ingredient of alcoholic beverages—**ethanol**, or **ethyl alcohol**, but it is often called just *alcohol*. Wine and beer have a relatively low percentage of alcohol, whereas whiskey, vodka, rum, and brandy may be as much as 50 percent alcohol.

The alcohols affect living things profoundly. Most alcohols are toxic, or poisonous; and ethanol is one of these, although less so than some. Sufficiently diluted and taken in small enough doses, it produces effects in the body that people label pleasurable and therefore seek—not without risk, but with a risk they consider acceptable.

Used to achieve these effects, alcohol is a drug—that is, a substance that can modify one or more of the body's functions. Ethanol happens to be the most widely used—and abused—drug in our society. It also happens to be the only legal, nonprescription euphoria-producing drug.

WHY PEOPLE DRINK

Drinkers will give lots of reasons why they drink alcohol: to celebrate, to unwind, because they like the taste of alcoholic beverages, because it's the custom. Young people drink because peer pressure demands it or because they think drinking shows their maturity. Still younger people use it as a way of rebelling against authority. In any case, like other addictive drugs, alcohol produces euphoria: heightening mood, relieving pain, and releasing tension. Because it alters mood, alcohol can facilitate social interactions: taken in moderation, it can relax people and reduce their inhibitions. (Just what constitutes moderate drinking is discussed on page 156.)

The percentage of alcohol in distilled liquor is stated as **proof**: 100-proof liquor is 50% alcohol; 90 proof is 45%, and so forth. A **drink** is a dose of any alcoholic beverage that delivers ½ oz of pure ethanol:
    3 to 4 oz wine.
    10 oz wine cooler.
    12 oz beer.
    1 oz hard liquor (whiskey, gin, rum, vodka).

A drug is a substance that produces physical, mental, emotional, or behavioral change in the user. Euphoria is a sense of well-being and pleasure, a high. See Chapter 7.

CONSUMER CAUTION

The media project an image of the alcohol drinker as a member of a select clique, socially sophisticated, wearing expensive attire and moving through plush surroundings. Ads suggest that drinking expensive brands of wine, beer, and liquor shows affluence. Drinkers on television are smiling, healthy, beautiful, strong, and young. Such advertisements imply that everybody who's anybody is drinking, and you'd better jump on the bandwagon, too, if you want to be somebody.

Drinking alcohol can also be a way to belong to a group whose members share a particular interest. For instance, alcohol consumption has become associated with certain sports, partly through famous athletes' appearances in liquor advertisements. Such appeals cultivate an image that affects both fans and athletes. Athletes are sometimes destroyed early in their careers by alcoholism.

Forms of emotional appeal to drink alcohol have found their way into almost every area of life. Greeting cards and comedy routines make drinking and even drunkenness socially acceptable and funny. All such appeals have one thing in common: they suppress facts about the product and strengthen the emotional impulse to consume liquor. With alcohol, as with any other product, learning to recognize emotional appeals for what they are can help consumers distinguish fake from fact and decide whether they really want what is offered.

Emotional appeals are attractive, but they are not rational.

Alcohol's social effects can be beneficial. The experience of the staff at a hospital for the aging, where three-fourths of the male clients were incontinent (unable to control their bladders) and needed safety restraints to hold them in their wheelchairs is an example.* Needless to say, these clients became depressed. The staff decided to serve beer, cheese, and crackers six times a week in the late afternoon in hopes that this would improve morale and perhaps encourage the men to enjoy themselves and socialize more. Within two months, only one-fourth were incontinent, only 12 percent needed safety restraints, and most had become able to walk around unaided. Group activity more than tripled. The staff attributed the change to the "socializing" effect of the cocktail hour.[1]

Some evidence indicates that people who use alcohol moderately over a lifetime have a lower risk of heart attack and a longer life than either non-drinkers or people who drink to excess.[2] This may be so, not because of any direct physical effect that alcohol has on the body, but because of the life, full of friendships and social stimulation, that such people often enjoy.[3] A person who relaxes with friends at intervals may suffer less stress, either from tension at work or from social isolation, and thereby sustain fewer of the life-shortening effects of stress. Of course, a person can learn to live such a life without alcohol, but in a drinking society, the two may often be found together.

So using alcohol in **moderation** appears to be a key to gaining the benefits from alcohol without incurring intolerable risks. Just what does this mean? No one exact amount of alcohol per day is appropriate for everyone, because people differ in their tolerance levels, but authorities have attempted to set a limit that is appropriate for most healthy people: not more than three drinks a day for the average-sized, healthy man or two drinks a day for the average-sized, healthy woman. This amount is supposed to be enough to produce euphoria without incurring any long-term harm to health. Doubtless some people could consume slightly more; others could definitely not handle nearly so much without significant risk.

Anyone could quarrel with this definition of moderate drinking. People who oppose the use of any alcohol at all could argue that there is nothing moderate whatever in taking three drinks a day for a lifetime, and medical evidence indicates that, indeed, harm to health can result from this level of intake. Habitual heavy drinkers could argue that three beers between, say, noon and midnight is *light* drinking and that six might more appropriately be called moderate. The important things to understand are that a wide range of drinking styles falls between total abstinence and alcoholism; that the most danger lies at the extreme of excessive alcohol consumption, and that the more a person drinks, the closer to that dangerous extreme the person is. Each person must monitor and evaluate his or her own drinking behavior. Terms that describe people who drink are in the margin, together with the definitions used here for them.

How *much* people drink is not the only relevant question. Other important questions are the *reasons* for their drinking and the *consequences* of it. This chapter's Life Choice Inventory helps to make the distinction between social drinkers, people who drink because they are psychologically dependent on alcohol, and those who are physically addicted.

Terms that describe drinkers:

moderate drinker: a person who does not drink excessively; that is, one who does not behave inappropriately on drinking occasions because of alcohol's influence and whose health is not adversely affected by alcohol over the long term.

social drinker: a person who drinks only on social occasions. Depending on the amounts of alcohol such a person consumes, the person may be a moderate or problem drinker.

problem drinker: a person whose drinking is causing social, emotional, family, job-related, or other problems; a person on the way to alcoholism. Other terms for this kind of drinker: **alcohol abuser, pre-alcoholic drinker.**

*The hospital described here is the Cushing Hospital, near Boston.

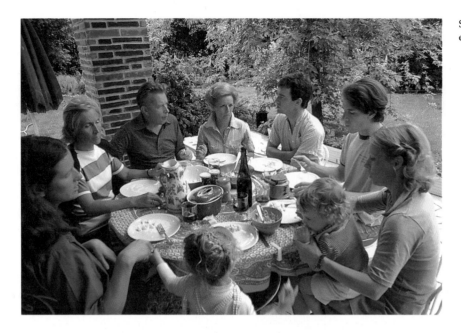

EFFECTS OF ALCOHOL ON BODY AND MIND

The drug alcohol has both short- and long-term effects, and they differ depending on whether the dose is moderate or excessive. To use alcohol without harm, the drinker needs to know just how it acts on the body.

Moderate Drinking, Immediate Effects

Alcohol affects every cell of the body. It is a special molecule in many ways. It is extremely small, as molecules go. It can move fast, and it can mix with both fatty and watery substances. This means that it meets with no barriers in the body; it can go anywhere.

From the moment a person swallows it, alcohol is active in a multitude of ways. From the stomach and intestines it moves rapidly into the bloodstream, and from the blood it enters every cell. Within minutes after the first sip of a drink, ethanol is affecting the brain, muscles, nerves, glands, and the small blood vessels of the skin. It also passes through an extensive bed of capillaries in the liver, the only organ equipped with enzymes for metabolism of alcohol—that is, equipped to convert it to harmless waste substances you can excrete. The liver goes to work on it right away, but can handle only about one drink an hour. If a person drinks faster than this, the excess keeps recirculating, affecting all the cells.

The effects the drinker is most conscious of, naturally, are those that result from its action on the nervous system. Alcohol acts first on some of the brain's fine-tuning inhibitory nerves—those that usually set limits on behavior. A person slightly under the influence of alcohol will talk or laugh more loudly and gesture more vigorously after these controls are released. The loud buzz of animated conversation that you start to hear half an hour into a pleasant cocktail party reflects this effect.

The inhibition-releasing effect of one drink has given people the impression that alcohol is a stimulant. It is not; it is a depressant. With the help of alcohol a person can enjoy social stimulation, but the molecule itself never

Alcohol meets with no barriers in the body; it can go anywhere.

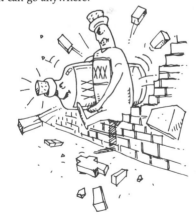

LIFE CHOICE INVENTORY

What is your drinking style? Some people drink primarily for social reasons. They may or may not drink to excess. Some drink for psychological reasons—for the mood change alcohol induces; they may be or may become psychologically dependent on alcohol. Some drink because they are physically addicted.

For each statement, circle the number that describes how often you feel that way about drinking. Answer every question.

I am the type of person who:	Always	Frequently	Occasionally	Seldom	Never
1. Drinks to be socially accepted.	4	3	2	1	0
2. Drinks to be more myself.	4	3	2	1	0
3. Feels more comfortable at a party when drinking.	4	3	2	1	0
4. Downs (gulps) my alcohol beverage.	4	3	2	1	0
5. Has had memory loss (blackout) during or after drinking.	4	3	2	1	0
6. Drinks when depressed, frustrated, or angry.	4	3	2	1	0
7. Accepts a drink when pressured by friends.	4	3	2	1	0
8. Has gotten into fights or arguments when drinking.	4	3	2	1	0
9. Feels more superior when drinking.	4	3	2	1	0
10. Drinks when I am bored.	4	3	2	1	0
11. Feels more popular when relaxed with alcohol.	4	3	2	1	0
12. Likes to drink alone.	4	3	2	1	0

Scoring: Be sure you answered all 12 questions. Add up the numbers you have circled, as shown here (numbers refer to question numbers). The higher your score on any index, the more likely you are dependent on alcohol in that way:

1 + 3 + 7 + 11 = Social Dependence Index.
2 + 6 + 9 + 10 = Psychological Dependence Index.
4 + 5 + 8 + 12 = Physical Dependence Index.

SOURCE: Adapted from an inventory contributed by Professor Martin Turnaver, Radford University, Radford, Virginia. Original source unknown.

stimulates any process within the body. In fact, it acts like anesthetics such as ether or chloroform. Alcohol is a poor choice among anesthetics, though; like heroin, the zone between unconsciousness and death is too narrow for safety. It does not reliably keep people under, and yet it can kill them. (It is still used in emergencies, when no better anesthetic is available.)

Soon after a few sips of alcohol, the drinker can feel it warming the skin. Nerves normally keep skin capillaries constricted to prevent heat loss by radiation, but alcohol relaxes these controls. It also disturbs sleep and reduces the ability to perform mental tasks requiring concentration. The brain helps shut out extraneous stimuli, but alcohol puts this function to sleep, leaving you undefended against distraction.

Another early effect of alcohol in the brain is to sedate the cerebral cortex (see Figure 8–1), where conscious thinking takes place. The drinker loses

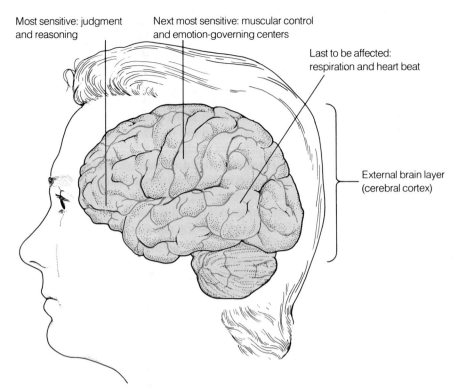

Most sensitive: judgment and reasoning

Next most sensitive: muscular control and emotion-governing centers

Last to be affected: respiration and heart beat

External brain layer (cerebral cortex)

FIGURE 8–1 Alcohol's Effects on the Brain

Alcohol is rightly termed an anesthetic, because it puts brain centers to sleep in order: first the cortex, then the emotion-governing centers, then the centers that govern muscular control, and finally the deep centers that control respiration and heartbeat.

certain kinds of consciousness, including consciousness of unpleasant recent events, worries, insecurity, discomfort, and pain. Simultaneously, the brain's speech and vision centers are being narcotized.

As the blood alcohol content rises, it affects deeper brain centers—among them, the center that inhibits the awareness and expression of emotions. Thus the person expresses love, joy, sorrow, anger, and hatred more easily than before.

Responsible social use of alcohol means achieving and maintaining a blood level high enough to enjoy the mood-heightening effects but low enough to prevent loss of control. The way to do this is to consume exactly as much per unit of time as the body can destroy in that time (as mentioned, about one drink an hour), so that you maintain a plateau.

Excessive Drinking, Immediate Effects

With increasing doses, behavior becomes unpredictable. People may act against their own desires and wishes, because their consciousness of those desires and wishes is now gone. Against all reason and judgment, a person may pick a fight; or a man and a woman may engage in sexual intercourse; or a person may attempt a dangerous physical exploit—with painful or even tragic consequences. The reason these things can happen is clear from the map of the brain in Figure 8–1: the person's judgment would prevent the behavior, but the judgment center has been put to sleep.

Judgment also would tell the person not to have another drink—but again, judgment is anesthetized. This is why a person may go on to drink to the point of passing out. The person no longer has the ability to perceive the need to stop. Next, speech, vision, and coordination are disabled and you might think judgment would tell the drinker not to drive—but at this point, drinkers cannot tell that they should not drive. Everyone has seen the out-of-control driver, weaving back and forth on the highway, out of touch with the cues that show how fast to go and how to steer. Lacking the perception that classifies the risks as life-threatening, the driver may be more entertained than frightened, though.

With still more drinking, the conscious brain is completely subdued, and the person passes out. Table 8–1 shows the blood alcohol levels that correspond with progressively greater intoxication.

While these events are proceeding, the drinker's body is processing alcohol as fast as it can, and internal responses are occurring, too. Alcohol is a toxin, and the body protects itself against ingested toxins in several ways. For one thing, straight alcohol stings as it goes down and triggers the choking reflex that keeps the drinker from swallowing too much at a time. A second protective device is the stomach, which rejects a too-large dose. The drinker vomits and expels at least part of the dose before it can be absorbed. What alcohol does get into the blood is metabolized or excreted by other body systems as quickly as possible.

Alcohol has a multitude of effects on a person's nutrition, some of which occur after only one or a few drinks. For one thing, alcohol depresses the appetite, reducing food intake. For another, it irritates the stomach lining. The more alcohol the stomach is exposed to, the greater this irritation and consequent damage (you know how alcohol feels on irritated skin). Normally, a day's abstinence repairs the damage done by the previous day's few drinks.

The less food the stomach contains, the more rapidly alcohol enters the bloodstream. This is why a person who drinks alcohol on an empty stomach can feel the effects on the brain within a minute. By the same token, if you want alcohol to trickle into the body rather than flooding it suddenly, eat first, then drink.

Alcohol entering the stomach and intestines diffuses rapidly into the bloodstream unless food is present to slow down its absorption. From there, it proceeds directly to the liver, which filters the blood before releasing it to the rest of the body. The liver's location at this point on the map of the circulatory system guarantees that it gets the chance to remove toxic substances before they reach other body organs such as the heart and brain,

TABLE 8–1   Effects of Different Alcohol Doses

Blood Alcohol Level (%)	Effect
0.04	Increased heart rate
0.06	Impaired judgment
0.10	Blurred vision, slurred speech, impaired coordination
0.30	Drunkenness, loss of control
0.40	Unconsciousness
0.50	Amnesia, eventual death

NOTE: Data are for an average-sized person under ordinary circumstances. Effects vary greatly from person to person, from day to day, and from one circumstance to another.

but the liver itself faces a hazard. Given too much of any toxin, the liver is the first organ to be damaged.

The liver possesses a set of enzymes that can metabolize alcohol and other drugs. Like all enzymes, they are made of protein, and like all body proteins, they are degraded when a person fasts. Fasting for as little as a day can reduce the rate of alcohol metabolism by half. Drinking on an empty stomach thus not only lets the drinker feel the effects more promptly, but also brings about higher blood alcohol levels for longer periods of time and increases the effect of alcohol in anesthetizing the brain. The drinker who does not know the risks of drinking on an empty stomach may be in for a dangerous surprise.

While in the system, alcohol causes some vitamins to be destroyed, excreted, or both. The person who drinks 300 calories of empty-calorie alcoholic beverages not only loses the nutrients that might have been delivered by 300 calories of food taken instead but loses more nutrients besides.

Whenever alcohol is being metabolized in the body, some is used as fuel and some is converted to fatty acids. Fat accumulates in the liver during a single night of drinking and begins to interfere with the distribution of nutrients and oxygen to the liver cells. Some research conducted on this process, using beer-drinking fraternity brothers on a college campus, showed that more fat could accumulate in the liver in a single night of heavy drinking than the body could clear away in a single day. People who drink as heavily as these young men were doing, and who do so every night, will therefore experience progressive accumulation of fat in their livers, even if they eat well and are otherwise strong and healthy. If drinking episodes are so close together that the liver can't recover between times, then the fat-stuffed liver cells stop functioning and liver disease develops—as described in the section on long-term effects of excessive drinking later in this chapter.

Drinking, Driving, Accidents, and Violence

Drinking slows reactions. Drinking before and while driving is the single greatest hazard on the road. Of all fatal automobile and motorcycle accidents occurring on the roads today, about half involve alcohol. The hazards associated with drinking and driving have prompted states to pass laws that forbid driving under the influence of alcohol. Under these laws, it is a punishable offense to be **DWI** (driving while impaired) or **DUI** (driving under the influence of alcohol or any other abusable substance). The influence of alcohol is considered proved if the driver's blood alcohol level is 0.10 percent, but DWI is established using tests of coordination and can occur at blood alcohol levels as low as 0.04 percent or even lower. Lobby groups such as MADD (Mothers Against Drunk Drivers) and SADD (Students Against Driving Drunk) are putting pressure on legislators to make the laws stricter, because they have lost too many cherished sons, daughters, and friends to alcohol-related accidents on the highways.[4]

Even after the blood alcohol level has fallen back to zero, a drinker cannot drive safely for several hours. Even moderate drinkers are advised not to drive the morning after an evening of drinking. They may feel fine, but their driving ability may still be impaired by as much as 20 percent—a finding based on research on moderate drinkers aged 19 to 38.[5]

Not only auto accidents, but all accidents, are more likely when people overconsume alcohol. Violent crimes are, too: most are committed by people

The **breathalyzer test** is used to determine blood alcohol level. About 10% of the alcohol in the blood is excreted through the breath, so the amount of alcohol in the breath is an indirect measure of that in the blood.

who have drunk heavily enough to produce blood alcohol levels from 0.10 to 0.30 percent. (With levels higher than that, people pass out.) Remember, these people are not necessarily violent people to begin with, but under alcohol's influence, they become violent. Violent behavior attributed to alcohol misuse accounts for one-third to two-thirds of all murders, assaults, rapes, suicides, assaults in the home, and child abuse.[6]

The Hangover

The hangover—the awful feeling of headache pain, unpleasant sensations in the mouth, and nausea that one has the morning after drinking too much—is a mild form of withdrawal. (The worse form is a delirium with severe tremors that warns of a danger of death and demands medical management.) Hangovers are caused by several factors. One is the toxic effects of **congeners**, other ingredients that accompany the alcohol in alcoholic beverages. The congeners in gin are different from those in vodka, which in turn are different from those in bourbon or rye whiskey. So if one particular kind of liquor produces a hangover, it's possible that another may not. However, this is only one of several factors that produce hangovers, and mixing or switching drinks will not prevent them if too much is drunk.

Dehydration of the brain is a second factor: alcohol not only causes the body to lose water, but actually reduces the brain cells' water content, too. When they rehydrate the morning after, nerve pain accompanies their swelling back to their normal size.[7] Another contributor to the hangover is **formaldehyde**, a chemical familiar as the stuff medical labs use to preserve dead animals. Figure 8–2 shows where it comes from.

For the headache pain, unpleasantness in the mouth, and nausea of a hangover, simple-minded remedies like the following clearly will not work: vitamins, tranquilizers, aspirin, drinking more alcohol, breathing pure oxygen, exercising, eating, or drinking something awful. No matter what you attempt to do, time alone is the cure for a hangover. The problem comes simply from drinking too much. Drink less next time.

Long-Term Effects of Excessive Drinking

The reason some people can drink for years and not suffer accelerating damage is that they stay within the limits of their recovery systems. The damage done by each bout of drinking is repaired in the interval before the next bout. Long-term drinking in excess of those limits wreaks havoc with the body. It causes the greatest damage in one person's heart, another person's pancreas, and another person's brain, but it always affects all organs and organ systems to various extents.

Probably the most common disease to occur among abusers of alcohol is liver disease. The liver converts alcohol to fat and excessive drinking for even one night starts to fill the liver cells with fat. If time between drinking bouts is not sufficient to permit this fat to be transported away to storage sites, then the fat-stuffed liver cells stop functioning, the liver cells die and harden, and function is lost forever.

Since the liver is a crossroads for all nutrients in the body, its injury results in many side effects. Foremost among them is high blood pressure, which sets the stage for heart damage and creates the serious risk of stroke. With prolonged heavy drinking, protein deficiencies develop, too. Eating well or

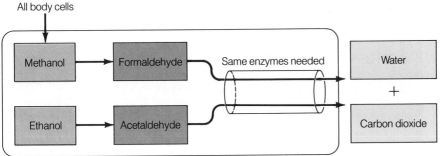

FIGURE 8–2 The Hangover

During the metabolism of excess alcohol, formaldehyde accumulates. It comes from *methanol*, an alcohol produced constantly by normal chemical processes in all the cells. Normally, a set of liver enzymes converts this methanol to formaldehyde and then a second set immediately converts the formaldehyde to carbon dioxide and water, harmless waste products that can be excreted. But the same liver enzymes that do this are needed to process ethanol 20 times over methanol. Both alcohols are metabolized without delay until the load of *acetaldehyde* becomes too great for its enzyme to handle at that point, formaldehyde starts accumulating and the hangover begins.

even taking supplements of protein, vitamins, and minerals does not protect the drinker from such malnutrition; one has to stop drinking alcohol for complete protection. Synthesis of some important immune system proteins also slows down, weakening the body's defenses against infection. Synthesis of fats speeds up, increasing their availability for deposit in the liver, arteries, heart muscle, and other places where they interfere with function. Thus alcohol has direct toxic effects, independent of the effect of malnutrition, on all body organs. An adequate diet cannot protect the heavy drinker against organ injury.[8]

Nerve and gland tissues are particularly sensitive to alcohol. The brain shrinks, even in people who drink only moderately.[9] Prolonged drinking beyond an individual's capacity to recover can cause severe and irreversible effects on vision, memory, learning ability, and other functions.[10] Prolonged drinking in combination with poor nutrition causes major brain diseases.

Alcohol abuse also increases the risk of cancer of the mouth, throat, esophagus, rectum, and lungs.[11] Abusing alcohol also causes failure of the pancreas; some people develop diabetes from alcohol abuse.[12]

Other long-term effects of alcohol abuse:

- Ulcers of the stomach and intestines.
- Deterioration of the muscles, including the heart muscle.
- Blood abnormalities.
- Kidney damage; bladder damage; prostate gland damage.
- Skin rashes and sores.
- Deterioration in the testicles and adrenal glands, leading to feminization and sexual impotence in men.
- Failure of the ovaries and early menopause in women.
- Lung damage leading to flu, pneumonia, tuberculosis.
- Adverse reactions to drugs in combination with alcohol.
- Psychological depression.[13]

Then there are the risks to the fetus carried by a pregnant woman who abuses alcohol—the longest-term risks of all. The effects of **fetal alcohol syndrome (FAS)**, which include mental and physical retardation and birth defects, last a lifetime. Chapter 12 describes FAS in more detail.

In short, alcohol abuse is globally damaging to health. Even social drinking is associated with an increased risk of death from all causes; social drinkers who drink to excess are at risk even though they may never appear drunk.[14] The great weight of evidence is against alcohol for its health effects; the only points in its favor seem to be the social benefits we mentioned at the start of this chapter. There we addressed the question of why people drink.

Perhaps an even more important question is, how can alcohol-dependent people stop drinking?

■ THE WAY BACK: STRATEGIES FOR RECOVERY

Alcohol is the best known of all the drugs on which people become dependent. We also know a great deal about recovery from alcohol dependence. Some aspects of the struggle to recover from dependency are specific to alcohol, but many apply to all drugs.

Recovery from dependency occurs in stages. First, the dependent person has to stop denying and "own" the problem, then quit using the drug and (usually) get help, and then "stay quit." It's simple—simple, but not easy, and few people make it. Estimates of the success rate in alcoholism recovery programs range from 1 in 3 to 1 in 33. Success rates depend, among other things, on the quality of the program and on the length of time the person stays in treatment.

Depending on your relationship to the problem, you may have any of several roles to play in the recovery process. Let's assume you are an onlooker—a spouse, another family member, or a helping agent such as a counselor or a member of the clergy. During the active drinking phase, the most important thing you can do is *not* enable the person to escape the problems resulting from excessive drinking.

Don't Enable

Enabling behavior was defined and described in Chapter 3. An enabler is a rescuer, a person who tries to save the alcohol abuser from the consequences of his or her behavior. The role of rescuer seems noble, but in the case of alcoholism, it blocks recovery. By paying the price for the alcohol abuser, the enabler disconnects the learning process that would otherwise take place: the alcohol abuser does not have to face the music as long as the enabler is around. Enabling takes many different forms—coming up with money when it's owed, helping make excuses ("I'm sorry to have to tell you this, Boss, but my spouse is sick today"), doing the other person's work. Enablers can be family members, sometimes called **co-dependents**, or so-called helpers outside the family (clergy, physicians, counselors, lawyers, and others). A support group for co-dependents, similar to Alcoholics Anonymous for alcohol dependent people, is Al-Anon, which can help enablers learn how not to get in the way of recovery.

Rules to eliminate enabling include the following:

■ Maintain a context of personal concern. (Convey the message, "I care about you. I object to your behaviors, but I see you as a worthwhile person.")
■ Be prompt. Speak as immediately after each episode as possible.
■ Point out the behavior, but do not attack the person. (Do say, "You got drunk last night"; don't say, "You are a no-good, worthless drunk.")
■ Be specific; name and describe behaviors; don't judge. (Do say, "You fell and broke the standing lamp"; don't say, "You made a fool of yourself.")
■ Reflect as a mirror would do. ("Your eyes are red; your hands are shaking.")
■ Don't analyze the other person's personality. (Don't try to explain why the person is behaving in a certain way.)

- Don't pacify the person; such action negates feelings of helplessness that are leading the person to say important things. (Do say, "Go ahead and cry. Here's a tissue"; don't say, "There, there, it'll be all right.")
- When you are angry, cool off before you confront the person who exhibits inappropriate behavior. (Don't let the other person "make" you angry; that's letting yourself be controlled. *You* make you angry, by assessing the situation in an irrational way. Change your assessment, as suggested in Chapter 3.)

Beyond these strategies, co-dependent should go about living and enjoying their own lives to the best of their ability, minimizing the other person's influence on their happiness. The alcohol problem is not their problem. They cannot solve it, change it, take it away, or assume responsibility for it; but they do have the responsibility for their own lives.

Recovery

The progression back to normality from alcohol addiction may take years, if the damage done by alcohol has progressed for years and every aspect of life has been affected. The way back is characterized by its own sequence of events. Over weeks, months, and years, the person stops drinking, becomes able to sleep, regains appetite, begins to function better socially, returns to functioning on the job, and regains health. It's hard, and not everyone succeeds.

Giving up a drug is a grief experience. For reasons the nondependent person cannot possibly fathom, the person is extremely attached to the substance alcohol and cannot imagine life without it any more than you can imagine life without the person you most dearly love. It is a friend, a lover, a comfort, even a god. To give it up requires going through several stages. An early one is denial. Another is bargaining. Then come alternating anger and guilt, and finally acceptance. The person giving up a dependency who goes through these stages deserves the respect to which any grieving person is entitled.

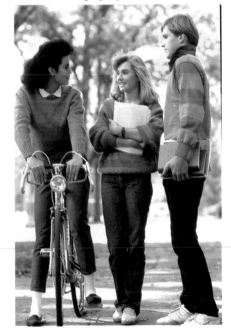

Honest talk helps people face problems.

It helps to put the person in touch with other people who have recovered. No one is so persuasive in assisting a person recovering from substance abuse as one who has been through the experience and succeeded. The worldwide self-help recovery group Alcoholics Anonymous (AA) is based on this principle. In AA, thousands of people have helped one another recover from alcoholism without cost or publicity. The AA program is particularly effective because it takes a positive approach—12 steps to recovery that promote spiritual growth and culminate in the person's actively helping others.* For drug dependencies, comparable groups exist, such as Narcotics Anonymous (NA).

In the beginning of the recovery process, the ex-user is "dry"; only later does the person become "sober." The person who is dry is going without the substance but craving it, and doesn't enjoy life without it. The person who is sober actually prefers life without the substance.

*AA and NA are listed in most telephone books under "AA," "NA," "Alcohol," and "Narcotics." The world address of AA is P.O. Box 459, Grand Central Station, New York, NY 10017.

HOW TO DRINK, HOW TO REFUSE, HOW TO GIVE A GREAT PARTY

Just as the only sure method of birth control is not to engage in sexual intercourse, so too, the only way to be completely protected against excessive drinking is not to drink at all. Those who choose to drink need to learn to handle drinking well, while those who choose to abstain need to learn to do so with ease.

Those who succeed in drinking moderately drink at appropriate times and in appropriate settings only. They limit their intake, and they enjoy being in control. Among the skills they report they've had to learn are the following:

- "I decide in advance how much I'm going to drink. If it's BYOB (bring your own bottle), I take only two drinks with me."
- "If they're serving beer by the pitcher, I still order it by the glass. I read a report that ordering beer by the pitcher tends to double a drinker's intake."[15]
- "I eat before and during a party and then I still drink slowly."
- "I allow time to metabolize the alcohol I've drunk before I drive home."
- "I sip my drinks; I add ice cubes or water; and I drink water if I'm thirsty."
- "I use fruit juices for mixers. They meet my calorie need and keep my blood sugar up."
- "When I want dessert, I eat ice cream. A pina colada has too many calories."
- "Now and then I skip a round. I don't accept drinks I don't want."
- "I go slowly with unfamiliar drinks."
- "If I need sleep, I sleep—I don't drink. If I need to relax, I relax—I don't drink."
- "I know my capacity, and I don't exceed it."[16]

A 103-year-old skier is reported once to have told the *New York Times*: "The secret to long life is to stay busy, get plenty of exercise, and don't

Life without the substance may be better.

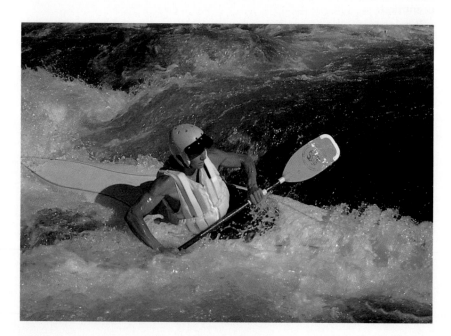

drink too much. Then, again, don't drink too little." To a younger person just starting to abuse alcohol, the skier might have gone on to point out that when people drink heavily, they are seeking the same positive feelings they once experienced from drinking more moderately. They may not realize that alcohol, taken in large doses, becomes a depressant and that their drinking behavior is self-defeating. Enjoyment may lead to health, but excess does not.[17]

Those who choose not to drink have every right to make that choice. The choice is personal, it is yours, and it is no one else's business. A perfectly legitimate statement is: "I don't drink because I don't want to drink." Nevertheless, some social groups give people a hard time for refusing to participate in drinking, because it is a shared experience. Pointers offered to the nondrinker by one source include the following:

■ Don't apologize.
■ Expect others to respect your choice.
■ Respect the drinker's choice to drink.[18]

Learning to serve alcohol responsibly is useful, for both social and legal reasons. At least one state has passed laws that hold a host accountable for alcohol-related accidents or damage caused by the host's guest. Learning to give enjoyable parties that don't include alcohol is worthwhile, because such parties are becoming increasingly popular with students, social organizations, and members of the business community.[19] This chapter's Strategies box offers suggestions on how to give a great party.

If a friend has drunk too much, you can't hasten the return of sobriety by taking your friend for a walk. The muscles have to work to walk, but since they cannot metabolize alcohol, they cannot help clear it from the blood. Time is the only thing that will do the job; each person's blood is cleared of alcohol at a steady but limited rate.

⊛ STRATEGIES: How to Give a Great Party

To give a great party:

1. Keep the cocktail hour short and the music turned down. (Music that makes it impossible to talk makes people drink more.)

2. Provide plenty of snacks with drinks. Don't serve drinks too early or too generously, and don't offer refills too often.

3. Be careful about whom you ask to tend bar. (Problem drinkers tend to push drinks at people.)

4. Offer nonalcoholic beverages so people can pace themselves.

5. Make nondrinkers feel accepted. (They may be pilots, surgeons, alcoholics, Moslems—whatever their reason for not drinking, it's their business.)

6. If you notice someone drinking too fast, offer that person coffee. (He or she will usually get the hint.)

7. Limit alcohol consumption by providing drinks with filling calories like punch or sangria. (If anyone's expectations for strong drinks are dashed by this, don't take it personally. Their disappointment is a reflection on their drinking problem, not on your hospitality.)

Nor will it help to give your friend a cup of coffee. Caffeine is a stimulant, but it won't help metabolize alcohol. The police say ruefully, "A drunk who drinks a cup of coffee won't get sober but may become a wide-awake drunk."

Other suggestions for dealing with someone who is intoxicated:

- Don't respond to emotions stirred by drink.
- Do show concern.
- Allow or withhold another drink based on your judgment, not your friend's.
- Take your friend's car keys away.

For someone who has had too much to drink, we repeat, time is the only real cure. One-half pint takes 10 hours to leave the system, and a person needs 24 hours to sober up completely after having passed out. Let such people sleep, don't let them drive, and never offer a drink for the road.[20]

You may have heard the story of the country woman who kept saying "Amen!" as the preacher ranted about one sin after another; but when he got to her favorite sin, she whispered to her husband that the preacher had "quit preachin' and gone to meddlin.'" We've tried to stick to scientific facts, so the only "meddlin'" we will do is to urge you to look again at Figure 8-1, the drawing of the brain, and note that judgment is affected first when someone drinks. A person's judgment may set the limit at two drinks, but the first drink may take that judgment away. The failure to stop drinking as planned, on repeated occasions, is a danger sign that indicates the person should not drink at all.

STUDY AIDS

1. Describe factors that promote people's drinking.
2. Identify a positive effect of moderate alcohol use.
3. Describe how one or two alcoholic drinks immediately affect the body and mind.
4. Describe the hazards associated with drinking too much too fast.
5. Identify some of the long-term effects of alcohol abuse on health.
6. Distinguish between enabling behaviors and those that force substance-dependent people to face the consequences of their own behavior.
7. Describe strategies for getting help for alcohol problems.
8. Describe the behaviors of a responsible drinker or host.
9. List ways to refuse alcohol without offending the host.

GLOSSARY

alcohol: a class of chemical compounds. The alcohol of alcoholic beverages, *ethanol* or *ethyl alcohol*, is one member of this class.

alcohol abuser: see *problem drinker*.

breathalyzer test: a test of the alcohol level in a person's breath, which is proportional to the blood level of alcohol.

co-dependent: a member of the family of a person dependent on a drug. Co-dependents have a tendency to become enablers.

congeners (CON-jen-ers): ingredients in alcoholic beverages, other than the alcohol itself, that confer flavor and other properties and that may have irritating effects on the nervous system either alone or in combination.

drink: with respect to alcoholic beverages, the amount of a beverage that delivers ½ ounce of pure ethanol—12 ounces of beer, 3 to 4 ounces of wine, or 1 ounce of 100-proof liquor.

DUI: driving under the influence (of alcohol). See *DWI*.

DWI: driving while intoxicated with alcohol or driving while impaired by any abusable substance—a crime by law. Intoxication is defined by blood alcohol level (a level of 0.10 percent in most states). Impairment is defined by measures of coordination or driving skill regardless of blood alcohol level.

ethanol (ethyl alcohol): see *alcohol*.

fetal alcohol syndrome (FAS): a cluster of birth defects including irreversible mental and physical retardation and a characteristic set of facial abnormalities in children born to mothers who abuse alcohol during pregnancy.

formaldehyde: a substance that accumulates during excessive alcohol consumption and contributes to the hangover.

moderate drinker: a person who does not drink excessively; that is, one who doesn't behave inappropriately because of alcohol's influence and whose health is not adversely affected by alcohol over the long term.

moderation: with respect to alcohol use, consumption of an amount of alcohol sufficient to produce euphoria without causing harm to health: not more than two drinks a day for the average-sized, healthy woman or three for the average-sized, healthy man.* See *drink*.

*Food and Nutrition Board, National Research Council, National Academy of Sciences, *Toward Healthful Diets*, as reprinted in *Nutrition Today*, May/June 1980, pp. 7-11. Another nutritionist defines moderation as 10% of calories from alcohol energy, which translates roughly to about two drinks per day for the average woman and three drinks per day for the average man. J. McDonald, Moderate amounts of alcoholic beverages and clinical nutrition, *Journal of Nutrition Education*, 14 (1982): 58-60.

pre-alcoholic drinker: see *problem drinker*.

problem drinker: a person whose drinking is beginning to cause social, emotional, family, job-related, or other problems; a person on the way to alcoholism. Other terms for this kind of drinker are *alcohol abuser* or *pre-alcoholic drinker*.

proof: a term used to describe the percentage of alcohol in a distilled liquor. 100 proof means 50 percent alcohol, 90 proof means 45 percent, and so forth.

social drinker: a person who drinks only on social occasions. Depending on the amounts of alcohol such a person consumes, the person may be a moderate drinker or an alcohol abuser.

QUIZ ANSWERS

1. *True*. Alcohol is a drug; it can modify one or more of the body's functions.

2. *True*. A person who drinks two drinks every day may be a moderate drinker.

3. *False*. It is more likely to make a person giggly, foolish, and careless.

4. *True*. Alcohol is a depressant drug; it slows people down.

5. *False*. Alcohol does not have to be digested; it is immediately absorbed into the blood.

6. *False*. Driving is impaired at blood alcohol levels lower than 0.10 percent.

7. *True*. Drinking alcohol kills brain cells.

8. *False*. Small amounts of alcohol harm body organs, but not beyond repair.

9. *False*. Muscles do not metabolize alcohol, and walking does not affect the rate of alcohol metabolism.

10. *False*. Coffee can wake up, but not sober up, a drunk.

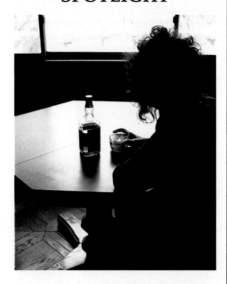

Alcoholism, the Disease

Alcoholism is one of the nation's most serious health problems. About two-thirds of all U.S. adults drink—a total of some 100 million people—and of these, about one in every ten is dependent on alcohol. The annual cost to the nation, including work time lost to alcohol abuse, is estimated in the tens of billions of dollars, and the rate of alcoholism is on the rise.[1]*

What does this mean in terms of people like ourselves?

If you live in a statistically average community, and you have 150 adult acquaintances, then 100 of them drink. Of these, about half are primarily beer drinkers, 40 drink primarily hard liquor, and 10 drink primarily wine. Ten of these people, regardless of what they drink, fall victim to alcoholism. In many settings, up to half of all people with alcoholism are female. Teenagers have a higher alcoholism rate; one in every five teenagers (aged 14 to 17) is already becoming dependent on alcohol.[2]

Surely, alcoholism can't be that common.

Many people would rather not see the problem of alcoholism. In fact, people can choose not to see it; they can convince themselves that it doesn't exist, or that it is a minor problem. Such blindness is even found in hospitals, where physicians list on clients' charts many illness caused by alcoholism without ever mentioning it as the root cause. Depending on the hospital, anywhere from 33 to 95 percent of all patients may be there because of alcohol-related illnesses—including diseases of every body organ, broken bones, and emotional problems. Whenever the problem underlying any of these diagnoses is alcoholism, this has to be dealt with first. And to deal with alcoholism, we have to know what it is.

*Reference notes are in Appendix D.

What is alcoholism?

Many misconceptions attached to the term *alcoholism* need to be corrected. First of all, alcoholism is not related to the kind of beverage drunk. Second, it is not defined by how much is drunk. Nor is alcoholism tied to a particular age. It is not always obvious. It is easy to hide, even well into the advanced stages. People have been amazed to learn that a good friend, whom they have respected and thought of as a fully functioning member of society, has reached a late stage of alcoholism before they discovered it.

To be drunk is not the same thing as to be a person with alcoholism. Anybody can get drunk, simply by drinking too much alcohol; but that does not necessarily signify alcoholism. (It may, but you would have to use other criteria to make the diagnosis.)

How is alcoholism diagnosed, then?

The diagnosis of alcoholism is usually made by the person with the problem. This is important to understand, because one of the key features of alcoholism is denial. Someone else may recognize that a person has a problem with alcoholism, but until the person has accepted that fact, nothing can be done. A person may recognize and own the disease by way of a self-assessment quiz such as the one shown in the accompanying box. A person who has to answer yes to three or more of the questions is on the way to alcoholism.

You have told me what alcoholism is not. Now, please tell me what it is.

As defined by the American Medical Association (AMA), the American Psychiatric Association (APA), and other authorities, alcoholism is a disease, briefly described as a dependence on alcohol. It is chronic, progressive, and potentially fatal, characterized by tolerance, physical

IIII Self-Test for Alcoholism

Score one point for each "yes" answer.

1. Do you feel you are not a normal drinker? (By *normal* we mean you drink less than or only as much as most other people.)
2. Do friends or relatives think you are not a normal drinker?
3. Are you unable to stop drinking when you want to?
4. Does your wife, husband, a parent, or other near relative ever worry or complain about your drinking?
5. Have you ever attended a meeting of Alcoholics Anonymous?
6. Has drinking ever created problems between you and your wife, husband, a parent, or other near relative?
7. Have you ever gotten into trouble at work because of drinking?
8. Have you ever neglected your obligations, your family, or your work for two or more days in a row because you were drinking?
9. Have you ever gone to anyone for help about your drinking?
10. Have you ever been in a hospital because of drinking?
11. Do you ever feel guilty about your drinking?
12. Have you ever been arrested for drunken driving, driving while intoxicated, or driving under the influence of alcoholic beverages?
13. Have you ever been arrested, even for a few hours, because of other drunken behavior?

A score of 0 or 1 indicates no alcohol problem; 2 indicates possible alcoholism; 3 or more indicates alcoholism. This test is highly accurate but is for screening purposes only. Final diagnosis should be made by an alcoholism expert.

SOURCE: Michigan Alcoholism Screening Test (MAST), developed by Dr. Melvin L. Selzer of the University of Michigan, as cited in Test shows alcoholism, *Tallahassee Democrat*, 29 October 1975, p. 10. There are longer tests, but this short one is valid, detecting from 94% to 99% of people with alcoholism.

MINIGLOSSARY

alcoholism: a disease characterized by dependence on alcohol.
blackout: temporary retrospective amnesia, characteristic of the person with alcoholism after a period of drinking.

and the *condition*. Consider the person worthwhile, even while you may oppose what the person *does*. Use language that reflects this attitude: speak of "the person with alcoholism," not of "the alcoholic." After all, if treatment is successful, the person may recover. It is probably not correct to think alcoholism can be cured; but certainly the disease is treatable, and it can be arrested, as long as the person steers clear of alcohol. The person is not "an alcoholic" any more than the person with diabetes is "a diabetic" or the person with cancer, "a canceric."

How can I tell whether a person is becoming alcohol dependent?

A key step along the way to alcoholism is the beginning of **blackouts**—episodes of amnesia. Some authorities say that blackouts are the single most useful diagnostic feature of alcoholism. This statement is open to question, but blackouts are certainly characteristic of people with alcoholism.

Are blackouts the same thing as passing out?

No. In fact, they bear no resemblance to passing out. A person who has had too much to drink may lose consciousness; that is passing out. A person having a blackout, in contrast, may show no external signs of it whatever. The person functions normally, although drinking, but the next day is unable to remember anything that happened beyond a certain point the day before.

An example may help make this clear. Susan eats dinner with her

dependency, and organ damage caused directly or indirectly by alcohol consumption.[3]

The sequence of symptoms is well defined. Alcoholism typically progresses from the first drink, usually in the teens, through increasing involvement with alcohol, to a point where alcohol comes to dominate the person's life, damaging family and friendships, work life, and physical health. Full-blown alcoholism typically takes from three to ten years to develop after heavy drinking has begun. Less time is required, though, if the abuser is young, and some teenagers are clearly already alcohol dependent.[4]

What sorts of people contract alcoholism?

Just as people with diabetes or cancer come in all sizes, shapes, and varieties, so do people with alcoholism. The disease is no respecter of income, education, social class, or physical attractiveness. The person you most admire from a distance is just as likely to be dependent on alcohol as the person you most despise. One does not have to be morally degenerate to be susceptible to alcoholism; one is just susceptible to alcoholism.

For this reason, it is useful to make the distinction between the *person*

family and then sits down at the sewing machine with a drink by her side, to make a dress. She finishes the first drink, goes and gets a second one, and continues making the dress. Several hours later she has had five drinks, has finished the dress, has ironed it and hung it up in the closet, has put away her sewing machine, and has gone to bed. The following morning she remembers nothing beyond the time when she started to sew. To see what she has done, she has to go back and look around. She finds the completed dress in the closet and a half-empty bottle in the cabinet.

As you can see, a person's behavior can be entirely normal during a blackout. Of course, some dire thing may happen instead. Rather than simply having completed a dress, Susan might have taken the car, gone out to buy another bottle, and killed someone on the way. The following morning, as before, she would have awakened completely unaware of what had transpired the previous evening. A dent and some blood on the front of her car might have been her first clues to the previous night's events.

The occurrence of blackouts often marks a turning point for people on their way to alcoholism. The disease of alcoholism can progress far beyond blackouts, but people can stop drinking at any time along the way. The beginning of blackouts is an excellent place to stop.

Chapter 9

Smoking and Smokeless Tobacco

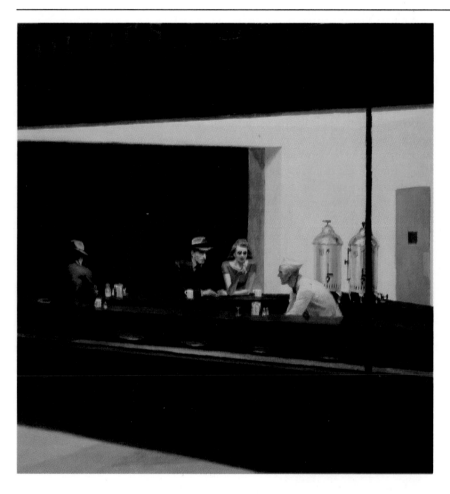

FOR OPENERS . . .

True or false? If false, say what is true.

1. After someone has started smoking, enjoyment is the reason he or she continues to smoke.
2. One of nicotine's chief effects is to elicit the stress response.
3. Because it is taken into the lungs rather than eaten, nicotine reaches the brain in a rush.
4. A sign of nicotine withdrawal is an inability to concentrate.
5. The people in the same room as a person who is smoking are forced to inhale the same substances the smoker does.
6. The way smoking harms health is to cause lung diseases.
7. In emphysema, the lungs first become damaged, not because people can't breathe in, but because they can't breathe out.
8. Smoking impairs people's ability to remember things.
9. Smoking wrinkles the skin.
10. One effective way to reduce the risk of cancer from smoking is to switch from cigarettes to chewing tobacco, snuff, or a pipe.

(Answers on page 189.)

Undeniably, smoking brings some people pleasure. Otherwise they wouldn't do it, because, as nearly everyone knows, a host of health hazards come along with it. This chapter discusses the smoker's viewpoint first and then goes on to ask if smokers should quit, how to quit, and how to help the quitter. It tries to present all the facts about smoking, both pro and con, with honesty. The evidence, though, is one-sided—con.

The green leaf of the tobacco plant may be beneficial to health in some ways. Tobacco paste is said to relieve the swelling caused by insect bites. Commercially manufactured tobacco spray has been reported to help heal bruises.[1]* But when people turn the green leaf into smoking or chewing tobacco, they alter its chemistry and its health effects.

WHY PEOPLE USE TOBACCO

The pursuasive power of the tobacco industry is clear. Its advertisements associate tobacco use (by suggestion) with stereotypes that undermine people's individuality, but people don't always see through them: handsome, macho cowboys; successful executives; sexy and dynamic-looking women. Young people, searching for role models, are often taken in. Imitating these models, they may adopt their habit of smoking or chewing (or drinking or whatever else they do). They may then show off their own sophistication, enticing their peers into the same habit. A person whose mind is open to using tobacco begins by trying it once. That one time may be followed by another, and in a short while, because nicotine is a powerfully addictive drug, the person becomes a user for life.

Statistics on smoking are impressive. Each day, 5,000 children light up for the first time—some of them only seven or eight years old, in a hurry

*Reference notes are in Appendix D.

Tobacco farmers make the effort to produce high-quality green tobacco.

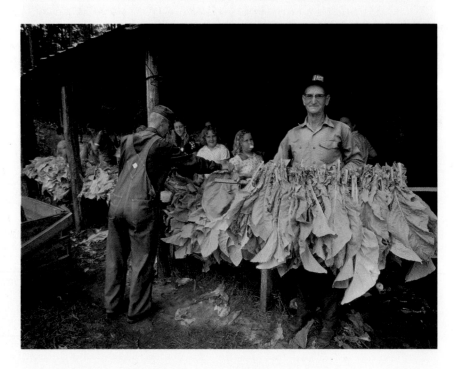

to grow up. Millions of teenagers are smoking.[2] About half of all adults smoke or have smoked at one time or another; only one in four succeeds in quitting. Once a symbol of prestige for the white male, smoking now is widespread among all races, all across the world. In this country, it is as much a habit of women as of men.[3]

A folder written by young people for young people describes how smokers rationalize their choice to smoke: I'm young now—I can quit later. I don't inhale—smoking can't hurt me. Smoking makes me look grown-up and mature. I smoke filter cigarettes—that will protect me. My parents smoke, all my friends smoke—why shouldn't I. If I don't spend the money on cigarettes—I'll spend it on something else. It keeps me from biting my nails. It keeps me from eating. It gives me something to do when I'm mad/bored/hurt/unhappy/restless.[4] Each of these reasons may be invalid, but the new smoker believes them.

Why do people keep on using tobacco? The first taste of a cigarette or other smoking material is, to most people, a noxious experience. Smoke or chewing tobacco in the mouth tastes unpleasant, and the body reacts to tobacco smoke inhaled into the lungs as to any smoke—by coughing to expel the foreign, unwelcome substance. If this were all there were to it, no one would get hooked. Yet smokers keep coming back for more, mainly for the effects of the drug **nicotine**, to which they have developed an addiction. The 350,000 premature deaths *per year* caused by cigarette smoking exceed all other drug and alcohol abuse deaths combined, seven times more than all automobile fatalities per year, and more than the combined American military fatalities in World War I, World War II, and the Vietnam war. More than 60 percent of these yearly deaths represent persons who became addicted to nicotine as adolescents, before the age of legal consent.[5]

Nicotine has multiple effects on the body, especially affecting the major communication networks (the nervous and hormonal systems), the circulatory system, and the digestive system. It stimulates stress hormone secretion, so it speeds up the heart and raises the blood pressure; it changes the brainwave pattern; and it calms the nerves. It reduces anxiety, increases tolerance to pain, facilitates concentration, dulls the taste buds, and reduces hunger. Depending on the pattern of use, it arouses or calms the smoker. Nicotine acts on many different brain centers, so it does different things for different people.[6] There are thus many reasons why people use tobacco, so there is no one way to help everyone stop.

About the stress hormones, see "The Stress Response," pages 28–29.

Because it is taken into the lungs rather than eaten, nicotine reaches the brain in a rush. The dose affects the user noticeably, but even more noticeable are the effects of withdrawal as the dose wears off: a slowed heart rate, reduced blood pressure, nausea, constipation or diarrhea, a headache, irritability, restlessness, anxiety, drowsiness, inability to concentrate, and a craving for another dose.[7]

For many users, the next dose is taken in order to avoid the letdown from the last one—a pattern revealing that they are addicted to tobacco. The addiction becomes so strong that they are unable to quit even in the face of obvious physical complications—about which we say more in a moment.

Psychological dependence is another reason people continue to use tobacco. Nicotine both increases pleasure and reduces pain. Smoking furnishes an excuse, in a busy routine, to take a break and relax. It seems to facilitate lively conversation. It gives immediate relief from small stresses. A person who is embarrassed and doesn't know what to say can light a cigarette. A

The tobacco companies know that once they've got you started, they've got you hooked.

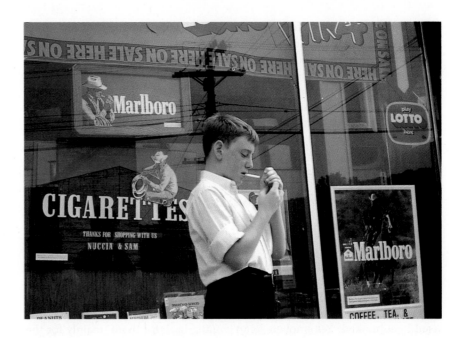

person who is angry and needs to cool off before speaking can pack a pipe. For these and many other reasons, people use tobacco. But they pay a price.

HEALTH EFFECTS OF SMOKING

Anything burned releases a multitude of chemicals not present in the original raw material. The harm brought on people by smoking is primarily from the *burning* ingredients of cigarettes—of which there are thousands. The most harmful ingredients are the **tars**, which are similar to the tars used on roads. These are notorious **carcinogens**, known to be responsible for most cases of lung cancer and for cancers of many other organs. They are also primarily responsible for **emphysema**, another major disease of the lungs.

Many other ingredients in cigarettes also harm smokers. Cigarette manufacturers select from an array of some 1,400 additives to enhance the appeal of their products, some of which, when burned, can form carcinogens. Some of the ingredients in cigarettes are company secrets, so scientists cannot conduct research on their effects. Perhaps a first step toward finding out the risks will be to insist that the industry disclose the ingredients in cigarettes.[8]

The smoke that reaches smokers is a little different from the smoke that reaches those in the room with them. The **mainstream smoke** from a cigarette is the smoke that passes through the cigarette and then enters the smoker's lungs; the **sidestream smoke** is the smoke that enters the air from the burning tip of the cigarette. Clearly, when people smoke, they are inhaling a multitude of compounds they don't normally breathe, many of which are harmful. Naturally, the organ most affected by smoke is the lungs.

The Lungs

A diagram of the lungs appears in Figure 9–1(a). The lungs oxygenate blood that then goes to the body. Every cell has to breathe; the lungs transmit oxygen to the cells so they can stay alive.

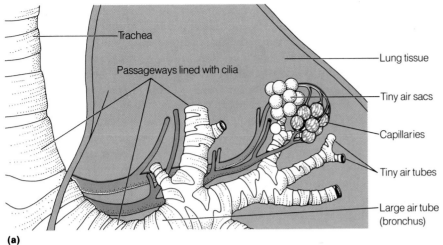

Trachea

Passageways lined with cilia

Lung tissue

Tiny air sacs

Capillaries

Tiny air tubes

Large air tube (bronchus)

(a)

Trapped air

Tiny air sacs have merged, forming a large rigid air pocket.

①
②
③

Pressure

(b)

FIGURE 9–1

(a) Normal lung. Tiny sacs at the ends of the air passageways permit release of the body's carbon dioxide into the air and recharging of the blood with oxygen from the air.

(b) Emphysema. Here, air sacs have burst to form a single, rigid, balloonlike pocket (1). The tiny air tube leading to this portion of lung tissue opens to bring in air but then closes under pressure from the surrounding tissue so that the air is trapped (2). The capillaries are breaking down (3).

The lungs are huge, compared with the heart, and they fill the chest. Their bright red-pink color and bubbling, seething sounds tell you that they are full of blood and air. To perform their life-sustaining work, the lungs draw in air deeply and, like a sponge, soak up oxygen and squeeze out carbon dioxide. Healthy **bronchi**, the major breathing tubes leading to each lung, are lined with cells coated with liquid, slippery **mucus** and little waving hairs (**cilia**). The mucus catches particles and bacteria that would otherwise lodge in the lungs, and the cilia sweep the mucus in a constant stream, up and out. Cilia also line the **trachea**, the windpipe, and they sweep the mucus all the way up to the throat.

Smoking damages the lung tissue in many ways. The tars in cigarette smoke make the mucus coat abnormally thick and also inhibit the action of the cilia so that they become sluggish in sweeping out the accumulated debris. Irritation builds, making the smoker feel like coughing; but each puff on a cigarette paralyzes the cilia for a while, so the smoker feels *less* irritation. The need to cough feels like a need to smoke; the very thing that harms also soothes.

Ultimately, particles from smoke collect to such an extent in the lungs that they form a visible black residue much like the accumulation of oil and tar on the underside of a car. A person examining the lungs can *see* that they can not exchange gases as efficiently as they did formerly.[9]

Some people who smoke ultimately get one or more chronic diseases of the lungs, such as **bronchitis** or emphysema. Bronchitis is familiar to most people as inflammation of the bronchi, which become infected and clogged with heavy mucus; the irritation causes deep, harsh coughing.

Emphysema does not strike every smoker—only those who are born with a genetic susceptibility to it, mostly men. Nor does it strike only smokers; people who live in smoggy cities or who are exposed to polluted air for other reasons (for example, coal miners or workers in smoky factories) may get it, too. But smoking is a major contributor to emphysema, and anyone who has seen exactly how the disease affects the lung tissue will never forget it. At present, no reliable method exists to determine who is susceptible to emphysema.[10]

Figure 9–1(b) shows lung tissue damaged by emphysema for comparison with the normal tissue. As you can see, the normal tissue is intricately laced

bron-KITE-us, em-fih-ZEE-muh

Bronchitis, emphysema, and other diseases of the lungs are often termed **chronic obstructive lung disease** (**COLD**), because they interfere with breathing.

with multitudes of tiny, bubblelike air sacs. A tiny air tube leads to each little sac. As the lung expands, the sac expands and draws air in through the tube. As the lung deflates, the air is squeezed back out.

In emphysema, the air sacs lose their intricate structure and merge to make large, empty pockets of air. (This is much like what happens when 50 tiny soap bubbles merge to form one big bubble.) These rigid, bulging pockets put pressure on the tubes that conduct air to and from them. As the lung expands, the pockets still draw air in, but as the lung deflates, the stiffened tissue around the air tubes shuts them down so that air can't escape. Bubbles of air are trapped in the lungs; they burst and tear lung tissue, making the pockets larger and more rigid and creating more pressure.

The merging of the sacs also greatly reduces the surface area of the lungs available to absorb oxygen. Thus not only does emphysema make it hard to breathe but also each breath delivers less oxygen to the person panting for it.

You can get some idea of what it is like to try to breathe with emphysema-damaged lungs if you run up a long flight of stairs and then clamp a wet towel over your nose and mouth. You are out of breath, your chest is heaving, but you cannot get enough air. The person with emphysema pants for oxygen 30 times a minute at rest, compared with the normal adult's 20 times, but never gets the satisfaction of taking a deep breath. It's a crippling, depressing, debilitating condition. It ruins the quality of life, and ultimately it kills. Death in emphysema is from slow suffocation—or from heart failure, because the heart muscle itself is deprived of oxygen at the same time it is being given the signal to pump harder because of a low level of oxygen in the blood.

Another disease of the lungs—cancer—is much more common in smokers than in nonsmokers. The carcinogens in cigarette smoke cause cancer not only in the lungs but also in the nose, lips, mouth, tongue, throat, and esophagus. Some of them get into the bloodstream and travel elsewhere in the body, so they can cause cancer in any other organ as well; smokers have higher rates of bladder, pancreatic, and kidney cancer than nonsmokers (see Table 9–1). Combined with alcohol, smoking greatly increases the risk of cancer of the esophagus. In fact, cigarette smoking is the major single cause of cancer mortality in the United States.

Smoking combined with certain environmental factors creates a far greater hazard than smoking alone. For example, asbestos by itself constitutes a cancer hazard; asbestos workers are 5 times more likely to contract cancer than are members of the general population. Smokers who do not work with asbestos are 10 times more likely. But people who both smoke and work with asbestos are 50 times more likely to contract lung cancer. Unfortunately, more than half of all asbestos workers smoke cigarettes.[11]

Smoking is responsible for more than one-fourth of all U.S. cancer deaths—for over 41 percent of cancers in men and for 14 percent of all cancers in women.[12] Lung cancer has now surpassed breast cancer as the leading killer among cancers in women, who are the victims of an "epidemic of smoking."[13] Smoking inflicts on blacks the highest rates of lung cancer of any population group in the country, 40 percent higher than whites'.[14]

Smokers know that they are risking lung cancer, but many believe that if they contract it, it can be caught in time for their lives to be saved. Unfortunately, by the time a cancerous spot in the lung is only a millimeter across—just large enough to be seen on an X ray—it is already too late to stop it. (Chapter 17 offers more on cancer.)

TABLE 9-1 The Risks of Smoking

Disease	Smokers' Increase Their Risk of Dying by:*
Lung cancer	7 to 15 times
Throat cancer	5 to 13 times
Oral cancer	3 to 15 times
Esophagus cancer	4 to 5 times
Bladder cancer	2 to 3 times
Pancreatic cancer	2 times
Kidney cancer	1 ½ times
Heart disease	1 ½ to 3 times
Emphysema and other chronic airway obstructions (excluding asthma)	10 to 20 times
Peptic ulcer disease	2 times

*A person who smokes one pack of cigarettes or less per day assumes the risks at the lower end of the spectrum. Those who smoke more than a pack a day assume risks at the higher end. Most important, *the smoker assumes risks of all these diseases at the same time.*

SOURCE: Adapted from American Council on Science and Health, *Smoking or Health: It's your Choice,* January 1984 (a report available from the American Council on Science and Health, 97 Maple St., Summit, NJ 06901).

The Heart

Smoking puts the heart in a quadruple bind. It creates four concurrent effects:

■ Nicotine speeds up the heart rate. The smoker's heart requires more oxygen than does the nonsmoker's heart.

■ Smoking raises the blood pressure, and the heart has to push blood around the body against this pressure. This increases the heart's work load.

■ Simultaneously, smoking reduces the amount of oxygen the blood can carry. Every time the smoker inhales, the blood receives a dose of **carbon monoxide**. The carbon monoxide combines with the protein hemoglobin in the red blood cells to form **carboxyhemoglobin**. This reduces the red blood cells' ability to transport oxygen and the heart's oxygen supply.

■ Nicotine also damages tiny particles in the blood, called **platelets**, and makes the formation of clots more likely than normal. When clots lodge in arteries that feed the heart muscle, they cause death of portions of that muscle—heart attacks. When they lodge in arteries that feed the brain, they cause death of parts of the brain—strokes.

In short, the two major ingredients of cigarettes, nicotine and tars, damage the body's two major life-support systems. Nicotine increases the heart's need for oxygen; tars reduce the lungs' ability to supply it. (Chapter 16 offers more on heart disease.)

Other Effects of Smoking

Smoking affects other organs besides the lungs and the heart. In fact, it affects every organ adversely. It:

■ Shuts down circulation in capillaries, causing cold hands and feet and wrinkling of skin; in some cases, limb amputation becomes necessary.[15]

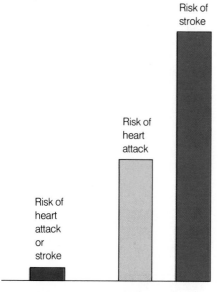

FIGURE 9–2   Smoking and Oral Contraceptives

A woman who smokes and takes birth control pills is 10 times as likely to suffer a heart attack and 20 times as likely to have a stroke as a woman who does neither.

Risk of stroke

Risk of heart attack

Risk of heart attack or stroke

Women who neither smoke nor use oral contraceptives

Women who smoke and use oral contraceptives

- Increases risks of ulcers and makes dying from ulcers more likely.[16]
- Increases the body's drug tolerance so that larger doses are needed for illness and pain, and vaccinations may be ineffective.[17] Oral contraceptives and smoking together increase risks of heart attack and stroke (see Figure 9–2).
- In pregnancy, deprives the developing fetus of oxygen, resulting in smaller babies, premature births, spontaneous abortions (fetal death),[18] and increased risk of infant death.[19]
- Interferes with estrogen production in women, causing early menopause, increased bone loss, and osteoporosis.[20]
- Reduces oxygen supply to the brain, impairing memory.[21]
- Thickens mucus, increasing the risk of chronic **sinusitis**, infection of the sinuses, which can spread to the brain and spinal cord.
- Suppresses immunity, making colds and flu likely.
- Interferes with normal sleep. (Quitters sleep better within three nights of quitting.[22])
- Delivers radiation to the chest. (Smoking one and a half packs of cigarettes a day for one year delivers radiation equal to 300 chest X rays.[23])
- Increases the likelihood of abnormal sperm production.[24]
- Causes progressive hearing loss in low sound frequencies.[25]
- Causes increased **plaque** formation on the teeth, with accompanying gum (periodontal) disease.[26]

Beyond all these effects is the matter of personal appearance. Besides wrinkling the skin, smoking causes bad breath and yellows the teeth. The smell of smoke clings to the smoker's hair, clothes, dwelling, and car, so people who find the smell unpleasant want to avoid both the person and the surroundings. Then, too, the economic cost is not inconsiderable. The heavy smoker may spend from $500 to $1,000 a year on the habit.

Finally, there is the danger of fire. Fires started by dropped or carelessly discarded cigarettes cause thousands of deaths and injuries each year.[27]

CONSUMER CAUTION

With addictive substances, advertisers know that once they've got you started, they've got you hooked.

Smoking, the very habit children need most to be warned against, is promoted to them as something that will make them grown up, cool, and "in." Robert Keeshan, TV's Captain Kangaroo, remembers as a 17-year-old U.S. marine being told by his buddies that if he did not smoke cigarettes, he was not a real marine. "I wanted to be just like John Wayne," he says, "and so I started smoking cigarettes. It took me 25 years to grow up and break the habit."[29]

Advertisers promote smoking to children because they know that a child who becomes addicted will be a paying customer for a long time—possibly, for life. They know how to make smoking seem attractive, too. What could be more enticing to a child, than the thought that a single magic bullet (cigarettes) could confer all the most admired characteristics of adulthood? Even adults fail to see through such subtle come-ons as cigarette brand names that reflect carefully chosen images—Slims, Kool, Satin, More, Eve, Vantage. A suggested warning on cigarette packages might be the following: "TEENAGERS: Smoking is addictive. Never starting means never having to try to quit."

Altogether, smoking is the single greatest cause of preventable death in the United States today.

Despite the seemingly obvious hazards smoking presents, many smokers are totally unaware that it increases risks. One poll showed that 13 to 17 percent of smokers don't know that cigarette smoking is hazardous at all, even though cigarette packages carry warnings. Especially distressing is that nearly half of all teenagers are unaware that nicotine is an addictive drug. Children see adults smoking and think that smoking is OK.[28]

Suppose you couldn't quit using tobacco but you wanted to reduce your risks. Could you improve the odds of retaining your health by switching to low-tar, low-nicotine cigarettes? It depends, of course, on how many you smoke after you switch. Studies of smokers who made this switch have shown that some compensate for the reduction of tar and nicotine by smoking more cigarettes, smoking to a shorter butt, puffing more frequently, or inhaling more deeply. Others, however, truly cut down.

Pipe smoking is an alternative many people consider. True, pipe smokers tend to have lower rates of lung cancer, emphysema, and heart disease than do cigarette smokers, because they don't inhale as much smoke, but they are susceptible to cancers of the lips and tongue. People who switch from cigarettes to pipes tend to inhale more smoke and thus have higher blood levels of nicotine than people who have smoked only pipes.[30]

Quitting altogether is clearly the best alternative. The sooner, the better, too. The degree of recovery from cigarette smoking is related to the total number of cigarettes smoked before stopping.[31] However, reducing the number or the strength of the cigarettes smoked is preferable to doing nothing. The less a person smokes, the smaller the risks. Every cigarette counts.

■ SECOND-HAND SMOKING

The spouses of cigarette smokers have a 60 percent higher risk of lung cancer than the spouses of nonsmokers.[32] Living or working with a smoker produces measurable impairments in lung function.[33] Second-hand smoke worsens heart disease, lung disease, allergic symptoms, asthma, and sinus conditions. It irritates the eyes, especially if contact lenses are worn, and it causes headaches, dizziness, and nausea. In children, it doubles the risk of pneumonia or bronchitis (up to age one), causes permanent lung damage, and brings on asthma attacks. And for the pregnant woman who lives with a smoker, there are even more severe risks to her fetus. It increases stillbirths (babies born dead). It causes more newborns to die in the first six weeks of life. It causes more newborns to be of small size (a health risk). It doubles the risk of birth defects, and it impairs mental and physical development of children up to age 11.[34]

The harm to passive smokers comes from sidestream smoke, which contains 40 known carcinogens as well as other compounds. One of its gases is carbon monoxide, and in a closed room with smokers, this may raise the amount of carboxyhemoglobin in a nonsmoker's blood fivefold. A non-smoking section in any closed space contains just as much carbon monoxide as the smoking section, because carbon monoxide is a gas and diffuses rapidly and freely. Improved ventilation could abolish such effects, but many environments, including workplaces and airplanes, are less than ideally ventilated. Thus many nonsmokers feel that they have no realistic alternative but to demand that smoking not be permitted in environments they share.

Chapter 14's Spotlight deals with fire prevention and escape.

SURGEON GENERAL'S WARNING: Smoking causes lung cancer, heart disease, emphysema, and may complicate pregnancy.

SURGEON GENERAL'S WARNING: Quitting smoking now greatly reduces serious risks to your health.

SURGEON GENERAL'S WARNING: Smoking by pregnant women may result in fetal injury, premature birth, and low birthweight.

SURGEON GENERAL'S WARNING: Cigarette smoke contains carbon monoxide.

Nonsmokers' rights associations have sprung up in many localities in recent decades.* Thanks to their efforts, nonsmoking areas now exist in restaurants, some airlines permit no smoking on flights of a certain duration or no smoking whatever, and many businesses do not allow smoking in their workplaces.

As an individual, if you object to people's smoking near you, you have the opportunity to practice asserting yourself. Without being aggressive or insulting to the smoker, simply say, "Please don't smoke. It bothers me."

▩ SMOKELESS TOBACCO

Some people use **smokeless tobacco** products—snuff or chewing tobacco. Snuff dipping is placing and retaining a pinch of finely ground or powdered tobacco between the gum and cheek, where it gradually releases its nicotine. Tobacco chewing is chewing a "quid" (a chunk of leaves torn from a wad of cured tobacco) to moisten it, and then stowing it in the cheek.

Smokeless tobacco products produce the same dependency as smoked products, because they deliver the addictive drug nicotine just as cigarettes

*The national U.S. organization is Americans for Nonsmokers' Rights, 2054 University Ave., Suite 500-H, Berkeley, CA 94704. The Canadian organization is the Non-Smoker's Rights Association, 455 Spadina Ave., Suite 426A, Toronto, Ontario M55 2G8, Canada.

▐▐▐ Tobacco and Profits

The tobacco industry is big business and represents immense financial interests, not only in the United States, but all across the world, too. Here are some of the facts on the worldwide marketing of tobacco:

▪ Taxpayers' money supports the tobacco industry. Without tax dollars it could not exist.

▪ The government gives out millions of dollars every year to support the growth of more tobacco than U.S. consumers can use. The excess is sold abroad.

▪ In other countries, too, the government supports tobacco production, and uses taxpayers' dollars.

▪ To cure a mere acre and a half of tobacco, the producers have to burn wood for six days. Each 300 cigarettes cost one tree. As a result, massive deforestation and soil erosion are taking place wherever tobacco is cured—for example, in Kenya and Tanzania.

▪ Less-developed countries produce tobacco at the expense of their own people's nutrition. Millions of acres of farmland have been diverted from food production to tobacco production in countries where food has to be imported. Labor for the production of tobacco is needed in spurts, diverting it from farms where it is needed continuously. As a result, food crops are neglected and fail, while laborers are out of work between times of working on tobacco crops.

▪ In less-developed countries where tobacco is marketed, sold, and smoked, people are now experiencing an epidemic of smoking-related diseases.

SOURCE: Adapted from C. B. Popescu, The Third World: Marlboro Country's final frontier, *ACSH News and Views*, May/June 1984, pp. 6-7.

do. A typical advertisement for a smokeless tobacco product suggests: use this sparingly at first, because it will irritate the gums. Increase exposure gradually over time, because, it takes time to get accustomed to strong products and large doses.[35] This introduction to new users is just like the initiation offered by dealers in illegal drugs.

Snuff dipping is associated with cancerous tumors in the nasal cavity, cheek, gum, and throat. Tobacco chewing incurs a *greater* hazard of mouth cancer than does tobacco smoking. Some two dozen studies are now on record documenting hundreds of cases of mouth and throat cancers associated with smokeless tobacco products.[36] The dentist who examines a person's mouth for signs of oral cancer looks for **leukoplakia**—whitish or grayish patches of cells that form in the mouths of tobacco chewers and tend to become cancerous. They develop where the tobacco is held.[37]

Less lethal drawbacks to tobacco chewing and snuff dipping include bad breath, discolored teeth, and a reduced sense of smell and taste. Tobacco chewing also makes the gums recede, wears the tooth surfaces, and destroys the supporting bones, making loss of teeth in later life likely.

■ THE DECISION TO QUIT

Quitting smoking is a major and difficult undertaking. Of people who still smoke, nine out of ten would like to stop but say they "can't."[38] Yet over 30 million people in the United States have quit in the last 20 years or so, and many teenagers, especially teenage girls, are deciding not to start. The next section speaks to "you," to personalize the presentation. It is addressed to smokers, but it might apply to the users of smokeless tobacco as well.

How to Quit Smoking

First of all, take plenty of credit for your decision; you are leaving many weaker souls behind. Quitting smoking is notoriously hard to do; you've decided to kick a powerful addiction. Congratulate yourself; and don't be hard on yourself for having been a smoker.

People seek enjoyment naturally. It is no reflection on you that you would like to continue smoking after having tasted the pleasures of it. Plan to give up the pleasures you have enjoyed, but to substitute others—healthful ones, this time—to take their place. Analyze your smoking style to find out what kinds of pleasures smoking gave you. This chapter's Life Choice Inventory enables you to identify the ones you especially value—stimulation, handling the cigarette, relaxation, or others. When you quit, pay special attention to meeting those needs in other ways. If you smoke for *stimulation*, try brisk walking or other moderate exercise. If you score high in the area of *handling*, toy with a pen or pencil, try doodling, or play with a coin, a piece of jewelry, or plastic cigarettes. If you smoke for *relaxation*, substitute healthful snacks or beverages, chewing gum, or social or physical activities. If your score suggests your habit is driven by psychological dependence, isolate yourself completely from cigarettes until the craving is gone—or use nicotine gum as described later in the chapter. If you are smoking out of habit, it may be easy to quit if you can break your habit patterns. Become aware of each cigarette you smoke. Ask yourself, "Do I really want this cigarette?" You may be surprised at how many you do not want.

SMOKELESS TOBACCO WARNINGS:
WARNING: This product may cause oral cancer.

WARNING: This product may cause gum disease and tooth loss.

WARNING: This product is not a safe alternative to cigarettes.

loo-koh-PLAKE-ee-uh

✳ Strategies for giving up smoking

To succeed in quitting:

✳ Take credit for your decision to quit.

✳ Don't be ashamed of having been a smoker.

✳ Plan your strategy.

LIFE CHOICE INVENTORY

Why do you smoke? Circle one number for each statement. Important: ANSWER EVERY QUESTION.

		Always	Frequently	Occasionally	Seldom	Never
A.	I smoke cigarettes to keep myself from slowing down.	5	4	3	2	1
B.	Handling a cigarette is part of the enjoyment of smoking.	5	4	3	2	1
C.	Smoking cigarettes is pleasant and relaxing.	5	4	3	2	1
D.	I light up a cigarette when I feel angry about something.	5	4	3	2	1
E.	When I have run out of cigarettes, I find it almost unbearable until I can get more.	5	4	3	2	1
F.	I smoke cigarettes without being aware of it.	5	4	3	2	1
G.	I smoke cigarettes to stimulate myself, to perk myself up.	5	4	3	2	1
H.	Part of the enjoyment of smoking a cigarette comes from the steps I take to light up.	5	4	3	2	1
I.	I find cigarettes pleasurable.	5	4	3	2	1
J.	When I feel upset, I light up a cigarette.	5	4	3	2	1
K.	When I'm not smoking, I am very much aware of it.	5	4	3	2	1
L.	I light up a cigarette without realizing I still have one burning in the ashtray.	5	4	3	2	1
M.	I smoke cigarettes to give myself a lift.	5	4	3	2	1
N.	When I smoke a cigarette, part of the enjoyment is watching the smoke as I exhale it.	5	4	3	2	1
O.	I want a cigarette most when I am comfortable and relaxed.	5	4	3	2	1
P.	When I feel blue, I smoke cigarettes.	5	4	3	2	1
Q.	I crave a cigarette when I haven't smoked for a while.	5	4	3	2	1
R.	I've sometimes found a cigarette in my mouth and don't remember putting it there.	5	4	3	2	1

LIFE CHOICE INVENTORY

How to score:

1. Enter the numbers you have circled for each question on the lines below.

___ A	+	___ G	+	___ M	=	___	Stimulation.
___ B	+	___ H	+	___ N	=	___	Handling.
___ C	+	___ I	+	___ O	=	___	Pleasure/relaxation.
___ D	+	___ J	+	___ P	=	___	Crutch/tension reduction.
___ E	+	___ K	+	___ Q	=	___	Craving/psychological dependence.
___ F	+	___ L	+	___ R	=	___	Habit.

2. Add up your scores. For example, the sum of the numbers on lines A, G, and M gives you your score on Stimulation; lines B, H, and N, your score on Handling, and so on. Scores can vary from 3 to 15. Any score 11 or above is high; any score 7 or below is low. The higher your score, the more important this source of satisfaction is to you.

SOURCE: Adapted from Test III of the Smoker's Self-Testing Kit developed by Daniel H. Horn, Ph.D., and originally printed by the National Clearinghouse for Smoking and Health, U. S. Department of Health, Education, and Welfare, HEW Publication no. (NIH) 79–1822, 1979. The wording of the test interpretation has been edited.

⊛ **Commit yourself.**

Now, commit yourself. There are two ways to quit—tapering off or quitting cold turkey (all at once). A way to taper off is to start smoking each day an hour later than you did the day before. Another is to take up a fitness activity that will squeeze out the smoking; in fact, such a choice can even lead someone to quit without initially having intended to do so. The person takes up jogging, discovers that smoking limits endurance, cuts down on smoking, experiences the reward of improved performance, and ultimately cuts out smoking altogether. Another motivator is to start spending time with someone who doesn't smoke or to take a job in a nonsmoking company. The more time you spend not smoking, the more apparent the rewards will be.

⊛ **Seek support.**

⊛ **Tune in to the immediate rewards.**

Tapering off works well for some people, but most are more successful quitting cold turkey, because the hard part is over with more quickly. Two weeks after quitting, people who quit cold turkey have fewer and less intense cravings for cigarettes than do those who quit by cutting back gradually. The Strategies box offers suggestions to help you quit smoking.

Once you've stopped smoking, start noticing the immediate rewards. At first, you will be keenly conscious of the craving to resume smoking. You will have to fight the temptation to light up again. Tuning in to the pleasures of *not* smoking will raise the odds in favor of success. Quitters list small and big pleasures:

- I can breathe again—deep breaths of clean air.
- I don't have to carry cigarettes and matches wherever I go.
- The guilt is gone. I can look my friends and family members in the eye.

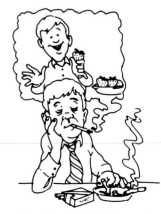

Imagine the pleasures of being smoke-free.

✳ STRATEGIES: How to Quit Smoking

To quit smoking:

1. Promise not to smoke at all for a week, even if the sky falls. More than a week is too much to handle; less makes it too tempting to fall back.

2. Inform everyone who is close to you. This puts your reputation at stake; you will lose face if you break your word.

3. Get a friend to quit with you. Make a friendly wager, agree to celebrate each week, call each other, or agree on other ways of giving each other support.

4. Ask for special consideration at first, in case you're irritable (or get your health care provider or a friend to ask in your behalf). You'll need it.

5. Keep busy—very busy—in whatever way you can. After two weeks, you can begin to relax and let down your guard.

6. If you do smoke, don't smoke just one. Smoke a whole pack in rapid succession; make yourself sick with smoking so that you will want to quit again.

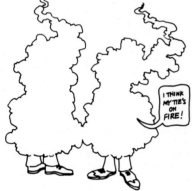

Another reward is that you don't burn holes in your clothes any more.

✳ **Develop alternative pleasures.**

- Foods taste better, and I can smell flowers again.
- My clothes and hair don't smell like smoke anymore.
- I don't get out of breath so quickly when I walk.
- I can talk on the phone without panicking if my cigarettes are out of reach.
- There are no dirty ashtrays around me.
- I'm not going to burn holes in my clothes anymore.

No matter why you decided to quit, what makes you persevere is that you feel better after only two or three days: better physically, and better about yourself.

Whenever you crave a smoke, breathe deeply. Pantomime the smoking process. Relax. You can have all the pleasures of smoking a cigarette, except the cigarette. You may find that what you really want is a moment of relaxation.

By the time the immediate pleasures have become routine, the new habits substituted for smoking should begin to bring pleasure. When you feel like reaching for a smoke, reach for the radio instead, or for the telephone, to make a date with a friend. Take up some form of exercise that will get your heart and lungs in shape. Great pleasure comes from the rapid improvement in fitness that occurs early in a training program for the person who is out of shape.

If you can't make it alone, or if you don't choose to, you can get help. Classes are offered by Smokenders, the American Cancer Society, the American Lung Association, and the American Heart Association. A class can help you identify your smoking style and tailor your quitting strategy accordingly.

You may be afraid that if you quit, you will gain weight. Some people actually lose weight, but most quitters do gain—for two reasons. One is psychological: smoking is an oral behavior, and to cope with the stress of giving it up, some smokers turn to another oral behavior: eating. The other reason is physiological: the enzymes that store fat are less active in smokers,

CHAPTER 9 ■ SMOKING AND SMOKELESS
   TOBACCO

and they resume normal activity when smokers quit.[39] You have some alternatives to prevent the gain:

- Diet at first, until your smoke-free life and weight have both stabilized.
- Drink lots of liquids, especially water, sparkling water, iced tea, diet beverages, and low-calorie fruit juices, in place of smoking.
- Eat sweet fruits and low-calorie vegetables instead of candy.
- Exercise—it will help to keep your weight down.

If you do gain a few pounds, it's worth it, to give up cigarettes. Once you are secure in being an ex-smoker, you can take off the weight; Chapter 5 offers more on how to do this. Others have done it; you can, too.

Nicotine-containing gum is an aid available to smokers as a stepping-stone to freedom from smoking. This gum, which can be obtained by prescription only, is designed to deliver the same amount of nicotine as two or three cigarettes. The user makes a firm commitment to stop using cigarettes and to chew the gum instead, at the rate of about six to eight pieces a day. The instructions say to chew each piece slowly, making it last a half-hour or more, thus delivering nicotine to the body at a steady rate. After several weeks of using the gum, you will have lost all the habits associated with smoking: handling the cigarettes, lighting them, puffing on them, and so forth. Now (the theory goes) it will be relatively easy to taper off the use of the gum, since nicotine addiction is the only problem left. Nicotine-containing gum proves successful in a significant number of cases.

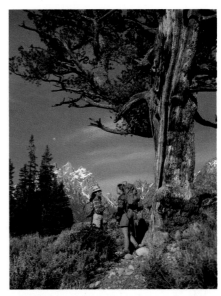

Develop alternative pleasures: try breathing clean air.

✳ Get help, if you like (see Chapter 3).

✳ Adopt weight control strategies if necessary.

How to Help the Smoker Quit

If you are a sympathetic bystander who wants to help a smoker quit, you must realize that smokers can quit only when they are ready. You cannot force them to quit. The key to effective helping is "tough love"—a term borrowed from alcoholism treatment. The idea is this: if you really care about a person, you will not keep quiet about a dangerous habit. Assert yourself. Confront the person. At the same time, show that you care, and make the distinction clear: it is the behavior you reject, not the person. Communicate your concern about the risks of the behavior. Express your dislike of the habit itself. Offer whatever information comes your way on the effects of smoking and the benefits of quitting. Identify reasons appropriate to the listener: tell the teenager, for example, that smoking impairs sports performance and that it is unattractive.

Do not be surprised, though, if the smoker cannot "hear" what you are saying. The person is committed to smoking, at least at present. The person ignores health warnings, giving only lip service to their existence: "Yes, I know." Still, speak up. Display information all over the place on the perils of smoking. Once ready, the person will pick it up, and it will reinforce the decision to quit.

Employers can help by prohibiting smoking on the job or refusing to hire smokers at all. This may seem unfair, but it is legal. Studies show that smokers take more breaks and are absent from work more often than nonsmokers.[40] Magazines, films, and other mass communicators can help by refusing to advertise tobacco—a decision that takes courage, because advertising is so profitable. Even children can help, by asking parents who smoke to stop.

Next time someone asks, "Mind if I smoke?" tell the truth.

Opposition to the marketing and sales of tobacco has been mounted by many organizations—cancer societies; medical, lung, and heart associations; and others. The American Council on Science and Health has raised the public's consciousness of the power of the tobacco industry, for example, by pointing out which magazines advertise cigarettes.* These magazines, because they accept cigarette advertising money, are under pressure by the advertisers not to publish information on the hazards of smoking, a phenomenon the council calls "the conspiracy of silence."

Many agencies share in working toward the goal of a smoke-free society by the year 2000. Many communities have passed no-smoking ordinances, and laws on advertising are getting stricter. Although many people still smoke and many young people are still starting, numbers of both are diminishing. The only group that opposes this trend is, of course, the tobacco industry.

In aggressively marketing tobacco, the industry is doing what any industry must do to be successful: maximizing profits and developing markets to foster its own growth. But because to expand the market means to persuade more people to smoke, and this compromises their health, an ethical problem exists. Those interested in promoting health must directly oppose the tobacco industry's interests and become deaf to their promotional appeals.

*Write to the Council at 47 Maple St., Summit, NJ 07901.

STUDY AIDS

1. Describe how people get started smoking, why they continue, and why they find it hard to quit.
2. Describe the effects of nicotine on the body and the sensations associated with withdrawal.
3. Describe some of the immediate effects of smoking on the lungs, the heart, and other organs.
4. Itemize some of the many long-term health hazards associated with smoking.
5. Describe the major health hazards smoking presents to women who smoke.
6. Cite some evidence that associates second-hand smoking with harm to health.
7. Compare the risks of cigarette smoking with those of pipe smoking, tobacco chewing, or snuff dipping.
8. Name some of the early rewards that can motivate a person to persist in the effort to quit smoking.
9. Describe strategies smokers can use to succeed in quitting and strategies people who care about them can use to help them quit.

GLOSSARY

bronchi: the large airways leading to the lungs, depicted in Figure 9–1.

bronchitis (bron-KITE-us): a respiratory disorder characterized by irritation and inflammation of the bronchi, with thickened mucus and deep, harsh coughing.

bronkhos = windpipe

carbon monoxide: a gas formed when oxidation or burning of carbon compounds is not complete enough to form the normal waste product, carbon dioxide. See *carboxyhemoglobin.*

carboxyhemoglobin (car-BOX-ee-HE-mo-gloh-bin): a compound formed when carbon monoxide combines with hemoglobin, interfering with hemoglobin's normal role of carrying oxygen. (See Chapter 4 for *hemoglobin.*)

carcinogen: a cancer-causing agent.

carcino = cancer
gen = gives rise to

chronic obstructive lung disease (COLD): any disease that interferes with breathing; also known as *chronic obstructive pulmonary disease (COPD).* Bronchitis and emphysema are examples.

cilia: waving, hair-like structures that cleanse the bronchi.

emphysema (em-fih-ZEE-muh): a disease of the lungs in which many small, flexible air sacs burst and form a few large, rigid air pockets; as a result, the lungs' absorbing surface is reduced, and breathing is both difficult and ineffective.

emphusan = to blow in

leukoplakia (loo-koh-PLAKE-ee-uh): whitish or grayish patches in the mouth that develop in response to exposure to tobacco and indicate a probability that cancer will follow.

leuko = white
plakia = patches

mainstream smoke: the smoke that flows through the cigarette and into the lungs when a smoker inhales.

mucus (MYOO-cuss): a slippery secretion produced by cells of the body's linings that protects the underlying tissues.

nicotine: an addictive drug present in tobacco.

plaque (PLACK): a buildup of material on a surface. Dental plaques build up on tooth enamel; arterial plaques accumulate in arteries. See Chapter 16 for more about arterial plaques.

placken = to patch

platelet (PLATE-let): a tiny particle in the blood, important in blood clotting. Damaged platelets also play a role in arterial plaque formation (see *plaque*).

platelet = little plate

sidestream smoke: the smoke that escapes into the air from the burning tip of a cigarette (and may then be inhaled by the smoker or by someone else). See also *mainstream smoke.*

sinusitis (sign-us-EYE-tus): infection of the sinuses, spaces in the bones of the skull.

smokeless tobacco: tobacco used for snuff or chewing rather than for smoking.

tar: one of a class of chemical compounds present in (among other things) tobacco. Burning tars contain many carcinogens.

trachea: the wind pipe; see Figure 9–1.

QUIZ ANSWERS

1. *False.* The main reason for continuing to smoke is addiction to nicotine.

2. *True.* One of nicotine's chief effects is to elicit the stress response.

3. *True.* Because it is taken into the lungs rather than eaten or injected, nicotine reaches the brain in a rush.

4. *True.* A sign of nicotine withdrawal is an inability to concentrate.

5. *False.* The smoker inhales the substances in both mainstream smoke and sidestream smoke; the people in the same room inhale only the sidestream smoke.

6. *False.* Lung disease is only one of the many negative effects of smoking on health; smoking also causes heart disease and many other ills.

7. *True.* In emphysema, the lungs first become damaged, not because people can't breathe in, but because they can't breathe out.

8. *True.* Smoking impairs people's ability to remember things.

9. *True.* Smoking wrinkles the skin.

10. *False.* The risks of cancer of the mouth and throat are greater for people using smokeless tobacco products and pipes than they are for cigarette smokers.

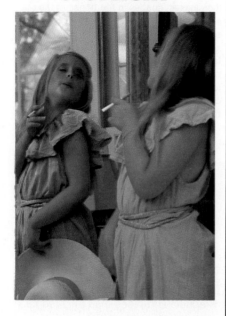

Tobacco Advertising and Ethics

Should tobacco companies be free to advertise products that harm people? The tobacco companies, of course, say yes—but the federal government is beginning to consider banning most tobacco advertising.

How do the tobacco companies state their case?

The tobacco companies argue that banning tobacco advertising would violate the Constitution's First Amendment, covering freedom of the press, which is central to the democratic way of life. They say that when all viewpoints are expressed, consumers may judge for themselves what may be harmful to them. But opponents of tobacco advertising argue that the state should take this burden from consumers, because they cannot be expected to judge wisely for themselves.

If a person writes something that causes harm to another person, does freedom of the press still protect the writer?

Yes, but exceptions do exist. One is slander: the publication of false statements that damage another's reputation. Freedom of the press was intended to protect the right to express opinions, but it does not give the right to publish false information about, and injure, another.

Tobacco advertising is not slander, but it certainly injures people. Tobacco ads make no health or safety claims, though, so they cannot be accused of telling lies. They "only" harm the smoker's health. Philip Morris USA even sponsored a contest that gave away $80,000 in prize money to the writer who wrote the best essay defending cigarette companies' rights to advertise their products.[1]* Philip Morris says virtually any ban on advertising is a threat to the most basic right of Americans to exchange ideas.

*Reference notes are in Appendix D.

What is the opposition's point of view?

The opposing view is represented by groups such as the New York-based antitobacco activist group Doctors Ought to Care (DOC). In response to Philip Morris's essay contest, DOC started a contest of its own. It offered $1,000 to the essayist who could best answer the question, "Are tobacco company executives criminally responsible for deaths caused by their products?"[2]

Wow. One minute you're talking about publishing false opinions and the next, you're talking about killing people. Is that question being debated seriously?

Yes, it is. The legal question of whether tobacco companies are liable for smoking-related deaths has been brought into focus as evidence piles up that, without doubt, smoking is responsible for many deaths from cancer and other diseases. Does a smoker who was influenced by tobacco ads to begin smoking have the right to sue a tobacco company for the costs of a major illness caused by smoking? Can the family sue the company if the smoker dies of that illness?

Wait a minute. It isn't possible to prove that smoking has caused a lung cancer death, is it?

That's right, and until 1988, no one suing a tobacco company for health complications had ever been awarded damages. Then the case of Cipollone vs. Philip Morris broke new ground.[3]

After smoking for 40 years, Rose Cipollone, of Lakehurst, New Jersey, died of lung cancer in 1984. Her husband filed charges claiming that Philip Morris and other tobacco companies were negligent and liable for her lung cancer. Cipollone's attorneys obtained access to the tobacco companies' confidential files, which detailed their incriminating public relations strategies. The companies had covered up what they knew about the dangers of smoking, stifled research into a safer cigarette, and unethically influenced public opinion.

The court awarded damages to the Cipollones, finding that the companies had conspired to conceal and misrepresent information on the dangers of smoking. U.S. District Judge H. Lee Sarokin wrote: "The evidence presented . . . permits the jury to find a tobacco industry conspiracy, vast in its scope, devious in its purpose, and devastating in its results."[4] The judge also stated that the companies conspired to "refute, undermine, and neutralize information coming from the scientific and medical community," and the companies tried to "confuse and mislead the consuming public in an effort to encourage existing smokers to continue and new persons to commence smoking."

The results of this case were expected to influence at least 100 similar cases pending at the time. This is in marked contrast to earlier legal history: after World War II, fewer than 10 cigarette liability cases ever went before a jury until the Cipollone case was tried.[5]

Why was it so difficult to sue in the past?"

As you saw from the statistics in the chapter, smoking greatly increases the number of deaths from many kinds of diseases, so clearly it does cause individual cases of disease. But some deaths from those same diseases arise among nonsmokers, too— so it may be impossible to say whether a particular instance of disease was caused by smoking. The person might have been one of those people who would have contracted the disease anyway.

That makes the case of smoking deaths different from, say, accidental deaths caused by negligence in building maintenance. If an elevator cable breaks and Mr. C falls to his death,

his family can sue the company for negligence. But suppose seven out of ten smokers die of lung cancer, and Mr. C is among them. Two would have died of cancer anyway, even if they had not smoked. The family cannot prove that Mr. C was one of the five whose deaths were caused by smoking; he might (though less probably) be one of the two who would have died of lung cancer anyway.

This legal problem arises whenever statistical responsibility can be proved, but direct, individual responsibility cannot be. It makes suing difficult, not only for smokers, but also for people whose illnesses and deaths are caused by industrial pollution where responsibility for individual illnesses or deaths can't be pinpointed.

While the legal question is being debated, can individuals do anything to cut down on the harmful influence of tobacco advertising? Must newspapers and magazines accept tobacco ads?

No, and many magazines have already taken action—they no longer accept tobacco advertisements, because they believe it is unethical to do so. (This is a brave action, for advertising money is essential to the survival of the magazines.) Among publications that do not accept tobacco money are the *Reader's Digest*, the *New Yorker*, *Good Housekeeping*, *National Geographic*, and *Scientific American*. The result is that fewer people in their readerships are influenced to use tobacco, and these magazines are completely outside any legal question of liability from readers who are harmed by tobacco.

How would people harmed by tobacco go about holding the tobacco companies responsible for that harm?

DOC first wants to convince lawmakers that smoking does cause deaths. It is conducting a campaign in which, each time a smoker dies of

lung cancer, coronary artery disease, emphysema, or any other tobacco-related illness, the health care provider sends a black-bordered announcement of the death to the client's senator or representative. The announcement reads: "Dear _____ , I wish to inform you that one of your constituents, who was a patient of mine, has died. The death was due to the following disease: _____ . This person was a smoker. Tobacco smoking is the major avoidable cause of this disease." DOC even suggests that the health care provider fill in the brand name of the tobacco product used, suggesting to lawmakers that "not only was it tobacco that killed them, it was Marlboro, made by Philip Morris."[6]

DOC, by informing legislators, will have made its point that smoking does cause deaths, and it will have influenced lawmakers to at least consider the possibility that tobacco advertising should be banned or severely restricted. A similar campaign, conducted in England in 1984, was effective in generating discussion and debate that led to stringent restrictions on tobacco advertising.[7]

So the question of how the First Amendment should be interpreted is open.

Yes. The question is still being debated. If someone writes something that influences you to take action, and that action harms your health, the law perhaps should protect you from harming yourself. Where the harm is to the pocketbook, except in cases of slander, the position the courts have held up to now is "caveat emptor"—let the buyer beware. But that position assumes that buyers are adults, supposedly capable of protecting themselves. In the case of tobacco ads, the people influenced are often children, incapable of making the necessary judgments to protect themselves. Furthermore, the harm is not only to financial well-being but to health and life as well.

Chapter 10

Intimacy, Pairing, and Commitment

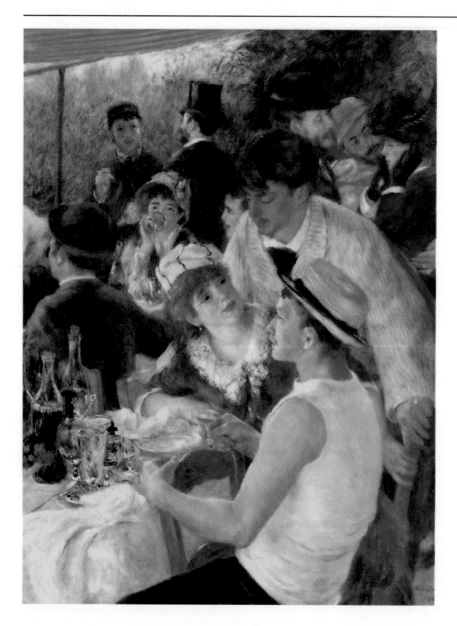

FOR OPENERS . . .

True or false? If false, say what is true.

1. People are sexual beings from puberty to old age.
2. Normal sexual activity is preferable to masturbation, for health's sake.
3. The need for nonsexual touching, kissing, and holding may be more essential to well-being than orgasm.
4. The master organ of sexual response in a man is the penis.
5. Orgasm is a reflex, similar to the jerk of the leg when the knee is tapped.
6. Both men and women have orgasms while dreaming.
7. The majority of sexual problems respond to simple treatments.
8. Giving too much can ruin a relationship, just as taking too much can.
9. Love conquers all, so long as you love completely enough.
10. The key to a lasting marriage is love.

(Answers on page 212.)

What first comes to mind when you think of **sex** may be the sex organs—but sex is expressed in all the body parts: hair, skin, eyes, lips, and body structure. And what first comes to mind when you think of **sexuality** may be sexual intercourse, but intercourse is only one aspect of sexuality. Sexuality is a part of the total personality from birth to death, whether or not a person is engaging in sexual activity. Your behaviors reflect your sexuality, including the way you walk, the way you hold things, and the ways you talk to and touch others. Even your thoughts, feelings, values, self-concept, and ideas about others are strongly tied to sexuality, as is the way you choose a life partner. Every relationship you have helps to define your sexuality. Sexuality affects the young, the old, the handicapped, all races, all sizes—all people.

A force so pervasive is worth pondering. This chapter looks at sexuality from many angles—from the anatomy and physiology of sex to the development of a long-term love relationship.

BIOLOGICAL SEX

The figures at the start of this chapter will help you understand sexual body parts and processes. The organs involved are often called sex organs, but they are really controlled by signals originating in the brain's **pituitary gland**. Figures 10–1 and 10–2 show the male internal and external organs, and Figures 10–3 and 10–4 show the female internal and external organs.

An abundance of terminology is associated with sexual anatomy and physiology. To break it into manageable blocks, the terms associated with male sexuality are presented in their own Miniglossary (page 195) and those associated with female sexuality, in theirs (page 195). The chapter Glossary defines other terms related to sexuality.

A few terms refer to both male and female sexual anatomy and physiology. The **genitals** are the external sex organs in both. The **gonads** are the sex glands—testes in males, ovaries in females. The **gametes** are the cells produced in those glands—sperm in males, ova in females. **Erection** is the aroused state of the penis and clitoris when they fill with blood in response to sexual stimulation; **orgasm** is the sexual climax, accompanied by sensa-

FIGURE 10–1 Anatomy and Physiology of the Male Reproductive System

The *testes (testicles)* produce the hormone *testosterone* (tes-TOSS-ter-own), which is essential for the continuous production of *sperm* cells.

The testes are surrounded by a tough-skinned sac, the *scrotum*, which contains muscles that contract and relax to bring the testes closer to, or farther away from, the body in order to regulate their temperature.

When sperm mature, they travel to a storage place, where they remain until ejaculation takes place. Then the storage organ contracts and propels the sperm into a conducting tube, the *vas deferens*. This tube also contracts, propelling the sperm on their way outside the body. On the way, the sperm combine with fluids from glands to form the mixture, *semen*, that leaves the penis. A single ejaculation yields about a teaspoon of semen, containing approximately 400 million sperm.

(The penis's external anatomy is described in Figure 10-2 and associated text.)

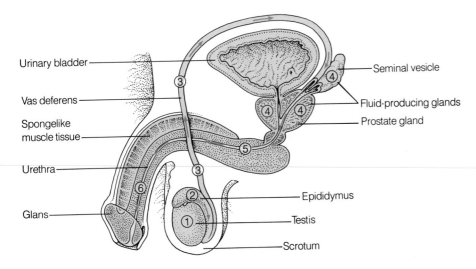

Urinary bladder
Vas deferens
Spongelike muscle tissue
Urethra
Glans

Seminal vesicle
Fluid-producing glands
Prostate gland
Epididymus
Testis
Scrotum

193

tions of pleasure, that occurs in both males and females during sexual activity. **Ejaculation** is the process by which the male expels sperm during orgasm. These events are described more fully later.

The monthly cycle of the female is known as the **ovulatory cycle**, because it is the cycle that leads to **ovulation** (the production of an ovum) each month, and also as the **menstrual cycle**, because it includes **menstruation** (the shedding of the uterine lining) each month.

Hormones govern the development of the sex organs and characteristic structures. Before birth, the **primary sex characteristics**, such as the penis in the male and clitoris in the female, develop from common fetal structures. The final differences are dictated by whether male or female hormones are present in the uterine environment. Later on, in adolescence, those same hormones trigger the development of the **secondary sex characteristics**: enlargement of the genitals, appearance of pubic and other body hair and of facial hair in men, development of breast structures in women, development of muscle bulk in men, widening of the pelvis in women, and so on.

If hormones govern physical characteristics, do they also influence behavior? Animal studies support the idea. Researchers believe that the male hormones produce a permanent physical change in parts of the brain responsible for sex behavior in rodents. However, it is impossible to say how much, if any, of the research on animals applies to human beings, and the question remains open.

Society guides people in choosing gender-related behaviors. The characteristics deemed by society to be appropriate for people of each sex are **gender roles**. The characteristics that a person internalizes are that person's **gender identity**, part of the self-concept. Growing up in our society, you may have learned:

■ Which external cues are sexual. The sight of an unclothed person may evoke physical sexual arousal, but only because you have learned to respond that way. In other societies, where nudity is the norm, viewing nakedness does not cause arousal.

■ How to discern and use sexually suggestive behavior. A warm smile and gentle touch from your parent you may interpret as parental love; the same behavior from a classmate you may interpret as flirting and become

FIGURE 10–2   External Male Organs

The *glans* of the *penis,* which is the most sensitive to pleasure, normally retracts beneath a sheath of skin, the *foreskin.* In some males, this sheath has been cut away (circumcision). The scrotum is the double-pouched sac that contains the testes, already shown in Figure 10-1.

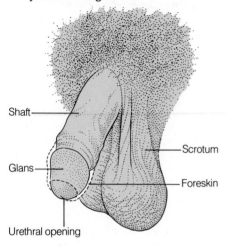

Shaft

Glans

Scrotum

Foreskin

Urethral opening

Primary sex characteristics:
 Genital organs, chromosomes, hormones.
Secondary sex characteristics:
 Males—facial hair, deep voice, muscle development, body hair.
 Females—breasts, fat pads, widened pelvis, body hair.

FIGURE 10–3   Anatomy of the Female Reproductive System

The *ovary* releases an *ovum* in close proximity to the gently grasping "fingers," or fringe, on the end of the *fallopian tube,* which draws the ovum in and propels it into the tube. The tube is lined with cilia, which sweep the ovum along to the *uterus.* There, if fertilized, the ovum will implant itself in the prepared lining. If not fertilized, it will be shed through the uterine opening (*cervix*) into the *vagina* together with the material of the uterine lining. The ovaries also produce hormones: *progesterone* and *estrogens.*

(See Figure 10-4 for the external female organs.)

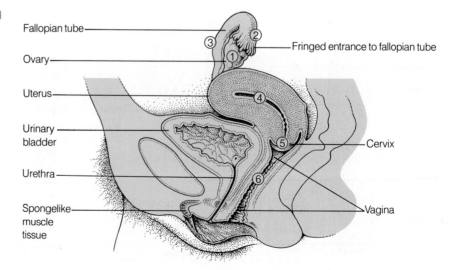

Fallopian tube

Ovary

Uterus

Urinary bladder

Urethra

Spongelike muscle tissue

Fringed entrance to fallopian tube

Cervix

Vagina

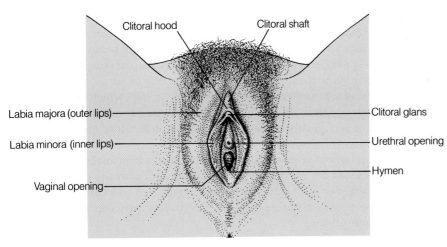

Clitoral hood
Clitoral shaft
Labia majora (outer lips)
Labia minora (inner lips)
Vaginal opening
Clitoral glans
Urethral opening
Hymen

FIGURE 10–4   External Female Organs

Two sets of ridges, the *labia,* enfold the other female organs. The labia border the vaginal opening and join together over the *clitoris,* forming its *foreskin.* The visible *glans* of the clitoris is just the tip of a rod-like structure that is made up partly of spongelike muscle tissue that becomes erect when stimulated. The clitoris is highly sensitive because it contains a tremendous number of sensory nerve endings. In young girls, a thin, fragile membrane, the *hymen,* partly covers the vaginal opening. Once thought to be "proof of virginity," the membrane may rupture at the first time of sexual intercourse, but is now known to often disintegrate during early life owing to exercise or use of tampons.

MINIGLOSSARY of Female Terms

For general terms relating to sexual and reproductive function, see the Glossary, page 211.

cervix (SER-vix): the neck of the uterus, which protrudes into the vagina; the cervix provides an opening for sperm to travel from the vagina into the uterus and through which menstrual flow and the fetus emerge. Its appearance is something like that of the glans of an erect penis.

   cervix = neck

clitoris (CLIT-uh-rus): the primary organ that receives pleasure sensations, as does the penis in men.

estrogens: hormones produced in the ovaries that promote the development of the secondary sex characteristics in young females and regulate the ovulatory cycle. Estrogens are produced also, in lesser amounts, by the adrenal glands of people of either sex.

fallopian (fah-LOH-pe-un) **tubes:** a pair of tubes opening near the ovaries that connect into the uterus; they convey the gametes (ova and sperm cells) toward each other. Fertilization usually takes place within these tubes.

foreskin: a sleeve of skin that covers the tip of the clitoris. Also called the *hood.*

glans: the tip of the clitoris.

   glans = acorn (shape)

hymen (HIGH-men): a thin membrane that partially covers the vaginal opening in early life.

   humen = membrane

labia (LAY-bee-uh): a set of liplike structures in the female external genital organs. The *labia majora* are the larger, more external ones and are covered with pubic hair; the *labia minora* are the two thin folds that lie between the labia majora.

   labium = lip

ovary (OH-vah-ree): one of the two female gonads, which produce female hormones and mature ova.

   ovarium = egg

ovum (OH-vum; plural **ova**) The female gamete, a single egg cell.

progesterone (pro-JESS-tuh-rone): a female hormone secreted by the ovaries.

uterus (YOU-ter-us): the organ in females that contains and nourishes the young before birth. Also called *womb.*

vagina: the muscular tube-shaped organ of the female that surrounds the penis in intercourse, conducts semen into the uterus, and serves as the passageway for menstrual flow and for birth.

   vagina = sheath

MINIGLOSSARY of Male Terms

For general terms relating to sexual and reproductive function, see the Glossary, page 211.

foreskin: a sleeve of skin that covers the tip of the uncircumcised penis. *Circumcision* is surgery to remove the foreskin of the penis usually performed shortly after birth; it may aid cleanliness, although opinions on this point vary.

glans: the tip of the penis.

   glans = acorn (shape)

penis: the male external genital organ, including the shaft, glans, and internal structural base, analogous to the clitoris in females.

scrotum (SCROH-tum): the double pouch that contains the testes.

semen (SEE-men): the fluid ejaculated from the penis that carries sperm.

   semen = seed

sperm: the male gamete.

testicle or testis (plural, **testes**): one of the two male gonads, which produce male hormones and sperm cells.

testosterone (tes-TOSS-ter-ohn): a hormone produced by the testis that regulates the production of sperm and promotes the development of the secondary sex characteristics in young males. Produced also, in lesser amounts, by the adrenal glands of people of either sex.

vas deferens (vas DEF-er-ens): the duct in the male through which the sperm are propelled during ejaculation.

   vas = duct

aroused or repelled. Also, you may have learned when and how to use such behaviors with others.

■ With whom you may and may not engage in sexual behavior. The limits are usually defined by sex; age; family relation; marital status; and perhaps affiliations such as race, religion, and economic or social class.

■ What sexual acts are acceptable for you. We "know" which of the possible sexual acts are right or wrong because they are learned from peers and, more or less explicitly, from books, movies, television, and a variety of other sources.

■ When and where you may and may not engage in sexual activity. In our society, closed doors, privacy, and waiting until after the children's bedtime are the norm. In other societies, parents and children may all share the same room or hut and sexual intercourse between parents is not considered private.

■ How to interpret your sex behavior—as having fun, procreating, giving in to lust, or expressing love. These distinctions may be difficult to make, because, in this society, the two sexes receive different messages as to what is permissible.

All of these norms are yours to choose from. You can accept them, reject them, or adjust them to suit yourself. A strategy that works is to accept those that ease your way in society, with the awareness that norms change and that you can help them change if you so desire.

▨ SEXUAL ACTIVITY

People share relationships with others for all sorts of rewards: companionship, recreation, intellectual growth, and many others. Sexuality pervades relationships, and sexual activities may become a part of the sharing (committment in relationships is addressed in a later section). At the same time, sexual activity is biologically designed for reproduction—even if the participants have no such intention. Part of learning how to use sexuality in a health-promoting way is learning how to control its reproductive function, the subject of the next chapter.

Masturbation and Sex Play

A person's first sexual relationship is with self. When you enjoy physical sensations, a sexual component is usually involved—it is **sensuous** to stroke your own skin. The same pleasure, taken a step farther, is **masturbation**. Children's natural playfulness and curiosity leads to exploring their sexual organs, and they learn to masturbate. Sometimes, they may share this experience. Early experiences such as these do not predict homosexuality in either sex.

Masturbation does not end when people grow up. Many sex therapists recommend masturbation to clients as a way to find out what sorts of stimulation please them. Later, they can communicate such information to their sex partners.

All sorts of problems have been attributed (falsely) to masturbation. In itself, masturbation does no harm; the guilt it may evoke, however, can injure the self-concept and create problems in sexual functioning.

Sex Play

One type of interpersonal sexual expression is **sex play** (sometimes called **petting**); it is shared sexual stimulation that does not include **sexual intercourse**. An advantage of sex play is that it is not goal oriented—the focus is on the pleasure that each partner can give the other. The word *petting* conveys the image of tenderly caressing something that is cherished—and that is what sex play is. It is common among people who are not engaging in intercourse, and it is a part of **foreplay**, the mutual pleasure-giving that precedes intercourse.

Sex play is useful for learning about the sexual response of another person and for communicating one's own sexual needs. We hear a lot about sex among adolescents, implying sexual intercourse, but most young adolescents do not engage in sexual intercourse—they pet.* In homosexual couples, sex play may be the preferred sexual behavior. (Much of this section applies to all people; a later section discusses homosexuality specifically.)

Naturally, touching gives pleasure. The skin is rich in sensory nerve endings, which transmit sexual pleasure along nerve fibers to the ultimate receptor, the brain. To many people, touching—hugging, kissing—meets an emotional need for closeness that is fulfilling in itself, whether or not intercourse follows. The need to be touched may be even more basic than the need for sex.

Kissing stimulates especially sensitive receptors, the lips. Kissing styles differ, but whatever the style, almost everyone in modern societies kisses.[1] Kissing may play a role in the development of a chemical bond between people; it may be that special substances, different for each individual, are exchanged when people kiss. These chemicals are thought to assist one person's recognition or acceptance of another.[2] Some kisses are not related to sex but are an expression of nonsexual affection or love.

Many people enjoy nipple stimulation. In our society, women's breasts are given great status as sexual organs and men's nipples are often overlooked. Usually, the nipples respond to the touch of the fingers or tongue by becoming erect. As with all sex play, breast and nipple stimulation can be preparation for intercourse or orgasm or an end in itself.

Caressing the genital organs is a form of sex play. This may lead to orgasm, it may lead to intercourse or oral stimulation of the genitals, or it may be an end in itself. Some couples engage in sex play often, interspersing it with other everyday activities. Sex therapists often recommend such play for people whose pleasure is diminished by "goal seeking"—the expectation that orgasm must occur.

People stimulate each other's genitals by using hands or mouth or by rubbing the genitals against each other. Manual stimulation consists of using hands and fingers to rub the penis or the clitoris, the two analogous organs of sexual response. Generally, a man's penis is stimulated by stroking, rubbing, and caressing of the shaft and glans, and sometimes with stimulation

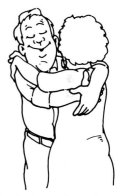

The need to be touched may be even more basic than the need for sex.

---

*One reliable source reported that fewer than than 20% of female adolescents aged 15 had ever had sexual intercourse; about 25% of 16-year-old females had done so; and 40% of 17-year-olds, 45% of 18-year-olds, and 55% of 19-year-old females had had sexual intercourse. Percentages for males are a little higher. M. Zelnik and J. F. Kantner, Sexual and contraceptive experience of young unmarried women in the United States 1976 and 1971, *Adolescent Pregnancy and Childbearing: Findings from Research*, NIH publication no. 81-2077, 1980, pp. 43-81.

*Reference notes are in Appendix D.

cun-ih-LING-gus, feh-LAY-she-oh

of the scrotum as well. A woman's clitoris may be stimulated directly by rubbing, stroking, and caressing, or it may be indirectly stimulated by stroking of the entire upper genital area. A woman may also enjoy the sensation of one or several of the partner's fingers stimulating her vagina, but for most women, sexual pleasure is situated in and around the clitoris, with or without vaginal stimulation.

Oral stimulation—**cunnilingus** or **fellatio**—is useful as sexual expression when intercourse is undesirable for one reason or another, as in the later stages of some pregnancies. The mouth and tongue are soft, warm, motile, and moist, and they can stimulate the penis or clitoris gently and sensitively.

Sex play usually results in intense sexual stimulation, with erection (stiffening) of the penis and **engorgement** (swelling) of the clitoris and labia. Lubricating fluids begin to flow within the vagina. Fluid moves down the man's urethra, neutralizing the acid left by urine and creating a safe environment for sperm. A drop or so of this fluid leaves the penis. It may contain live cells, including sperm. This presents a risk of infection and of pregnancy, because the fluid may contain agents of sexually transmitted diseases (see Chapter 15) and because sperm are equipped to find their way through the uterus into the fallopian tubes, even from the external genitalia.

Chapter 11 explains avoiding pregnancy through birth control. Chapter 15 presents details about sexually transmitted diseases and how to avoid them.

If sex play is continued, orgasm may occur within a few seconds, a few minutes, or an hour or more, depending on the individuals and the activity. Sometimes people purposely postpone orgasm to make the pleasure last.

It is sometimes difficult to tell another person about your own desires or to listen openly, without defensiveness, to someone else's needs. The suggestions in this chapter's Strategies box may help to break the ice and open communication.

 Strategies: Talking about Sex

To communicate sensitively about sex:

1. Tell your partner that you would like to talk about your sexual interaction, and ask for suggestions about the best place and time to do so. That way, the idea is already familiar when the two of you actually start talking. Bringing up the topic may be the hardest part.

2. Say, "I most like it when you . . . ," not "You are wrong to . . ." People react most positively to messages about what you like, not what they do wrong.

3. Be open to honest criticism. Accept joint responsibility. Disappointing sex is usually a two-way street.

4. Bring up only the issues most important to you, only when they are consistently a problem.

5. Stay sensitive to nonverbal communication about preferences. People don't always say aloud what they want.

6. Talk often to understand the changing needs of your partner. A sexual relationship is a growing, changing interaction.

7. Talk to a sex therapist or counselor to help break the ice at first. Once the lines are open, future discussions may be easier.

SOURCE: Several of these ideas were suggested in W. H. Masters, V. E. Johnson, and R. C. Kolodny, *Human Sexuality*, 2nd ed. (Boston: Little, Brown, 1985), pp. 332–333.

Intercourse

Sexual intercourse is a simple act in a physical sense, but it becomes a complex interaction, because individuals bring to it their moods, motives, physical states, expectations, self-concepts, and everything else that makes them unique. People must be sensitive to perceive the messages that intercourse conveys. For those who learn such sensitivity, intercourse is a rich medium for communication. In fact, how well a couple's sex life is doing is usually related to the state of the nonsexual relationship—a healthy sex life is typically surrounded by a healthy relationship. Intercourse is a way to communicate tenderness, love, and a sense of unity. It can also communicate unaddressed grievances, whether or not people want them known.

Usually, people bring with them a combination of motives for intercourse: the desire to relieve sexual tension, gain emotional intimacy, have fun, become pregnant, or numerous others. Negative motives also exist: to build up ego (scoring); to reduce negative feelings (grief, depression, loneliness); to gain peer acceptance; to reduce pressure from partner; to pressure partner into premature commitment; to rebel against authority; to take revenge on someone else. Table 10–1 shows how a person with any motive might try to influence a partner to have intercourse or not to have it.

TABLE 10–1   Ways People Influence Sexual Encounters

Strategy	Definition
Reward	Giving gifts, providing services, and flattering the person in exchange for compliance.
Coercion	Punishing or threatening to punish noncompliance by withdrawing resources or services.
Logic	Using rational, but not moral, arguments to convince the person to have or avoid sexual intercourse.
Moralizing	Telling the person that it is a legitimate or socially sanctioned right to have or avoid sexual intercourse.
Information	Telling the person whether or not sex is desired in a straightforward, direct manner.
Manipulation	Hinting at sexual intention by subtly altering one's appearance, the setting, or the topic of conversation.
Body language	Using facial expression, posture, closeness or distance, and gestures to communicate sexual intentions.
Deception	Using a strategy for having or avoiding sex that relies on giving the person false information.
Relationship conceptualizing	Influencing a person by talking about the relationship and indicating concern for the date's feelings, promise to marry to obtain sex, or promise of sex to get married.
Seduction	Having a definite, step-by-step plan for getting a date to have sexual intercourse, focusing on sexually stimulating the person.

SOURCE: Adapted from N. B. McCormick, Come ons and put offs: Unmarried students' strategies for having and avoiding sexual intercourse, *Psychology of Women Quarterly* 4 (1979): 194–211. Copyright © Human Sciences Press, New York. Reprinted with permission of the publisher.

Ideally, no one would have sexual intercourse for motives other than pleasure, love, and the desire to share intimacy. The kind of intercourse described here is that between two loving people.

The act of intercourse itself consists of a man's and a woman's positioning their bodies so that the woman's vagina can receive the man's penis; the two move together in a thrusting, grinding, or other motion that brings them sexual sensation and pleasure, usually ending with the man's orgasm. The woman's orgasm may have occurred before the man's, or simultaneously with it, or it may occur afterward. Along with the contact between vagina and penis, people use hands, fingers, arms, lips, or any other parts of their bodies to stimulate each other in desired ways with appropriate timing. This additional stimulation might be viewed as a continuation of sex play.

People usually have intercourse in one of five positions: with the man on top, with the woman on top, with both lying on their sides face to face, with the man behind the woman, or with the partners sitting face to face. Each of these positions has many variations, and people may experiment to find what pleases them. Different positions offer different advantages, such as face-to-face communication, ease of hand contact with genitals, freedom of movement, or possession of control. A couple needn't choose just one and use it over and over; positions preferred by each should be used often. Position is only one aspect of intercourse among many that demand clear, accurate communication between partners. Others include level of desire, preferences in foreplay, readiness for intercourse, and timing of orgasm.

The Stages of Sexual Response

Sexual response begins with desire, which is a complex interplay of several factors. One is a person's perception of whether the time, place, and partner are appropriate. Others are the person's psychological state and physical need for sexual expression.

Some people think of sexual responses as a series of push-button reactions—"If I do this, then that will happen." That attitude treats complex human beings like machines. Sexual interest is to some extent stimulated by the different, the unexpected; routines can become boring. The mystery of sexual response lies in the complex human brain—the true master sex organ. The four phases of the sexual response cycle are common to both partners: **excitement**, **plateau**, orgasm, **resolution**. These stages are listed as a sequence, but they may occur with different timing and in different orders. They may differ in kind from person to person and may even vary in the same person from time to time.

The description that follows centers on the primary organs of sexual response, the clitoris and penis, but pleasurable feelings also arise from many other locations in the body. Some body parts are believed to be especially capable of receiving sexual sensation—the penis, clitoris, lips, buttocks, breasts, and so on—and these have been named the **erogenous zones**. Stroking these zones may add to sexual pleasure, but people's entire bodies can become pleasure-receiving. Repetitious stimulation of any sensitive body part can cause numbness or become irritating after a while. The key to knowing how to give pleasure is in perceiving and heeding the partner's signals.

The most easily observed event of the excitement phase is penile erection, that is, the stiffening of the normally soft penis as its spongelike muscle tissue fills with blood trapped by obstruction of the veins that normally conduct the blood out of the penis. During the excitement phase, the testes elevate and enlarge, the scrotum tightens, and the penis releases a drop of fluid. The tissues of the clitoris and labia engorge, and the vaginal lining becomes coated with smooth, slippery lubricating fluid. The uterus tilts upward, elongating the vagina in what is called the **tenting effect**.

If stimulation continues, the person moves into the plateau phase. This phase includes constriction of the lower third of the vagina, further expansion of the vagina, further enlargement of the penis, and possibly a deepening of its color. The testes, and possibly the breasts, enlarge. The clitoris withdraws under its foreskin to protect the sensitive glans from direct friction, which would be painful at this time; the clitoris still responds when stroked through this protective layer of skin.

In both men and women, the nipples become erect and sensitive, especially if stimulated, and a sex flush (a pink rash) may appear on the face, neck, or chest. Blood pressure, pulse rate, and breathing rate increase; voluntary and involuntary muscles contract in preparation for orgasm.

Orgasm is a reflex, an involuntary response that occurs automatically after appropriate and sufficient stimulation. In women, orgasm involves involuntary rhythmic contractions of the uterus, the outer portion of the vagina, the anus, and the surrounding muscles. Orgasm usually lasts about 30 seconds and is accompanied by sensations of intense pleasure. In men, there is first an expulsion of about a teaspoonful of semen from its storage places (ejaculation). The orgasm that follows involves rhythmic contractions of the penile muscles that push semen out through the urethra. During orgasm, the blood that has engorged the penis, clitoris, vagina, and labia is forced out of the veins by the muscular contractions. Orgasms may be short or long, intense or mild; they differ more among individuals than between the sexes.

Orgasm is the peak of sexual pleasure; the resolution phase offers further pleasure of its own. Resolution is the reversal of the physical changes of arousal—tensed muscles relax, congested blood vessels and swollen tissues return to normal, and normal color returns within a few minutes. The period is usually characterized by feelings of well-being sometimes called the **afterglow**.

Orgasm sometimes occurs in men and women during sleep, especially accompanying sexy dreams. Men most often report having such orgasms, called **nocturnal emissions**, or **wet dreams**. It is not uncommon for women to have orgasms while dreaming, too. Some people may never experience them.

Problems and Strategies

Some people experience times of inability to enjoy sex, even though they may wish to. A few have a lifelong history of such inability, and most people experience at least some difficulty at some time during their lives. Normally, people take it in stride—it goes away by itself, but sometimes, lack of enjoyment of sex may become a problem known as **sexual dysfunction**.

Many people experience interference with arousal from no apparent physical cause. Arousal may be slowed or sexual desire may be lacking, or the person may even fear sexual activity. Of course, almost everyone has times of disinterest in sexual activity, but when disinterest or other problems cause distress to the person or harm a relationship, they may be worth attention. Most cases are treatable.[3]

In men, the problem may show itself as an inability to achieve or maintain an erection. In women, the most common complaints are lack of orgasm during intercourse and lack of sexual excitement.

Although some women achieve orgasm from the stimulation of intercourse alone, many do not. Some reasons for this have been suggested.[4] In men, the stimulation to the penis is direct and continuous throughout intercourse, but a women's clitoris is frequently not stimulated sufficiently for orgasm to occur. The penis may not exert enough pressure in the right places. Also, the change in shape of the vagina may move sensitive areas out of reach of the penis. Or it may be that a woman's plateau stage is longer than a man's; if so, a change in timing may facilitate the woman's achieving orgasm by intercourse alone. Alternatively, manual stimulation of the clitoris during intercourse usually produces orgasm.

Perhaps the most easily corrected causes are physical. Many disease states reduce the capacity for sexual response, and control of them often reverses the sexual dysfunction. Treatment of the underlying cause usually removes the problem. Men who have conditions that are not reversible may find a workable option in surgery to install one of a number of implanted devices that create rigidity in the penis.

Use of drugs (the medical kind, as well as alcohol and others) can cause temporary dysfunction. Endorphins in the brain may have a regulating effect on sexual appetite; people with a reduced sex drive have been found to have endorphin levels higher than other people's.[5] It could be that euphoria-producing drugs raise the endorphin levels in the brain and reduce sex drive in habitual users.

When the cause of sexual dysfunction is other than physical or chemical and cannot be resolved through communication, sex therapy may be useful. Sex therapy is a largely unmonitored field, however, and anybody can adopt the title of sex therapist. To find one of the relatively few who have adequate credentials:

■ Contact a university or hospital that has a sex clinic.
■ Check the credentials of the therapist.*
■ Look for a graduate degree in the specialty of sex therapy and postgraduate training.[6]

*The professional organizations to look for are the Society for Sex Therapy and Research (SSTAR) or the American Association of Sex Educators, Counselors, and Therapists (AASECT).

CONSUMER CAUTION

When things go wrong in sex, there are no quick fixes.

When people have problems as personal as sexual problems are, they may be reluctant to seek help from others. It is tempting to turn first to a product. A warning is in order, though—no secret compound, no exotic ingredient, and no food or nutrient can enhance or restore sexual vitality. The substances called **aphrodisiacs** do not work, and they may be dangerous. Many are strong stimulants, hormones, or depressants. According to the Food and Drug Administration, all claims for over-the-counter aphrodisiacs are false, misleading, or unsupported by scientific evidence.[7] Chances are that failing sexual responses, like most other messages from the body, need time, energy, and attention.

Legitimate therapists do not use sexual contact in therapy. Therapists do ask intimate questions about experiences to find the reason for the dysfunction.

Here are some self-help strategies. First, make sure you are physically healthy and that all the health habits covered in the first nine chapters of this book are under control. Also, be sure that communication between you and your partner is open and honest. Make your needs, fears, and hopes known.

Next, have a sexy time with your partner, but with the agreement that neither of you will have orgasm. As the days go by, sexual activity will become more and more desirable and therefore more likely. In addition, use the relaxation techniques described in the Strategies box of Chapter 2 for a few minutes before sexual activity to help make the transition to the sexual way of responding. Once relaxed, pay attention only to sensation, and let conscious thought go. In other words, let tomorrow's worries wait for tomorrow—or at least until later. Stress has no place in sexual activity. Your sexual response is important. You are entitled to it, so expect and enjoy it.

HOMOSEXUALITY

History has shown that **homosexuality** has been around for a long time; it has been both endorsed and denounced, but it has never been eliminated. Today, the general view of it is negative, a view that springs from prevailing religious teachings. Homosexuality is a sin in most Christian and Jewish doctrines. A high rate of AIDS among homosexuals has fueled this view.

Homosexuality, although not deemed a mental illness, has been assigned a status of abnormality by a consensus of the scientific community, which considers **heterosexual** orientation normal. In this society, people attempt to control homosexuality by passing laws against it and by trying to cure it as they would a physical or psychological illness. Laws forbid certain sexual acts, the so-called **sodomy** laws. The homosexual person is neither criminal nor sick, though; such labeling comes from people who cannot tolerate others who are different from themselves.

Homosexuality may seem clear-cut at first glance—orientation toward same-sex partners. But for those who think further, the subject becomes more complex. Do homosexual acts identify homosexual people? Or is just fantasizing about same-sex partners enough? In fact, homosexuality seems to exist on a continuum, with most people having a certain degree of both homosexual and heterosexual orientation.

People can also be **bisexual**. This is not the same as feeling warm and physically affectionate with members of both sexes; most people feel that way. Rather, bisexuality is being sexually attracted to members of both sexes. About 25 percent of men in the United States and about 10 to 15 percent of women are bisexual by that definition. Some people who marry and have heterosexual relationships later discover that they have a preference for members of the same sex and develop homosexual relationships as well. In addition, many people who call themselves homosexual have reported being aroused by opposite-sex individuals. They, too, are bisexual. Still other people are **asexual**, meaning that they are sexually attracted to neither sex.

If you tried to identify "the" homosexual lifestyle, you couldn't do it. Homosexual people's lifestyles differ just as lifestyles of heterosexual people do. They are uncommitted, married, secretive, open, prostitute. They are

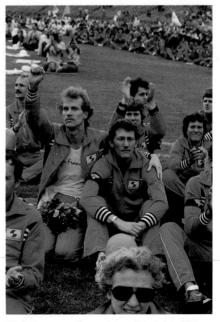

Within some communities, homosexuality is the norm.

Steps to establishing active homosexuality (as reported by males aged 20 to 25):

1. Suspecting.
2. Labeling feelings as homosexual.
3. Labeling self as homosexual; associating with others who are homosexual.
4. First love relationship.

SOURCE: Adapted from R. R. Troiden and E. Goode, Variables related to the acquisition of a gay identity, *Journal of Homosexuality* 5 (1980): 383–392.

lawyers, dentists, grocers, accountants, and everything that heterosexuals are, except where blockades have been put up by people who fear them.

Many such blockades exist. For example, some people fear that homosexuals may harm children, so they exclude them from jobs where they would have contact with children. (Sometimes homosexual parents' own children are taken away because the parents may be deemed "unfit.") They may be denied insurance, memberships in organizations, or other privileges solely because of their sexual orientation. Legal battles for the rights of homosexuals have begun to bring about slightly more openness about their plight and a few more legal rights within the larger society, but they are still an oppressed group.

Homosexuals sometimes form communities which serve as an escape from an oppressive society, and more than that, as a source of identity and support. Homosexual people need the same things from relationships that heterosexual people do: love, caring, trust, affection. Growing up homosexual is not easy. The messages are loud and clear—homosexuality is bad, perverted, and sinful. To develop a positive self-image and maintain self-esteem is difficult. Acceptance by a community gives people the feeling of belonging that is essential to self-esteem.

LOVE

No matter who you are or what your sexual orientation, goals, or life situation, you need close relationships with other people. It is important to share even simple daily life events with someone else, to reflect your life in their understanding. It is important to talk about problems, hear other opinions, and ultimately come to some resolution or agreement. People who live without such relationships more often suffer poor mental and physical health than do people who maintain them.[8]

Besides close relationships with friends, most people want a special relationship—namely, **love**. You can read love's description in poetry, see its reflection in art, observe the emotion glowing in the eyes of a person who is describing a loved one. You can also study it objectively (to a point) for a deeper understanding of its essence. But what is love?

What Love Is

Love is an emotion, a strong feeling that you can experience but that you cannot force to happen through conscious effort. Liking is a conscious activity, and it is not as powerful as loving; you like a person who has qualities that you respect or value. You may like different people for different qualities: one, for appearance; another, for wisdom; still another, for a lively sense of humor. Love, though, includes feelings of emotional attachment and a unique closeness with another person; **intimacy** is essential to love.

Intimacy is often equated with sexual behavior, and indeed, sexual behavior involves intimate physical acts. But another type of intimacy is an essential ingredient of love—psychological intimacy. People can be strangers and be sexually intimate; only people who love each other in some way can be psychologically intimate as well. Psychological intimacy means sharing your true mind and true feelings with another person, without hiding, without deceit; love requires that. Ideally, communication between lovers is free, simple, natural, honest, without artificial responses contrived to create an effect. To communicate in this way, you have to feel good about revealing the person you really are; that is, your self-esteem must be high.

An intimate relationship takes time to develop and does so in stages. First, people meet, like each other, and develop compatibility, a level of understanding. Next, through honest responses, they begin revealing themselves to each other. If they feel inclined to go on, they next become mutually dependent, developing habits that require each other's presence. For example, the couple may attend movies and critique them together. Once the pattern is established, going alone may seem lonely. As the relationship develops, emotional needs are met: to confide and to be trusted, to support and to be encouraged. The relationship may, but need not, lead to commitment to each other.

Love does not always progress along this smooth path. Relationships have different potentials. One that appears at first to be a love relationship might become instead a rewarding friendship; another friendship might blossom into love.

A new love relationship makes everything seem wonderful: "love is blind," or the lovers are "looking through rose-colored glasses." Such love is exhilarating beyond description, but the strength of feelings does not predict whether the relationship will last. In those that do last, though, this stage gives fond memories and the momentum to get through hard times.

As the relationship begins to move past the first stages, a letdown ensues in which reality makes itself evident. The partner has failings that can no longer be ignored. Nor should they be, because recognizing them is the path to growth. The relationship itself is no longer as rewarding as it was; of course, nothing could compare with the excitement of that initial stage of love. If this predictable but nonetheless rocky period can be weathered, with each partner's accepting the shortcomings of the other, the partners can gain the security of knowing that they are a couple. They trust each other to be accepting, because the true self of each, complete with faults, has been seen by the other. The practical aspects of love are among the best predictors of the success of a long-term relationship, and this chapter's Life Choice Inventory examines some of them.

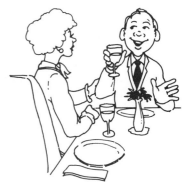

Love is an honest state and thrives on clear vision.

What Love Is Not

Love is specific in its requirements, and several things prevent its growth. Love cannot tolerate a contrived image of the partner. To romanticize, or imagine that the partner has nonexistent qualities, is to prevent love from becoming real. Love requires honesty and clear vision. Similarly, **infatuation** is not love. *Infatuation* is passionate, all-consuming preoccupation with the object of desire. It is often mistaken for sexual devotion, but it is different in that it quickly fades. It leads people to do things they ordinarily would not consider (such as lover's leap suicide). Luckily, infatuation's short life allows for recovery of reason in time to prevent disasters.

Old myths often detract from love. The myth that "love conquers all" may lead people to ignore a partner's real self in the belief that if love is strong enough, the partner will become the perfect mate. "You only love once, and when you meet him or her, you'll know it" leads people to ignore a rich selection of real-people partners who may not be princes or princesses but who aren't toads either. Real people become lovers; fairy tales are useful for lulling young children to sleep.

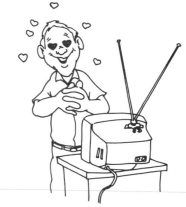

LYNDON WAS INFATUATED WITH SOAP OPERA QUEEN DAHLIA BOBBAY....

Infatuation is an excited state, and thrives on illusion.

LIFE CHOICE INVENTORY

Will your relationship last? Differences of opinion will pepper an otherwise bland relationship with challenges—but they can also destroy the relationship. It helps to know ahead of time where the major differences will be. The more of these questions you and your proposed partner agree on, the more likely your relationship will be a lasting one.

Money

1. Should each of us work? Should one stop working after children come?
2. Should we keep all our money in a shared bank account? If so, who should pay the bills? If not, who should pay which bills?
3. What should the limits be on use of credit cards?
4. Who decides on "big" purchases?
5. Should we follow a written budget? How closely?
6. If one of us wants to do something more rewarding personally than financially, will that be all right?
7. If one of our careers requires a move, will that be all right with the other?
8. How much of our income should we save, invest, and spend on insurance?
9. Will we own the home, car, and other property jointly? If not, who will hold the titles?

Children

1. Do we want to have children? How many? When?
2. Should children's needs be put before our needs?
3. How much money shall we save for, or spend on, children's education, recreation, and other options?
4. Who should discipline the children, and how—by physical punishment or withholding of privileges?

In-laws

1. How close is each of us to our families? Will it be important to see them frequently?
2. Is each of us willing to receive advice from the other's parents?
3. Can we or should we accept financial help from our families? How much, for what, from which family?

Religious Traditions

1. Are our religious beliefs compatible? If not, can we each live with the other's different beliefs?

2. Does either of us feel strongly that the other must attend religious services?
3. Should children be raised with particular religious beliefs?
4. Should religious practices be part of every day's routine? How will religious holidays be spent?
5. How much money, energy, or time should we spend on religious and charitable organizations?

Sex

1. Is sexual intercourse before marriage forbidden, permitted, or endorsed? For both of us or only one?
2. How often will each of us want to have intercourse? When, where, and under what circumstances?
3. Should each person be willing to have sex if the other wants it? Can each express desire freely to the other?
4. Is nudity acceptable around the house?
5. Is it important to each of us how the other dresses?
6. Is it acceptable to each of us if the other flirts?
7. How much of a display of affection is appropriate in public?

Miscellaneous

1. Is profanity acceptable? Under what conditions?
2. Is alcohol drinking acceptable? Is occasional drunkenness acceptable? How much of our money should be spent on alcohol?
3. Is drug use acceptable?
4. Is smoking acceptable? Under what conditions?
5. Should underage children be allowed to drink or smoke?
6. How should each of us behave in the home? Should we be available at all times to each other, or should we each have time alone or for projects of our own?
7. Should both of us go to bed at the same time? Who should get up first?
8. Who should do the shopping? Cook meals? See to repairs? Clean the bathroom?
9. How important is reading?
10. Should each of us be willing, if asked, to tell each other everything we think, feel, and do?

Certain mental attitudes destroy love. Someone who consistently tries to do more for a partner than what is realistic is a **martyr**. Martyrs may try to be understanding no matter what (while hiding hurt or angry feelings), may help the partner grow (while neglecting their own growth), may always go along with the other (while never stating a preference). Actually, the martyr may feel less than equal to the partner. Eventually, martyrs get angry if they are constantly overlooked.

MAR-ter

A person who tries to control a partner by underhanded means is a **manipulator**. Manipulation can be verbal, nonverbal, or both. A common verbal technique is sarcasm—saying the opposite of what you really mean in a contemptuous or mocking way ("Oh, well excuse *me!*" when you are sure it is the other person who needs excusing). Inducing guilt is another ("You're making me so upset that I can't work or even sleep at night anymore!"). A nonverbal technique is pouting or sulking, one person's visible attempt to change another's behavior without directly saying what the problem is. A more subtle kind of manipulation uses both words and actions—feigned helplessness. A person who detests, say, washing the car or cooking may lavishly praise the other's ability to wash the car or cook ("Oh, you're so much better at it than I am!") while making feeble gestures that indicate an inability to perform the task. Manipulation can take many forms, but it is always an attempt to manage others in a devious, underhanded way.

Martyrs and manipulators are just two examples of people who believe that if they were to let their real selves show, they would not be loved. Before love can grow between two people, both must feel that, even with their faults honestly displayed, they are worthy of love. That is, they must have high self-esteem. Self-esteem begins in childhood, thanks to nurturing parents, but it is never too late to develop it, and it is absolutely necessary for love.

■ SINGLEHOOD

Today many people choose to remain single—because they want to postpone marriage, because they choose not to marry, or because they haven't yet found the right partner. Many women are delaying marriage in order to develop careers. Single life is on the increase and is becoming more accepted.

People often stereotype single people: they view them either as living in the free-and-easy fast lane or at the opposite extreme—lonely, depressed, withdrawn. Actually, singles experience life's ups and downs as everyone does. Researchers have reported that single women, especially those who live alone, are psychologically better off than are married women, reporting higher self-esteem, less irritation, and less stress.[9] On the other hand, it seems that married men fare better than single men on the same scales. It may be that the costs of traditional marriage roles outweigh the benefits for women, whereas for men the opposite is more often true.[10] Singles, whether men or women, share some special concerns.

Single people need other people. Those who have developed strong social support networks are healthier than their more isolated peers.

Single people have another concern: how to meet their sexual needs in a society that officially sanctions only marriage for sexual activity. Some people choose to abstain from sexual activity. Religious teachings influence some to take such a stand, and it can be a positive choice. Other times the decision

Relationships with self and world are experienced most intensely in solitude.

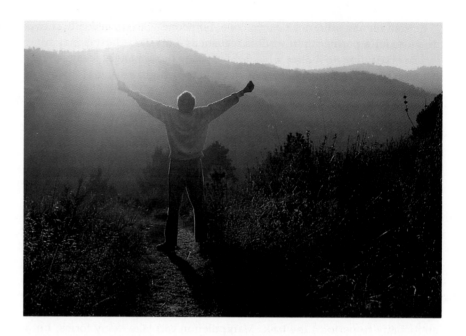

may be based on the old **double standard** that says sexual acts outside of marriage are acceptable for men but not for women.

Other single people choose not to abstain. People often choose sexual intimacy as a way to deepen relationships or explore others' sexual styles before marriage. Some people choose to have sex without love or affection, often when they are between meaningful relationships, not as a permanent choice. Overall, married people seem to be happier with their sex lives than single people are, while single people report having more partners.[11]

COMMITMENT

Anyone who chooses to embark on a long-term monogamous relationship is required to do something extraordinary—make a **commitment** to another person. A commitment is a promise to take on a long-term obligation, made in the face of many choices, with the knowledge that all will not always go well. In relationships, commitment is considered by some to be the highest form of maturity.[12]

The choosing of a life partner is a tricky business, and many people choose wrongly. To form a long-term, intimate bond that truly satisfies both partners involves more than simply the wish to do so. Psychologist Carl Rogers conducted a study of couples who had formed various types of bonds and attempted to define the ingredients that accounted for success.[13] Here is what he found:

It is not enough to say, "I love you" or "We love each other." We may mean what we say, but these statements easily change into "I thought I loved you" or "We thought we loved each other." It is also not enough (or it is a mistake) to say, "I commit myself wholly to you and your welfare." This can lead to a submergence of self that is fatal to the partnership. Nor is it enough to say, "We will work hard on our marriage"; work alone is insufficient. "We hold the institution of marriage sacred" or "We pledge ourselves to each other until death do us part" are also not enough; witness the statistics on divorce after such pledges. People also break up even when they feel deeply bound through their children.

So what *does* hold a partnership together? Rogers finally arrives at this statement:

We each commit ourselves to working together on the changing process of our present relationship, because that relationship is currently enriching our love and our life and we wish it to grow.

Every word in this statement is significant; the marginal glossary shows what they mean. "When dedication and commitment are defined in [this] manner, then I believe they constitute the cradle in which a real, related partnership can begin to grow," Rogers says.

These are among the rewards of a successful relationship: enjoying the other person, working out a lifestyle that suits both people, allowing the freedoms the other most needs, and meeting some of the other person's most important needs. Independence is important, too. The person who finds ways to meet many needs outside the paired relationship will be most successful at pairing. Recall the needs described in Maslow's scheme (Chapter 3). You cannot realistically ask your partner to provide total security—whether emotional, financial, or physical. You must stand on your own feet and provide your own security. You, yourself, are the only person you will never leave or lose. The person who is most independent is most ready to become interdependent.

Meanings of words in Rogers's statement:
Each—we are both doing it.
Commit—we won't back out.
Working—it takes work, and we are willing to do it.
Together—it is cooperative, not one for the other, but each with the other.
Changing—we know we cannot keep it as it was in the beginning; we have to take the risk of changing.
Present, currently—it is not that we promised each other long ago that we would do this; we are doing it now.
Enriching—the rewards are also present; we feel them today.
Grow—we see the process of change as necessary and desirable.

Marriage

Did you ever wonder what happened to Cinderella and the Prince after they married? Did they really live happily ever after? Probably the most destructive concept associated with marriage is that this could possibly be the case. Marriage is never the *end* of the story, as in fairy tales. It is the beginning. The plot thickens.

What comes to mind when you hear the word **marriage**? "It's common knowledge," you may say, "everyone knows what marriage means." And indeed, almost everyone agrees on a few things. The assumptions that most marriage partners agree on are called the **marriage premises**:

PREM-iss-ez

1. The relationship is permanent, or at least permanence is something the partners are willing to work for.
2. The partners will be mutually primary to each other. No other relationship will have a higher priority.

The first premise, permanence, distinguishes marriage from all other pair relationships. Dating and even living together usually do not possess the permanence of marriage. The other premise of marriage, primariness, varies more in its meaning to individuals. Often, people equate primariness with sexual **monogamy**; the partners have sexual relations only with each other. Other people define primariness in other ways. (See *marriage* in the chapter Glossary.) In any case, maintaining primariness throughout married life demands conscious effort; investments of time, care, and patience; and even personal sacrifice.

Before they marry, people would do well to look honestly at their own expectations. Clearly it is essential to establish what a potential partner means when the word *marriage* comes up.

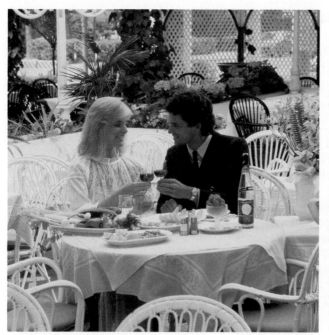

In a fantasy marriage, people live happily ever after.

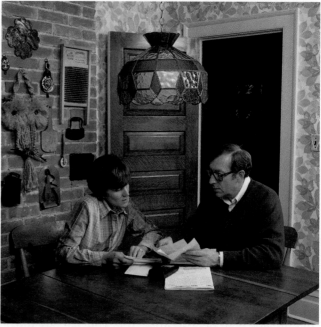

In a real marriage, people work things out.

Working through Conflict

Partners may think that anger and conflict have no place in a "happy" committed relationship and so may deny their negative feelings. In reality, every pair experiences conflicts, and how they handle them can determine whether their relationship grows or dies.

Destructive things happen when feelings of anger are not addressed. People who keep them inside find other, unhealthy ways of dealing with the feelings, such as engaging in compulsive behaviors (drinking, drug abuse, overeating, or gambling). Alternatively, they may start talking to the wrong people about their anger instead of telling the one who needs to know—the partner. Psychosomatic illness may develop, as may psychological disorders such as depression.

Instead of directing the anger inward, the person may express it inappropriately and destructively. The person who chronically criticizes, nags, or uses sarcasm may feel as if the anger is getting out in the open, but it is really just aimed to hurt the other, not to cure the problem. More subtle forms of attack are sabotage (messing up the other's plans), anger displacement (being rude to, or angry at, in-laws or children), or verbal abuse of the mate. In some cases, the angry person engages in spouse abuse—physical violence against the mate.

Some people believe (falsely) that mild episodes of physical aggression can release tension and help to "clear the air." Actually, partners and family members withdraw farther away in response to such displays. Assertion, not aggression, is the path to clear air (see Chapter 3). Equally useless are tactics to evade issues, such as leaving when disagreement arises, refusing to talk, not taking the other seriously (he's just had a hard day/she must have her period), or not giving the other time to respond. Evading quarrels by saving up hurts is useless—they come spilling out in a confusing mess at some later date.

Developing and maintaining intimacy is hard work. One must grow, oneself, and encourage the other to grow. One must drop harmful attitudes and not blame the other for one's own shortcomings. One must give the partner unconditional acceptance as a fully human, and therefore worthwhile, person. One must learn to understand how the partner views other people and life events and accept and empathize with those views.

STUDY AIDS

1. Explain in what ways male and female reproductive systems are similar and how they differ.
2. Define the terms *masturbation* and *sex play*, and describe what contributions these activities make to adult sexual activity.
3. List the four phases of sexual response in men and women, and identify some of the characteristic physical changes that accompany them.
4. List some common sexual problems, their possible causes, and strategies to help overcome them.
5. List the steps to active homosexuality.
6. Describe the progressive stages in the development of love.
7. List myths and attitudes that prevent the development of love.
8. Discuss the special concerns of the single person.
9. Define *commitment*.
10. Explain how a person's emotional health provides a framework for successful pairing.
11. List destructive ways of dealing with conflict, along with their constructive counterparts.

GLOSSARY

For terms relating to sexual and reproductive anatomy and physiology, see the Miniglossaries on page 195.

afterglow: the pleasure of the resolution phase of the sexual response.

aphrodisiac (af-roh-DIZ-ee-ack): a substance reputed to excite sexual desire. Actually no known substance does this, but many claim to do so.

   Aphrodite = the Greek goddess of love

asexual: having no sexual inclinations.

   a = without

bisexual: being sexually oriented to members of both sexes.

   bi = two

coitus: see *sexual intercourse*.

commitment: a decision to embark on a long-term monogamous relationship with another person, without a guaranteed outcome.

copulation: see *sexual intercourse*.

cunnilingus (cun-ih-LING-gus): oral stimulation of a woman's clitoris and labia.

   cunnus = external female genitalia
   lingere = to lick

double standard: a tradition that gives certain freedoms to one group but not to another. An example: the tradition that gives men sexual freedoms that women do not have.

ejaculation: the discharge of semen from the penis during a man's orgasm.

   ex = out
   jaculari = to throw

engorgement: swelling. With reference to the sexual response, the sex organs' filling with blood preparatory to orgasm.

erection: the state of a normally soft tissue when it fills with blood and becomes firm. Both penis and clitoris can become erect.

erogenous (eh-ROJ-eh-nus) **zones:** areas of the body especially sensitive to sexual stimulation—the penis, clitoris, nipples, lips, and others.

   eros = sexual love
   gen = giving rise to

excitement: as used to describe a stage of sexual intercourse, the early stage.

fellatio (feh-LAY-she-oh): oral stimulation of a man's penis.

   fellare = to suck

foreplay: activity that precedes intercourse, in which each partner gives pleasure to the other.

gamete: a mature cell produced for the purpose of reproduction—sperm cells in men, egg cells (ova) in women.

   gamein = to marry

gender identity: that part of the self-concept influenced by the meaning ascribed to being male or female.

gender role: the role assigned by society to people of each sex.

genitals: the external organs of the reproductive system—the penis and scrotum in men; the labia and clitoris in women.

   genitalis = to beget

gonad (GO-nad): a primary sex organ; testis or ovary.

   gonos = procreation

heterosexual: sexual orientation to persons of the opposite sex.

   heteros = other

homosexuality: sexual orientation to persons of the same sex, popularly called *gay* orientation or, in women, *lesbianism*.

   homo = same

infatuation: unreasoning, temporary passion or attraction for another person.

   fatuus = foolish

intimacy: the state of being very close and familiar, as in deep friendships, sexual relationships, and committed love relationships.

love: affection, attachment, or devotion.

manipulator: a person who tries to control others by underhanded means.

marriage: the institution that joins a man and woman by contract for the purpose of creating and maintaining a family. See *marriage premises*. Marriages may take several forms. In a *monogamous marriage* the partners have sexual relations only with each other. A *closed marriage* permits neither social nor sexual relations outside the marriage. An *open marriage* permits social and sometimes sexual relations with partners other than the spouse. A *utilitarian marriage* is a practical relationship that meets people's practical needs. An *intrinsic marriage* is based on psychological intimacy without regard for practical considerations. A *group marriage* is any marriage involving more than two people.

marriage premises (PREM-iss-ez): the assumptions of a marriage that the relationship will be permanent and that the partners will be primary to each other.

martyr (MAR-ter): a great and constant sufferer.

masturbation: rubbing, stroking, or otherwise stimulating one's own genitals.

menstrual cycle: the monthly fertility cycle, directed by hormones, that prepares the uterus to receive a fertilized ovum. The monthly shedding of the uterine lining is called *menstruation*.

mens = month

menstruation: see *menstrual cycle*.

monogamy (moh-NOG-uh-mee): a term used to refer to sexual exclusivity in marriage and other relationships.

mono = one

nocturnal emission: the emission of semen during sleep. See *wet dream*.

nocturnus = night

orgasm: the climax of sexual excitement that typically occurs during sexual intercourse. Several such climaxes in rapid succession are called *multiple orgasm*.

ovulation (AH-vyoo-LAY-shun): the release of an ovum from the ovary.

ovulatory cycle: the monthly ripening of an ovum.

petting: see *sex play*.

pituitary gland: the master gland of the hormonal system, located in the brain. The hormones it produces control other glands, including the gonads.

plateau: literally, a high, flat place. In sexual intercourse, the plateau phase is the period of intense physical enjoyment preceding orgasm.

primary sex characteristic: one of the anatomical characteristics that distinguish the sexes at birth—primarily, the sex organs.

resolution: in sexual intercourse, the stage of relaxation that follows orgasm.

secondary sex characteristic: one of the anatomical sex characteristics that develop during puberty, including the male's deep voice, the female's breasts, and the characteristic body hair on both.

sensuous: related to the experience of pleasure through the senses.

sex: the sum of the differences between males and females that serve the purpose of permitting and promoting reproduction.

sex play: physical expression of affection and sexual desire that does not involve sexual intercourse; hugging, kissing, fondling; also called *petting*.

sexual dysfunction: impaired responses of sexual excitement or orgasm due to psychological, interpersonal, physical, environmental, or cultural causes; formerly called *impotence* in men and *frigidity* in women.

sexual intercourse: the reproductive act between the sexes. The term *intercourse* means connection or communication of any kind—talking or trading, for example. Sexual intercourse between human beings is termed *coitus* (CO-ih-tus); between animals it is termed *copulation* (cop-you-LAY-shun).

copulare = to join together

sexuality: the collective characteristics that mark the differences between male and female people.

sodomy (SOD-oh-me): unnatural sex acts, as defined by a particular society, especially anal and oral sexual activity.

tenting effect: vaginal expansion caused by the upward tilting of the uterus during the excitement phase of sexual arousal.

wet dream: unconscious, solo orgasm that occurs during sleep. In males, it is accompanied by ejaculation.

QUIZ ANSWERS

1. *False*. People are sexual beings from infancy on.

2. *False*. Masturbation is normal sexual activity, and it is sometimes preferable to other forms of sexual activity, for health's sake.

3. *True*. The need for nonsexual touching, kissing, and holding may be more essential to well-being than orgasm.

4. *False*. The master organ of sexual response (in both men and women) is the brain.

5. *True*. Orgasm is a reflex, similar to the jerk of the leg when the knee is tapped.

6. *True*. Both men and women have orgasms while dreaming.

7. *True*. Most sexual problems respond to simple treatments.

8. *True*. Giving too much can ruin a relationship, just as taking too much can.

9. *False*. Care in choosing whom to love is essential; no amount of giving of self can turn discord into harmony.

10. *False*. Love alone is not enough; success takes commitment from both people's working together on the relationship.

SPOTLIGHT

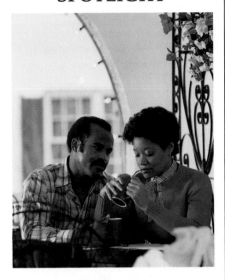

Gender and Power

Chapter 10 has described relationships between people in terms of love. Within all human relationships, though, people give and take. Power is the element that determines who does the giving and who does the taking, to what extent, and under what circumstances.

The word *power* makes me think of one person pushing another around. Is that what you mean by power in relationships?

Yes and no. Several different types of power in relationships exist. One type, coercive power, uses fear of punishment. When this type of power is used, one person submits to the other's will because he or she fears retaliation, such as physical harm, withheld affection, withheld sexual gratification, or withheld money. But this type of power may also be based on the opposite expectation—one person submits because he or she expects to be rewarded. In both cases, the punisher or the rewarder holds the power, because that person can evoke the other's "giving"—behaving the way the power-holder wants. Another kind of power comes simply from the belief that such power exists—for example, that the husband has the final say or that the wife has a right to be supported financially. Power differentials are often agreed on unconsciously by both partners. Both the powerful and the powerless can gain from the roles. But people don't always act on the power they have—one may defer to the other for the sake of reaching an agreement.

How does one person submit to the other's will?

Examples are life decisions such as whether to have children, where to live, who leaves a job to accommodate the career advancement of the other, or whether to make a major purchase. Other decisions may deal with everyday matters—who does the dishes, the financial recording, the bathroom cleaning, or the landscaping of the yard.

How are these things decided?

Two types of power structures exist in relationships, the **traditional** power structure and the **egalitarian** power structure. Traditional power is so named because it fits the stereotyped system of gender roles in which men have more power than women in important issues—spending leisure time, spending money, picking friends, and having sexual relations—while women are permitted to decide on minor issues such as colors and styles of furnishings and appliances.

Gender roles aside, the person who needs the relationship less is in the position of power. That is, if one person has a rich field of options for dates and careers, and the other has fewer options, the partner with more options wields over the other the power of being freer to leave the relationship. Traditional male and female gender roles give males more options—they have more career opportunities, chances to initiate relationships, and independence. Traditionally, women have been afforded fewer opportunities and hence less power. Further, one person may simply know more, or be perceived as knowing more, about a certain topic and so be empowered by agreement to act on it. As women become better educated, their options become more numerous, and they gain power.

Does pregnancy affect a woman's power? Those stories of husbands running out in the night for pickles and ice cream make me think so.

Women do enjoy a certain special status during pregnancy, but pregnancy and childbearing temporarily lessen a woman's power by making support from the relationship more essential to her well-being. Her power returns to its original level as the children grow and become less dependent themselves.[1]*

What if I want a relationship that gives equal power to both people?

Today, some men and women are working to share power equally in their relationships. They have few role models to guide them, only their own honest commitment to their mutual well-being. They share equally the responsibility for earning income, and they value each career on its own merits, not on the basis of which person is holding it. Other tasks are equally shared—one partner may specialize in cooking while the other may clean up, but these jobs are not dispensed according to sex.

*Reference notes are in Appendix D.

That sounds harmonious. Does it work?

Yes, for people who are willing to work at it. When partners share life with such a side-by-side orientation, they report greater personal happiness, fewer unshared areas of life, more common experience—greater intimacy. They also enjoy greater financial and domestic independence and more free time spent together. Egalitarian relationships are emerging as a workable alternative to the traditional power structure.[2]

I keep reading that women are actually still doing most of the household work in these so-called equal relationships. Is that true?

Although the great majority of both men and women say they would like to share equal power, their actual behaviors more often reflect a traditional power structure. This shows that while conscious attitudes may be changing, old gender role teachings and family models persist and overwhelm conscious desires.[3]

Equality aside, isn't it still true that the man and the woman in a relationship should have different qualities?

Actually, it seems that most of today's college-age men and women describe desirable mates in much the same terms. Both have a few stereotyped expectations, but mainly both say they want a mate who is:

- Independent.
- Skilled in business.
- Outspoken.
- Self-confident and ambitious.
- Not easily influenced.
- Active, adventurous, and worldly.
- Interested in sex.
- Able to make decisions easily.
- Persevering.
- Interested in science and math.
- Outgoing.
- Intellectual.
- Superior feeling.
- Emotional.
- Grateful.
- Home oriented.
- A person with a strong conscience.
- Creative.
- Understanding, considerate, and tactful.
- Needful of approval.
- Excitable in major crises.
- Fond of art and music.
- Capable of feeling hurt.
- Helpful to others.
- Religious.
- Fond of children.

Just a few years ago, people saw many of these traits as exclusively male or female. Now, they see them as desirable *human* traits—those that typify the kind of person people want to marry.[4]

Conception, Infertility, and Family Planning

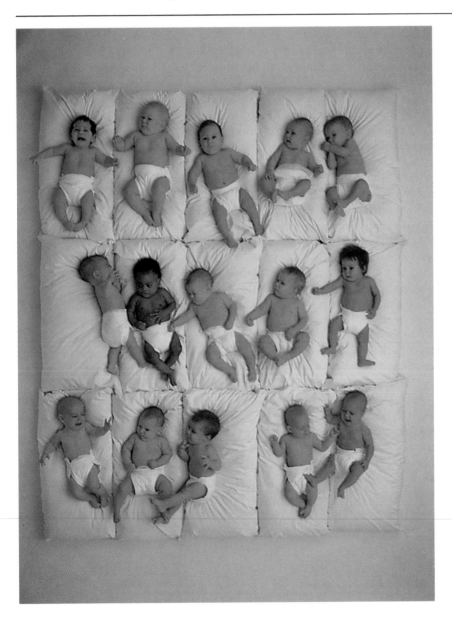

FOR OPENERS . . .

True or false? If false, say what is true.

1. If a couple does not conceive in a year of trying, chances are slim that they ever will.
2. Contraception can help make healthy babies.
3. Of ten sexually active couples using no contraception, nine become pregnant within one year.
4. You can find the perfect contraceptive method, as long as you first obtain all the facts.
5. Sterilization operations involve lengthy, complex surgical procedures.
6. You can be completely protected against pregnancy, if you use a contraceptive method correctly at each time of sexual intercourse.
7. When an unplanned pregnancy occurs, a woman has three choices: to become a parent, to have an abortion, or to give birth and give the baby up for adoption.
8. Most women who have abortions suffer from mental illness eventually.
9. Both abortion clinics and hospitals provide safe abortion services.
10. Most abortions could be avoided if all sexually active couples who do not wish to produce a child would begin now to use contraceptives.

(Answers on page 232.)

The event that starts a whole new human being takes place in a single moment. The event described here is **conception**.

CONCEPTION AND INFERTILITY

In a woman with normal **fertility,** an ovum, tinier than the period at the end of this sentence, has grown ready for **fertilization** about once every month since she began menstruating in her teens. A man of normal fertility has produced millions of microscopic sperm cells a day since puberty. Upon sexual intercourse, sperm swim up the vagina, propelled by their long, whipping tails, and attach to the surface of a waiting ovum. One sperm finally enters, triggering an instantaneous change in the ovum's surface so that no more sperm can penetrate. The new cell that forms is a **zygote.** If conditions are right, the zygote imbeds in the uterine wall **(implantation)** and begins to develop. Only about 40 percent of all zygotes actually implant and develop; the other 60 percent fail to implant or are dislodged later, expelled from the uterus into the vagina and lost from the body.[1*]

The events of pregnancy and birth are presented in Chapter 12. The next sections are about getting the timing right—**family planning**. This first section addresses the couple who want to have a baby right away.

Conception can be a thrilling event for people who want to have a baby. Most people have no trouble conceiving. Of sexually active couples who use no preventive measures, 90 percent conceive within one year with no conscious effort. They can, however, plan more precisely when to conceive by using the **fertility awareness method**—a method that also can be used in planning not to conceive.

An ovum lives for only 12 to 24 hours. For fertilization to be accomplished, sexual intercourse must occur within a time limit—living sperm must arrive in time to meet the mature ovum as it travels toward the uterus. Sperm can live quite well for a few days within the female reproductive tract, so they can get there first and wait. Intercourse within a few days before ovulation can produce a pregnancy.*

A couple who uses fertility awareness to conceive has sexual intercourse more frequently during or before ovulation. Methods to determine the time of ovulation include recording menstruation days on a calendar, measuring daily body temperature, observing changes in vaginal secretions, or a combination of these. Family planning centers offer help in learning to use these fertility awareness methods both to conceive and to prevent conception.

An at-home test kit for ovulation can be purchased over the counter. The test is expensive in comparison with the standard fertility awareness methods just mentioned. It is useless for preventing conception.

If a couple engages in sexual intercourse with the right timing, but conception still does not take place, the problem may be **infertility**. Its causes are many and varied, and they occur with equal frequency in men and women.

Diseases can render people infertile. A cause common among women is **pelvic inflammatory disease (PID)**, an infection that spreads throughout

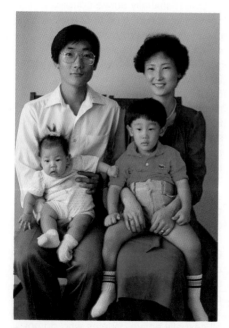

Family planning means getting the timing right.

*Reference notes are in Appendix D.
*The exact life span of sperm within the female reproductive tract is not known, but scientists think it is in the range from at least 24 hours to as long as five days.

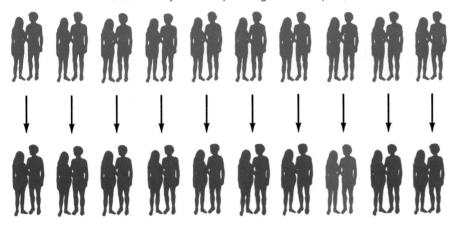

Of ten sexually active couples using no contraception,

Nine become pregnant within one year.

The odds favor conception when sexually active people use no contraception.

the fallopian tubes. Another condition, called **endometriosis**, develops when the cells of the inner lining of the uterus, the endometrium, escape into the abdominal cavity, tubes, and ovaries, where they adhere and grow, causing scarring.

In men, the mumps affects the testes and sometimes leaves them infertile. So does the more common problem of testicular varicose veins. Physical trauma, malnutrition, some medicines, substance abuse, reproductive tract abnormalities, inadequate production of sperm or ova, and even mild infections in both men and women also bring about infertility.

If a couple is unsuccessful in attempts to conceive for more than about a year, it may be time to seek a medical diagnosis. Even then, about half of all such couples succeed in conceiving with no treatment if they simply keep on trying.[2]

The treatment of infertility depends on the cause. In the case of an anatomical problem that interferes with conception, surgery may help. A woman who produces too few ova might be treated with **fertility drugs**. These drugs call forth the hormones, or are themselves the hormones, that force the ovaries to mature and release ova. No doubt you have heard of women bearing four or five children at once after taking such drugs. What happened was that the drug dose made four or five ova ready for fertilization simultaneously. (This outcome can't be avoided; the same drug dose in another woman would be just right.) Multiple births of this magnitude almost never happen except when fertility drugs are used.

If a man produces insufficient numbers of sperm per ejaculation, the couple can be helped to conceive by **artificial insemination**. In this procedure, the man's semen from many ejaculations is collected and stored in a cup to be fitted over the woman's cervix at the time of ovulation. If this fails, a fertile man other than the prospective father may become a **sperm donor**.

If the woman is infertile, the couple may elect to hire a **surrogate mother**. This is a woman who agrees to be artificially inseminated with the husband's sperm, bear the baby, and surrender it to the infertile couple. Surrogate motherhood may sound good in theory, but in practice it is full of legal, ethical, and emotional uncertainties; hence, it is seldom employed.

An experimental measure is **in-vitro fertilization**. The name "test-tube babies" is given to children conceived this way, although only the fertilization takes place in a test tube; the fetus grows in the mother's uterus. The procedure is a complicated, expensive surgical process, and produces pregnancy only one-fourth of the time, but hundreds of babies have been conceived this way.

While conception is difficult for some, it is all too easy for the majority of sexually active couples. With timeless patience, nature has perfected the reproduction of living things, guarding and improving the carriers of life in each new generation. People set themselves a tough task when they try to control their own fertility through family planning.

Anyone now having sexual intercourse but using no means of contraception is indicating a wish to have a child. A person has much to consider in committing to this choice. Almost every aspect of life is touched by the choice of whether to reproduce. An extreme case is that of the adolescent mother. By deciding to carry an unplanned pregnancy to term, a girl alters 50 to 90 percent of the rest of her life.[3] She becomes isolated from her peers. Her educational and subsequent career or job opportunities dwindle. She incurs physical risks and so does her infant. Both may not be healthy. Ultimately, she is likely to support more children than her peers who bear children later. She will be preoccupied with securing food and shelter instead of attending to personal growth (recall Maslow's hierarchy from Chapter 3).

Fertility's power also touches adults. Surprise pregnancies are not uncommon, and a person who has had one or more may fear sexual activity itself. When unplanned pregnancies occur, careers may end, relationships may falter, and even spiritual beliefs may be compromised. Part of Chapter 12 is dedicated to helping people make the decision whether to raise a child. Anyone who is not ready, and who is sexually active, should opt for **contraception**.

THE CHOICE OF FAMILY PLANNING

Although it may sound preposterous, contraception is good for babies—for one important reason: people can use it while cultivating lifestyle practices that maximize their chances of having healthy babies. Another benefit of using contraception in family planning is that parents can choose how many children to have and when to have each one.

Contraception is a controversial subject. Some people's religious convictions forbid its use; other people would like to legislate its use for everyone who is sexually active. This chapter takes the position that the choice is personal; it presents the facts people need to make choices as informed consumers.

Contraception is not for women only. It is a shared human responsibility that accompanies the personal pleasure of sexual intercourse. No one should ever assume that a partner will take care of it. The topic should be open for discussion. Appropriate concern about contraception is a sign of commitment to the partner. Further, open communication about it can not only help the couple find a suitable method but also tends to enhance their closeness, promote lasting sexual pleasure, and strengthen the relationship.

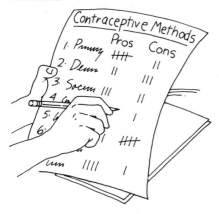

Whether to use contraception, and which form to use, is for people to decide for themselves.

Contraception and **birth control** are often used to mean the same thing, but contraception comes first. Contraception means to prevent conception—or to interfere with its result immediately afterward. The term *birth control* should be reserved for prevention of births— that is, a larger concept including both contraception and **abortion**. This chapter distinguishes between the two terms.

Where to Get Help with Contraception

Before choosing a method of contraception, a person is wise to consult with a physician, physician's assistant, or nurse practitioner. The professional will be able to check for unsuspected health problems and give education as well as a prescription when one is needed.

Planning centers and other resources such as student health services or county health departments furnish services much the same as those offered by private physicians and at a reasonable cost. (Many centers use a sliding fee scale based on income.) These facilities often also provide free contraception counseling to individuals or couples, and most also have special help clinics for teenagers. Counseling in all federally funded clinics and in many private ones is strictly confidential for adults; minors who go to federally funded clinics are not afforded confidentiality, and their parents may be notified. Planned Parenthood is privately funded and maintains strict confidentiality, regardless of the client's age.

Religious organizations sometimes offer counseling services for people with concerns about sexuality, pregnancy, and other issues as well as contraception. One such organization is Catholic Alternatives.

If you choose to seek contraception assistance from one of these sources, make an advance appointment. These organizations are made up of individuals, and not every counselor is the right one for every person. If you should feel uncomfortable with one counselor, ask to see someone else. The professionals are concerned with your welfare and will schedule you to speak with several different people if you wish.

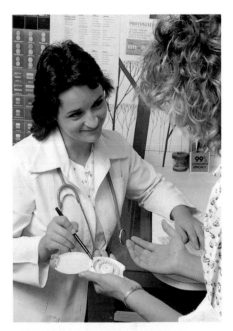

Before choosing a method, obtain adequate information.

Choosing a Method

No contraceptive method is perfect. The person choosing a method has to face that fact. To obtain the advantages of one method, a person has to be willing to accept disadvantages that invariably accompany it. For that reason, it is important to decide which features are indispensable and which disadvantages are acceptable. This chapter's Life Choice Inventory asks questions to help people decide which methods they might find most suitable. Table 11–1 can help you pick based on the effectiveness of the methods.

First, though, a few words about effectiveness and side effects will lay some groundwork. Different estimates of effectiveness may be cited for the same contraceptive method, because different researchers take different approaches. One approach is to assume every couple will use the method perfectly and to measure only the failure rate of the method itself. This approach produces **laboratory effectiveness** data: statements of how well the method would work if 100 couples used it perfectly for a year. The other approach is to answer the question, How many *typical* users out of 100 become pregnant while using contraceptive X for one year? The answer gives an estimate of **user effectiveness**. If, in real life, 8 women out of 100 become pregnant using a method, then that method's user effectiveness is 92 percent, no matter how perfectly the device is supposed to work. This chapter lists both effectiveness ratings whenever possible. Giving only one might be misleading.[4]

The lists of side effects that may result from using each method also need explanation. Some of the lists are long and sound threatening, but remember, a drug company has to report side effects even if they occur only once in

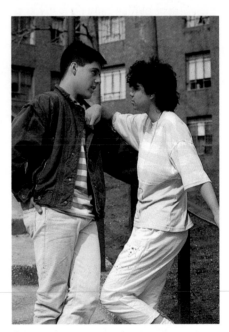

Open communication about contraception promotes both wise planning and closeness.

every million users. Before you start to worry about the dangers of contraception, remember that carrying a baby to term entails risks that are considerably greater than those incurred by using any contraceptive method except one (the Pill, for a woman who smokes). In fact, driving down the street is more likely to injure your health.

LIFE CHOICE INVENTORY

Which method of contraception is most suitable for you? The questions below point out matters to consider in sorting out your priorities. Ask the following questions regarding each method of contraception. The more "Yes" responses that apply to a particular method, the more appropriate the method is for you.

1. *Possible obstacles to use:*
   If necessary, are you willing to use a method that requires you to touch your genitals? _____
   Are you willing (and will you remember) to use the method every time you have intercourse or to stay on a daily schedule? _____
   Would you find it acceptable to interrupt foreplay to use contraception? _____
   Does your partner accept the idea of interrupting foreplay to use contraception? (You may face a conflict in which you want to protect yourself and please your partner but find that you cannot do both.)
   Are you and your partner without fear or aversions to the method being considered? _____

2. *Locus of control:*
   Does the method allow the control to be with the person you want it to be with? _____
   If you have to rely on your partner, is your partner reliable? _____

3. *Privacy and confidentiality:*
   Does the method give you the confidentiality you need? _____ (If you would rather keep your contraception strictly your own business, choose a method that does not require having devices or products on hand.)

4. *Reversibility:*
   Is the method appropriate for your future family goals? _____ (If you and your partner feel that you have enough children, you may wish to consider a permanent form of contraception.)

5. *Frequency of intercourse:*
   Will you be able to use the method consistently with your frequency of intercourse? _____ Does the method provide protection when you need it, without excessive protection when you don't? (Does it fit your lifestyle?)

6. *Noncontraceptive benefits:*
   Would this method provide a health benefit, other than contraception, that would make you favor it? _____ (For example, condom use protects against sexually transmitted diseases (see Chapter 15); birth control pills might make an irregular menstrual period regular.)
   Is the method in keeping with your and your partner's your religious beliefs? _____ (If not, contact an organization of your religious group for counseling.)

7. *Cost:*
   Is the method affordable? _____ (Most county health departments provide free or low-cost contraceptive drugs and devices.)

8. *Medical side effects and risks:*
   Is the method medically safe for you? _____

9. *Physical limiting factors:*
   Has this method always prevented pregnancy for you when you've used it in the past? _____ (If no, choose another method.)

10. *Effectiveness:*
    Is the effectiveness of the method consistent with your needs? _____ (If pregnancy would be unacceptable, you may choose a highly effective method, if pregnancy would be acceptable, you may choose to use a less effective method. You and your partner may want to discuss how you feel about abortion or raising a child in case your method should fail.)

SOURCE: Based primarily on information in R. A. Hatcher and coauthors, Choosing a contraceptive: Effectiveness, safety, and important personal considerations, in *Contraceptive Technology* (New York: Irvington, 1984), pp. 1–18.

TABLE 11–1 Standard Birth Control Methods Accepted or Rejected on the Basis of Effectiveness[a]
Circle yes or no for each method.

Method	Effectiveness If Used Perfectly (%)	Effectiveness in Typical Users (%)	Factors to Consider	Acceptability to You (circle one)	
Abstinence	100	Unknown	Chance of pregnancy within a year in a person who does not abstain is 90%.	Yes	No
Oral contraceptives (combination pill and minipill)	99.5 99	98 97.5	Users who find it easy to take pills regularly use the method most successfully.	Yes	No
Intrauterine device (IUD)	98.5	95	The device can be expelled without the user's awareness; pregnancy may occur with the device in place.	Yes	No
Spermicides	95 to 97	82	Users who follow directions exactly use the method most successfully.	Yes	No
Diaphragm with spermicide	98	88	Successful use requires proper fit and following instructions exactly.	Yes	No
Vaginal contraceptive sponge	95 to 98	83 to 90	Users who follow directions exactly use the method most successfully.	Yes	No
Condom	98	90	High quality condoms are most protective; improper use or leakage of sperm makes failure likely.	Yes	No
Condom with spermicide	99.5	98	Users must follow directions exactly. Poor-quality condoms or leakage of sperm prior to use makes failure likely.	Yes	No
Fertility awareness	80 to 95	76	Ovulation is unpredictable. A high degree of training, skill, and dedication is required.	Yes	No
Male sterilization	99.85	99.85	Successful, except if the user has intercourse before sperm are absent from semen or if spontaneous repair occurs (very unlikely).	Yes	No
Female sterilization	99.96	99.96	Pregnancy is likely only if spontaneous regeneration occurs.	Yes	No

[a]Effectiveness ratings may vary depending upon how the method was studied—in the laboratory or in real life. Laboratory ratings, because they exclude the mistakes people make, are higher.

THE STANDARD REVERSIBLE METHODS

This section briefly discusses each of the birth control methods. The amount of information given here about any method does not reflect its desirability, but only its complexity.

The first method is **abstinence**. Occasional pregnancies do begin because a single drop of semen, deposited near the opening of a woman's vagina, has permitted sperm to travel to meet a mature ovum. Assuming no such contact, however, abstinence is 100 percent guaranteed. It is the choice of many people, especially young ones. Many people share this preference because of lack of a suitable partner, fear of pregnancy or disease, or personal or religious values.

It takes courage to decide to abstain from sexual intercourse and willpower to maintain the decision in the face of social pressures to be sexy, look sexy, and act sexy. Abstinence is sometimes a temporary decision until marriage or other conditions make an appropriate relationship possible.

Many women choose **oral contraceptives**, popularly known as the Pill. Approximately one-third of all women aged 30 and under and one-tenth of women aged 30 to 39 use oral contraceptives.[5]

There are two types of oral contraceptives: the **combination pill**, which contains synthetic versions of the hormones estrogen and progesterone (the synthetic version is called **progestin**), taken for 21 days of each month; and the **minipill**, which contains only progestin and is taken continuously. The ovaries produce estrogen after ovulation. The rise in estrogen suppresses ovulation until after the next menstruation. The estrogen in the combination pills prevents pregnancy the same way, by suppressing ovulation. A woman may still ovulate during her first month on pills, and should use a backup method of contraception during this time.

The minipill contains no estrogen, and most of its effects take place in the uterus itself. The progestin in the minipill makes the mucus surrounding the uterine opening (cervix) less penetrable to sperm and also may deactivate sperm cells. Progestin also interrupts the normal preparation of the uterine endometrium so that a zygote may not implant. Taking pills is not the only way to introduce progestins into the body: some contraceptive devices release the drugs directly into the uterus or vagina, and in other countries, women can receive a shot of progestins that lasts for three months.*

Years ago, pills contained much more estrogen than they do now. Low doses of estrogen do not always stop ovulation, so the newer low-dose tablets rely on the effects of progestin as a backup to prevent pregnancy.

Some pills, the **triphasic oral contraceptives**, offer combined hormones in the lowest doses that stop ovulation. On pill schedules used previously, such low doses often caused menstrual irregularities in the women who took them. The triphasic pills, though, deliver the hormones in three levels throughout the cycle, an improved schedule. This scheme prevents ovulation and promotes more regular menstrual cycles.

The effectiveness of any type of pill depends on regular and correct use. It is imperative to ask questions of the prescribing physician or counselor to clear up any confusion about how the pill works and how to use it. If a woman forgets to take her pill for a day or more, she should use a backup method of contraception for the remainder of that pill cycle.

Abstinence effectiveness = 100%.

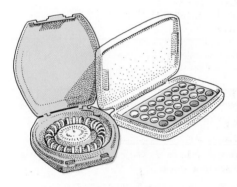

Oral contraceptive effectiveness:
 Combination pills, laboratory rating = 99.5%.
 Combination pills, user effectiveness = 98%.
 Minipill, laboratory rating = 99%.
 Minipill, user effectiveness = 97.5%.

*Among devices that release progestin are intrauterine devices (IUDs) and vaginal rings. The shot is Depo Provera.

All oral contraceptives present side effects, ranging from common nuisances to rare, life-threatening conditions. They may include tenderness of the breasts, emotional depression or fatigue, nausea or vomiting, skin conditions, weight gain or loss, stopping of menstruation, unexpected vaginal bleeding, increased frequency of vaginal yeast infections, higher levels of sugar and fat in the blood, decreased sex drive, headaches, and fluid retention. Among the rare conditions are diseases of the heart, kidney, liver, or gallbladder; stroke; benign tumors of the uterus; and blood clots that can lodge in vital organs and cause death. Women who use the Pill are strongly advised not to smoke, because smoking, together with use of the Pill, increases the risk of heart attack or stroke (Chapter 9 mentioned this effect). Early warnings are almost always evident before complications become serious medical emergencies, so women who take oral contraceptives should report to their physicians any of the symptoms listed in the margin. Not all side effects are negative. For example, oral contraceptives can help to regulate irregular menstrual periods. They have also been associated with decreased risk of certain cancers.[6]

Report these symptoms:
  Abdominal pain.
  Chest pain.
  Breathlessness.
  Headaches.
  Blurred vision or loss of vision.
  Leg pain.

The minipill produces fewer and less severe side effects than the combination pill; hence, women who experience side effects when they take the combination pills may successfully take the minipill. Of course, the minipill has possible side effects of its own, including menstrual disorders and, less often, headaches.

Most women who use the Pill experience no side effects at all. Of those who experience minor side effects, many find that the discomfort goes away after about three months. Others need only to switch from one brand of pill to another (the prescribing physician can advise about this possibility).

It is important to be aware that depression, a relatively common side effect, may take some time to develop; the user may not realize that it is associated with oral contraceptive use. When moodiness, sadness, or irritability is not brought on by explainable events and does not improve after several months, pill users should suspect the pills and ask their physicians for another type.

CONSUMER CAUTION

The Pill affects a woman's nutrition status, and users may wonder whether they need to take supplements to compensate. However, the Pill *increases* blood levels of iron and copper, so that women who take it may need less of these two minerals. On the other hand, the Pill interferes with the body's use of two vitamins, folacin and vitamin B_6. Deficiencies of these produce anemia or emotional depression in some users.

Vitamin companies use these findings to promote the taking (and buying) of all sorts of supplements, often recommending them instead of what the person urgently needs—a balanced diet of whole foods. The companies may be telling the truth about a woman's increased need for nutrients, but the response they advocate benefits them, not her.

Ads may state the truth, but consumers must evaluate its significance.

A woman who believes she may be pregnant should not take the Pill, because it increases the risk of defects in the fetus. In fact, a woman who decides to become pregnant and is using oral contraceptives should wait at

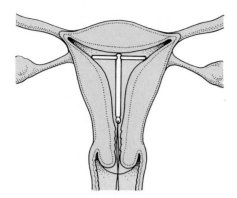

IUD effectiveness:
Laboratory rating = 98.5%.
User effectiveness = 95%.

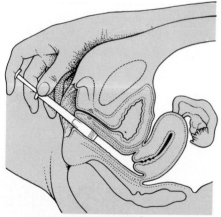

Spermicide (foams, creams, jellies, and suppositories) effectiveness:
Laboratory rating = 95 to 97%.
User effectiveness = 82%.

least two months (some health care providers suggest six months to a year) after stopping use of the Pill and use another method of contraception.

Less widely used, especially recently, but still popular among some users is another for-women-only contraceptive method: the **intrauterine device,** or **IUD.** The IUD is a small plastic or plastic and metal object that is inserted into a woman's uterus. A tiny nylon thread hangs from the IUD through the cervix into the vagina as an indicator that the IUD is in place and as an aid to removal.

The IUD is intended for long-term use and is not appropriate for repeated insertions and removals, such as between pregnancies in a growing family. The mechanism of action of the IUD is not fully known, but one theory is that the IUD makes the uterine environment hostile to sperm or to zygotes and prevents implantation. Progestin-containing IUDs slowly release this synthetic hormone into the uterus, making it an even more unfavorable environment for sperm and zygotes. The IUD may be inserted up to five days *after* unprotected intercourse and still prevent pregnancy.

Pelvic inflammatory disease (PID), which can lead to sterility, is a complication of IUD use—rare, but still four times more common in IUD users than in nonusers.[7] One IUD, the Dalkon shield, was produced years ago, and thousands of women had it inserted before it was found to be of faulty design. By that time, many women had suffered PID; for some, permanent sterility or even death had resulted from using the device.[8*] The company voluntarily recalled the product and discontinued its production, but thousands of women sued the company, and hundreds more have attempted to sue producers of other IUDs as well. Many manufacturers of IUDs have determined that they no longer can afford the legal costs of defending their products and so have discontinued making them. Companies that still produce them require clients to sign statements indicating that they are aware of the risks before insertion.

Sperm-killing or sperm-immobilizing products, the **spermicides,** can be inserted into the vagina just before intercourse. These are available over the counter as foams, creams, jellies, sheets, or suppositories—some preloaded in disposable applicators, some in aerosol cans with reusable applicators, some as preformed inserts, and some in other forms. These contraceptives are **barrier devices**—they interpose a physical and chemical barrier between sperm and ovum at the opening of the uterus. Most do not last long—only half an hour or so—and therefore must be inserted just before each occasion of sexual intercourse. Some people find that spermicides act as a local anesthetic and inhibit sexual response.

The **diaphragm** is another barrier device. It is a circular metal spring or ring fitted with a shallow cup of thin rubber that the user fills with spermicidal cream or jelly. The device is folded for insertion into the vagina; once inside, it gently springs open to cover the cervix. The diaphragm bars sperm from entering the uterus and acts as a holder for spermicide.

To fit a diaphragm, the health care provider measures a woman's vaginal interior and prescribes the size that ensures an all-important proper fit. (Some women may be tempted to borrow a diaphragm "just to try it" before going in to be fitted themselves. This is a mistake, because the likelihood that a borrowed diaphragm will fit properly is slim indeed.)

*Anyone still using a Dalkon shield should have it removed immediately.

The user of a diaphragm can insert it up to six hours in advance of intercourse and so avoid the inconvenience of last minute preparation. Some sources recommend that if the diaphragm is left in place for more than about two hours before use, an additional application of spermicide should be inserted into the vagina. The diaphragm must be left in place for at least six hours after intercourse and then removed as soon as convenient within 24 hours. The user should store her diaphragm as instructed and check it periodically for holes or other defects by holding it up to the light. It has a limited life span.

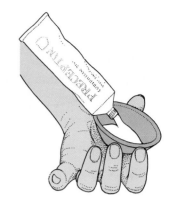

Similar in principle to the diaphragm is the vaginal contraceptive **sponge**. The sponge is a disposable product, currently available as "Today." It resembles a diaphragm in shape but is made of thick sponge rubber and comes equipped with a woven handle to facilitate removal. The sponge contains a spermicide that is activated when it is moistened with water. A bowl-shaped indentation fits over the cervix and helps hold the sponge in place.

The sponge can be inserted anytime before sexual intercourse and gives continuous protection for 24 hours thereafter, with nothing more to do, even for repeated intercourse. Like the diaphragm, it must be left in place for at least six hours after intercourse and then should be removed as soon as convenient.

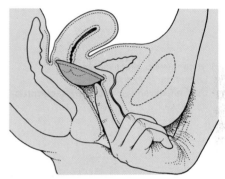

The **cervical cap** is similiar to the diaphragm in use and effectiveness and is available by prescription. The cap is a flexible, cuplike device about an inch and a half in diameter that is fitted by a physician to cover the base of the woman's cervix. Like the diaphragm, the cap is a holder for spermicide. It differs from the diaphragm in that it is smaller, more durable, and can be worn for 48 hours, compared with 24 hours for the diaphragm. Since the cap fits tightly and rarely leaks, the repeated use of spermicide before intercourse is unnecessary.

Diaphragm with spermicide effectiveness:
  Laboratory rating = 98%.
  User effectiveness = 88%.

Cervical cap effectiveness:
  Average effectiveness = 82.6%

In a very few instances, a dangerous kind of bacterial poisoning known as **toxic shock syndrome (TSS)** has been associated with diaphragm, sponge, and cervical cap use.[9] (Toxic shock syndrome was linked more often with the use of a brand of tampons that has now been removed from the market.) Because of the risk of toxic shock syndrome, it may be wise to avoid using the diaphragm or sponge during a menstrual period and to always remove it after no longer than 24 hours. The early warnings of TSS resemble other conditions, so users of tampons, diaphragm, or sponge should be suspicious of and report diarrhea, fever, muscle aches (flulike), and skin rash resembling a sunburn.

The **condom** is a disposable barrier device whose effectiveness in preventing the transmission of AIDS has brought it widespread attention. Its usefulness as a barrier to disease is discussed in Chapter 15. It consists of a thin sheath of rubber or processed lamb tissue that is rolled over the erect penis before intercourse. There are many varieties, shapes, and colors, but all work the same way—they collect semen, sometimes in a small pouch at the tip of the condom, and retain it for disposal.

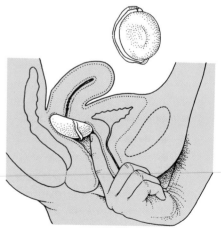

When being applied, the condom should be left rolled up as it comes from the wrapper and placed loosely on the glans of the erect penis. The condom is gently and slowly unrolled down to the base of the penis, while the thumb and index finger of one hand hold the condom's tip to create a reservoir for the semen. The condom should not be stretched tightly over the glans—it could break during intercourse. Some condoms are coated with lubricating jelly or powder on the outside to reduce friction in the vagina. For maximum

Sponge effectiveness:
  Laboratory rating = 95 to 98%.
  User effectiveness = 83 to 90%.

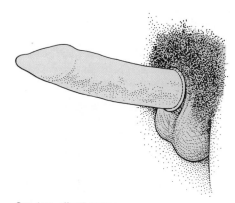

Condom effectiveness:
  Condom, laboratory rating = 98%.
  Condom, user effectiveness = 90%.
  Condom with spermicide = same as combination pill—98%.

Rhythm method effectiveness:
  Laboratory rating = 77-89%.
  User effectiveness = unknown, but probably lower.

Withdrawal effectiveness:
  Laboratory rating = 84%.
  User effectiveness = 77%.

The word *douche* is pronounced "DOOSH."

effectiveness, when a man uses a condom, the woman should use a vaginal spermicide. Alternatively, he can choose to use condoms that come with spermicide already applied to them.

The condom must be in place before any contact occurs between the penis and the vagina, because as mentioned, fluid that contains sperm is released even before intercourse begins. If the condom is applied too late, even if before orgasm, effectiveness drops dramatically. Condoms vary in quality; vending machine varieties break easily, and the more expensive ones are recommended.

A condom will slip off a penis that is not fully erect. A man who uses one must withdraw from contact after intercourse, and a man who tends to lose penile erection during intercourse should not rely on a condom for contraception.

The **rhythm method**—mentioned earlier as the fertility awareness method—uses neither drugs nor devices. It is available to anyone, but training by professionals is necessary for people to use it successfully. Even the most comprehensive, technically correct references warn people that merely reading about the method is insufficient to enable them to use it successfully to prevent conception.*

Other methods of contraception are being developed. Some are available in other countries, some are in the research stage, but none is as well researched as those just presented. Lack of government support, fear of lawsuits, and modest profits from new products slow progress in contraceptive technology.

■ METHODS NOT RECOMMENDED

Popular belief often endorses contraception strategies other than those just described. One idea is that pregnancy can be prevented by using a method that involves neither drugs nor devices—the **withdrawal method**, also known as **coitus interruptus**. It is just what it sounds like—the man withdraws his penis from the vagina before he ejaculates, taking care that his semen is not deposited in, at, or near the vagina.

This method often fails to prevent pregnancy because the man finds it difficult to withdraw his penis when he is near orgasm; he feels an urge for deeper penetration at that time.[10] Even if everything else goes as planned, live sperm from the fluid at the tip of the penis may have already entered the vagina. Withdrawal is slightly better than no method at all, but it still allows 23 women out of 100 to become pregnant in one year of use. It is not recommended for individuals who are serious about preventing pregnancy.

Throughout history, women have attempted to wash out or kill sperm after unprotected intercourse by using **douches** of such preparations as lemon juice, carbonated beverages, vinegar, or even hazardous chemicals such as turpentine. Most douches used today are the over-the-counter variety and are not intended for contraception; also their use is associated with PID. In any case, vaginal douches after sexual intercourse are not effective for preventing pregnancy. The fluid may wash sperm up the cervix as easily

*For more information about fertility awareness methods, consult the latest edition of R. A. Hatcher and coauthors, *Contraceptive Technology* (New York: Irvington). Most libraries have this book, which contains the explicit instructions needed by the person who wants to use the method.

as washing them out. Effectiveness in actual users is reported at 60 percent—meaning that within a year, 40 out of every 100 women who rely on this strategy will become pregnant.

Still another strategy not recommended for contraception is **lactation**. It is true that when a woman is breastfeeding an infant, the likelihood that she will ovulate is reduced—but unfortunately, there is no way she can know for sure. Lactation is an important means of child spacing throughout a population, but it is unreliable as a contraception method for any individual woman.

IRREVERSIBLE METHODS: STERILIZATION

In direct contrast to the approaches just discussed, **sterilization** is a highly effective contraceptive method—in most cases, irreversible. Each year, millions of people choose to be rendered permanently infertile, and the number is increasing—in fact, sterilization is the leading contraceptive method in the world. As of 1982, 32 percent of married couples in the United States had chosen sterilization, and the total worldwide was about 90 million.[11]

The choice to be sterilized is highly personal. No one can count on being able to reverse it later. For the person who desires temporary, reversible contraception, sterilization is not appropriate. (This does not mean, though, that sterilization is 100 percent effective; in rare cases, the ends of the tubes that are surgically severed find each other and grow back together, restoring fertility.)

People have a legal right to choose sterilization and also a legal right not to be sterilized against their will. Federal regulations state that the person to be sterilized must be at least 21 years of age, receive counseling, give written consent, and wait 30 days after that.

The simplest and most common sterilization procedures are **vasectomy** in men and **tubal ligation** in women. The vasectomy is a procedure that involves making one or two tiny incisions in the scrotum and severing the vas deferens, through which the sperm travel to become part of the semen. The procedure takes about half an hour and may be performed under local anesthesia in a physician's office. The incisions are so tiny that vasectomies are called "Band-Aid surgery." The vasectomized man continues to produce sperm, but they are reduced in number, and they are absorbed by the body rather than being released into the semen. Interruption of the production of sperm has no effect on the production of testosterone.

Vasectomy does not affect a man's ability or desire to have intercourse, although his fear of the surgery may do so. Sometimes a man needs a brief period of adjustment after the operation before he is sure he desires and enjoys sexual intercourse as much as he did before. Thereafter, many men report increased enjoyment, because they need not fear their partners' becoming pregnant.

Vasectomy is a low-cost, one-time procedure. It permits the man to resume normal activity within a day or so, although he must use another form of contraception for a few days until tests show no sperm left in his semen. Ejaculation and orgasm are normal. Pain is minimal although soreness should be expected for a day or so; side effects are rare.

For a woman, a tubal ligation often can be performed on an outpatient basis at a hospital or clinic. Commonly referred to as "tying the tubes," the ligation is a procedure in which the surgeon cuts and seals the fallopian

To review the anatomy of the reproductive organs while reading the next section, see Figures 10–1 through 10–4 in Chapter 10.

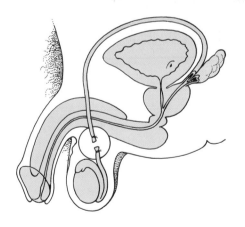

Vasectomy effectiveness:
Laboratory rating = 99.85%.
User effectiveness = 99.85%.

CHAPTER 11 ■ **CONCEPTION, INFERTILITY, AND FAMILY PLANNING**

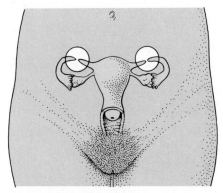

Tubal ligation effectiveness:
Laboratory rating = 99.96%.
User effectiveness = 99.96%.

laparotomy (LAP-uh-ROT-oh-mee)
laparoscopy (LAP-uh-RAHS-koh-pee)

tubes. This permanently prevents passage of ova from the ovaries to the uterus. The operation can be performed with either a local or general anesthetic and leaves a tiny scar on the abdomen, in the navel, or in the vagina.

Tubal ligation may be accomplished by one of several procedures. **Laparotomy** is an incision in the abdomen; the **minilaparotomy** (like the vasectomy, sometimes called "Band-Aid surgery") is a small abdominal incision; in a **laparoscopy**, the surgeon makes two smaller incisions, one to accommodate a viewing instrument and one through which the tubes are severed. After the operation, the woman continues to menstruate and ovulate as before; when the ripe ovum is released, it is reabsorbed by the body. (Another, different procedure, the **hysterectomy**, is the removal of the uterus, and although this major surgery produces sterility, it is not usually performed for contraceptive purposes.)

▮ CONTRACEPTIVE FAILURE AND ABORTION

Failure of contraception is not unusual. Any method of contraception may fail, especially if it is imperfectly used. Talking about a method's failure rate may bring impersonal statistics to mind, but consider the numbers in human terms—they refer to real women who have become pregnant despite efforts to prevent it.

When you read that a certain method is 97 percent effective, that may make you think that it almost completely prevents unwanted pregnancy, but a look at some numbers can be enlightening. If the adult, fertile female population of the United States were 100 million (it's close to that number) and if all of these women were using one of the most effective methods of contraception and using it correctly, 3 million women would still become pregnant each year. Of course, in real life, not all fertile women use contraception, even those who wish to avoid pregnancy; and those who do often use it incorrectly.

Actually, over 4 million women in the United States alone face unwanted pregnancies each year. Considering that each woman's fertility lasts 30 years or more, it is clear that the chance of any woman's being included in the total for at least one of those years is strong indeed. A woman with an unwanted pregnancy may be the victim of failed contraception, rape, or sexual abuse; she may be young or old, poor or rich, a student, a professional, a blue-collar worker, or a housewife. Each of these women may face the difficult decision of whether to have an abortion or continue the pregnancy.

The first decision for a woman who suspects that she is pregnant is how to confirm or allay her suspicion. Chapter 12 provides information on pregnancy testing, but a warning is in order here. Because abortion is an issue on which many people have strong feelings, a woman may encounter pressure if she is tested for pregnancy in an agency that advocates a particular choice. Most local health departments offer free or low-cost tests without accompanying advice.

Imagine you have received news of a positive pregnancy test. (If you are a man, imagine that you are involved in an unplanned pregnancy.) If you have a hard time imagining the decision you would make, you may be sure that it is even harder under the physical and emotional stress of a pregnancy. Remember from Chapter 3 ("Emotional Health") that decisions mean weighing your feelings, judgments, and values; in the case of abortion, feelings, judgments, and values often conflict with one another. Besides those problems, pregnancy causes hormonal changes that can affect mood and physical well-being. The pregnant, unmarried woman may also be experiencing guilt, anger, embarrassment, concern for feelings of parents or partner, and dread of others' reactions to the news.

Of women with unwanted pregnancies, 90 percent make the decision to abort or to carry through the pregnancy within 12 weeks. Of the abortions, half are performed by the 8th week, and almost all the rest by the 12th. Of the women who decide to give birth, most adjust to the event and make the child welcome. Others make the child available for adoption.

A variety of support services are available to a woman who is struggling to decide whether to keep the baby or give it up for adoption, and whether to marry the father. These decisions are best made with the support of people who can help the woman accept herself and her decision.

The conflict that people face when considering terminating an unwanted pregnancy centers around a basic question. Which is more important, the embryo that is developing inside the woman, or the quality of the future child's and the woman's own life? Almost everyone has mixed feelings about the issue.

Heated political battles rage between groups that support legal abortion and groups that oppose it. Members of both seek to do what they believe is right, but both groups include extremists. A person who goes to a facility that opposes abortion stands a chance of being served by people of extreme bias. Other, more professional facilities, such as Planned Parenthood centers, value the person above all else and strive to help the woman decide what action best suits her or her family. Objective counseling can be a great help in deciding how to handle an unplanned pregnancy. Action must be swift, however; delays increase the woman's risks, whether she ultimately continues the pregnancy or has an abortion. If an abortion is delayed, the procedures become more complex; if prenatal care is delayed, the health of the fetus, as well as that of the woman, may be compromised.

Agencies are available to help women who choose to carry their unplanned pregnancies to term. Such agencies usually keep up-to-date lists of resources designed to meet the needs of women with problems such as abandonment by family or father of the child, poor health, insufficient income, lack of emotional support, and many others.

Many such agencies are associated with political organizations called pro-life or right-to-life. They hold strong religious or moral convictions against abortion. They may be supported by religious groups and may include religious teaching in their counseling. They can be especially helpful when a woman wants to continue a pregnancy but is unable to pay for the needed services. Services vary from place to place, but they can include free pregnancy testing; group counseling; medical care before, during, and after the birth; housing; adoption services; maternity and infant clothing; and day care.

For those who choose abortion, most abortion clinics offer services such as free or low-cost pregnancy tests, preabortion counseling, examinations, standard preoperative blood tests, and abortions. Importantly, they also provide postabortion contraception advice. They also offer emotional support, often in the form of individual or group counseling for women, men, or couples.

The Politics of Abortion

In the United States' early years, abortion was legal. At the time, however, medical techniques were too primitive to perform abortions safely, and many women died from the procedure. The government did what it could to protect these women, by making abortion illegal. Still, people performed abortions, illegally, often for outrageous fees.

Women who sought abortions received treatment at the hands of crudely trained or untrained people. The operations were performed with unsanitary hooks, knives, or coat hangers, and the women received no medical care afterward. Infection, permanent disability, and death were likely.

Today, because the procedure is legal, it is safe and usually uncomplicated. It is performed in sanitary facilities by trained personnel. Indeed, the number of unwanted children born since the legalization of abortion has decreased dramatically.

The pendulum has been swinging back and forth—from making abortion illegal, to legal and free, to legal but expensive—and it may swing back to illegal again. Whether it is legal or not, however, many women will continue to choose this course.

The abortion facility a woman chooses should have the same degree of professionalism as any other medical facility.[12] The physical surroundings should be clean, the staff should be courteous, postabortion contraception information and prescriptions should be provided, and the woman should be afforded privacy. If any of these conditions is lacking, or if a woman feels uncomfortable for any reason, she should look elsewhere. Remember, walking into a medical office is not an obligation to be treated there.

Abortion methods vary according to the length of the pregnancy.* Abortions that take place early in pregnancy require no anesthesia, or local anesthesia only; they are routine for the medical staff and are well tolerated by most women. Those performed later in pregnancy require general anesthesia and surgery. In all surgical abortions, the first step is to widen the opening of the cervix to allow access of medical tools. In early abortions, up through 13 weeks' gestation, a thin, hollow tube is inserted into the uterus, suction is applied, and the contents of the uterus are vacuumed out in a process called **vacuum aspiration**.

Between 13 and about 16 weeks, an abortion requires a more direct technique, because the pregnancy has progressed to a point where suction alone cannot remove all of the uterine contents. A large-diameter vacuum tube is needed which requires that the cervix be dilated enough to accommodate it and other tools used for removal. This operation is known as a **D and E** (dilation of the cervix and evacuation of the uterus). A similar procedure, the **D and C** (dilation and curettage), involves scraping the uterus with other tools.

Medical methods are an alternative to surgery for abortions after 13 weeks of gestation. Chemicals are administered to induce labor: prostaglandins and solutions of salt or urea may be injected directly into the sac surrounding the fetus, and a labor-inducing hormone* may be administered to the woman.

The physical risk of abortion is much lower today than in the past. The procedures still carry some slight risk, however, especially late in pregnancy. Generally, early abortion (during the first three months) carries a risk to the woman's life only slightly higher than that posed by contraception, and both contraception and abortion up to 16 weeks carry much less risk than pregnancy and childbirth.[13] Some question remains, however, about whether late abortions have long-term effects on fertility and on the outcomes of future pregnancies.

Fees for early abortion around $250 are common (late 1980s). Although much lower than the thousands of dollars women used to pay for illegal abortions, these fees are still too much for some people to pay. Limited funding of abortions for the nation's poor makes the service unavailable to estimated tens of thousands of the very women who are least financially able to bear and care for unplanned children. Abortion is costly, but not when the cost of raising a child to maturity is weighed against it.

This year, about four out of every 100 women of childbearing age will choose to have an abortion.[14] Chances are you know one or two of them, whether you realize it or not. Until contraception is 100 percent effective, until every sexually active person uses it when appropriate, and until rape is wiped out for all time, one of these four women will still have to face the

---

*An invaluable reference that describes abortion techniques and procedures in detail is R. A. Hatcher and coauthors, *Contraceptive Technology* (New York: Irvington). Look for the latest edition.
*The hormone is oxytocin.

choice every year. The other three could be spared this emotional and physical stress if they would begin, now, to use a reliable method of contraception and continue using it faithfully and correctly every time they had sexual intercourse.[15]

STUDY AIDS

1. Describe the events of conception.
2. Define the term *fertility*, and discuss its significance in people's lives.
3. Define the term *family planning*, and describe two of its benefits.
4. List some common causes of infertility and actions to correct them.
5. Describe the person who should be using contraceptives.
6. Describe the information that should be given to a person who wanted to know where to get contraceptive help.
7. Describe accurately the various contraceptive methods.
8. List and describe ten elements to be considered when selecting a contraceptive method.
9. Evaluate the safety and effectiveness of several contraceptive methods.
10. Identify factors that lead to unplanned pregnancies, and list the alternatives for action.
11. State advantages of making an early decision about whether to terminate an unwanted pregnancy or continue it.
12. Describe methods for both early and late abortions.

GLOSSARY

abortion: a general term meaning a pregnancy that ends before the fetus is viable outside the uterus. A *spontaneous* abortion is a miscarriage; an *induced* or *therapeutic* abortion is one brought on by medical means. In *septic* abortion, the uterine lining and contents have become infected, a dangerous condition. See also *D and C*, *D and E*, and *vacuum aspiration*.

abstinence: refraining from sexual intercourse, a 100% effective contraceptive method.

artificial insemination: a means of achieving pregnancy without intercourse, in which semen is mechanically introduced into the vagina.

barrier devices: contraceptive devices that physically or chemically obstruct the travel of sperm toward the ovum. These devices are also called *noninvasive* methods, because they do not alter other body processes with drugs or devices.

birth control: any method used to control the number of children born. See also *contraception*.

birth control pills: see *oral contraceptives*.

cervical cap: a cuplike barrier device that fits over the cervix and holds spermicide against the uterine opening.

coitus interruptus: see *withdrawal method*.

combination pill: an oral contraceptive containing estrogens and progestin.

conception: fertilization, the union of ovum and sperm that starts a new individual.

condom: a barrier device consisting of a sheath worn over the penis during intercourse to contain the semen and/or prevent transmission of sexually transmitted disease.

contraception: any method of preventing conception. The term *birth control* is often used as a synonym, although technically, it refers to methods of preventing birth as well as of preventing conception.

D and C: the abbreviation for *dilation* (alternate spelling *dilatation*) *and curettage* (scraping), a type of abortion.

D and E: the abbreviation for *dilation and evacuation*, a type of abortion.

diaphragm: a barrier device consisting of a dome that fits over the cervix and holds spermicidal cream or jelly against the uterine entrance to block the passage of sperm.

douche (doosh): a stream of fluid directed into the vagina, useful in certain disease conditions but ineffective as a contraceptive.

endometriosis (EN-doh-mee-tree-OH-sis): invasion of the abdominal cavity by the mucous membrane lining the uterus.

family planning: limiting the number and spacing of children according to the wishes of the couple rather than leaving them to chance—accomplished by birth control.

fertility: ability to produce and expel gametes sufficient for reproduction.

fertility awareness method: a method of predicting or discerning ovulation, which includes charting of a menstrual calendar, body temperature, and observations of mucus. The method can be used either to plan conception or to prevent it.

fertility drugs: hormones that induce the production and release of gametes, or chemicals that induce the body to synthesize such hormones.

fertilization: the fusion of an ovum and a sperm.

hysterectomy: removal of the uterus.

implantation: the event in which a zygote embeds itself in the wall of the uterus and begins to develop, during the first two weeks after conception.

infertility: inability to produce gametes and/or offspring.

intrauterine device (IUD): a device inserted into the uterus to make conditions hostile to sperm or zygotes, preventing conception or implantation.

in-vitro (in-VEE-troh) **fertilization:** a laboratory procedure in which fertilization takes place outside the body. *In vitro* means "in the test-tube," as opposed to *in vivo* (in VEE-voh), which means "in the body."

laboratory effectiveness: the percentage of women protected from pregnancy in a year's time by a contraceptive method or device under ideal experimental conditions. See also *user effectiveness*.

lactation: the production of milk—sometimes inappropriately relied on as a contraceptive method.

laparoscopy (LAP-uh-RAHS-koh-pee): surgical sterilization of women that employs a viewing device (a laparoscope) and is performed through two small abdominal incisions.

laparotomy (LAP-uh-ROT-oh-mee): a general surgical term referring to the opening of the abdomen; a surgical sterilization of women performed through an abdominal incision.

minilaparotomy: a surgical sterilization of women using a tiny abdominal incision.

minipill: a progestin-only oral contraceptive. See also *combination pill* and *oral contraceptives.*

oral contraceptives: pills containing synthetic hormones that disrupt the female menstrual cycle and prevent ovulation; used to prevent conception, often called *birth control pills.*

pelvic inflammatory disease (PID): a dangerous infection of the female reproductive tract, resulting in scarring of the fallopian tubes, temporary or permanent sterility, and possibly death.

progestin: synthetic progesterone, used as a contraceptive drug.

rhythm method: see *fertility awareness.*

sperm donor: a man chosen to donate semen for artificial insemination.

spermicide: a chemical that kills or immobilizes sperm, used in several barrier contraceptive devices.

sponge: a barrier device similar to the diaphragm that fits over the cervix and releases spermicide when moistened with water.

sterilization: the process of rendering people infertile, usually by surgical severing and sealing the vas deferens or fallopian tubes.

surrogate mother: a woman who undertakes to bear an infant for another person.

toxic shock syndrome (TSS): a dangerous group of symptoms brought on by a toxin produced by bacteria within the vagina that breed in menstrual blood when it is prevented from flowing out. The syndrome has occurred with prolonged tampon retention and in diaphragm users during the menstrual flow.

triphasic oral contraceptives: birth control pills of low hormone content, administered in three phases over the menstrual cycle.

tubal ligation: surgical severing and sealing of the fallopian tubes to sterilize women.

user effectiveness: the percentage of typical women users protected from pregnancy in a year's time by a contraceptive method or device. See also *laboratory effectiveness.*

vacuum aspiration: vacuuming of the uterus, a type of abortion.

vasectomy: surgical severing and sealing of the vas deferens to sterilize men.

withdrawal method (coitus interruptus): a technique in sexual intercourse of withdrawing the penis from the vagina just before ejaculation.

zygote: the product of the union of ovum and sperm, so termed for two weeks after conception. (After that, it is called an *embryo.*)

QUIZ ANSWERS

1. *False.* Many couples conceive without treatment if they just keep trying, and most others can be helped to conceive through simple medical means.

2. *True.* Contraception can help make healthy babies.

3. *True.* Of ten sexually active couples using no contraception, nine become pregnant within one year.

4. *False.* No contraceptive method is perfect, and to obtain the advantages of one method, a person must be willing to put up with its disadvantages.

5. *False.* Sterilization operations are safe and simple.

6. *False.* All contraceptive methods fail occasionally, no matter how conscientiously they are used.

7. *True.* When an unplanned pregnancy occurs, a woman has three choices: to become a parent, to have an abortion, or to give birth and give the baby up for adoption.

8. *False.* Very few women suffer lasting effects from abortions.

9. *True.* Both abortion clinics and hospitals provide safe abortion services.

10. *True.* Most abortions could be avoided if all sexually active couples who do not wish to produce a child would begin now to use contraceptives.

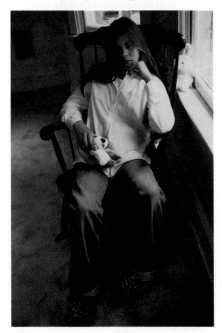

Why People Don't Use Contraception

Many individuals consciously choose not to use contraception. They may cite moral, religious, or personal reasons for this choice, or their culture may encourage large families and discourage contraception. However, enormous numbers of unplanned pregnancies end in abortions or unwanted births each year, and most of these result from simple failure to use adequate contraception by people who made no conscious choice. In fact, some people may avoid the decision altogether. But as mentioned in the chapter, not choosing to use contraception is a choice to have a child.

Why would people decide to take such a chance?

Emotional immaturity and fear are two powerful reasons. People in their teen years are especially prone to avoid the contraception decision because of real or imagined parental disapproval, embarrassment, lack of information, or failure to perceive the connection between sexual intercourse and pregnancy. Fears may lead people to rely on misinformation offered by friends or lovers rather than to seek out facts from reliable sources. Such people may find planning a contraceptive strategy an uncomfortable task because it implies that they anticipate engaging in sex-

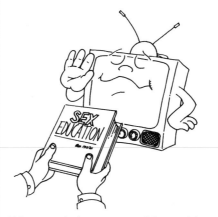

Television shirks its responsibility to deliver sex education.

ual intercourse. The assumption seems to be that sex is great, but nice people don't plan it—it "just happens." If they used contraception, it would destroy this illusion. People who wrap themselves in this illusion can pretend to lead lifestyles in keeping with traditional values but still get what they want. Using contraception makes a statement—that the person is sexually active. However, so does pregnancy, and our society has a high rate of unwanted pregnancies.

What is it about our society that promotes so many unwanted pregnancies?

The mass-communication media are at least partly responsible, because they do not educate. The media offer abundant sexually oriented material depicting bedroom scenes and other sexual images, but seldom do they show couples pausing in their passion to use contraception. When such scenes do occur, they are usually humorous ones that demean the act. Television makes practically nonstop sexual suggestions to its audience, and yet networks do not advertise contraception. Magazines use sexy images to sell everything from automobiles to zebra-striped underclothes—everything, that is, except contraception. In fact, romance novels and many movies and television programs do much to reinforce the attitude already mentioned: an unwillingness to own one's sexual behavior.

The media thus use as heroes and heroines people who serve as poor role models. They are not in control of their sexuality, and they are not responsible for it. Also, their lives are unrealistic: even though they often are swept off their feet by overwhelming passion, they never get pregnant, and they never get sick. They never, in other words, have a price to pay.

The attitudes of sexually active teenagers, when studied, seem sensible enough. They often feel that they should postpone sex or use contraception; or at least, they say they do. Their behaviors, however, are like those of media role models—out of touch with reality. Many sexually active teenagers who say they *should* use contraception also say they did not, the last time they had intercourse.[1]* It is as if they had no comprehension of the potential consequences of their behavior—as if getting pregnant were as likely as the sky's falling and they were equally helpless in the face of both.

When people do use contraception, what factors influence them to do so?

Four things have been observed. The more a woman embraces her own normal sexuality, the more likely she is to use contraception.[2] The more a couple care about each other, the more likely they are to protect each other with contraception.[3] The older and more sexually experienced they are, the more likely they are to use effective contraception.[4] And the more they see pregnancy prevention as a shared responsibility, the more likely they are to use contraception.[5]

What about sex education? Doesn't that help?

Ideally, parents would be the primary sex educators, but they sometimes withhold, or do not have, accurate information. To make sure that this information is not withheld from children, society needs to provide these facts through its regular information-delivery route—the school system. In societies that do furnish meaningful sex education with whole-hearted community support, teenage pregnancies drop. Combined with freely available, sub-

*Reference notes are in Appendix D.

sidized birth control for teens, such sex education contributes to a substantial drop in the number of teenage pregnancies and in the number of abortions. The United States and other countries, on the other hand, are experiencing increases in teenage pregnancies and abortions.[6]

But sex education is only part of the solution. Research has indicated that the young people most likely either to delay sexual activity or to use contraceptives when they do become sexually active are those whose parents have discussed sex with them.[7] To promote a responsible attitude toward contraception, an attitude shift needs to take place within individual families and within society as a whole. Right now, our society promotes the sex act itself without promoting a responsible attitude toward it. If teenagers continue to receive the same clearly hypocritical messages they have been getting, we should not be surprised when they continue to experience unwanted pregnancies.

It strikes me that part of the reason people don't take responsibility for contraception is that they have no sense of the price they'll pay.

That's right. An attitude common among sexually active teenagers is typified by the statement, "If I have a baby, I'm sure someone will take care of it. The father will marry me; or my parents will help; or I'll be an adult, then, so it'll be OK." In fact, teenagers may trust that pregnancy must be all right or else it wouldn't happen. They may have no consciousness that they alone may be left to carry the responsibility for the child during all the years of dependency and even, possibly, may have to carry the responsibility for the child's children. The latter can happen because early childbearing runs in families.

I've also heard some people say they think that contraception will lessen their sex drive. Where would such a notion come from?

Some people mistakenly think that contraception will reduce their sexual appetite or performance because it reduces their chances of pregnancy. Actually, research shows that when contraception is used, sexual drive and performance remain the same for both sexes and sometimes even increase in response to the removal of the weighty fear of pregnancy.

Some people who seem to know everything there is to know about contraception still don't use it. Why?

That's the most puzzling question of all. People can read and hear the facts so often that they become old hat, they can take classroom tests on the material and pass them with high marks, and yet chances are high that when the moment of decision arrives in real life, they will choose to ignore everything they know. Impulse, indecision, inconvenience, insecurity with the partner—only individuals can pinpoint the reasons for their own reluctance to use contraception.

Also, part of the reason may be that people haven't yet learned to face facts and recognize probabilities. People can develop a false sense of security: when one episode of unprotected sexual intercourse does not produce pregnancy, they "learn" that they do not need to worry, they may fantasize that they are immune to pregnancy. Unfortunately, the odds stack up: as mentioned earlier, 90 percent of normal sexually active couples who do not use contraception will become pregnant within one year. It is a sign of maturity to understand that what happens to "other people" also can happen to "me."

Chapter 12

Pregnancy, Childbirth, and Parenting

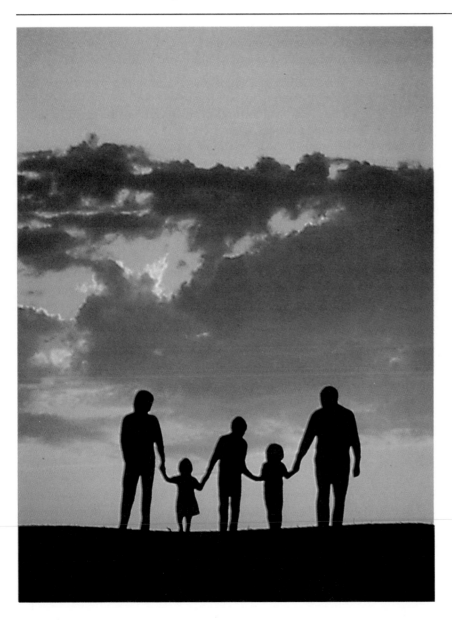

FOR OPENERS . . .

True or false? If false, say what is true.

1. The lifestyle choices a man has made in the days and weeks before he impregnates a woman can affect the development of the baby-to-be.
2. A woman may have a menstrual period even after she becomes pregnant.
3. Home pregnancy tests are completely unreliable.
4. Sometimes, spontaneous abortions occur without a woman's even knowing she has been pregnant.
5. Pregnant women can continue most exercises as vigorously as ever, as long as they are comfortable doing so.
6. Smoothing cream or oil on the abdomen will prevent stretch marks.
7. No matter what a pregnant woman eats, her baby's needs will be met, even by drawing nutrients from her own body.
8. False labor is a warning sign that a pregnant woman is likely to have a miscarriage.
9. A woman's eating poorly before and during her pregnancy may harm the health of her grandchild.
10. Probably the single most important task in parenting is to instill in the child a strong selse of self-esteem.

Answers on page 256.

The decision whether to have a child is sometimes based on unrealistic ideas.

When people become parents, they change their lives irreversibly. In the past, in all probability, the likelihood of *not* having children hardly entered anyone's mind, but today it is more of an option.

DECIDING TO BEAR OR ADOPT CHILDREN

The decision whether to have a child is influenced by self-image, spiritual beliefs, and personal needs, including some unconscious needs. It is also affected by outside pressures, such as spouse needs, or parents' or friends' expectations. Among the unconscious influences on the decision are:

■ Childhood memories or romantic fantasies of what families are like.
■ Wanting to experience being parents.
■ A desire to live on in someone else (a parent says, "She's got my nose!").
■ A feeling that children bring hope for the future.
■ A desire to participate in the human chain.
■ A need for companionship and love.
■ Wanting to demonstrate love and commitment to one's spouse.

The decision to raise a child has vague and mysterious dynamics, but the answers to some down-to-earth questions are relevant, too. Most are forms of a single question: How would it affect my life if I had a child to raise? After all, children are "forever," even more so than marriage partners.

To get an idea how "forever" children are, young people considering parenthood can try the following exercise. Borrow a basketball and carry it home. Don't put it down. Carry it from place to place, even to the bathroom. Bathe it every day. Keep an eye on it at all times. Sleep with it. Set your alarm for 2 A.M., and get up to check the basketball. Never let it out of your sight unless you can obtain the agreement of another person to tend it as you are doing. Try this for a week, and you will get some sense of what it would be like to have responsibility for the care of a child.

This chapter's Life Choice Inventory highlights questions you and your partner would be wise to ask yourselves before choosing to embark on the long process of bearing or adopting and raising a child. You and your partner should answer these questions and be aware of each other's answers to them. If you are contemplating becoming a single parent, you should think hard about the questions that involve reliance on a partner. If you are considering becoming a stepparent, many of these questions apply to you, too. All kinds of families raise children, of course, not just the traditional type of **family** (see the definition of *family* in the end-of-chapter Glossary).

Chances are, no one will be able to answer all the questions with perfect confidence that all will go well. Life is not like that—there is no perfect time to have a child. But now that you have faced the trade-offs, you should be better able to answer yes or no to parenthood with realistic expectations.

If your answer is yes, one possible route to parenthood is to adopt. People may choose adoption because they want to offer a home to a homeless child or because they have been unable to conceive and bear a child. Adoption is not quick; it requires persistence, patience, and the willingness to work with an agency. Such agencies may seem to "sit in judgment," but they take seriously their responsibility of matching parents and children. They do ask questions about people's private lives, but only so that they can be sure the match is a good one.

LIFE CHOICE INVENTORY

Are you ready to have a child? The answers to these questions will help you decide.

1. How will having a child affect your job or career? It is hard to work full-time and be a full-time parent, too.
2. Someone has to be aware of the child's whereabouts and needs, 24 hours a day, for 15 or so years. During the hours that you can't do it, will your partner do it? If not, who will?
3. If your partner should become unwilling or unable to continue carrying the responsibility of parenthood, are you prepared (or can you get prepared) to carry it by yourself? Accidents happen.
4. How will having a child affect your relationship with your present or future partner? Will your partner be willing to share your attention, energy, and love with another human being who will be very important to you?
5. Are you and your partner equally enthusiastic about becoming parents? A partner who is unwilling may withdraw emotionally from both you and the child.
6. Where will you be able to get help (for example, baby-sitters, parents of playmates, or relatives) when you need to get away? You cannot raise a child without help.
7. Will you be willing to give up much of your free time to devote yourself to the needs of a child? Will your partner? Children limit your freedom to play.
8. Do your finances allow for proper prenatal and newborn care? Pregnant women, new babies, and new mothers have needs that cost money in addition to the costs of the birth. Can you meet more needs on less income for a while?
9. Are you willing and able to invest your financial resources for years in the well-being of your child? The cost of raising a child to adulthood varies widely according to family income, personal choices, and location, but on the average, the cost in the late 1980's was between $75,000 and $150,000.
10. Do you know your chances of having a child with a hereditary disease? If not, get genetic counseling before making your decision.
11. How well would you be able to adjust to raising a less-than-perfect child? Parents always run a small risk of having a handicapped child, even if they follow all of the rules before and during pregnancy.
12. Are you willing to make a new baby the center of attention? The new family member will most certainly grab the spotlight, and you may feel neglected because the baby gets more nurturing than you do.
13. In deciding to become the parent to a second or later child, will you be able to stretch your physical, emotional, financial, and other resources that much farther? In some ways, two children are as easy to raise as one; in others, they are harder.
14. Have you vented anger and frustration on pets or children in the past? If so, wait to have children until you receive help in learning to redirect hostility—important in stopping the pattern of child abuse.

Babies of nonwhite races are usually the easiest to adopt, as are the homeless children of certain other countries. Babies with some sort of inborn problem are also more available for adoption than normal babies, and parents who adopt such infants must be prepared to give them special care and sometimes extensive medical treatments. Still, adoptive parents of such children usually say they were glad to give the extra care required.

Foster parenthood, too, offers an opportunity to care for children with special needs. Foster children need homes but may not be able to stay permanently. Such children are usually older than adoptive children and may have had a less-than-ideal home life. Many have emotional or other problems. Opening your home—and life—to them is an especially challenging choice, but it is also rewarding.

PREGNANCY

Let's say you have decided to bear a child. The foundation for a healthy pregnancy is laid far in advance. When someone decides, ''Yes, I'm ready to have a baby now,'' that person is in an excellent position—free to make choices that will give the baby-to-be every possible advantage. For example, for at least three months before pregnancy, both prospective parents should be free from drugs of all kinds—over-the-counter medications; prescription medications; and mind-altering drugs, including alcohol.[1]* Only on the physician's advice should any medicines be continued. During the three months prior to conception, the gametes—the ovum of the mother and the sperm of the father—go through a maturing process that includes cell division. Any substance that interferes with cell division can affect those new cells in this vulnerable stage. A newly recognized fact is that the man's health habits before conception, as well as the woman's, are important.

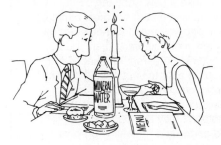

Both prospective parents can prepare in advance for a healthy pregnancy.

Both prospective parents should be well nourished. Malnutrition may affect the development of the gametes, or it may disturb the hormone balance necessary for conception, especially in women.[2] Before pregnancy, a diet that follows the guidelines presented in Chapter 4 would well cover the nutrient needs of the prospective parents (diet during pregnancy is discussed later).

When a woman whose nutrition has been inferior becomes pregnant, she may not have the nutrient stores she needs to produce a healthy baby. Historical records of babies who were conceived during the last few weeks of famines but whose mothers had adequate food during their pregnancies show clearly that full nutrient stores *before* pregnancy are essential to the health of the infant. A baby conceived after a time of famine is at a greater disadvantage, even if its mother eats well throughout her pregnancy, than a baby conceived during a time of plenty and then affected by famine throughout its fetal life.[3] Equally at a disadvantage is the infant of a woman who chooses a poor diet in order to lose weight, or who snacks on candies, high-fat snacks, and soda pop. If pregnancy is in her future, she should develop healthy eating habits now. She also should be exercising, so that once pregnancy is confirmed, she can continue at the same level as before pregnancy.

Many chronic health problems, such as diabetes, can also cause adverse effects during pregnancy. A woman must seek medical help for such conditions to be sure that they are well under control before she becomes pregnant. To prevent contagious diseases, vaccinations should be brought up to date at least three months before conception.

Determining Pregnancy

Long before any tests are taken, a woman may suspect that she is pregnant. A typical sign is a missed menstrual period, but that is not always an accurate indicator. A more accurate indicator is subtle color changes in the cervix and outer genital area, which darken with a bluish cast. Another sign is that the breasts may become tender and full and the nipples may darken. A chemical test can also confirm that a woman is pregnant. Several such tests are available. Some use urine, some blood, but they all rely on detecting one of the many hormones present during pregnancy, **human chorionic gonadotropin (HCG)**. Home pregnancy test kits are available and are widely used. Un-

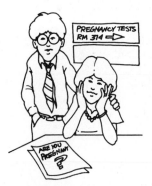

Only an accurate test can resolve immense suspense.

*Reference notes are in Appendix D.

fortunately, many times the instructions may not be clear or the results may be hard to interpret; the tests also have a high error rate and must be repeated to ensure accuracy.[4]* The two main advantages to the home test are immediacy and privacy.

Fetal Development

The first division of the zygote takes place within a day after fertilization, even while it is still traveling toward the uterus through the fallopian tube. (Sometimes the two new cells become detached at this stage and produce **identical twins**. In contrast, if two eggs had been released and fertilized at the same time, the result would have been **fraternal twins**, not identical twins.)

Meanwhile, the zygote becomes embedded in the uterine wall. During the weeks following fertilization, cell division goes on, with each new set of cells dividing again to create many smaller cells. These cells sort themselves into three layers that eventually form the various body systems.

At the same time, a new organ grows within the uterus—the **placenta**, shown in Figure 12–1. Two associated structures form. One is the **amniotic sac**, a sort of fluid-filled balloon that houses the developing fetus. The other is the **umbilical cord**, a ropelike structure containing fetal blood vessels that extends from the fetus's "belly button" to the placenta.

The placenta is a sort of pillow of tissue in which fetal and maternal blood flow side by side, each in its own vessels. The mother's blood delivers nutrients and oxygen to the fetus across the walls of these vessels, and carries fetal waste products away to be excreted by the mother.

The placenta is a highly metabolic organ with some 60 enzymes of its own. Much like muscles, it uses energy fuels to support its work of actively gathering up maternally produced hormones, nutrients of all descriptions, large protein molecules such as antibodies, and other necessary items and forcing them into the fetal bloodstream. It also produces and releases into maternal blood an array of hormones and other substances that maintain pregnancy and prepare the mother's breasts for lactation. It is essential that the placenta develop normally if the developing fetus is to attain its genetic potential. Should it break down, no alternative source of sustenance is available.

The period of embryonic development registers astonishing physical changes. The number of cells in the embryo doubles approximately every 24 hours. In comparison, this rate slows to only one doubling during the final 10 weeks of pregnancy. The embryo's size changes very little, but the events taking place are momentous. From the outermost of the three layers of cells, the nervous system and skin begin to develop; from the middle layer, the muscles and internal organ systems; and from the innermost layer, the glands and linings of the digestive, respiratory, and excretory systems. At eight weeks, the embryo is only a little more than an inch long, but already has a complete central nervous system, a beating heart, a complete digestive system, well defined fingers and toes, and the beginnings of facial features.

Thereafter, in the fetus, each organ grows to maturity with its own timing. Each organ has certain **critical periods** during its growth—critical in the sense that the events taking place during those times can occur only then and not later. If cell division and the final cell number achieved are limited during an organ's critical period, that organ will fail to reach its full genetic

*Accuracy of home pregnancy tests ranges from about 45% to 89%.

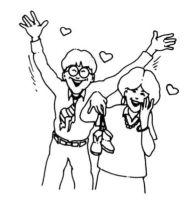

"We're pregnant!"

FIGURE 12–1   The Placenta

Maternal blood vessels

Fetal arteries and veins

Pool of maternal blood

Umbilical cord

Placenta

Umbilical cord

Uterine wall

Many details are already there at eight weeks.

The names given to the stages of **gestation**:
  From fertilization through week two: **zygote**.
  From the second through the eighth weeks: **embryo**.
  From the ninth week through the end of pregnancy, usually the 40th week: **fetus**.
The term of pregnancy itself is often divided into thirds, called **trimesters**.

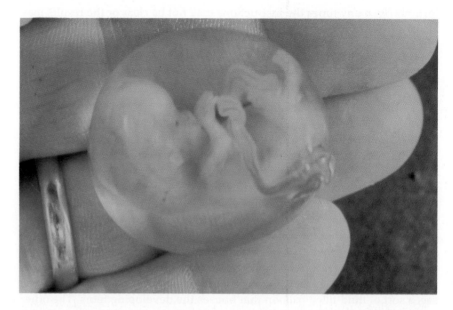

potential and later will not function optimally; later recovery is impossible. Thus if exposure to a harmful chemical, a nutrient deficiency, or other insult occurs during one stage of development, it will affect the heart; if it occurs at another stage, it will affect the developing limbs. Pregnancy, then, is clearly a time for a woman to be especially careful to take care of her health.

The brain and central nervous system are the first organ system to reach maturity in the developing fetus. For several weeks, during a critical period, the fetal brain increases by 100,000 cells a minute. Nutritional deprivation or chemical insults during this time are especially devastating to the brain.

Spontaneous Abortion and Ectopic Pregnancy

Approximately 10 percent of all zygotes fail to implant in the uterus; of those that do implant, 50 percent are shed in spontaneous abortion (see *abortion* on page 231).[5] Spontaneous abortion is a natural and expected part of fertility; it prevents imperfect embryos from becoming full-term infants or occurs when a woman's uterus is unable to support a pregnancy.

Most spontaneous abortions take place early, with no more sign than a heavy menstrual flow. The hormonal transition from pregnancy back to the nonpregnant state may depress a woman's mood, and she may not even know why.

Spontaneous abortions late in pregnancy resemble the experience of birth and carry greater hazards. Infection may start in the uterus and spread through the fallopian tubes into the abdominal cavity, leading to a dangerous generalized body infection (septic abortion).

Another dangerous condition is **ectopic pregnancy**, in which the zygote implants in the fallopian tube or in the abdominal cavity instead of in the uterus. This can happen when passage to the uterus is blocked, when certain infections exist, or when an obstacle such as an IUD is present in the uterus. No tissue except the uterus can safely support a pregnancy, and surgery is required to terminate ectopic pregnancy.

The premature termination of a pregnancy often corrects an abnormality that needs correcting. Even so, a woman may feel grief as intense as if a child had died.

Warning signs to report to the health care provider:
  Discharge of water or blood from the vagina.
  Severe headaches.
  Uncontrollable vomiting.
  Loss of consciousness.
  Sudden swelling of feet, hands, or ankles.
  Chills or fever.
  Abdominal pain.
  Frequent, burning urination.
  Failure to urinate.
  Blurred vision or other vision disturbances.

The Woman's Experience

Gina doesn't want to go out after work any more. Her pregnancy barely shows, so the baby cannot weigh that much. Paul, the young father-to-be, wonders if she is acting. He doesn't realize that the changes one can see from the outside are trivial compared with the dramatic internal events taking place in Gina's body. She is producing more blood; her uterus and its supporting muscles are increasing in size and strength; her joints are becoming more flexible in preparation for childbirth; and her breasts are growing and changing in preparation for lactation. The hormones that mediate all these changes may influence Gina's brain and mood and make her sleepy. She may be having problems with constipation, shortness of breath, and frequent urination. She may also be experiencing morning sickness (actually nausea at any time of the day or night) which varies from woman to woman and from pregnancy to pregnancy within the same woman. (Sometimes, nibbling on small meals throughout the day helps.)

Gina needs fitness now, just as she did before, so that her body will recover quickly after childbirth. Most types of exercise are acceptable as long as the abdomen is protected against injury and the level of activity is not greater than before pregnancy. Thus conditioned joggers, sports players, and swimmers can continue their activities. Swimming is ideal, because it allows the body to move freely with the water supporting its weight, instead of its own muscles, joints, and ligaments straining to do so. Exercising in the heat is ill advised: high body temperature has been associated with birth defects. Prolonged hot baths, saunas, steam rooms, and hot whirlpools should be avoided, too. Sexual activity need not change because of pregnancy, except for medical reasons. At no time is orgasm harmful, nor will it induce labor.

Late in pregnancy, the skin over a woman's abdomen, buttocks, and breasts may stretch to the point where scars form. The tendency to develop these "stretch marks" runs in families. This may be controlled by keeping weight gain within the normal limits. The stretched skin can be partially repaired by a plastic surgeon, but only if the pregnancy is certain to be the last one.

Some general rules for exercise during pregnancy:

Stop exercising if you feel overheated.
Drink plenty of fluids before you exercise.
Avoid exercising in hot, humid weather.
Protect the abdomen from injury, especially in games like baseball or basketball in which accidents are likely.
Discontinue any exercise that causes discomfort.
Do not exercise while lying on your back after about the fourth month.
Do not allow your heart rate to exceed 140 beats per minute.

241

The subject of stretch marks leads to one of the most important elements of a woman's pregnancy—namely, her feelings about it. Most pregnant women today enjoy their changing bodies. They feel strong. They willingly adopt sound eating habits and conscientious self-care. A few may fear the weight gain necessary in pregnancy and need to know that it is not permanent.

Many folk myths have been inflicted on pregnant women through the centuries. They usually run something like this: "If you lift a box up to a shelf, or go outside in the rain, or look at the full moon, then your baby will be born with birth defects." Those tales are especially destructive, because they point a finger of blame at the woman who has a baby with problems and she may take upon herself unearned guilt. In such a case, counseling can be a help.

Gina should ignore folk myths and practice relaxation techniques to relieve stress. Animal studies have shown that stress causes alterations in embryonic nerve cells and changes their genetic potential.[6] Stress may also affect later mating behavior in animals.[7] An outpouring of stress hormones into the maternal blood is thought to reduce blood flow and oxygen supply to the fetus and is suspected of causing birth defects. It is important that other people be sensitive to the pregnant woman's needs for emotional security and welcome her pregnancy with her.

Advice to Paul: Treat Gina with respect for the monumental adjustments she is making. Give her extra love and understanding to bolster her in making them. And Gina, keep Paul informed about how you feel. Encourage him to share his feelings, too. Pregnancy is a landmark event for the relationship, so experience it together. You'll be laying a strong foundation for the shared parenthood ahead.

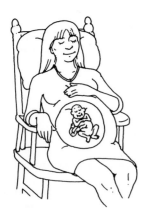

Relaxing for two.

Nutrition during Pregnancy

Earlier, we said that prepregnancy behavior can affect the outcome of pregnancy. This especially holds true for nutrition. If the mother's nutrient stores are inadequate early in pregnancy, then the placenta will be adversely affected during the critical period of its development and will never reach the full size necessary to deliver optimum nourishment to the fetus. The infant will be born small and may get a poor start in life. As a result, a girl child may grow up ill equipped to store sufficient nutrients to support a normal pregnancy, and she, in turn, may bear a poorly developed infant. Thus a woman's poor nutrition during or before pregnancy can have an adverse impact not only on her child, but on her *grandchild*:[8]

Grandmother
poorly nourished (before and during pregnancy)
↓
Mother
(even if well nourished before and during pregnancy)
↓
Infant
(poor health)

Malnutrition during pregnancy not only can reduce infant brain cell number but also can impair every organ and every body system.

The pregnant woman must gain weight—ideally, about 25 pounds. A teenager or a grown woman who is underweight to begin with should gain about 30 pounds, and an obese woman should gain at least 15 pounds. The average baby will weigh 7 1/2 pounds, and all the other pounds are accounted for by the growth of the mother's uterus, blood, and breasts, and the accumulation of fluid that surrounds the fetus. Even if overweight, a woman should not diet until after the baby's birth unless medically indicated.

Nutrient needs during pregnancy are greater than at any other time. When the baby is born, its body will contain bones, muscles, blood, and other tissues made from nutrients the mother eats. If she does not eat enough nutritious food, her own body tissues will have to make up some of the deficit, and she and the fetus will both fall short of having their needs fully met. It used to be thought that a woman could eat carelessly during her pregnancy without worrying that this would hurt her fetus, but that is not true: both will suffer deficits to varying extents, depending on the nutrient. All women need professional advice on supplements; many need added iron—but not too much, because iron salts in supplements interfere with the absorption of zinc. Some may need folacin; deficiencies during pregnancy are relatively common. Some may need fluoride, depending on the quality of the local water supply.

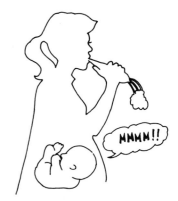

Eating for two.

Energy needs during pregnancy increase less than nutrient needs do. To meet nutrient needs without overconsuming calories, a pregnant woman must choose foods whose nutrient contributions are high relative to their calorie amounts—that is, nutrient-dense foods, the same ones that dieters are advised to select. A balance similar to that of the Four Food Group Plan (Chapter 4) is recommended, but with more servings, especially of milk.

High-Risk and Low-Risk Pregnancies

Some pregnancies are riskier to the life and health of the mother and fetus than are others. In the United States, the rates of such illness and death are still relatively low, but increasing. Table 12–1 (page 244) identifies some factors that correlate with fetal illness and death. Many of them are easy to control once they are discovered—an argument for early prenatal examination and care. All the risks rise whenever community programs supporting maternal and child health are cut and fall whenever support is restored.

A **low-risk pregnancy** occurs in a woman to whom none of the risk factors identified in Table 12–1 apply. The more factors that apply, the higher the risk. Even a **high-risk pregnancy**, once identified, can be managed to minimize risk. For example, a woman known to have diabetes can be closely monitored to ensure that the disease is under control throughout the pregnancy; a woman who develops **pregnancy-induced hypertension** (formerly called **toxemia**) should be similarly treated.

Pregnancy among teens is a special problem. Both pregnancy and childbirth carry greater risk for the young teenaged mother than for a mother in her 20s.[9] Compared with babies of other mothers, newborns of teens more often suffer from disease and die before their first birthday.[10] It seems that a young, growing teen cannot meet the physical needs of both the fetus and herself, so both suffer. Also, a teenage pregnancy tends to perpetuate a cycle of early childbearing and poverty throughout generations.

A risk associated with older age at pregnancy is bearing a child with Down's syndrome. A Down's syndrome child is born with a host of physical and mental abnormalities and may also, years later, develop Alzheimer's disease, a brain-crippling condition that robs people of their mental and physical functioning.[11] The condition arises when the original fertilization event delivers a particular abnormal distribution of genetic material to the

TABLE 12–1 Factors Affecting Pregnancy Outcome

Factor	Effect on Risk
Maternal height and weight	Too low and too high increase risk.
Maternal malnutrition	Nutrient deficiencies increase risk.
Socioeconomic status	Deprivation increases risk.
Lifestyle habits	Smoking and drug and alcohol abuse increase risk.
Age	The youngest and oldest mothers have the greatest risk.
Previous pregnancies	
Number	The more previous pregnancies, the greater the risk.
Interval	The shorter the interval, the greater the risk.
Outcomes	Previous problems predict risk.
Maternal health factors	
High blood pressure	A condition known as *pregnancy-induced hypertension*—formerly known as *toxemia*—increases risk.
Rh factor in blood	(see text).
Chronic diseases	Diabetes, heart and kidney disease, and others increase risk.

SOURCE: Adapted from R. G. Newcombe, Nonnutritional factors affecting fetal growth, *American Journal of Clinical Nutrition* 34 (1981): 732–737.

first cell, and subsequent divisions of that cell pass the defect on to every cell of the child's body. Factors that may raise the chances for Down's syndrome are:

■ Maternal age over 35.
■ Paternal age (it is thought that up to 20 percent of cases are due to genetic material contributed by the father).
■ Radiation exposure.
■ Previous Down's conception.
■ Maternal inability to spontaneously abort imperfect zygotes and embryos.[12]

Of these, parental age is most certain. Medical science has improved the odds so that today, with appropriate prenatal care and tests such as **amniocentesis**, the overwhelming majority of babies born to parents of any age are normal.

It used to be true that any pregnancy after about age 35 was classified high risk. Aside from Down's syndrome, older women also have more failures of conception and more early spontaneous abortions than younger women do. This might be because of hardening of the uterine arteries, which cuts down the blood supply to this organ.[13] Even so, once established, pregnancies in older women who receive adequate prenatal care usually go smoothly and carry risks much the same as those younger women face.[14]

If a mother does not obtain corrective treatment for a problem, she may give birth to a **low-birthweight** baby. Low-birthweight infants, defined as infants who weigh 5 1/2 pounds or less, are of two types. Some are **premature**; they are born early and are the right size for the number of days they have spent in the womb. Others have suffered growth failure in the uterus; they may or may not be born early, but they are **small for date**.

Bearing a small, full-term infant may not be a catastrophe; a small mother may give birth to a small, normal, alert, and healthy baby. But often, a small-for-date baby is one who is likely to get sick or die early in life. Its birth is more likely to be complicated by problems during delivery than a normal baby's birth. Such a baby also is likely to be too weak to nurse effectively or to cry to win its mother's attention. It can therefore become an apathetic, ignored baby, and this compounds the original problems. Statistically, birthweight is a potent indicator of an infant's future health status.

About 1 in every 15 infants born in the United States is a low-birthweight baby, and about a quarter of them die within the first month of life.[15] Worldwide, it is estimated that a sixth of all live babies are of low birthweight; more than 9 out of 10 of these are born in the developing countries.[16] Most of them are not premature but are full-term babies; they are small because of malnutrition and disease.

Some infants are born with **congenital** abnormalities—*congenital* meaning "from birth." Some of the abnormalities are inherited diseases; others are anatomical abnormalities known as **birth defects**. Abnormalities can arise from three causes: genetic inheritance, adverse physical or chemical conditions before or during development of the fetus, or accidents during childbirth. Down's syndrome, already described, is an example of faulty genetic inheritance. Among the adverse uterine conditions that cause disease are environmental toxins, drugs, and especially alcohol, as discussed in the next section. Accidents during childbirth include any event that cuts off fetal life-support systems before it can obtain oxygen and nourishment on its own.

con-JEN-ih-tal

When all other conditions are perfect, the odds of giving birth to a child with such an abnormality are small; most children are born normal. Certain abnormalities run in families, however, and for members of those families, the risks are greater. A **genetic counselor** can advise a family on the odds for a healthy baby and provide counseling.

Environmental Hazards

For a baby to be born normal, not only must its genetic inheritance at conception be correct but two other conditions must also be met. Its environment during development must be healthy, and its birth must be free of complications. (A later section deals with childbirth.)

Environmental agents that cause birth defects are **teratogens**. They may damage developing organs directly, or they may act indirectly by limiting the supply of oxygen or nutrients to the fetus. Many teratogens act on the genetic material of the dividing cells—the instructions that determine how development will come out. Since each cell of a developing embryo or fetus is dividing rapidly to become many cells, the damage multiplies with every division, drastically altering the final, completed organ of which they are a part.

teh-RAT-oh-genz

Among teratogens are many drugs, including alcohol; and prescription drugs such as **thalidomide** and **diethylstilbestrol (DES)**; environmental contaminants and household products,* radiation; compounds in spoiled foods;

DYE-eth-il-STILL-bes-trahl

*A woman who doubts the safety of a chemical should call the Pregnancy/Environmental Hotline of the National Birth Defects Center at (617) 787-4957; toll-free in Massachusetts: (1-800) 322-5014.

and even megadoses of some nutrients, especially of vitamins A, B₆, C, and D, and the mineral iodine. A well-known example of a teratogenic disease is German measles virus, or **rubella**. If contracted during early pregnancy, rubella causes fetal malformations, especially cataracts that result in blindness. Rubella does not yield to medical drugs; it has to be prevented in advance. Luckily, people develop permanent immunity to it after one exposure or after vaccination.

Most drugs of abuse disturb fetal development.[17] Their teratogenic effects are still under study; some of the known ones are listed in Table 12–2. Excessive alcohol consumption can cause irreversible brain damage and mental and physical retardation in the fetus—**fetal alcohol syndrome (FAS)**, already mentioned in Chapter 8. The damage of FAS can occur with as few as two drinks a day, and its most severe impact is likely to be in the first month, before the woman may be aware of her pregnancy. During the first month of pregnancy, the fetal brain is growing at the rate of 100,000 new brain cells a minute. Oxygen is indispensable to this growth, and a sudden dose of alcohol can halt the delivery of oxygen through the umbilical cord. Even a few minutes of such exposure can have a major effect on the brain and nervous system of the fetus.

Can the pregnant woman drink alcohol at all then? Experts debate the exact amount that could turn out to be safe, or at least do minimal damage. Clearly, three ounces of alcohol a day is too much, even if the woman stops drinking immediately after she learns that she is pregnant. Two ounces a day during pregnancy is enough to bring on the symptoms of FAS, and recent evidence suggests that even two drinks *a week* may be associated with miscarriages. The accumulating evidence has led even the most conservative medical organizations to take the position that women should stop drinking

---

TABLE 12–2 Some Teratogenic Effects of Drugs of Abuse Seen in Infants

Drug	Effect
Amphetamines	Suspected nervous system damage; behavior abnormalities
Barbiturates	Newborn withdrawal lasting up to six months
Cocaine	Uncontrolled jerking motions; paralyzation; depressed interactive behavior; poor organizational response to environmental stimuli; permanent mental and physical damage
Marijuana	Short-term irritability at birth
Opiates (including heroin)	Immediate withdrawal in the newborn; permanent learning disability (attention deficit disorder)

SOURCE: For all but cocaine, adapted from D. E. Hutchings, Prenatal opioid exposure and the problem of causal inference: Current research on the consequences of maternal drug abuse, *NIDA Research Monograph Series* 59 (Washington, D.C.: Government Printing Office, 1985), pp. 6–19. Cocaine information from I. J. Chasnoff and coauthors, Cocaine use in pregnancy, *New England Journal of Medicine* 313 (1985): 666–669.

as soon as they *plan* to become pregnant. It is important to know that a woman who has already drunk heavily during the first months of pregnancy can still prevent some damage by stopping drinking during the later months.

The choice to take an occasional drink during pregnancy is personal; no doubt that there is a level of alcohol tolerable to the fetus, but it is still unknown what that level might be. If the choice were ours to make, we'd opt for a healthy baby. We'd give up the pleasures, even of wine with meals, for the duration of the pregnancy, and celebrate with champagne (once) after the baby's birth.

Pregnant women also should not smoke. Smoking limits the delivery of oxygen and nutrients to the growing fetus; the more a mother smokes, the smaller her baby will be and the greater the risk of retarded development and complications at birth, sometimes lasting throughout childhood. In addition, **sudden infant death syndrome (SIDS)**, the sudden, unexplained death of an infant, has been positively linked to the mother's cigarette smoking during pregnancy[18] and even to smoking in the household.[19] Finally, the Surgeon General has concluded from the abundant evidence now available that maternal cigarette smoking causes death in otherwise healthy fetuses and newborns.[20]

Some claim that pregnant women should give up coffee, tea, and colas because of the caffeine they contain, but most studies suggest that the caffeine equivalent of a cup or two of coffee or tea is well within safe limits.[21] Some questions have been raised about the overuse of saccharin, too—but too much attention given to these relatively safe practices might distract from what is really important. There would be little point in a woman's giving up saccharin and continuing to smoke two packs of cigarettes a day.

Like chemicals, radiation of certain kinds can harm cells; it penetrates them and disrupts the genetic material. One way a fetus might be exposed to such radiation is through X-rays. If X-rays should become necessary, the woman who knows or suspects that she is pregnant should inform all medical personnel. They may then choose to use smaller amounts of radiation or to postpone the procedure. Even routine dental X-rays should be postponed, if possible.

The teratogenic agents discussed here are only a few of thousands that we are exposed to every day. However, the odds of being affected by such agents are small. The body's ability to tolerate adverse influences and to repair damage inflicted by harmful agents is phenomenal, particularly when it is well nourished. Thus the overwhelming majority of babies are born normal.

STRATEGIES to Avoid Harmful Influences

To protect a healthy pregnancy:

- **Avoid drugs, smoking, and alcohol.**
- **Use moderation in other things.**
- **Avoid environmental toxins.**
- **Skip unnecessary X-rays.**

BREASTFEEDING OR FORMULA FEEDING

The woman who plans to breastfeed her baby should think ahead during pregnancy. No elaborate or expensive preparation is necessary; babies have been breastfed successfully for generations. Still, she might enjoy reading one of the many available handbooks or taking a class on breastfeeding. She would be wise to form a support system of family and medical team members.

Under most circumstances, a woman can choose freely between feeding breast milk or formula, knowing that both are equally beneficial in supporting growth of the infant. But if the infant is premature, if the family has little economic support, or if other factors act to the baby's disadvantage, then breastfeeding is the preferred choice, especially at first. The earliest secretion from the breast, **colostrum**, contains factors from the mother's blood that help make the infant immune to the diseases prevalent in the environment. Breast milk that comes in later in the first week contains immune factors too, and the infant is receptive to them. Thus, breastfeeding has nonnutritional advantages, especially in the first few weeks or months.

Drugs the mother takes can be secreted in breast milk. If they are likely to affect the infant, then weaning to formula is necessary. Drug addicts, including alcohol abusers, are capable of taking such high doses that their infants become addicted. Most prescription drugs, however, do not reach nursing infants in large enough quantities to harm them. A mother with an ordinary cold can go on nursing. The infant will catch it from her anyway, if susceptible, and may be less susceptible thanks to breast milk's immunologic protection than a formula-fed baby would be.

A pregnant woman may sometimes hesitate to consider breastfeeding because she has heard that environmental contaminants may enter her milk and harm her baby. If this is the case, the decision whether to breastfeed might best be made after consultation with a health professional—possibly a dietitian familiar with the local circumstances. The choices a woman makes about her lifestyle, her nutrition, and her environment, will help determine whether her pregnancy ends with a happy event—the birth of a normal baby.

CHILDBIRTH

If you could look into the uterus just before birth, you might notice that the fetus seems to be breathing. It is practicing, readying its lungs for the endless succession of breaths that will support life for some 70 or more years to come. The fetus may suck its thumb; its tiny hands may grasp the umbilical cord; and it wakes, smiles, kicks, rolls over, stretches, sleeps, and dreams. The pregnant woman is aware of these activities. When the fetus kicks, it is she who is kicked. When she feels tiny rhythmic movements, she may recognize them as fetal hiccups. A fetus who is active in the womb will probably be an active infant and child, too.

As the time for birth nears, conditions become cramped in the tiny quarters, and the head turns downward and fits snugly into the mother's pelvis, an event called **lightening**. The mother feels relief from the pressure on her cramped stomach, heart, and lungs, and she can breathe and eat more easily. Her body feels lighter, although the weight shift can cause her lower back to hurt. Walking is harder, and increased pressure on her bladder makes her urinate more frequently.

Near term, the mother may perceive mild contractions of her uterus and think that labor has begun. Termed **false labor** by some, mild contractions are common throughout later pregnancy. A more descriptive name might be "warm-up contractions," because they indicate that the muscular uterus is getting ready for the hard work ahead. The cervix is softening, and the uterus is practicing for the birth that will follow.

Labor begins as the woman's hormones, including **oxytocin**, cause the muscles of her uterus to contract powerfully and rhythmically. Thereafter, labor proceeds by stages (Figure 12–2). In the first one, the **dilation stage**, the cervix dilates until the baby's head can pass through it, while the contractions become more and more powerful and closer and closer together.

The stages of labor:
    Dilation—the cervix dilates.
    Expulsion—the infant is born.
    Placental stage—the placenta is expelled.

Before birth.

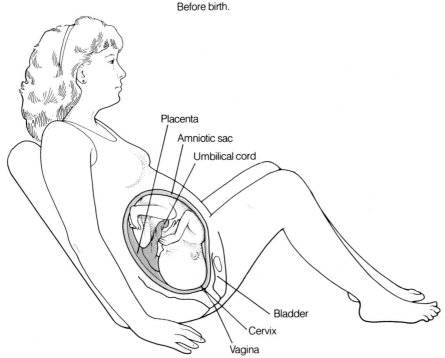

Placenta
Amniotic sac
Umbilical cord

Bladder
Cervix
Vagina

FIGURE 12–2 Childbirth

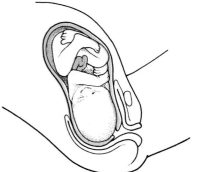

Dilation. The cervix has begun to widen.

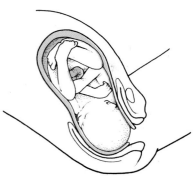

End of dilation. The amniotic sac has broken; the cervix is fully dilated.

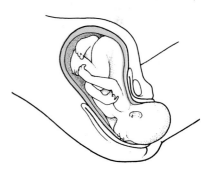

Crowning and expulsion.

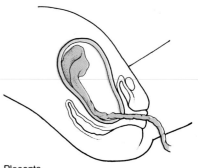

Placenta

Then a transition occurs, bringing on the still more powerful contractions of the **expulsion stage**, in which the baby's head starts to emerge from the birth canal (**crowning**), the amniotic sac breaks (if it has not broken already), and the baby is born. Sometimes, a small incision, an **episiotomy**, is made to widen the vaginal opening to prevent tearing of tissue during birth. The final stage, the **placental stage**, consists of several final contractions that expel the placenta.

Nearly all babies dive into the world headfirst. Rarely, **breech births** occur, in which feet or hind end or other body parts are born first, the head last. About half of these few cases pose no extra problems; a birth attendant is able to maneuver the fetus into a position that allows normal delivery.[22] However, the attending health care professional may decide to perform a surgical birth, or **cesarean section**. General or local anesthesia may be used; the physician makes an incision through the mother's abdominal wall and uterus and lifts the baby and placenta out through the opening. The operation is relatively safe for both mother and baby, but recovery for the mother requires more healing and takes longer.

Childbirth is more than just a series of stages; it is an experience. The woman feels the wavelike contractions and pain that begin at the top of the uterus and sweep downward, pulling and stretching the opening of the cervix. Labor bears an appropriate name—it is the hardest of all physical work, and the woman cannot rest until it is finished. Full dilation of the cervix may take just a couple of hours or more than a day. At the end of the dilation stage the woman feels the baby's head slip downward through the cervix, and when the amniotic sac breaks, she feels the warm fluid escaping. During the expulsion, the woman experiences a sensation she has at no other time—the urge to bear down and push the baby through the vagina. Then she hears the baby give a small cry.

Many people have false impressions of the events of childbirth, mostly from the fictions of Hollywood that picture tortured, helpless women requiring someone to rescue them by "delivering" the baby and then inflicting a sharp slap on the tiny newborn. In reality, women in labor are not victims who need saving; they are women who are working to the maximum and who will deliver babies with or without help. And the brand-new individual is greeted with kindness. The attendant uses a gentle suctioning device to remove fluid and start the baby breathing. The medical staff may pause to treat the eyes with a drug to prevent infection and to test the baby's responses to stimulation, breathing, heart rate, movement, color, and muscle tone before the child and parents meet face to face. The result of such testing is the **Apgar score**, which can predict problems. Soon after the testing, the baby may begin to feed at the mother's breast even before leaving the birthing room.

After delivery, recovery begins immediately. As the infant nurses, the hormone of labor, oxytocin, is released and stimulates both the flow of milk and the contractions that shrink the uterus from a pregnancy size of over two pounds to the prepregnancy size of about three ounces. Blood and fluid continue flowing for several weeks in what is similar to a long menstrual period.

The woman may have sexual intercourse after her health care provider has said she may safely do so, after incisions have healed (about one month). The couple should use a contraceptive if they don't want another baby right away, because pregnancy can occur even if the woman is breastfeeding her infant.

Exercise may speed recovery. A woman can resume exercising as soon as it is comfortable, usually two to three weeks after delivery. It is generally safe to continue exercising at the level maintained during pregnancy for the first four weeks or so and to gradually increase the level, if desired; but the woman should adopt the strategies listed in the margin.

✸ STRATEGIES
for Post-Pregnancy Exercise:

For a few weeks after the birth:

✸ Exercise regularly, at least 3 times a week.

✸ Don't compete in sports.

✸ Avoid outdoor activities in hot, humid weather.

✸ Use smooth stretches, not jerky motions (joints and ligaments are softened by the hormones of pregnancy).

✸ Avoid deep stretches—don't push yourself too far. Warm up well before each session, and cool down afterward with gentle stretches.

✸ Avoid jarring motions or fast-reaction activities (again, because joints are unstable).

The end of childbirth is the beginning of new life—for everyone.

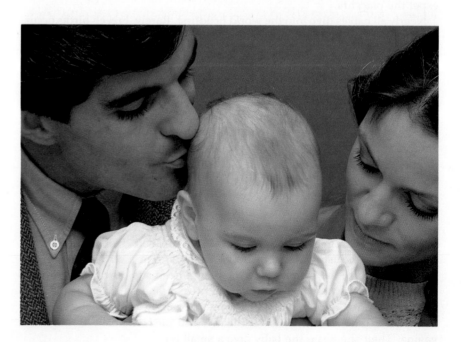

At delivery, the mother normally loses all the weight associated with the fetus and the placenta, but she retains the fat she necessarily gained during pregnancy. Breastfeeding can draw on these fat stores and help the woman lose weight. Even without breastfeeding, many women lose these pounds within a few weeks or months, but it may take some effort to do so.

Some women feel depressed after giving birth, feel like crying, or are unable to sleep. Such discomforts may result from the sharp changes in hormone levels after birth or from simple exhaustion caused by the baby, who doesn't yet sleep for long stretches. New fathers, too, sometimes experience this **postpartum depression**, or "blues." Cutting back on all but essential activities and spending a few weeks alone with family sometimes helps to ease the adjustments.

The time after childbirth brings changes for everyone in the household. Not only is there a new baby to care for; there are new roles to play. Suddenly, a woman is a mother, a man is a father, an only child a sibling. All these changes seemingly happen overnight, and everyone may be a bit uncertain in playing the parts at first. Slowly, a new routine sets in, and the new ways become as comfortable as the old ones were. But what routine is best? Now that you have children, what do you do with them?

THE ELEMENTS OF PARENTING

Parenting is a skill that can be learned. While it is true that almost everyone has had a model to follow—that of their own parents—most people would do well to learn more about the needs of children. Doing what comes naturally in this regard may not always be best for the child.

In the worst case, parents whose own childhoods included physical or psychological **child abuse** tend to become abusive themselves whenever their own needs are not met. Some may even sexually abuse their children.

Child abuse, of course, is illegal, and you can help prevent it. If you should confront a suspected case of sexual or other abuse of a child, believe the child. The majority of children's reports of such situations are truthful. Seek expert help, support, and counseling for the abuser. You can report child abuse anonymously: check the "Abuse Registry" in the front of your phone book for a toll-free number. The rest of this section is about optimal parenting, the kind that parents would choose to give if they knew how.

Parenting is not a one-way process. It is not just adult people acting on little ones; children contribute to it, too. Some parent factors are:

- The parents' age—older parents have a more positive attitude about parenting.[23]
- Expectations—parents who have realistic expectations of what babies are like from the beginning are better parents.[24]
- Parental family experience—parents will nurture, neglect, or abuse their children as their parents did.
- Sensitivity—parents who can accurately "read" their babies form the best relationships with them.[25]

Some child factors are:

- Responsiveness—a baby who responds easily and positively to parents establishes greater closeness to them.

- Physical appearance—normal babyish features elicit a perception of cuteness and a nurturing response from adults.[26] Babies who have physical handicaps may not elicit such responses; children who do not live up to parental expectations are more likely to be abused than others.
- Birth order—parents' expectations change with each child's birth. Those born first receive most of the attention, and parents expect them to be more dominant and responsible, whereas later children are seen as more social.[27]
- Sex—the sex of the baby influences how adults respond (see Chapter 10).

A parent supports all of a child's developmental needs—physical, psychological, and social.

Physical needs are easy to identify. From infancy until they are financially able to stand alone, children need food, clothing, play activities, school equipment, the company of other children, transportation to wherever these resources are, health care, and medical care. Parenting manuals offer the details on these topics. Other vital aspects of parenting are listed in this chapter's Strategies box.

⊛ STRATEGIES: Guide for Effective Parenting

If you want to practice the skills of a nurturing parent, try these suggestions:

1. Foster self-esteem by responding to the child as an individual, without comparisons to others. Rejoice in the child's uniqueness.

2. Meet the young infant's needs consistently to establish trust and, later, independence.

3. Interact with the infant affectionately and often to begin the process of socialization.

4. Stimulate the baby's senses to develop intellectual capacity.

5. Give toddlers' experiences that use each of their senses.

6. Try to view the world as they experience it, and allow them the freedom to discover what the world is like on their own. Keep them safe, but don't overprotect.

7. To develop language, talk to toddlers; listen to them, and try to understand what they mean.

8. To develop intellectual capacity, watch to see what interests the child, and seize the opportunity to provide related experiences.

9. To enhance self-esteem, tell children through words and actions that they are special and loved for being themselves.

10. To advance the child's socialization, make sure the child has playmates, as well as playthings.

11. To promote further socialization, help children interpret social interactions among other people. Show them how to act in many situations, and praise them when they use social skills.

12. Be alert to learning differences and disabilities. Seek help.

13. Set limits and discipline children to help them feel safe and secure.

14. To strengthen problem-solving skills, cultivate curiosity, encourage experimentation and exploration, and allow children to work out their own solutions.

Early nutrition and physical stimulation are both important. The role of nutrition is easily explained: infants and children need essential nutrients to build the materials of which their bodies are made. (But it has been shown that adequate nutrition without love is not sufficient to promote optimal growth; given touching and attention, children grow better than they do otherwise.) Also, exercise is important. Children don't get enough exercise just by being children; in fact, the children of developed nations today are less fit, fatter, and more disease-prone than at any time in the past. Young children need physical activity, and it is up to adults to give them opportunities for it.

As for a child's psychological and social needs, look at Erikson's scheme of the development of children in Chapter 3, which is also a statement of the tasks for parents. They are to instill trust, to foster autonomy, to encourage initiative, to encourage industry—in other words, to nurture and shape the person who will finally emerge from the family as an adult, ready to assume the roles of a responsible member of society.

Probably the single most important task for the parent is to instill in the child a strong sense of self-esteem. As earlier chapters showed, the feeling that "I am OK, I am worthwhile" helps an individual to be effective in every area of life— relationships with others, work, play, contributions to the larger society. Giving love and attention consistently throughout the early years is vital to successful parenting; to balance this, it is equally vital to place limits on behavior— in other words, **discipline**. Having limits makes children feel safe and secure; Table 12–3 offers some strategies for effective use of constructive discipline.

TABLE 12–3 Strategies for Discipline and Guidelines for Effective Punishment

Discipline is most effective when you:	When punishment is needed:
1. Discipline yourself first. Live by the rules you set.	1. Be consistent about which behaviors are acceptable and which are not.
2. Include the child in decisions about limits and consequences.	2. Punish immediately. However, if you tend to be emotional, be sure not to administer punishments while you are upset.
3. Explain the reasons for the rules.	
4. Remove sources of trouble, or remove the child from trouble.	3. Do not use the "Wait until Father (or Mother) comes home" approach.
5. Redirect the child's behavior or energy in a safe direction.	4. Make the punishment proportional to the misbehavior. Use the minimum amount of punishment that will successfully accomplish your goal.
6. Let natural consequences teach the child, unless it would cause injury.	
7. Warn before punishing.	
8. Warn only once.	
9. Threaten only humane punishment that you are willing to administer.	5. Combine punishment with reinforcement for the correct response. This increases the effectiveness of both.
10. Give the child a chance to answer any accusations.	6. Be certain to keep the lines of communication open. Overreliance on punishment decreases communication, as children become afraid to confide in adults.
11. Punish as little as possible; communicate as much as possible.	
12. Love the child.	

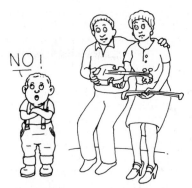

Children participate in their own development from early on.

Is parenting the only key to raising an emotionally healthy individual? Or, putting it another way, if a child turns out to be timid or overly aggressive, is this the parents' fault? Apparently not. To a great extent, temperament is inborn, and so long as parents do their best to provide the needed opportunities and physical supports, no blame can be assigned if children turn out differently from what the parents expect or want. Parenting is an opportunity to realize the potential that is there—but that potential differs from child to child, and no amount of effort on the parents' part will change certain inborn personality traits.

Furthermore, children participate in their own development from early on, making conscious choices about opportunities presented to them. Their own choices, to a great extent, determine the adults they will become.

Some common threads draw together all the theories of child development. Children are not miniature adults—that is, they think and reason in ways unique to children. Children develop in predictable stages, and each child proceeds through those stages at his or her own pace, depending partly on the child's own genetic resources and partly on the environment furnished by adults.

This chapter began with the decision of whether to have a child. Throughout, we have stressed the duties parents face in holding the needs of the developing person primary. Let us end with this: the work of parenting may be hard and long, but with it comes a reward that lasts a lifetime—the special love of a child. Those who plan ahead to meet their own and their child's needs can expect the parenting years to be joyful ones.

STUDY AIDS

1. Identify the unconscious motives that may lead people to think they want to have children.
2. List factors people should consider when they make the decision whether to have children, either by natural birth or adoption.
3. Advise a couple considering starting a pregnancy on health habits they should adopt or maintain beforehand.
4. Describe the normal events of healthy placental and fetal development.
5. Define the term *critical period*.
6. Explain the significance to later life and health of environmental influences on critical periods.
7. Explain what makes a pregnant woman feel different during pregnancy.
8. Indicate what a pregnant woman needs to know about exercise.
9. Give an example of how malnutrition impairs fetal development.
10. Describe wise food choices for the pregnant woman.
11. Define low-risk and high-risk pregnancies.
12. Describe some of the special problems of the pregnant teen-aged girl.
13. Define the term *teratogen*.
14. State some effects of tobacco smoke, alcohol, other drugs, and chemicals on the outcome of pregnancy.
15. List some of the advantages of breastfeeding.
16. List the stages of labor, and state what occurs in each one.
17. List some concerns of the woman recovering from childbirth, and suggest ways of handling them.
18. Identify the goals of disciplining children, and describe effective discipline techniques.
19. Describe what you can do when you suspect someone of child abuse.
20. Describe three aspects of a child's developmental needs to parents must attend.

GLOSSARY

amniocentesis (AM-nee-oh-cen-TEE-sis): a test of fetal cells drawn by needle through the abdomen from the liquid-filled amniotic sac at about 15 to 17 weeks' gestation. Fetal cells can then be analyzed for chromosomal abnormalities. A less painful and safer procedure, *chorionic villus sampling*, provides similar information at 11 weeks gestation.

centesis = to puncture

amniotic (am-nee-OTT-ic) **sac:** the "bag of waters" in the uterus, in which the fetus floats.

Apgar score: a system of scoring an infant's physical condition right after birth, based on heart rate, respiration rate, muscle tone, response to stimuli, and color.

birth defects: anatomical abnormalities present in an individual from birth.

breech birth: a birth in which the infant emerges otherwise than head first.

cesarean (sih-ZEHR-ee-un) **section:** surgical childbirth, in which the infant is taken through an incision in the woman's abdomen. (Alternative spellings: *cesarian*, *caesarian*.)

Caesar = the emperor Julius Caesar, who was born this way

child abuse: verbal, psychological, physical, or sexual assault on a child.

colostrum (co-LAHS-trum): a milklike substance rich in antibodies, secreted from the breast during the first several days after a woman has given birth, before milk appears.

congenital (con-JEN-ih-tal): present from birth.

con = with

genit = to bear

critical period: a finite period during development in which certain events occur that will have irreversible effects on later developmental stages. In a body organ, a critical period is usually a period of cell division.

crowning: the moment during childbirth in which the crown of the baby's head is first seen.

diethylstilbestrol (DYE-eth-il-STILL-bestrahl), or **DES:** a synthetic hormone preparation possessing the characteristics of estrogen; used in pregnancy to prevent miscarriage only when the benefit is deemed to outweigh the risk of subsequent vaginal abnormalities in a girl born of that pregnancy.

dilation stage: the stage of childbirth during which the cervix is opening, before expulsion of the infant begins.

discipline: the shaping of behavior by way of rewards and/or punishments to make it socially acceptable.

ectopic (ek-TOP-ick) **pregnancy:** a pregnancy in which the zygote has implanted and begun to develop in one of the fallopian tubes or elsewhere outside the uterus, a dangerous situation.

ec = out

topic = place

embryo (EM-bree-oh): the developing infant during the second to eighth week after conception.

episiotomy (eh-PEEZ-ee-OT-oh-me): a surgical incision made to prevent tearing of the vagina when it becomes apparent that the vagina cannot stretch enough to accommodate an impending birth.

episio = pubic region

tomy = incision

expulsion stage: the stage of childbirth during which the uterine contractions are actively pushing the infant through the birth canal.

false labor: warm-up contractions that many women experience before the contractions of the birth process; they stretch and thin the cervix in preparation for birth. Also known as *Braxton Hicks contractions*.

family: a group of people, related by ancestry or choice (such as marriage), whose roles in society are to parent children, function as an economic unit, provide intimacy to its members, and furnish a place in society for them. A *nuclear family* consists of parents and children, an *extended family* includes other relatives, a *traditional nuclear family* is a nuclear family in which only the husband works, a *dual-worker family* is one in which both parents work, a *single-parent family* is made up of children and one parent, and a *blended family* is one in which two single-parent families are joined. Nonbiological parents, acquired through parental marriage, are *stepparents*. Other units that function as families include pairs of friends, sisters or brothers living together, or pairs of homosexuals with or without children.

fetal alcohol syndrome (FAS): the cluster of symptoms seen in an infant or child whose mother consumed excess alcohol during her pregnancy; includes mental and physical retardation with facial and other body deformites. A subtle version of FAS is *subclinical FAS* that includes hidden defects such as learning disabilities, behavioral abnormalities, and motor impairments. Defined previously in Chapter 8.

fetus (FEET-us), sometimes spelled *foetus*: the developing infant from the ninth week after conception until birth.

fraternal twins: twins formed by the fertilization of two different ova by two different sperm. See also *identical twins*.

frater = brother

genetic counselor: an adviser who is qualified in several medical specialties (such as internal medicine, pediatrics, and genetics) to predict and advise on the likelihood that genetic defects will occur in a family.

gestation (jes-TAY-shun): the period from conception to birth; the term of a pregnancy.

gestatio = a carrying

high-risk pregnancy: a pregnancy characterized by indicators that point to a high probability of problems surrounding the birth, such as premature delivery, difficult birth, retarded growth, birth defects, and early infant death.

human chorionic (CORE-ee-AHN-ick) **gonadotropin** (go-NAD-oh-TROPE-in), or **HCG:** a hormone produced immediately after conception by the implanted zygote and the tissues surrounding it; the hormone detected in pregnancy tests.

identical twins: twins produced from a single fertilized ovum when the two daughter cells produced by the first division separate and develop into two individuals instead of remaining together and producing one individual, as they normally do.

lightening: the sensation a pregnant woman experiences when the unborn infant settles into the birth position.

low birthweight: a birthweight of 5 1/2 pounds (2,500 grams) or less, used as a predictor of poor health in the newborn full-term infant and as a probable indicator of poor nutrition status of the mother during and/or before pregnancy. Normal birthweight for a full-term baby is 6 1/2 pounds (3,000 grams) or more. See also *premature*.

low-risk pregnancy: a pregnancy characterized by indicators that point to a high probability of normal outcome.

oxytocin (ox-ee-TOCE-in): a pituitary hormone that stimulates the uterus to contract, thus initiating the birth process. It also acts on the mammary gland to stimulate the release of milk.

oxy = sharp

tocin = childbirth

placenta (plah-SEN-tuh): an organ that develops during pregnancy, in which maternal and fetal blood circulate in close proximity so that materials can be exchanged between them. See Figure 12-1.

plac = flat cake

placental stage: the final stage of childbirth, after the infant has been born, in which the placenta is expelled.

postpartum depression: the emotional depression a woman may experience after the birth of her infant, ascribed to changes in hormone levels. When a man experiences depression after the birth of his child, it is usually ascribed to changed life conditions.

post = after

partum = to part with, give birth

pregnancy-induced hypertension: a condition seen in pregnancy characterized by hypertension (high blood pressure) and protein in the urine. In serious cases, symptoms may include convulsions and coma. Pregnancy-induced hypertension was formerly called *toxemia* (tox-EEM-ee-uh). For more about hypertension, see Chapter 16.

premature: born before the end of the normal nine-month term of pregnancy. Some premature infants are of a weight *appropriate for gestational age (AGA)*; others are *small for gestational age (SGA)*, often reflecting malnutrition. The latter type are also called *small for date* babies.

rubella: an acute, infectious, contagious disease, especially dangerous to pregnant women because it can cause congenital cataracts and other malformations in their unborn infants.

  rubellus = red

small for date: see *premature*.
sudden infant death syndrome (SIDS): the unexpected and unexplained death of an apparently well infant, the most common cause of death of infants between the second week and the end of the first year of life; also called *crib death*.
teratogen (teh-RAT-oh-gen): a chemical or physical agent that causes birth defects.

  terat = monster

thalidomide (tha-LID-oh-mide): a drug given to pregnant women to relieve morning sickness—found to produce birth defects and no longer on the market.

toxemia: see *pregnancy-induced hypertension*.
trimester: one-third of the term of a pregnancy; a three-month period.
umbilical (um-BIL-ih-cul) **cord:** the rope-like structure through which the fetus's veins and arteries reach the placenta; the route of nourishment and oxygen into the fetus and of waste disposal from the fetus.
zygote: (also in Chapter 11) the product of the union of ovum and sperm, so termed for two weeks after conception. (After that, it is called an embryo.)

▦ QUIZ ANSWERS

1. *True.* The lifestyle choices a man has made in the days and weeks before he impregnates a woman can affect the development of the baby-to-be.

2. *True.* A woman may have a menstrual period even after she becomes pregnant.

3. *False.* Home pregnancy tests are often reliable, but for best results, they should be repeated.

4. *True.* Sometimes, spontaneous abortions occur without a woman's even knowing she has been pregnant.

5. *True.* Pregnant women can continue most exercises as vigorously as ever, as long as they are comfortable doing so.

6. *False.* Smoothing cream or oil on the abdomen will not prevent stretch marks.

7. *False.* If a pregnant woman eats a poor diet, she and her baby will both pay a price in health.

8. *False.* False labor is the normal, mild contractions of the pregnant uterus, and it does not signify an impending miscarriage.

9. *True.* A woman's eating poorly before and during her pregnancy may harm the health of her grandchild.

10. *True.* Probably the single most important task in parenting is to instill in the child a strong sense of self-esteem.

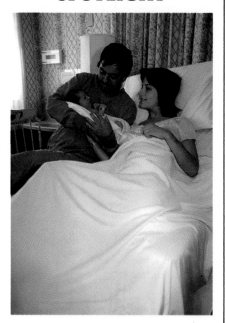

Birthing Styles

The successive stages of birthing occur more or less predictably for everyone, but each birth is also unique in terms of human experience. Each one has a character influenced by where it takes place, who attends, and how they interact. Once labor has begun, it proceeds relentlessly; you must decide in advance of labor's onset how things should be done. This Spotlight can help you to identify the issues that may be important to you so that you can plan ahead. (*You* refers to both men and women in this context, as pregnancy and childbirth are an experience shared by both.)

What sorts of choices do people have about giving birth?

Many of the choices have to do with location. How much the birth will cost, the degree of privacy and control, who can attend, and even which drugs will be used can all depend on where the birth takes place.

It seems as though most people go to the hospital to give birth, so it must be a good choice.

Many successful births take place in hospitals each year. Hospitals are reliable and available to most communities. Hospitals are fully equipped with sophisticated equipment to deal with emergencies, and so may be the only choice open to someone with, say, a high-risk pregnancy.

Hospitals have drawbacks, though. For one thing, they cost a lot. Hospitals specialize in illnesses, and the prices they charge must cover much more equipment and staff than is required at a routine birth, even if the facilities aren't used at a birth. Another concern: hospitals present risks of infectious diseases brought there by sick people. Further, the philosophy in a hospital may be to view the birth as a medical event rather than a family event, and so the staff may limit participation by family members.

I've heard that some women just stay home for the birth. Is this safe?

It can be, as long as the details are carefully worked out in advance. A home birth should be attended by a certified nurse **midwife** who works with a physician on call in case minor problems arise. For normal births, this option is safe and far less expensive than a hospital birth. People who make this choice gain privacy, comfort, and control over the birth.

The right attendant is an absolute must for home births. Today's certified nurse midwives are highly trained birthing specialists; they attend to the woman throughout labor and delivery, unlike busy hospital physicians who check on their clients only periodically. Midwives also employ such techniques as massage of the tissues surrounding the vaginal opening before birth. Such massages before and during birth relax the tissues enough to permit birth without tearing or cutting the tissues.

As for family attendance, in your home you make the rules, and invite whomever you please. A major drawback to home birth is that in the event of an emergency, an ambulance ride to the hospital can cost precious time.

Is there another alternative for people who want to share the birthing process?

Yes, there is a third alternative—a birthing center. In such a center, the environment is homelike and may offer comforts, such as a whirlpool bath (recommended by some to help the laboring woman relax). These centers usually allow family involvement, and respect the wishes of family members. A birthing center has a physician on call, and established emergency routines for fast transport, should the need arise. Although help may be swift, time is still lost in an ambulance ride to the hospital. Birthing centers are becoming so popular that some hospitals have opened their own on or near the hospital grounds, thus blending the advantages of each.

Births are sometimes portrayed as a woman's experience alone, and other times as a family experience where everyone attends. What roles should family members play?

There is no one answer to this question. It depends on family members' feelings and desires about being present. Some may want to attend throughout labor and birth, or may even want to "catch" the baby. Others may feel that they'd rather not be present, and this should be known and honored. Children, grandparents, or others may wish to be present, and the laboring woman may want them there. On the other hand, she may want more privacy than company, and her wishes should be respected. Whatever the family decides, they should check with the birth facility they choose, to make sure that regulations won't conflict with their desires.

Who determines what kinds of drugs are given during the birth?

To the degree that the standard policy of the facility is followed, where you are may affect what you get. For example, a traditional hospital may routinely administer a drug (a synthetic version of the hormone oxytocin) to speed labor by enhancing the contractions' strength and frequency. A midwife is more likely to hold the view that most labors gather strength at their own pace if left alone. The same is true of pain-killing drugs, but to a lesser degree. A woman *can* request drugs to help with pain, or she can refuse some or all of those offered, but it is difficult for a woman to make judgments of this kind while laboring.

Why would a woman refuse pain-killing drugs?

A trade-off exists between the drawbacks and advantages to pain-killing drugs used to ease labor. They dull the pain, but some have side effects, such as nausea or prolonged grogginess. Others affect the baby. Babies of mothers who receive certain drugs may be lethargic for several hours afterward, may have a slowed heart rate, and might require help to get started breathing. Also, the mother may wish to experience the birth without mind-altering drugs. A drug-free labor may require her to handle more pain, but her perception of the birth will be clear, and she will be awake to celebrate when the baby arrives.

How can a woman handle the pain without drugs?

Women who prepare ahead for the birth are in a better position to do so than those who "go in cold." Parents-to-be can take classes and prepare physically and mentally to take charge of the birth experience. One method, the **Lamaze method**, gives the woman the tools she needs—knowledge, relaxation techniques, and breathing control to speed the labor along and minimize pain. The classes teach men (or others) to assist the laboring woman—to massage her back or abdomen to relieve pain, to administer ice and other comforts as she needs them, and to keep her relaxed and on track. The name *natural childbirth*, sometimes given to such births, can be misleading. The method does not guarantee that the woman will need no drugs at all, but if well prepared, she will probably require smaller doses of drugs to achieve pain control. It is especially important for a

MINIGLOSSARY

midwife: a birth attendant. A *certified nurse midwife (CNM)* is a trained, credentialed health care professional who is part of the team that cares for mothers and their infants during normal pregnancy, labor, and childbirth.
Lamaze (lah-MAHZ) **method:** a method of childbirth in which the woman uses rhythmic breathing, relaxation techniques, and the help of a coach while giving birth.

woman who wishes to control pain with a method like Lamaze to choose the birth attendant carefully.

How can a person choose the right birth attendant?

First, the person should be college trained and certified in the specialty of birthing, as are nurse midwives and obstetricians. Beyond this, you should ask the birth attendant how often clients receive surgical births (the average for physicians is around 25 percent; midwives do not perform them, but call on backup physicians to do so). Ask how often they use episiotomies (physicians average 75 percent of the time, midwives less). Ask about their philosophy on drugs: Do they induce labor with oxytocin? Do they always give drugs for pain, give them on request, or avoid giving them altogether? Would the attendant allow pictures to be taken, if the parents wish to remember the birth this way? Clearing the air on these issues in advance will lay a foundation of trust to help ensure a joyful birth experience.

Mature Life, Aging, and Death

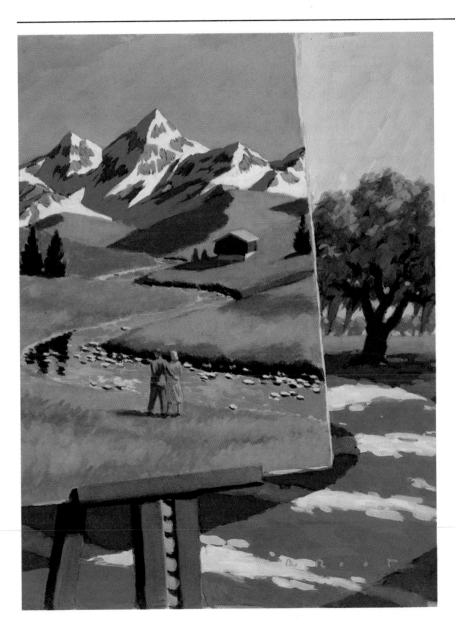

FOR OPENERS . . .

True or false? If false, say what is true.

1. People beyond their 20s generally enjoy life more than people in their 20s.
2. The happiest people are those who have experienced the fewest tragedies.
3. Most people's income is drastically reduced at retirement.
4. The maximum human life span has increased steadily over the past 100 years.
5. People should expect to lose their sex drives at around 50 years of age.
6. Mental confusion in older people is often preventable.
7. Most people can expect to spend their later years in nursing homes.
8. A hospice is a place where people can go to die.
9. No matter how grief-stricken you are at someone's death, you should be pretty well over it within a year.
10. After someone has died, it is best not to mention that person to a grieving survivor.

(Answers on page 276.)

Each person views life in his or her own way. Some people approach it with a rational plan for five, ten, or more years from now; for some, life is something of a sport, and the object is to "win" through accruing riches, power, and positions of leadership. Other people view their lives as an adventure of the unexpected, and they ride along in whichever way the wind carries them. Such people are free from being measured against preconceived scales, but they may feel out of control, and late in life they may look back to find they have not accomplished much to speak of. Philosophy aside, when people are asked about what is important in life, they most often mention happiness.

THE PURSUIT OF HAPPINESS

Psychologists usually study people who come to them for treatment, most times because of feelings of unhappiness. Recently, though, one researcher decided to study people who not only didn't have such problems but who were doing extraordinarily well. For the most part, the people who reported being happiest with their lives were people who did not subscribe to any rigid definition of success and who were not solely concerned about their own power or wealth. They were people who had defined success in light of their own values and who lived accordingly. They were working toward some larger goal, outside their immediate needs.

Characteristics of such people can be described this way:

- Their lives have meaning and direction.
- They handle life events in their own, sometimes unusual, ways.
- They rarely feel cheated by life.
- They have attained several long-term goals.
- They are pleased with their own growth and development.
- They love and are loved by a partner.
- They have many friends.
- They are cheerful.
- They can take criticism.
- They have no major fears.

What is more, the people who are enjoying life most are likely to be beyond their 20s, those who have lived through the fears and restlessness of youth. A high level of education is a factor in their happiness, as is enough money to cover life's basic needs.[1] They also know how to balance spontaneity with planning, so that their lives are neither tied too tightly to a mooring nor allowed to drift aimlessly. Their involvement in helping others is balanced with a healthy concern for self.

You may think that these people were born lucky, but most were not; most of the happiest people had already lived through at least one major life tragedy. They grew into their happiness, striving for it through their daily thoughts and actions. They faced up to the tasks of adult development as described in Chapter 3.

People who stay involved tend to stay happy.

*Reference notes are in Appendix D.

AGING

There is every reason to strive for a long life and to preserve health to support it, and more people are doing this successfully than ever before. The elderly make up the fastest growing segment of today's society, and if predictions are accurate, their numbers will continue to increase throughout this century and well into the next.

Expectations and Misconceptions

What life will be like when you are older depends largely on what you think it will be like. Your physical health matters; your financial success makes a difference; but your own expectations make an equal contribution to your future. One saying has it that "as the twig is bent, so grows the tree"—only, unlike a tree, you can bend your own twig.

Are you aware of your expectations of later life? (We were not, until we began to write of them.) Most people, without realizing it, carry an internal, unconscious stereotype, largely negative, of what it is like to be old—and then they become that way.

Many people are afraid of aging, so they try to deny that it is happening to them. Denial leads to prejudices and a psychological distancing from older people. Ageism is a unique form of prejudice, in that neither sex is excluded, nor is any social class, race, or religion. Everyone ages; people who are ageists are, therefore, prejudiced against *everyone*, including their own future selves.

People may not even be aware of their ageist views. Such ideas sneak into the unconscious mind via children's literature (the wicked *old* stepmother, mean *old* king), movies, television, and books. In language, we find only a handful of positive age-related expressions such as *mellow*, *mature*, and *worldly*—but they are balanced by at least 75 negative ones (*crotchety*, *granny*, *grump*, *fossil*).[2] In many portrayals of life, the elderly are subtly demeaned either by total exclusion from the scene or by being depicted as confused, helpless, bossy, or socially inept. To see whether you hold ageist views, try answering the questions in this chapter's Life Choice Inventory (page 262).

Most people are not openly hostile to people in their later years—they simply discount them. For example, they cherish a living myth of the golden years that envisions all old people in neat, white cottages, leading safe, undemanding lives with little stress. They think they are unable to work, free of emotional needs and desires, and unable to change. In reality, older people are an incredibly diverse group, and for the most part they are self-sufficient, socially sophisticated, mentally lucid, fully participating members of society who report themselves to be happy and healthy.[3] Their income is often drastically reduced upon retiring, and unless they have undertaken some careful planning many years in advance, their later years can be years of deprivation. Still, most people do plan ahead, and so almost half of the elderly need no financial assistance from the government.[4]

Many great intellectual and artistic achievements have been and are being produced by people in their 70s and 80s. Age does not automatically make one brilliant or philanthropic, and some people at 80 remain as immature as they were at 20. But to brush off the wisdom and perspective of the growing number of people who have experienced more life than anyone else is foolhardy.

LIFE CHOICE INVENTORY

What will the aging process be like for you? For each of the following questions, choose the answer that more nearly describes your expectations.

1. In what ways do you expect your appearance to change as you grow older?
   a. I expect to grow more and more wrinkled, lame, and unattractive.
   b. I expect to grow more and more radiant, confident, and attractive.
2. How fit do you expect to be at 70?
   a. I expect to be less fit than I am now.
   b. I expect to be very fit for my age.
3. What will be your financial status?
   a. I expect to be financially dependent on my family or the state.
   b. I expect to be financially independent.
4. What will your sex life be like? Will others see you as sexy?
   a. I expect my sex life to decline; other people will not see me as sexy.
   b. I expect to continue to be interested in sex; other people will see me as sexy.
5. Will you have many friends, only a few, or none?
   a. I will have only a few or no friends.
   b. I will have many friends.
6. What sorts of things will you do with your friends?
   a. I won't do much of anything with my friends.
   b. I expect to enjoy many, varied activities with my friends.
7. Will you be happy? Cheerful? Curious? Or will you be set in your ways?
   a. I will be set in my ways.
   b. I will be happy, cheerful, and curious.

Scoring: Your answers reveal not only what will probably become of you, but also what you think of older people. Count only your "b" answers:

7 "b" answers: Your attitudes are consistent with a rewarding and fulfilling later life.

5 or 6 "b" answers: You will be a happy older person, for the most part, but could be preparing better for old age in the areas in which you answered "a."

4 or fewer "b" answers: Unfortunately, you hold some ageist prejudices, and they may affect the quality of your own later life adversely.

The Aging Process

Although people believe that aging starts around 40 or 45, in reality, aging begins at birth. Until about age 20, aging takes the form of growth and maturing; after growth is completed, aging brings with it the gradual loss of youthful appearance and condition. Everyone ages, and many people are apprehensive about it. What is happening inside your body as you age? Research provides some answers.

Of course, all body organs age at the same rate chronologically; do they age at the same rate physiologically, too? Scientists have determined that the organs grow old together. That means that when your heart has reached a certain physiological age, your other organs will be at the same stage of aging.[5] By implication, if you live so as to slow the aging rate of one organ, such as your heart, lungs, or brain, all other parts of your body will benefit.

Within the different body organs, though, the cells have different aging patterns and life spans. Some blood cells live only three days or so; most nerve cells last for the person's lifetime. In a healthy older person, each cell lives on to the end of its normal life span in much the same fashion as in the person's younger years. As the person ages, though, the cells do change: they function less efficiently, they accumulate products not found in younger people's cells, and they lose some of their ability to reproduce.[6]

As to what exactly causes the aging process to occur, there are only theories. It may be that the genetic material contains instructions for aging or becomes damaged over the years and less able to produce functioning products. Another theory holds that ongoing chemical reactions lead to hormonal imbalances, enzyme malfunctions, and membrane deterioration over the years.

A person's **life span** is the *maximum* possible length of life that the person could reach, conditions being ideal. The person's **life expectancy** is the *average*, statistically predicted length of life. A person's life span is set by heredity, and for some, it is in the neighborhood of 100 years or more. Many people, however, do not live to their life span, owing to disease or accidents. Today, the life expectancy for men is about 71 years; for women, about 78 years.

Another term referring to length of life is **longevity**—the actual length of life observed in a person or family. Some people are blessed with extraordinary longevity, perhaps for a combination of hereditary and environmental reasons. You may have the impression that the life span is increasing, because people are living longer today than ever before. The life span (maximum) has not changed, however. What has changed is the life expectancy (average), primarily for two reasons. First, the rate of deaths from disease and accidents among the very young has declined: there are fewer young deaths to bring the average down. Second, medical advances are prolonging adults' lives so that they more nearly reach their maximum.

Many strategies have been proposed to extend human longevity, and many do not work. A scientific review of some 200 research studies concluded that none of the popular antiaging items listed in the margin had any life-extending effect except insofar as they caused caloric restriction

Strategies against aging that do not work:

The antiaging enzyme, SOD (superoxide dismutase).

Drugs that arrest deposition of aging pigment (names are Centrophenoxine, meclofenoxate, Clofenoxine, Lucidril, Helfergin, ANP 235).

Drugs that alter neurotransmitter levels (levodopa).

Stimulation of the immune system (coenzyme Q).

Antidepressant medication (Gerovital H3).

Youth steroid (DHEA, or dehydroepiandrosterone).

Antiwrinkle cream.

People have tried everything imaginable to delay or reverse aging. Years ago, the Spaniards sailed to the New World in search of the Fountain of Youth; today, people rush to buy products based on "new scientific breakthroughs" that promise to restore youth. Their motivation is the same: they want a miracle. Whenever many people desire something that is unobtainable, someone steps in with empty promises and useless products and wins a growing bank account for the effort.

Frauds that plague the elderly are not limited to the longevity hypes; old people are targets of many other schemes (described in Spotlight 1). Why are the elderly the targets for such deception? First, many of them have ready access to money—retirement funds, pensions, insurance policies, paid-up mortgages. Second, as people age, they experience more symptoms and may be frustrated by the medical profession's inability to help or unwillingness to take them seriously. They seek help where it is offered, proved or not. And as people get older, they may develop a "what have I got to lose" attitude about trying products that claim to prolong life or improve health. Money seems less important than even the slightest chance of a cure, and even brilliant, sophisticated people let themselves be bamboozled.

The combination of ready money with the chance for a miracle empties many people's pockets—even if the cost is high, the chance small, and the people smart.

without malnutrition.[7] Strategies that do work have more to do with lifestyle and less with pills and shots, as the reader of this book will not be surprised to learn.

What's Inevitable, What's Not

No magic can keep a person young forever. No matter what you do to prevent it, your body will age. You can, however, do quite a bit to slow the process of aging and maximize your health and enjoyment of life. One of the most important things you can do, according to the research review just mentioned, is to maintain appropriate body weight: obesity shortens life.[8] Aside from that, our discussion of chronological age versus physiological age in Chapter 1 identified the other keys to health maintenance in the later years. They were all of the health principles this book has emphasized—sound nutrition, adequate sleep, regular exercise, and avoidance of substance abuse. Much of the quality of the later years depends on the daily choices a person makes in youth and on the habits that become fixed as a result of those choices. Table 13–1 shows a sampling of age-related changes that can be prevented by continued exercise and other health-supporting habits.

Given wholesome choices, for each negative change that takes place as people age, a positive one seems to help compensate. For example, although older people are less able to recover physically from stress,[9] they seem to be more resilient psychologically—perhaps because they have seen more of life and have learned to adjust to unexpected turns of events.[10]

Another example: the immune system becomes less efficient at fighting off disease, but older people get infections less often than younger people do. Perhaps this is because they have developed immunity against many diseases.

Although people fear their sex lives will decline, people remain sexual beings until they die. The sex life changes, but it need not become less satisfying. "The only thing age has to do with sex performance is that the longer you live, the more you learn," says one happy older person. Physically, the reproductive organs diminish in size and function, but sexual activity itself helps to maintain a normal sexual response. Desire may remain unchanged.

In women, the later years bring **menopause**, in which monthly ovulation becomes irregular and finally ceases, as does menstruation, owing largely to depletion of estrogen. Estrogen depletion is also the cause of the periodic perception of warmth some women call hot flashes. Hot flashes are related to dilation of the blood vessels in the skin.

A major surge of bone loss (**osteoporosis**) takes place at the onset of menopause. Women whose calcium intakes and exercise levels have been insufficient to build skeletal reserves before menopause may lose bone material rapidly and become crippled with osteoporosis within a few years (see Chapter 4). To prevent the further depletion of bone material, as well as to counter some of the other effects of menopause, physicians often prescribe estrogen replacement therapy. Whatever risks this hormone may incur are far outweighed by its protective benefits.[11] In the younger years, though, the best prevention is an abundant calcium intake from food and exercise to cement the ingested calcium into place.

Take kindly the counsel of the years, gracefully surrendering the things of youth . . . Beyond a wholesome discipline, be gentle with yourself . . . Be careful, strive to be happy. *Desiderata*, found in Old St. Paul's Church, Baltimore, dated 1692, author unknown.

✳ **STRATEGIES**
for Growing Old Gracefully

To maintain health in later years:

✳ Maintain appropriate body weight.

✳ Consciously practice your stress-management skills.

✳ For women: see your physician about estrogen replacement therapy.

CHAPTER 13 ■ MATURE LIFE, AGING, AND DEATH

TABLE 13–1 Changes with Age: Inevitable versus Preventable

	You probably cannot change these:	You probably can slow or prevent these changes by exercising, maintaining other good health habits, and planning ahead:
Appearance		
Greying of hair	√	
Balding	√	
Drying and wrinkling of skin	√	
Nervous System		
Impairment of near vision	√	
Some loss of hearing	√	
Reduced taste and smell	√	
Reduced touch sensitivity	√	
Slowed reactions (reflexes)	√	
Slowed mental function	√	
Mental confusion		√
Cardiovascular System		
Increased blood pressure		√
Increased resting heart rate		√
Decreased oxygen consumption		√
Body Composition/Metabolism		
Increased body fatness		√
Raised blood cholesterol		√
Slowed energy metabolism		√
Other Physical Characteristics		
Menopause (women);	√	
Loss of fertility (men)	√	
Joints: loss of elasticity	√	
Joints: loss of flexibility		√
Loss of teeth; gum disease		√
Bone loss		√
Accident/Disease Proneness		
Accidents		√
Inherited diseases	√	
Lifestyle diseases		√
Psychological/Other		
Reduced self-esteem		√
Loss of sex drive		√
Loss of interest in work		√
Depression, loneliness		√
Reduced financial status		√

Menopause sets in early in women who smoke, and so does osteoporosis. This may be because smoking suppresses production of the hormone estrogen or because of toxic action of the ingredients of tobacco on the ovary.[12] Chapter 9 gave abundant reasons for abstaining from smoking; add these to them.

⊗ **Do not smoke. If you do smoke, quit.**

The **male menopause** is experienced as a gradual decline of fertility rather than the abrupt cessation experienced by women. In fact, some men retain fertility into their 80s. Testosterone production gradually decreases, as does sperm production. Hormones and testicular functioning may diminish, as may the need for sexual activity. The acuity of all of the senses, including the sense of touch, diminishes with age, so it may take more stimulation to reach orgasm. An older couple may actually enjoy sex more, because it allows more time for play and affection.

Physical prowess changes, too. Older muscles do not build up as quickly as younger ones do, so it takes longer and harder work to gain condition. Balanced against that, older muscles lose condition at a slower rate than young muscles do. Once fit, an older person who has to take a break from exercise will maintain condition longer, although he or she still should resume exercising as soon as possible. The more people exercise, the less likely they are to die of heart and lung diseases.[13] This does not mean for sure that exercise prolongs life, but it does enhance the quality of life and help keep you from dying before your time.

An older person's reflexes are slowed, and the joints may be less flexible than a younger person's. Activities should be adjusted to fit the body's changing abilities. The following words offer a wise strategy: "A former Olympic gold medal sprinter now walks. A once bone-bruising quarterback now plays golf and a little handball. Regular exercise is important, but equally important is whether you enjoy it. Go easy on yourself."[14]

Some changes take place in the brain and nervous system. Research has documented declines in five areas: reasoning skill, recall (memory), spatial sense, speed, and senses, but these are counterbalanced by increased wisdom and judgment.[15] People can adopt strategies to compensate for declines, such as learning to write things down so that they will not forget or allowing more time for certain tasks.

The mental confusion called **senility** is not always inevitable. Causes of mental confusion in older people are diverse—and most are preventable, only one (brain disease itself) is not. The preventable causes of mental confusion are:

■ Abuse of drugs, including alcohol; misuse or incompatibility of prescription drugs. Their effects can sometimes resemble those of strokes and seizures.

■ Accidents. Falls can cause concussions or bleeding that puts pressure on the brain, which surgery can relieve.

■ Poor vision and hearing. Both can cause confusion; both can be corrected or compensated for.

■ Malnutrition. Taste acuity, digestive secretions, and appetite diminish, while nutrient needs remain the same. Energy needs decrease, though, so older people need foods of high nutrient density.

■ Disease states. Diseases present different symptoms in older people than in younger ones. Tuberculosis, diabetes, meningitis, encephalitis, and even heart attack can all begin with confusion, rather than with obvious fever or pain. Many remediable brain problems—including nonmalignant tumors, small strokes, and seizures from epilepsy—can cause confusion.

■ Depression. Depression can slow down the mind in old people, as in the young. The distractedness that results may appear similar to senility, but the cause may be external—loss of family, friends, status, or income.

- Dehydration. The thirst signal may become faint. Drugs for high blood pressure can also cause dehydration. One of its major symptoms is confusion.
- Disuse. People do lose what they don't use. Practicing mental skills reinstates them.[16]

If an older person becomes confused, it is imperative to see that these causes are corrected first.

Here is an example of the way one of these factors, depression, can cause the symptoms of senility. A woman who invited her mother-in-law to live with her while the older woman waited for a place in a nursing home. The mother-in-law had exhibited the classic signs of senility—mental confusion, inability to make decisions, forgetting to perform important tasks such as turning off a stove burner—so the family had decided she needed institutional care. After several weeks in the daughter-in-law's home—eating meals with the family and enjoying social stimulation—she became her old self again and returned to her home. This story has been repeated with many variations and serves to remind us to seek a careful medical diagnosis before concluding that a person needs institutional care. What harm could there be in first trying home life, regular meals, and plenty of tender, loving care?

One presently incurable cause of confusion is **Alzheimer's disease**. The condition appears most often in people over 65 and is a major cause of death in that age group. It afflicts 30 percent of all those over 85. It starts as the loss of memory, progresses to inability to perform everyday functions, and then leads to the total inability to care for oneself. In the brain, the nerve pathways become tangled and blocked, cutting off the memory functions. Once it sets in, Alzheimer's disease is irreversible and progresses from mild confusion to extreme disability and death in a period of months or years. The person suffering from it usually requires a level of care beyond that which can be provided by family members.

Other unavoidable aspects of aging are financial and social losses. Being aware of this and preparing for it will enable you to weather losses more successfully than you might otherwise do. Financial planning is essential. Nearly everyone suffers a loss of income in the retirement years, aggravated by inflation. It is important to have set aside enough money for retirement—to have the home paid for or adequate income to pay the rent—and to have insurance to cover unexpected medical and other expenses.

Another form of preparation is planning an alternative living arrangement, should it become too difficult to continue carrying the responsibility for the present home. Only 5 percent of old people end up in nursing homes, but there are many alternatives between staying in a home alone and entering a nursing home. Rather than leave it to their children to decide for them where they will live, older people can decide for themselves.

However, financial preparation will not ward off the losses that take place in the emotional and social realm. These may be multiple. Old friends are lost because they die or move away; offspring move away also and may be too busy to write; income is lost upon retiring, as is status in the community. Loss of control of the environment also occurs, such as finding that the home that was to be a haven in retirement now sits in the middle of a high-crime area, or that the familiar shops and fruit stands have closed. The aging person can develop a feeling of deep loneliness as the familiar environment shifts. A loss of identity may accompany retirement or the death of a spouse.

✹ Drink eight or more glasses a day of water or other liquids, even if you aren't thirsty; don't forget.

✹ Practice using your mental skills. Keep on doing math, reading, following directions, writing, figuring things out, using your imagination, creating things.

✹ For the children of aging parents: provide or obtain the needed care and stimulation for them.

✹ Make financial plans. Be sure you can live on your income in the retirement years.

A working person can say, "I'm a farmer, a nurse, a manager." After retirement, that part of the self is gone. A married person might say, "My spouse is a golfer, an artist, a birdwatcher." When the spouse dies, that part of the self is gone. How can an old person meet new friends or find a new spouse?

The person who does not take positive steps to replace each loss can become gradually overwhelmed with loneliness and depression. Try to imagine how it would be to wake up tomorrow with all these changes having taken place at once. You have no one to report to, no deadlines, no place in particular to go. It might be wonderful to lie in bed for a day, or two, or three. But imagine that the days stretch into weeks or months, and still, nothing pushes you to do your best, expand your mind, or accomplish things. Add to this your lack of friends, your physical inability to pursue your favorite activities, and the strangeness of your environment. Changes creep up gradually on people as they age; it takes effort to remain aware of them and take measures to counter them.

You may think it's unnecessary for a person of 18 or 28 to confront the problems of loneliness and loss in later life, but such is not the case. Emotional and social health in the later years is built upon a foundation established in youth. To be happy when you are old, you need to practice happiness when you are young. Losses occur then, too. Learn to grieve over them and move on. Refill your life with new loves, new activities, new enthusiasms. Maintain a strong social support system. Keep reaching out; create a web of support so that as relationships are lost, others are gained.

Cultivate spiritual health, too. Delve into the meaning of life and how you can make it meaningful for others. Find ways to contribute your gifts, to leave something of value to those you care for. Keep working at projects that are meaningful to you. Growing is not for children only; it is a life-long enterprise.

✛ **Learn to adjust to constant change. Work at recovering from losses. Re-fill your life with new friends, new activities.**

✛ **Cultivate spiritual health. Consult your values, and make your life meaningful.**

Involvement of the old with the young benefits both.

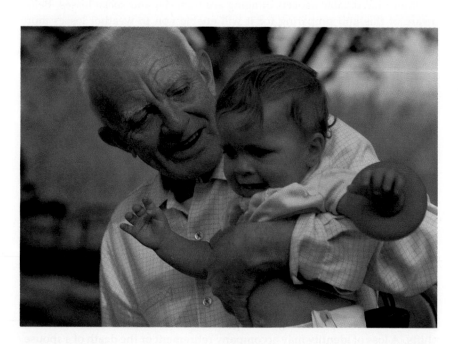

▨ DYING

No chapter on adult life would be complete without a discussion of the human experience of being mortal. We all die, and part of coming to grips with life is going through the process of other people's dying and preparing for your own death.

Fear of Death

Many people cannot stand to think of death. It is natural to fear death; all living creatures do. To express your fear is healthy: it shows a willingness to own and express emotion. Like all feelings, however, the fear of death can be changed into a more constructive emotion. The thought of death need not be morbid and depressing. After all, morbidity is in the mind of the thinker.[17] Death is a reality, but its effect on your spirits is your choice. To flee and hide from reality is unhealthy.

Consider this comfort: a sage once told a young person who feared death, "Have no fear. It is not you who will die. First you will age, aging will change you into someone other than who you are right now, and then that person will die." Alternatively, consider this view of death: it gives meaning to life. It gives you a task—to make something of your life within a limited time period. You have a deadline to meet. Whatever you want to accomplish in life, you must accomplish before you die. Whatever you start and can't complete within your own lifetime, you must pass on to others to carry on. Death has inspired towering works of art, and because you can pass on ideas and traditions to those who follow, it encourages you to make a heritage for your descendants.

The sage's answer may work for older people, but sometimes young people die, and it can be painful for them and their parents and friends to accept. Our society tends to view a child's death as a tragedy, but losing someone you love at an older age isn't any easier. All lives are meaningful, whether they are short or long. All are precious. To have lived, loved, and been loved is what matters, and even a child can come to see this, with understanding counsel. Children have been known to die peacefully and willingly, given the emotional support they need.

For those who live, it is a lesson in values to fully understand that children may die. Parents often feel as though their children are their possessions forever, and they may take them for granted or even begin to value material things more than they value their children. Each day when parents and children are reunited is a gift, not to be squandered worrying about cookie crumbs in the rug or milk on the couch. The knowledge that a loved one can be taken from you in a heartbeat is sobering; people who are so aware take opportunities to show the people they love, now, that they are cherished.

To get over the fear of death completely may be impossible, but people fear most the things they are unprepared to face. If you prepare for death, you will fear it less.

Preparation for Death

For one thing, make a will, and start thinking about life insurance. Half of those who die, die without having done so.[18] When they die, the state distributes their property according to its laws, and often the family loses much of it. Often much more goes in taxes than is necessary.

Even if you don't have any property worth mentioning, don't postpone this step for too long. Make a will before the time comes when dying without one would deprive the people you care about of what you would want them to have. A good time to make a will is when you first marry or become a parent. Even if you have little or no property at that time, assume you will have, and plan accordingly. Then when the thought of your death crosses your mind, that particular fear will be gone. You will have the comfort of knowing you have protected those you love from avoidable losses.

||| Allowing Death

If you want to die, should you be allowed to? If someone you love wants to die, should you let him? Should you help her? These are questions about **euthanasia**—one person's inducing another's death or allowing it to happen, out of humane motives. Needless to say, it is a controversial question whether, and how, one person should make decisions about another's death. Yet such decisions are faced daily, and not only by medical personnel.

A familiar case is that of the person who is terminally ill, is unconscious, has no hope of recovery, and requires machines to stay alive. The conventional medical treatment historically has been to do everything possible to prolong life, on the theory that where there is life there is hope. But many believe heroic measures to support life under such circumstances are a poor choice and that it would be preferable to take no measures or to discontinue them if they have been started.

If the latter choice is made, though, who should make it? A physician entrusted with the person's care? A nurse who has tended the person for a long time and knows the situation well? A family member? Who should keep watch over such decisions to see that they are made fairly? And who should establish the criteria by which the rightness or wrongness of such decisions should be judged?

The medical and court systems are working out answers to these questions, but many areas of uncertainty remain. In some cases, a court order is needed; in others, the physicians, together with the family and a hospital ethics committee, can decide without disobeying the law. In general, it is considered reasonable to consider terminating a person's life if:

▢ The person is clearly dying, anyway.
▢ The means necessary to prolong life would be painful or invasive.
▢ Those who know the person well are reasonably certain that the person would want such a choice to be made.

It is considered wrong to terminate a life if:

▢ The quality of life might conceivably be restored by the treatment.
▢ The treatment is not painful or invasive.
▢ The person would want his or her life prolonged.

As long as they follow these guidelines, medical personnel and the family are generally permitted to make decisions without obtaining court permission. The court is appropriately called in if the decision is urgent and if there is uncertainty about:

▢ The client's mental faculties.
▢ The probable outcomes with or without treatment.
▢ The consent of the client, spouse, or guardian.
▢ The good faith or interests of those making the decision.

Clearly, it helps if the person has earlier made a living will, and most states now honor such wills, although each state places restrictions on them. Examples of restrictions are that the will may be put in effect 14 days after diagnosis of a terminal illness and that witnesses must have been present at the signing.

When the decision has been made to deny or terminate treatment, the hard choices have not all been made. For example, the health care provider may have to decide whether to give treatments that relieve discomfort, such as water or oxygen, if they also prolong life. Perhaps the decision should rest on the purpose of the treatment with the guideline "If it provides comfort, give it."

SOURCE: Adapted from Legal considerations, in *Nursing Practice in the Care of the Dying* (Kansas City, Mo.: American Nurses Association, 1982), pp. 7-11.

For another thing, have adequate insurance. If you develop a serious illness, it may be too late to get insurance. Different kinds of policies are appropriate at different times in life and under different conditions. It is possible to be underinsured, but it is also possible to be overinsured.[19] Shop carefully and beware: the salesperson may not have your best interests at heart, because the desire for personal gain can contaminate the salesperson's motives. Chapter 18 provides insurance insight.

There are other ways to prepare for death. Strictly speaking, these are not health issues, but at some point you should also learn about the rights of hospital clients; the roles of coroners and medical examiners; the reasons for autopsies; the need for, and uses of, morgues; the various options for funerals; the possibilities for donating organs to the living; and the costs and paperwork involved in death.[20]

Some people fear that if they lose consciousness, other people will then have to decide what will happen to them. It is possible to prevent that situation from occurring: prepare and sign a **living will**. Such a document gives instructions stating exactly how you want to be treated, should you lose the ability to make decisions for yourself. Some people request that no measures be taken to prolong their lives, to avoid what they believe would be unnecessary grief and expense for their families. They may instruct their families to use no **life-support systems** after **brain death** has occurred, or they may even instruct their families to "pull the plug" if such measures have been started. Other people who fear that relatives won't have their best interests at heart may request the opposite—that *every* measure be taken to save their lives, regardless of expense. You need not linger if you do not want to—but it is important to take the responsibility for the decision, yourself. It's a heavy burden for someone else to make the choice for you— and in many instances, it is not permitted by law. An example of a living will is shown in Figure 13–1.

It is not even necessary to die in a hospital. Given the choice, many people prefer to die at home, using a **hospice** for support. A hospice is a support system especially set up for people with **terminal illnesses** and their families. The intent is to enable a person to be cared for at home by the family, and if appropriate, to die there.[21] If you are diagnosed with a terminal illness, discuss this possibility with your family, and learn where the nearest hospice facilities are available.

The key phrase of the hospice movement is "death with dignity," and the emphasis is on achieving quality in the dying person's remaining lifetime. People with terminal illnesses who are cared for at home experience more dignity and comfort, and their families have less difficulty in adjusting to the impending death.[22]

Hospice services are provided by a team of professionals, each attending to a different aspect of the dying person's care. A team typically includes physicians, nurses, and a psychiatrist or psychologist, and often social workers, clergy, and trained volunteers. The hospice has a twofold purpose: to make the dying person as comfortable as possible by controlling pain and distressing symptoms; and to offer support to the client and family—including psychological, social, and spiritual support. Care continues beyond the person's death into the bereavement period.*

*The address for the National Hospice Organization is Suite 307, 1901 North Fort Myer Dr., Arlington, VA 22209; the telephone number is (703) 243-5900. The National Consumer League publishes a booklet, *A Consumer Guide to Hospice Care*, by B. Coleman, February 1985, available from 600 Maryland Ave. SW, Suite 202-West, Washington, DC 20024.

To My Family, My Physician, My Lawyer and All Others Whom It May Concern

Death is as much a reality as birth, growth, maturity and old age—it is the one certainty of life. If the time comes when I can no longer take part in decisions for my own future, let this statement stand as an expression of my wishes and directions, while I am still of sound mind.

If at such a time the situation should arise in which there is no reasonable expectation of my recovery from extreme physical or mental disability, I direct that I be allowed to die and not be kept alive by medications, artificial means or "heroic measures." I do, however, ask that medication be mercifully administered to me to alleviate suffering even though this may shorten my remaining life.

This statement is made after careful consideration and is in accordance with my strong convictions and beliefs. I want the wishes and directions here expressed carried out to the extent permitted by law. Insofar as they are not legally enforceable, I hope that those to whom this Will is addressed will regard themselves as morally bound by these provisions.

DURABLE POWER OF ATTORNEY (optional)

I hereby designate _____ to serve as my attorney-in-fact for the purpose of making medical treatment decisions. This power of attorney shall remain effective in the event that I become incompetent or otherwise unable to make such decisions for myself.

Optional Notarization:

"Sworn and subscribed to

before me this _____ day

of _____, 19_____ ."

_____
Notary Public
(seal)

Signed _____

Date _____

Witness _____

_____
Address

Witness _____

_____
Address

Copies of this request have been given to _____

_____

FIGURE 13–1 Example of a Living Will

The most important way to prepare for death is spiritually. Study the meaning of life. Live now the way you will wish you had lived when you die. It's been suggested that you should live each day as if it were your last. This isn't a suggestion to be morbid but a reminder that, realistically, your time and the time of people you love is limited. As the end nears, savor the moments that remain. Let go of less important values; intensify your relationships with those dearest to you. Reconcile unmended friendships. If there are people who should know you love them, tell them. If there's a kindness you've been postponing doing, do it. Find and affirm value in life. All these preparations are things people can do while they're alive—now. They are ways of coping. They can help to make death less scary. This chapter's Spotlight discusses the concept of spiritual health.

FIGURE 13–1   continued

Grief

Grief at death is unavoidable and painful, but education about death may help people cope with it when it happens. Grief takes many forms. One form is felt when someone you know is going to die and you feel sad ahead of time. This is called anticipatory grief, and it can be hard to deal with. People naturally feel pity, anger, and even revulsion at the impending death of someone they love. It is human to want to avoid contact. It helps to know that.

Many people find it so hard to face the process of someone's dying that they miss out on many opportunities to give support. But remember, the person who has learned that death is coming is still the same person as before. If the person had lost a fortune, a home, or an opportunity, you would offer sympathy and love. Now that the person is facing the loss of life itself, doesn't it make sense to offer that same sympathy and love? It may be hard to do, but perhaps it's easier if you realize that there is no one right way to go about it. Your personal style is fine, whatever it is. If your habit has been to laugh and joke with the person, then laugh and joke now, too. After all, the person is alive and capable of responding to cheering company. If you tend to show sorrow easily, that's all right, too. Listen well, if the person wants to communicate. Let the person know you care in whatever way feels right to you. The thing not to do is to avoid the person: any kind of personal contact is better than simply writing your friend off before the end.

The most painful grief is easier to bear when people know, at least intellectually, that it will ease with time. People typically go through a series of stages of grief when facing death—their own, or someone else's. These stages were first described by Elizabeth Kubler-Ross, who spent many hours with dying persons during the 1960s and wrote a highly respected, humane book about them.[23] The stages in the acceptance of death are:

- Denial—"No, it can't be!"
- Anger—"Why me? It's too soon!"
- Bargaining—"I'll do anything; just let me live."
- Depression—withdrawal, loss of hope.
- Acceptance—"I am ready, now. It's all right."

The stages are experienced both by the dying person and by those nearby, and they are quite universal. It helps to know that you will experience these emotions, sometimes over and over again, in the process of coming to accept death. Not everyone goes through all the stages, however, and not everyone needs to express their feelings about them.

People can also handle grief better when they realize that they have something to *do* about it: they have "grief work" to do.[24] Our culture has some traditions that, though painful, help people come to terms with death. These include preparing the body, writing obituaries, notifying friends and relatives, conducting the funeral ceremony and burial, thanking donors of gifts and letters, and disposing of possessions. If people don't do this grief work, they are likely to grieve longer, to experience delayed grief reactions, or to experience later maladjustment.[25]

After someone has died, people often think it's best not to mention the dead person to the survivor. "I don't want to remind her," they think. "Let's stay off the subject. I don't want to stir up her grief." Yet the very opposite is more often advisable. After someone close has died, the memory is still very much alive. A person can't suddenly shut off all thoughts of someone they've loved. It actually helps survivors to know you're thinking of the person, too. You should mention the person when the thought crosses your mind. Bring back and share memories: "Sis would have enjoyed this," or "I thought of your mom today," or "Did I ever tell you about the discussion your husband and I had"—remarks like these let the grieving person know that you, too, remember and miss the one who is gone.

For as long as they occur to you, such comments are appropriate. Grief doesn't have a time limit. You may have heard that it takes about a year to get over someone's death. The tradition that a widow or widower should grieve for a year has some validity, for that permits every occasion throughout the year to pass, once, without the person with whom it had been shared earlier—religious holidays, birthdays, anniversaries, and all the rest. But grief can spring to the heart years after a loss and be felt as keenly as if the person had died just yesterday. It may never be completely gone, and if you care about the person who is grieving, you will be willing to share in those feelings whenever they arise.

It is considered unhealthy, though, to grieve without relief for an unusually long time over someone who has died. Sometimes people don't seem able to pull out of grief; they get stuck. Such people may need help, and it is not necessarily supportive in such cases to indulge their grief forever. There are grief counselors who can help people to complete their goodbyes and go on.

Attending the Dying

Birth attendants are professionally trained to assist at the start of life; ideally, people present at death should also be trained.[26] You need to know the signs of impending death and the comforts to offer the dying person. When you have things to do rather than stand helplessly by, it makes it easier to be present.

Everyone knows what it is like to be sick in bed and have to be cared for by others. The experience is the same for a person near death. For as long as the person is alive, you are tending a living person, not a dying person. Think of it that way, and you will know better what to do.

A person who is sick, weak, uncomfortable, and possibly in pain has little energy to give to the psychological task you may be facing. The person needs physical comforts: learn what they are and offer them.

The signs of impending death include glazed eyes, open mouth, cold skin, irregular breathing and pulse, and restless arms and hands. The process of dying usually progresses from the lower part of the body upward. Sensation is lost first in the lower extremities. Then control of the digestive system is lost, and it becomes useless to offer food. As long as the person can swallow, though, water helps—just a little at a time so that it won't cause choking. Keep the mouth wet, with a gauze wick if necessary. Be sure the person is not lying flat when facing upward, because water or even the tongue can fall back in the throat and cause choking. In other ways, too, you may perceive that the person is uncomfortable and needs to be helped to change position, bathed if sweating, helped to breathe, and so forth.

The restlessness of a dying person is often caused by the feeling of being too hot. People often don't realize this, because the skin becomes cold as circulation to the peripheral parts begins to cease. But inside, the person's body is hot, and the circulation is failing to radiate that heat away in the normal fashion. Fresh, moving air helps. Light is comforting; a dying person may ask to be allowed to lie in the sun, and dying people turn toward the light. Soothing music may help, but be sure it's of a kind the person doesn't dislike. And don't whisper nearby; speak audibly or not at all.

According to an authority on dying, it is always easy at the last. There is always an interval of perfect peace and often of ecstasy before death, perhaps because pain ceases. The words of people who could speak at the moment of death indicates that they experience no suffering at that point.[27]

Death itself is not an experience we go *through*. We go through life—up to the point of death. If we live as we intend to, then we are doing all we can—for choices that have to do with life are the only choices we are given to make.

STUDY AIDS

1. Identify the characteristics of people who are happy in later life.
2. Compare and contrast constructive and destructive views of aging and their effects on people's self-concepts and attitudes toward others.
3. Distinguish what is inevitable about the aging process from what is not.
4. Describe strategies to maintain a high quality of life into the later years.
5. List some preventable, reversible, and controllable causes of mental confusion in older people.
6. Itemize ways that people can prepare for death.
7. Explain what a hospice is and what services it performs.
8. Discuss the purposes of a Living Will.
9. Identify the stages of grief.
10. Explain how you would go about easing a person's transition into death.

GLOSSARY

Alzheimer's disease: a relentless, irreversible brain disease that occurs in some victims with increasing age; the final stage is complete helplessness and death.

brain death: irreversible and total cessation of function of the higher brain centers, reflected in a flat line recorded by the electroencephalograph, as opposed to the irregular wave pattern made by an active brain. Brain death is not mere sleep or unconsciousness but irreversible and total cessation of function. The *electroencephalogram (EEG)* is a recording of brainwaves, made by a machine, from electrodes attached painlessly to the scalp.

euthanasia (you-than-AY-zee-uh): allowing a person to die; sometimes called *mercy killing*. In *direct euthanasia*, an act is performed, such as pulling the plug on life-support equipment (which may be legal in some cases) or injecting a poison (which is illegal). In *indirect euthanasia*, a person is simply allowed to die; no action is taken to prevent death, such as instituting mechanical life-support measures, feeding, or the like.

eu = beneficial

thanatos = death

hospice (HOS-pis): a support system for people with terminal illnesses and their families, which helps the family to let the person die at home with dignity and in comfort.

life expectancy: the number of years an individual can realistically expect to live based on heritary and environmental factors.

life span: the maximum years of life genetically attainable.

life-support systems: a term used to refer to mechanical and/or artificial means of supporting life, such as machines that force air into the lungs or feedings given into a central vein.

living will: a will a person can make to indicate how he or she would like to be treated on becoming unable to make decisions (for example, in the event of brain death).

longevity: an individual's length of life.

menopause: cessation of ovulation and menstruation in a woman, due to advancing age. The equivalent in men is **male menopause**, the gradual decline in fertility and sexual desire due to advancing age.

osteoporosis (also in Chapter 4): adult bone loss.

senility: a general term pertaining to the weakness of mind and body occurring in old age.

terminal illness: an illness that is expected to end in death.

QUIZ ANSWERS

1. *True*. People beyond their 20s generally enjoy life more than people in their 20s.

2. *False*. The happiest people are those who have lived through at least one major life tragedy.

3. *True*. Most people's income is drastically reduced at retirement.

4. *False*. The maximum human life span has not changed, but the average life expectancy has increased steadily over the past 100 years.

5. *False*. People can expect to remain sexual creatures until they die.

6. *True*. Mental confusion in older people is often preventable.

7. *False*. Fewer than 5 old people out of 100 end up in nursing homes.

8. *False*. A hospice is an organization that offers support for families of people who choose to die at home.

9. *False*. Grief has no time limits, and can revisit a person years after a loved one has died.

10. *False*. It is best to speak freely of the life of someone who has died to a grieving survivor, whenever the thought of that person arises.

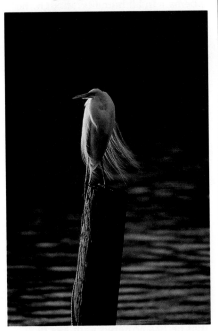

Spiritual Health

People have always contemplated the reason for their existence. Imagine, for a minute, someone standing alone on the globe looking out into the deep, dark recesses of space, asking, "Why am I here?" "What purpose do I serve?" "What is the reason for my existence?" Whenever people clear their minds of all other thoughts and look inside themselves and to the world to ask these questions, they are expressing a need for spiritual health.

"Spiritual health" sounds like a vague term to me. What is it? Is it the same as membership in a church or temple?

No—a spiritual person may, but may not, belong to an organized religious institution. Conversely, a person who belongs to an organized religious institution may or may not be a spiritual person. Spiritual health has been defined as "the ability to . . discover, articulate, and act on our own basic purpose in life; to learn how to give and receive love, joy, and peace; to pursue a fulfilling life; and to contribute to the improvement of the spiritual health of others."[1] The word *learn* is important in this definition, because it implies that the skills one needs can be acquired by effort.

I haven't heard much talk about the value of a spiritual life. It seems that our society focuses instead on making a lot of money.

Unfortunately, this is true. Recently displayed on a car bumper was a sticker that read, "He who dies with the most toys wins." This way of life equates value with material possessions and is pleasure centered. People who seek happiness through ownership and acquiring are locked into continual seeking *more* material things. Because possessions only bring fleeting pleasures, such people never have enough. Ultimately, materialism brings boredom and emptiness.

In contrast, living a spiritual life deemphasizes what we own. It values what we do and who we are. One person described all people as having a vacuum inside them that can only be filled by spirituality. A person who tries to fill this emptiness with possessions finds that they don't meet the need, and is left feeling empty.

Do you have to believe in God to have a spiritual life?

You have to believe in a power greater than yourself, although you may not choose to call it God. Some people call it love, peace, the unconscious mind, other people, psychic energy, nature, E.S.P., or the cosmos. This belief is a recognition that your own ability to make things happen is small in relation to a greater power that controls the universe.

What difference does it make if you believe in such a power?

It relieves you of the feeling that you have to manage your life entirely on your own. It relieves you of having to make all decisions consciously, relying on only your own strength. It lets you instead relax and trust things to come about with others' help, in natural ways, and without your conscious, solitary effort. That power may come from your own unconscious mind, from other people, or from some other unknown source.

Faith is an important part of spirituality: faith in a higher power, faith in other people, faith in yourself, and faith in life. Faith grows with the awareness that your basic needs will be met, not by your own efforts alone, but also from sources outside yourself. Recall the five basic needs identified by Maslow (Chapter 3): you will be helped to meet them all—your survival needs, your need for safety and security, your need to belong, your need for esteem, and your need for self-actualization.

Are there other benefits of spiritual health?

Yes, having spiritual health enhances the quality of life. It gives a person's life significance, value, purpose, and meaning. It brings the feelings of hope, peace, and contentment. In contrast, atheist existentialist philosophers believe the universe is impersonal and life's events are a product of blind chance. This view holds that since there is no higher power, life has no ultimate meaning. Therefore life is absurd and futile and people are miserable because they feel uncertain and insignficant. An existentialist life is cynical and pessimistic; a spiritual life is optimistic.

What does spiritual health have to do with health?

A person with spiritual health is also emotionally healthy. The person feels loved and is able to love. The person has high self-esteem, which is essential in coping with life's problems (see Chapter 3). The person relates well to self, others, and society, and acts as part of the environment, rather than in opposition to it (see Chapter 19's Spotlight). In addition, people with spiritual health often practice prayer and meditation, which have a relaxation effect and counteract the effects of stress (see Chapter 2).

That sounds like a religious way of life to me.

Yes; true religious life is as we have described. In fact, every one of the world's religions has that as its basis: "All religions imply in one way or another that human beings do not, and cannot, stand alone, that they are vitally related with and even dependent on powers in nature and society external to themselves. Dimly or clearly, they know that they are not independent centers of force capable of standing apart from the world."[2]

What about science and psychology? Don't they contradict this concept of spirituality?

No; in fact, the perception of a higher power has counterparts in psychology, in science, and even in fields like politics and sports. Psychologists, for example, use the term *ego* to describe the isolated individual, and *self* to describe the individual in touch with a higher power. *Ego* refers to a small part of the personality—the conscious part. *Self* refers to the whole personality, conscious and unconscious. According to one school of psychological thought, the Jungians, a large part of early life consists in developing the ego, but in later life the ego must "die" to the greater self. The loss of ego and the birth of the self is the successful outcome of the spiritual crisis of middle life, when one realizes the limits of one's own ability to control people and events. During that crisis, the personality is transformed—dying and being reborn as a Self that knows its limits, is fully and humbly human, and can love and experience joy and fulfillment.

Similarly, some of the world's greatest scientists have been deeply religious people. Even Charles Darwin, widely viewed as a scientist whose ideas opposed the conventional Christian perspective of his time, was profoundly humble, and said that it was impossible to conceive "that this grand and wondrous universe, with our conscious selves, arose through chance."[3] Lewis Thomas, a modern-day biologist, has written, "We are in trouble whenever persuaded that we know everything. . . . We humans are a profoundly immature species, only now beginning the process of learning how to learn. . . . We are aware of our consciousness, but we cannot even make good guesses as to how this awareness arises in our brains—or even, for that matter, that it does arise there . . . We do not understand why we make

music, or dance, or paint, or write poems." In all humility, though, he goes on to say, "Our place in the life of the world is surely not absurd. We matter."[4] Thomas devoted much of his life to making a scientific view of the the world and humankind spiritually meaningful to nonscientists.

You say that in politics and sports, too, people believe in the necessity for a spiritual life. Can you give an example?

There are many. A judge advised a college graduating class that one of the ways they needed to equip themselves for their lives as adults was to cultivate "a little basic faith." He quoted Adlai Stevenson, Jr., a governer and U.N. ambassador, as saying, "What a man knows at 50 that he did not know at 20 boils down to something like this: the knowledge that he has acquired with age is . . . not gained by words but by touch, sight, sound, victories, failures, sleeplessness, devotion, love . . . a little faith and a little reverence for the things you cannot see."[5]

In sports, too, top performers are often aware that to gain the edge in competition requires more than mere physical preparation, as important as that may be. Indispensable to top performance is a mental attitude born of some mysterious process beyond mere thinking. Zen Buddhist masters of swordsmanship teach their students how *not* to think, when they are finally ready to compete. As a Zen master put it, "Quit trying, quit trying not to try, quit quitting."[6]

You said that the skills one needs to lead a healthy spiritual life can be acquired by effort. What sort of effort did you have in mind?

One pair of authors identify these sources of spiritual energy, among others: love relationships, personal writing, prayer, solitude, and dreams. They say that without these, people "burn out." "The secret of recapturing energy lies in awareness of our authentic self, our feelings, needs, desires. Faith is likewise a key factor for recovery. . . . Faith gives us a sense of who really is doing the work, the loving."[7] It isn't an effort for us to love if we let it flow through us from a higher power, rather than feeling we have to generate it out of our own strength alone.

That's an inspiring thought.

Yes, and in fact the word *inspiration* describes exactly what this discussion is about: being filled (*in*) with the *spirit*.

What do you mean by "the" spirit?

Whatever spirit lifts you up when you are down—depressed, lonely, or exhausted. Your own name for it might be the best one to use—the spirit of love, of hope, or, a holy spirit. By whatever name, it is a spirit you need if you are not to be defeated by life's down side.

In saying the "spirit of love," do you mean human love?

Yes, certainly. Christians say that God's spirit is within every human being. Human love is the recognition and embracing of that spirit in others. Loneliness comes when we are cut off from this experience, and feel that we are neither loving nor loved enough. Part of learning to live a spiritual life is learning that we *are* loved enough, that we *can* love enough, even though we are only human.[8] To achieve this, we need to be willing to risk being known as we really are (intimacy) and to love another as that person really is (acceptance). Human love, realized this way, is one of the highest expressions of spiritual development.

How do the solitary occupations like personal writing, prayer, and dreams contribute to the experience of love?

These are ways of getting in touch with the sources of your inspiration—your higher power, and learning to love your *self*, as well as others. When you are fully comfortable with yourself, when you love yourself and love to *be* yourself, then you need not feel lonely even when you are alone.

How do you go about getting in touch with this higher power?

You have to abandon *conscious* effort, and allow time for your nonthinking, unconscious self. You accomplish this by:

- Less preoccupation with "doing things" and more ability to let things happen.
- Less attention to making decisions and more ability to let deepest desires well up to consciousness.
- Less reasoning and thinking and more intuition and freeing up of deeper regions of the psyche.[9]

A religious writer describes "The Golden Key" to harmony and happiness as the way to get out of any difficulty: "Stop thinking about the difficulty, whatever it is, and think about God instead."[10] Another way to say this is, "Don't be part of the problem, become part of the solution." "Let go and let God." Christians describe getting in touch with the higher power through prayer (speaking to God) and reading the Bible (listening to God). Christian faith emphasizes spending time alone with God.

Is that a description of prayer?

Yes, but it could equally well be called meditation or contemplation or relaxation or silence. These activities impart a unique energy to people, energy that they would not be able to obtain otherwise. One of our favorite ways of describing this energy is "the energy of attention." Whatever you give your attention to, is what your life will be about.[11] Whatever you think about all day describes you. If your thoughts are positive and constructive, then your life will be likewise. If your thoughts are pessimistic and defeatist, then your life will be likewise. Change your thoughts, focus your attention in a positive direction, and spiritual power will change your life.

That must be where the discipline comes in.

That is true. People have to train themselves to think positively. It takes practice, but it is worth it. One religious teacher wrote a book called *The Power of Positive Thinking*. He says the most powerful force in human nature is spiritual power: if you can believe, all things are possible.[12]

How can one go about training oneself to develop spiritual health?

There are as many different ways to go about it as there are spiritual and religious traditions:

- Attend a church or other religious institution of your choice; pay attention to the messages it conveys; and apply them in your personal life.
- Keep a journal of events, thoughts, feelings, prayers, dreams; this is a way of paying attention to your self.
- Pray and meditate on a regular basis.
- Read books suggested by your church or friends.
- Stay open, listen everywhere for messages about how to live your life. Keep your spiritual health in mind.
- Think of others as spiritual seekers, too. Cultivate humility and your sense of oneness with others.

The benefits of spiritual health are many. Human beings can reach their full potential only if they develop the spiritual side of themselves. Life is hardly worth living without joy, faith, and love. Spiritual health brings the peace that surpasses all understanding.

Accident and Injury Prevention

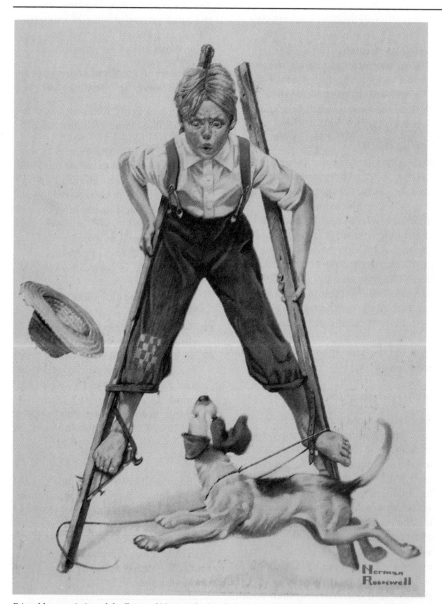

Printed by permission of the Estate of Norman Rockwell Copyright © 1919 Estate of Norman Rockwell.

FOR OPENERS . . .

True or false? If false, say what is true.

1. One out of every ten people suffers an injury every year.
2. The primary characteristic you need to prevent accidents on the road is driving skill.
3. Safety belts sometimes cause injuries, but more often, they prevent them.
4. Small children in cars need better protection than safety belts can offer.
5. Young people fall more often than older people do, because they are more careless.
6. A person climbing down a ladder should face the ladder.
7. Of all parts of the body, the head affects balance the most.
8. The Heimlich maneuver is a trick devised by German spies during World War II to get through barbed wire fences without injury.
9. You can injure your back picking up a feather.
10. The emergency telephone number in most parts of the United States is 911.

(Answers on page 295.)

Whatever age you are, you probably now know things you wish you had known sooner. But have you ever noticed how, when you try to warn others of what you have learned, they seem uninterested in your advice? Being careful is boring, and until accidents happen, they seem unlikely. If only people could learn to be careful enough to avoid getting hurt without losing spontaneity and joy in life! Most people, we hope, are willing to learn about the prevention of **accidents** once they realize how likely accidents are to affect them. Answering the questions in this chapter's Life Choice Inventory (page 282) can help you find out whether you are now skilled in accident prevention or whether you have more to learn.

We should note right away that not all accidents are preventable, of course. Some just happen. But many accidents are preventable; this chapter is about those that never have to happen.

This year, chances are that one out of every three people you know will suffer an injury. As many as 80,000 accidents a year are *preventable* accidents. Among them are tens of thousands of accidents that cause brain and spinal cord injuries leading to permanent disability. Injuries also claim young lives—more of them than any disease does.[1]*

Relatively little attention has been paid to this major public health problem. Figure 14–1 shows that many more years of life are lost to accidents than to heart disease and cancer, but look at the amounts of research money spent on those three health areas. Clearly, heart disease and cancer claim many more research dollars than does accident prevention. That is why we are choosing to devote a whole chapter of this book to accident prevention: it needs attention.

■■■ HIGHWAY ACCIDENTS

Nearly half of the accidents that take place are car accidents. Good drivers do not usually cause them, but they do have them—because some accidents

*Reference notes are in Appendix D.

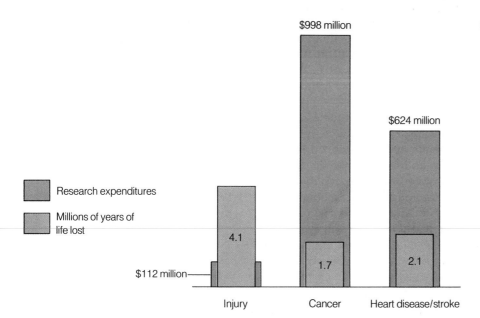

FIGURE 14–1 Loss of Life and Prevention Efforts, United States, 1985

Injuries cost many more years of life than cancer or heart disease, yet hardly any money is spent on research to learn how to prevent injury, while hundreds of millions of dollars are spent on cancer and heart disease research.

CHAPTER 14 ■■ **ACCIDENT AND INJURY PREVENTION**

LIFE CHOICE INVENTORY

How safety-conscious are you? Answer these questions to find out whether you are now doing all you reasonably should do to prevent accidents, or whether you have room for improvement in this respect:

1. I have taken a first aid course (or I have made plans to take one).
2. I have taken a driver education course (or I plan to take one before I drive).
3. When driving, I always slow down when approaching an intersection (or I am sure I will do this when I drive).
4. I always buckle my safety belt when driving or riding in a car.
5. I never drink or use drugs and then drive (or I am sure I would never do this).
6. I cross the street at crosswalks only; I do not jaywalk.
7. I keep my home (room) in order, with no objects or cords on the floor that people might trip on.
8. I have a stepladder, and I use it for climbing and reaching.
9. I have a fire extinguisher, and I keep it where I can get to it in case of fire.
10. I have planned an escape from my bedroom in case of fire.
11. I never smoke in bed (or I do not smoke).
12. I dispose of my trash regularly.
13. I have my community's emergency phone numbers right by my phone.
14. I can swim (or I have made plans to learn to swim).
15. I obey all safety rules around water and boats.
16. I read and heed all label directions on containers of chemicals and drugs.
17. Children would not be able to hurt themselves in my home (room).
18. I maintain all electrical equipment as instructed; I replace old cords and plugs.
19. I know how to avoid back injury when lifting an object, and I practice what I know.

Scoring: Give yourself 5 points for each yes answer.
90 to 95: You are a safety-conscious person.
80 to 85: You have a few more refinements to make on your choices.
70 to 75: You have some room for improvement.
65 or below: You need to improve your safety awareness and behavior.

---

are unpreventable. Until you have had one, it is hard to believe that such a thing is possible, but remember, accidents are not deliberate. You do not see them coming; you do not expect them; you do not have time to avoid them. Just think about the last time you cut yourself even slightly: you did not mean to. The trouble was, you did not see that it was about to happen. The control was not all in your hands.

Knowledge and skill are not sufficient to prevent car accidents; an equally important characteristic of the driver is attitude. Consider the attitudes of two different drivers. Attitude 1 is, "I'm invulnerable. I'm in control." A person with attitude 1 simply goes out and drives, unconcerned with potential hazards. Attitude 2 is, "The control is not all in my hands. I need to be aware of other drivers and watch for possible accidents about to happen." A person with attitude 2 drives defensively.

For an intelligent person to move from attitude 1 to attitude 2, no more is required than to grasp the way statistics translate into real-life events. Is the car you see approaching from the right going to run that red light? No, it's not. And the next car? No, it's not, either. In fact, the chances are only 1 in 10,000 that you will approach a green light at an intersection just as a car drives out in front of you.

So how long will it be before a car does run a red light just as you are driving through an intersection? If you pass through enough intersections (say, ten a day), then it will take a thousand days, on the average, for you to encounter this event. That is about once in three years. Thus if you

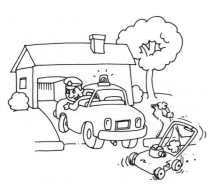
Knowledge and skill are not enough to prevent accidents.

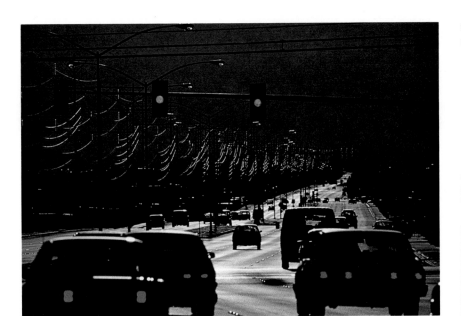

Sooner or later everyone has a close encounter at an intersection.

▌▌▌ Defensive Driving

The instructor of a defensive driving course warns the pupils: "At the end of this course you'll have an exam. It's a long exam. It's a tough exam. If you miss any one question, you'll fail it." But in the last class the instructor passes out no test pages, explaining, "The exam is outside this room. You start taking it when you get back in your car to drive home. It goes on for the rest of your life. Every time you get on the road, you're taking the test. And if you miss one question, you fail it."

accumulate a total of 30 years' driving experience in your life, it is almost inevitable that ten times in your life a car will unexpectedly pull out in front of you as you pass through an intersection. That it will happen once is virtually certain. You cannot know when, but it will occur. You can probably avoid collisions if you approach every intersection, all your driving life, with the expectation that a car may suddenly pull out in front of you. With that in mind, you will slow down, you will be ready to turn or hit the brake, you will be planning ahead to avoid colliding with the cars next to you and behind you. That is the spirit of defensive driving as it applies to one of hundreds of driving situations. Defensive driving saves thousands of lives each year.

Driver education courses reduce accidents, too. As a result, automobile insurance rates are lower for drivers who have had driver education courses.

Judgment is also essential to driving safety. The American Red Cross makes this point: "Driving skill and judgment cannot be separated; both are equally important in preventing accidents."[2] Driving skill comprises the person's ability to control the vehicle under all road conditions. Driving judgment is the driver's ability to anticipate or recognize a potential accident and to know how to avoid it. The effective exercise of both skill and judgment, the Red Cross points out, depends on the driver's *attitude*.

Part of the defensive driving attitude is self-defense against injury. A defensive driver uses a safety belt whenever driving and insists that passengers do the same. Some people claim that safety belts injure people in accidents—and they sometimes do, but far more often, they save lives. People must be persuaded to become as motivated as the person (call her Susan) who says she cannot even repark her car without first buckling her safety belt.

Susan explains that a driving instructor told her, "Think of your unprotected body flying through the air at 50 miles an hour and suddenly hitting a stationary car dashboard. When you are driving at 50 miles an hour, both your car and your body are moving *independently* at that speed. If the car hits something and stops, you'll keep flying at 50 miles an hour until *you*

Use a safety belt.

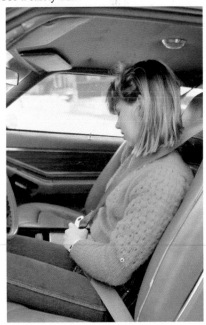

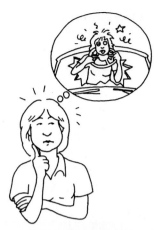

Your car will stop during a collision, but without a safety belt, your body won't.

hit something." A safety belt decreases a person's momentum as the car's momentum decreases, and it distributes the force of the impact across the body's strongest parts. Also, it keeps the driver behind the wheel and in control, able to prevent further collisions. Being thrown from the vehicle is *not* an advantage in a collision, rather, it increases the likelihood of fatality 25 times. Safety belts keep you inside and safe. Another piece of safety equipment is important: head restraints prevent whiplash injury.

Parents need to learn to protect their babies, too. Strap the baby into a certified child passenger carrier every time you ride in the car. Safety belts alone do not protect young children well enough.

The responsible driver also:

- Keeps track of the vehicle's condition—tires, windshield wipers, horn, lights, brakes, wheel alignment, steering mechanism, and all other systems.
- Maintains self-awareness of physical and psychological conditions and does not drive after drinking alcohol; after taking drugs that cause drowsiness; or when emotional, anxious, distracted, irritated, or tired.
- Wears corrective glasses if indicated.
- Adjusts speed, technique, and distance from other vehicles to different driving conditions. Keeps windshield, rear window, and mirrors clear.
- Obeys traffic signs and regulations; signals all turns and stops.
- Uses snow tires and/or chains when indicated.
- Watches for and anticipates pedestrians, joggers, and bicyclists.

All of these statements about attitude apply equally to motorcyclists. In addition, motorcyclists should learn and employ safety techniques specific to them (the highway patrol offers courses in these), and they should wear helmets, whether or not they are required by law to do so.

Vehicles used off the highway cause accidents, too. All-terrain vehicles seriously injure or kill thousands of users, including many who are not misusing them. They tend to tip over and land on top of their drivers; they are often sold to children; they are not safety tested; and often, no warnings are given at the time they are sold. Snowmobiles are dangerous for similar reasons and also because people use them for thrills rather than for transportation. In some states, no license is required to operate such vehicles, and children are allowed to do so without safety training, equipment, or supervision. The mounting accident and death rates are forcing some states to take action to regulate the use of such vehicles.

If you are nearby when an accident occurs and no one certified in **first aid** is available, you can sometimes assist the injured by following a few simple procedures outlined briefly in Appendix C. Note that to give truly effective first aid, you must take a course and become certified. Appendix C presents only stopgap measures to use until qualified help arrives.

▦ FALLS

Second to highway accidents, falls cause the most accidental deaths. Statistics demonstrate that for each person, sooner or later, one accidental fall will likely be a devastating one. The same attitude that prevents driving accidents works for falls: anticipation and defensive action against them can prevent them.

Most falls happen at home. To prevent slips and trips:

- Wipe up spills.
- Use nonslip floor wax.
- Secure small rugs—do not use them at tops and bottoms of staircases.
- Clean up snow in walking areas—use sand or salt on icy spots.
- Keep a safety mat in the bathtub and install handholds on the wall.
- Be careful in wet grass, especially with a power mower.
- Repair torn and frayed carpet promptly.
- Keep walking areas clear and the yard picked up.
- Keep stairs and hallways well lighted—install handrails.
- Flag all cables and lines such as wires holding up trees and flagpoles.

To prevent falls that occur when climbing or reaching:

- Use a sturdy ladder; do not use makeshift piles of furniture or boxes.
- Inspect the ladder before you use it.
- Never paint a ladder; paint hides structural defects.
- Reposition the ladder instead of reaching to the side from the top of it. Climb down, move the ladder, and climb up again.
- Position the bottom of a straight ladder not less than one quarter of its length away from the wall.
- Keep your hands free to grip the ladder as you climb. Hoist paint up when you get to the top, and wear your tools in a tool belt.
- Keep your body weight centered between the ladder rails.
- Face the ladder when climbing down.
- Hire an expert for high jobs, especially roof jobs. Or become an expert yourself. Use a safety belt and strong rope.

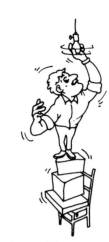

Plan climbs sensibly.

Special notes for special age groups: falls are the leading cause of accidental death and injury to older people, so be aware that physical coordination, agility, vision, and especially balance decline with age. Sudden motions affect balance the most—especially motions involving the head, which is heavy and can pull the whole body off center. Slow down and move with grace. For the other special age group, infants, falls from tables and bassinets are a frequent cause of injury. Do not look away from an infant in such a place, even for a moment.

BURNS

The third leading cause of accidental death is fires and burns. One-fifth of those who die are children, and four-fifths of the deaths caused by fire occur in the home. Fire prevention precautions are the topic of this chapter's Spotlight. Appendix C offers rudimentary tips for assisting burn victims; a class in first aid can give you more.

A special class of burns—chemical burns—damages eyes, skin, and lungs without fire. Read the labels of sprays, products that contain gases, and caustic compounds. Follow directions.

Other specifics to prevent fires and burns:

- Install fire extinguishers near danger spots where you can get to them.
- Keep a garden hose near a faucet.

- Use chemical fire extinguishers, never water, on electrical fires. Baking soda will safely smother a grease fire, so keep a box close at hand.
- Install adequate insulation around ovens, heaters, and fireplaces.
- Perform the required maintenance on heating systems.
- Dispose of trash immediately.
- Use only nonflammable cleaning fluids.
- Hang clothes well away from stoves or fireplaces.
- Supervise children playing near an open fire.
- Store matches in a metal container and out of reach of children.
- Be careful with hot tap water; it can cause scalds that require hospitalization.
- Do not smoke in bed or if you are sleepy; provide adequate ashtrays.
- Install home fire detectors.[3]

Finally, should a fire start, what will you do? Think now, because you need to know ahead of time what moves to make. The Spotlight tells you how to preplan your way out of burning buildings; one thing to carry in your head at all times is the emergency telephone number: 911.*

▰▰▰ SWIMMING AND BOATING ACCIDENTS

Drowning is the fourth leading cause of accidental death, and in the active age groups it is second only to highway accidents as a cause of accidental death. Most drownings occur when someone who can't swim falls into the water—often from a boat. Surprisingly, people who can't swim often put themselves in situations in which they may drown—and then do.

To reduce the risk of drowning:

- Learn to swim.
- Never swim alone or let others do so.
- Choose swimming places with discrimination.
- Protect pools with fences.
- Supply boats with flotation devices.
- Ease into the water when it is cold.
- Never play rough in or near the water.
- Swim only when you feel well, and do not swim if you have been drinking alcohol or using other drugs.

When diving, never dive where obstructions might lurk or where you don't know the depth; and do not overestimate your ability; do not dive too deep. It is also wise to have a boat accompany you on a distance swim and to get out of the water when lightning threatens. Except in emergencies, rely on your own swimming ability, not on inner tubes or floats.

If you see someone in trouble in the water, help by using the techniques described in Table 14–1. Only a trained lifeguard should attempt rescue by swimming out to the victim; a drowning person can easily overpower a novice and drown them both.

You may have heard that you should not swim until an hour after eating, to prevent stomach cramps. It is not necessarily dangerous to swim with a full stomach, especially if you exercise lightly. However, if you undertake an intense swimming workout after eating, you may indeed experience cramps, and they are just as likely to occur in your legs or arms as in your

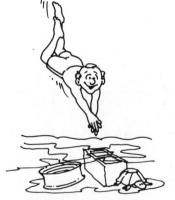

Don't dive where obstructions might lurk.

*This emergency number is used almost everywhere throughout the United States.

TABLE 14–1 Water Rescue Techniques

Even if you cannot swim, you can assist a swimmer who is nearby and in trouble. If the swimmer is near a dock or in a pool:

■ Lie flat on the dock or pool ledge; extend an arm or leg, towel, shirt, fishing pole, oar, or other object, and pull the victim within reach of the edge. Most pools have long-handled cleaning tools around that work well. If there is a lifesaving cushion or float nearby, aim carefully and throw it to the victim.

If the troubled swimmer is farther away than you can reach:

■ Wade into the water up to your waist, and extend an object or push a float or a board, or throw a rope where the victim can reach it.

If the victim fell from a boat, or you are in a boat:

■ Allow the victim to hang onto the boat or to an object you hold out.

If the victim is too weak to hold on:

■ Pull the victim into the boat carefully to avoid worsening any injuries.

If the victim fell through ice:

■ Push a ladder or other long object, tied with a rope at the bottom rung and secured, out to the victim or use ropes, poles, sticks, or a human chain to reach the person.

■ If the victim is too weak to hold on, a rescuer can crawl along the ladder to help.

SOURCE: Adapted from American Red Cross, *Standard First Aid and Personal Safety* (New York: Doubleday, 1979) pp. 249–253.

stomach. The reason may be that digestion requires energy and oxygen, robbing them from the hard-working muscles. You need not stay out of the lake altogether after a picnic—just take it easy while your stomach is full.

To ensure safe boating pleasure:

■ Do not operate boating equipment if using alcohol or other drugs.
■ Know your boat and the rules of the waterway.
■ Carry safety equipment: make sure there are enough Coast Guard-approved personal flotation devices for everyone, and do not rely on inner tubes or toys as flotation devices.
■ Load the boat reasonably.
■ Keep your weight low in the boat.
■ Tell shore personnel where you are going and when to expect you back.
■ If the boat upsets or fills with water, hang onto it (it will probably still float).
■ If the weather threatens, skip the trip.

▣ OTHER SPORTS INJURIES AND ACCIDENTS

Fitness-minded people talk a lot about **shin splints**, **stress fractures**, **tennis elbows**, and an assortment of other anatomical hobgoblins. The Miniglossary of Sports Injuries lists the injuries that are mentioned most often. These and other injuries can be avoided by following a proper program that builds fitness slowly. The only reason why marathon runners can run so far without joint damage is that they have built up their capacities slowly over a long training period.[4]

> **MINIGLOSSARY**
> **of Sports Injuries**
>
> **damaged cartilage:** a joint injury. Cartilage damage is especially troublesome in the knee.
> **shin splints:** damage to the muscles and supporting tissues of the shin region from stress, shock, or excessive demands. Such damage usually heals with rest.
> **stress fractures:** bone damage resulting from repeated physical force that strains the attachment between ligament and bone.
> **tennis elbow:** a painful condition of arm and joint, usually caused by excessive strain, as from playing tennis.

Supportive shoes designed specifically for a sport are important, too, especially in foot-jarring activities such as jogging. Going easy on downhill runs and jogging on soft surfaces will help prevent injury. In tennis, proper equipment and correct stroke techniques taught early in training can prevent elbow and arm damage. In aerobic dance, sudden bursts of high-impact movements have caused many injuries. Supportive footwear and resilient flooring (not concrete under carpet) can reduce the impact to the feet and legs. Low-impact aerobic programs that do not require leaps and jumps are probably safer.

A "weekend athlete," who is sedentary all week and then exercises vigorously on weekends, is inviting injury. At the extreme, the sudden exertion can tax a weak heart to a dangerous degree. More commonly, though, vigorous and sudden demands on out-of-condition muscles, ligaments, and tendons lead to sprains and strains. Such people could take on a regular program of fitness to develop the strength that safe weekend play demands.

Pain during activity is a signal that something is wrong. For example, if a jogger feels leg pain, a change of posture may be indicated. If the pain persists despite efforts to correct technique, stop the activity until the pain goes away and then try again slowly, increasing just a little at a time.

If you have injured yourself, you have two options: to go to a health care provider or to wait to see whether it clears up by itself. (If you are bleeding or badly hurt, of course, choose the former.) Again, pain is your guide. If the pain diminishes during the first few hours, chances are the injury is slight. If it increases or stays the same for several hours, you may have a more serious condition that requires attention. If any injury fails to clear up in two or three days, get medical help, but while you are waiting, here is what you can do: elevate the injured part, and place an ice pack on it for as long as you can bear it throughout the first day. The second day, use ice several times for short periods. The ice reduces fluid accumulation, soothes pain, and promotes healing. Never use heat at first. Tape and bandages are first aid measures. Use them only to reduce swelling in conjunction with rest, ice, and elevation. Do not use them to enable you to keep playing despite an injury.

Heat is a by-product of energy fuel breakdown, so muscles heat up during exertion; they are "burning" large amounts of fuel. To maintain a normal body temperature, blood penetrates the muscles and transports the heat to the skin, where the surrounding air and the evaporation of sweat can carry it away. On humid days, sweat does not evaporate well, heat builds up, and the body sweats copiously in an attempt to effect cooling. This excessive sweating can be extremely hazardous, because fluid and electrolyte losses beyond a certain point disturb cellular functioning and can even be fatal.

The body sends signals of distress, such as cramps, nausea, chest pains, or diarrhea, that warn of **hyperthermia**: **heat stroke** may be threatening. The most important preventive step is to stop the activity immediately, even if you must lose a competition. For the same reasons, it is unwise to exercise in a plastic or rubber suit in hopes of losing pounds. The waterproof material prevents evaporation, causing you to sweat excessively, and brings about a dangerous rise in body temperature. Similarly, too long a stay in a hot whirlpool bath, hot tub, or sauna can cause heat stroke. Pointers to avoid heat stroke: drink adequate fluid, recognize dangerous conditions such as high humidity and temperature, limit intentional exposure to heat.

In potential heat stroke weather:

- Wear lightweight, loose-fitting clothing.
- Drink several extra glasses of water in the hours before you exercise heavily.
- Replace water lost during the activity (Table 6–1 of Chapter 6 explained how).
- Recognize your body's distress signals, and heed the message to stop exercising—take a rest in the shade.

Whenever you jog, bicycle, or walk along the roadside, traffic is a hazard. Two-thirds of all pedestrian deaths and injuries occur when people are crossing or entering streets. Some drivers may not see you; some may be out of control. Be sure to exercise these precautions:

- Cross only at intersections or marked crosswalks; obey traffic signals.
- Whenever you walk, jog, or bicycle alongside the street, always keep right, following the flow of traffic.
- Wear bright, easy-to-see clothing; wear reflective strips or tape at night.

To avoid inhaling exhaust and pollutants from passing cars, try to stay at least 50 feet off major roads while jogging, running or biking; and avoid activity during rush hour. If your city has no bike or jogging trails, you might be able to contact the elected public officials, such as city commissioners, and ask how to start such a project.

RAPE

Rape is a violent sexual act against another human being. Overwhelmingly, rapists are men, and the victims are women of all ages or children of either sex. Rape is not the result of passion in the rapist, nor is it caused by seductive behavior on the victim's part; in fact, the only role that the sex

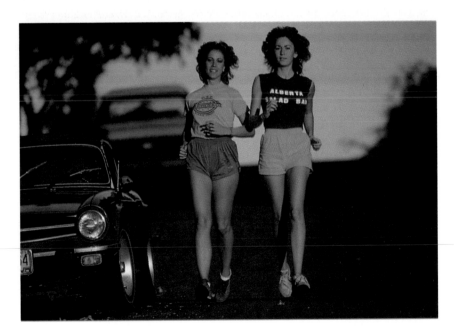

Run with a partner.

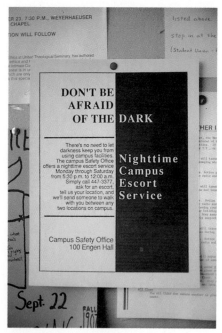

Use a rape-prevention service.

⊕ STRATEGIES: How to Protect Yourself against Rape

At home:

1. Keep your doors and windows locked. Use a dead-bolt door lock and a peephole to check visitors before opening the door. If a window can be opened, use a lock that keeps the opening to a maximum of five inches.

2. Verify the identity of men who claim to be salespeople, meter readers, and the like. Direct those who ask to use your telephone to the nearest pay phone.

3. Let no one except those you trust know when you are home alone.

4. Keep your shades drawn at night.

5. If you suspect that someone has broken in, do not go into the house alone.

6. Use only your last name on the mailbox and door.

7. Do not hide your key around the outside of your house; leave a copy with a trusted neighbor for emergencies.

8. Do not invite a man in, or go home with him, on your first or second date; wait until you know him very well.

In an elevator:

1. If a lone man of whom you are suspicious is in the elevator, do not get on.

2. Stand near the buttons and push as many as you can, including the alarm button, if someone bothers you.

3. If you are on your way up, do not ride down to the basement first.

In your car:

1. Make sure the car is in good working order and has plenty of gas.

2. Glance into the car, checking the seats and floor, before you get in.

3. Have your keys ready before you reach the car, get in quickly, and lock the doors.

4. If your car breaks down on the road, raise the hood, tie a white rag on the handle or aerial, and then get back into the car and lock the doors. Stay in the car and wait for the police.

5. Never pick up hitchhikers, and never hitchhike.

Some steps you can take to protect yourself outdoors are:

1. Stay alert to suspicious-looking people.

2. Use shopping bags and carts to free your arms for defense.

3. Stay on busy, well-lighted streets.

4. Make sure the street lamps on your block are working.

5. Have your keys ready before you get to your front door.

6. Carry a hatpin or stickpin in your hand.

7. At night, go with an escort and use a rape prevention service.

If efforts fail and you are attacked or approached:

1. Ring the nearest doorbell, if you are being followed.

2. Try to stall for time; someone may come along.

3. Scream "fire" (not "police," since others are then likely to avoid becoming involved), and pull a fire alarm box.

4. Break a window; someone is likely to respond to the noise.

5. Use your key or a stickpin to aim decisively for the attacker's eyes, temples, Adam's apple, or ears. Stab hard, without warning.

6. Try to disgust your attacker by urinating or by gagging yourself to induce vomiting. Tell him you have a sexually transmitted disease.

SOURCE: Adapted from Office of Justice Assistance, Research, and Statistics for the Crime Prevention Coalition, *How to Protect Yourself against Sexual Assault* (Washington, D.C.: Government Printing Office).

act plays in rape is that of a weapon. Rape is a violent crime with the intent to injure and humiliate the victim.

Rapists are usually unstable, aggressive men who have strong feelings of anger toward women. Often, the victim knows the attacker; it may be a relative, acquaintance, neighbor, repair person, or someone a woman is dating. Women can take steps to prevent some cases of rape, as this chapter's Strategies box shows.

POISONS AND RADIATION IN HOME AND WORKPLACE

People can be poisoned by swallowing, inhaling, injecting, or having skin contact with poisons. Many poisonings can be prevented by some simple precautions:

■ Read and heed all label directions.
■ Dispose of all chemicals and drugs you do not have to keep around and all old ones.
■ Keep chemicals and drugs out of reach of children and irresponsible people—under lock and key, if necessary (see box, "Preventing Child Poisoning").
■ Never store a chemical in a container that is used for food or drink; someone might mistake it for food or drink.

Poisons are also found in yard and garden plants, houseplants, and the like. Call the local agricultural department to learn which poison-containing plants grow or are sold in your area and what precautions to take. Also, ask about insects and animals you should watch out for.

A significant hazard from poisoning occurs in homes where people cannot see, feel, or smell it: slow poisoning due to repeated exposure to radiation and toxic substances within their own homes. The chief form of radiation

Preventing Child Poisoning

Children love to explore pretty bottles of pills and medicines; they also love to taste everything they touch. It is up to the adults around them—family members, visitors, babysitters—to keep dangerous items out of reach. The following list describes steps you can take to prevent child poisoning:

- Keep all household chemicals and medicines out of reach or locked up.
- If you are distracted from a job using such chemicals, carry them with you when answering the phone or door—do not leave them on the job site where children can get to them.
- Store items in their original containers, and especially do not use old food or drink containers—children may ingest the contents.
- Read labels on household chemicals, and reread them every time you use the products.
- Avoid letting children see you take medicine—they like to mimic what they see adults do.
- When giving medicine to children, call it medicine, not candy.
- Throw out unused medicines after the illness is over.
- Select OTC medicines and request prescription drugs in childproof containers.

that appears in many people's homes is from **radon**, a naturally occurring radioactive gas that seeps into homes from underground.[5]

In addition, many home-building and decorating materials contain toxic chemicals that, in tightly insulated homes, accumulate to cause hazards in indoor air. Particle board and plywood are preserved with one well-known toxic chemical, formaldehyde. Others abound in oil-based paints, varnishes, and polyurethane floor finishes; air fresheners, toilet-bowl cleaners, and moth crystals; newly dry-cleaned clothes; and even the hot water of a shower, if it comes from a chlorinated water source. Homes also often contain measurable levels of a number of pesticides. People exposed to high doses or repeated low doses of pesticides (including roach, flea, and termite killers in their own homes) may suffer impairment of their mental and physical capacities over the years. High-dose effects are easiest to demonstrate, but repeated low-dose effects also occur. Make sure your home is well ventilated; never stay in a closed space where you know or suspect that harmful chemicals may be in the air.

Other agents found in the home that act as stressors are noise, lights, dust and smoke from old heating devices, pet allergies, smokers' smoke, and many more. It is natural to feel safe in a cozy home, but do not be lulled into false security. Look at your home, now and then, as if you were encountering it for the first time. Take note of possible sources of trouble, and then correct them.

Like the home, the workplace should ideally be a hazard-free environment, but many workplaces are not, and workers are often not able to alter them. Many workplaces, by the nature of the work performed there, cannot be free of hazards. In industrial workplaces, for example, risks may include accidents; skin reactions and organ damage from injurious chemicals or

STRATEGIES to Protect Your Health in the Home or Workplace

For your own safety:

- **Study your home environment; improve its quality; correct hazards.**

radiation; lung damage from breathing toxic chemicals, including pesticides, gases, and dusts; hearing loss from excessive noise; and stress from job pressures, including the boredom of routine trivial tasks. These hazards can cause cancers, lung and heart diseases, birth defects, reduction or loss of the senses, injuries, and psychological problems.

People working in such places are responsible for learning what the hazards are, and their employers are responsible for informing workers about them. Workers are entitled to education and workplace changes to control hazards. Management should provide protective equipment and safety training, where necessary; and can also promote employee health by offering fitness programs that include exercise, stress management education, and screening for major chronic disease risks.[6] Employers are ultimately responsible for maintaining healthful and safe work environments, but it is well known that they do not always do so. Once they know the hazards, people may choose to avoid occupations that carry unacceptable risks or to take group action to demand appropriate treatment from managers, employers, and government.

⊛ **Learn the hazards associated with your occupation.***

⊛ **Avoid occupations that carry risks unacceptable to you.**

⊛ **Take group action to demand occupational safety and hazard control.**

▨ OTHER ACCIDENTS

Other accidents often arise from carelessness, and choking is one that can happen almost anywhere. To prevent choking, pay attention to what you are eating. Cut meat into small pieces, and take into your mouth only small forkfuls of any food. Do not attempt to speak or laugh with food in your mouth, and chew each bite thoroughly before attempting to swallow. Take particular care when eating round pieces of food such as grapes or cherry tomatoes—bite them with your front teeth to crush them. For small children, cut food into tiny pieces—even grapes and hotdogs should be cut before serving—or teach the child to bite them as adults do. Peanuts should be split open, and popcorn should not be served to small children, because it is light enough to be carried by the breath and round enough to lodge in the throat. If someone does choke, use the Heimlich maneuver to dislodge the particle from the throat. Appendix C gives a basic description of the maneuver, but you can best learn it in a first aid course.

Other accidents can arise from the careless use of tools, toys, and other devices. Most such accidents occur in the home. Work and leisure-time accidents add significantly to the number of deaths and injuries. To prevent them:

- Use sharp objects only for their intended purpose, handle them with care, and keep them out of the reach of children.
- Make sure that children's toys do not include sticks or articles that may break if the children fall (for example, bottles, glasses, or even some plastic toys).
- Do not allow children to play with fireworks.
- Mark large glass windows and doors so that everyone can see that they are not walk-through spaces.

*Write to OSHA: Office of Information and Consumer Affairs, Occupational Safety and Health Administration, Department of Labor, Room N3637, 200 Constitution Ave. NW, Washington, D.C. 20210. Telephone: (202) 523-8151.

- Evaluate as sources of injury all household appliances and equipment for work or play, including power tools, lawnmowers, and all electrical equipment.
- Follow the manufacturer's instructions carefully when using equipment.
- Unplug electric cords when equipment is not in use.
- Do not use electric appliances, such as hair dryers, around water, including the bathroom basin, tub, and other sinks.
- Instruct children not to play with or around television sets, electrical devices in the kitchen and bathroom, fans, power tools, household cleaning equipment, sewing machines, lawn tools, and other dangerous objects.
- Keep a neat house. Keep home, yard, garage, storage room, basement, and play areas free of trash and bottles.
- Clean up spills promptly to prevent slipping.
- Sweep up broken glass promptly. Discard cracked china and glassware. Children should always use nonbreakable dishes and containers; everyone should use them around tile and cement surfaces.
- Remove nails from boards in storage.
- Learn and obey all firearms safety rules.
- Keep guns and ammunition in separate places, each protected by lock and key.
- Do not allow children to play with any guns, including pellet and BB guns.
- Never load a gun until you are ready to shoot it. Assume that all guns you handle are loaded, even when you know they are not. Do not misuse blank cartridges; they can cause serious injury and even death.[7]

To avoid back injury while lifting an object, the Red Cross says:

- Plant the feet firmly and apart.
- Squat—do not lean—forward, keeping the back as straight as possible, and get a firm grip on the object.
- Lift slowly, pushing up with the strong thigh and leg muscles.
- Do not jerk the object upward or twist your body as you lift.
- To lower an object, reverse this procedure.[8]

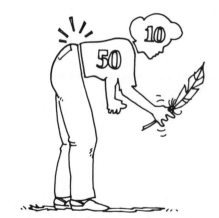

Your upper body is itself a heavy object.

Heavy objects are not the only ones that should be lifted this way. Your upper body itself is a heavy object, so whenever you bend over, you are asking your lower back muscles to hoist this weight. You can injure your back picking up a feather if you do it wrong.

Another threat, particularly for infants and older people, is **hypothermia**, a dangerous loss of body heat. During winter weather, the body can lose heat, especially through the head, neck, and feet. The person may not be aware of the drop in body temperature because age, illness, or drugs may have rendered them insensitive. The warning signs of hypothermia are mental confusion, cold or pale skin, bloated face, trembling, slow pulse, shallow breathing, and stiff movements. An oral temperature below 95 degrees Fahrenheit warrants medical attention; recovery is rare when the oral temperature drops to about 80 degrees Fahrenheit. People can get dangerously cold, and even die of hypothermia, at a room temperature as high as 65 degrees Fahrenheit, so wear socks and a hat if you feel chilly. Emergency measures for hypothermia are in Appendix C.

There are many more kinds of accidents, but the ones discussed here are considered most probable and therefore most important. The Red Cross book we have been referring to, *Standard First Aid and Personal Safety*, is also an invaluable reference; in fact, everyone should take a first aid course. Time is critical after an accident. Be sure that you know ahead of time how to call an ambulance, and memorize the locations of nearby trauma centers.

Earlier we showed that research on accident prevention is sadly lacking. Besides more research, major action on two additional fronts would help to reduce the toll accidents take every year. One is education: we need to teach safety in all settings to all segments of the population. The other is legislation: we have to adopt strong, enforceable laws to insist that people not endanger their own or other people's lives.

STUDY AIDS

1. Evaluate the likelihood of highway collisions for a person who does an average amount of driving.
2. List and describe the characteristics of the automobile driver who does the most to prevent highway accidents.
3. Describe why safety belts can prevent injury in the event of a highway accident.
4. List the duties of a responsible driver and motorcyclist.
5. List strategies to prevent the following kinds of accidents and injuries, and explain the rationale behind them:
   a. Falls.
   b. Fires.
   c. Drownings.
   d. Boating accidents.
   e. Sports injuries.
   f. Rape.
   g. Poisonings.
   h. Chokings.
   i. Miscellaneous accidents in the home.
6. Name areas of the body that are particularly vulnerable to injury, and describe ways to prevent injuries.
7. List the duties of a responsible pedestrian and those of a responsible jogger.
8. Explain why attitude is an essential component in preventing accidents of all kinds.
9. Describe which kinds of accidents pose the greatest risks to infants and which to older people.

GLOSSARY

accident: an unexpected and undesirable event; an unintentional happening. Many, though not all, accidents are preventable.
first aid: literally, aid given first or on the way to the hospital (although part of the training is knowing when to go and when not to go). Appendix C offers first aid basics.
hyperthermia: excess internal body temperature. Also called **heatstroke** or *sunstroke.*

hypothermia: a dangerous drop in internal body temperature.
radon: a naturally occurring radioactive gas that seeps into homes from underground.

QUIZ ANSWERS

1. *False.* One out of every three, not ten, people suffers an injury each year.
2. *False.* Skill is important, but attitude is equally important in preventing accidents on the road.
3. *True.* Safety belts sometimes cause injuries, but more often, they prevent them.
4. *True.* Small children in cars need better protection than safety belts can offer.

5. *False.* Older people are more likely to fall than younger people, because they are less coordinated.
6. *True.* A person climbing down a ladder should face the ladder.
7. *True.* Of all parts of the body, the head affects balance the most.
8. *False.* The Heimlich maneuver is a means of dislodging a particle caught in someone's throat.

9. *True.* You can injure your back picking up a feather.
10. *True.* The emergency telephone number in most parts of the United States is 911.

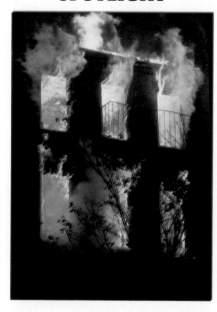

Fire Prevention and Escape

As mentioned, fires and burns are the third leading cause of accidental death in the United States. About 20 percent of those who die are children, and four out of five deaths caused by fire occur in the home. It is worth the time and space to offer some guidelines here on fire prevention.

That's fine with me. I already know most of the precautions, I think, but it never hurts to review them.

It's good to hear you say that. As with all accidents, the attitude of recognizing that fires are possible and the willingness to attend to safety precautions are the keys to prevention.

Multitudes of fires are caused by simple carelessness in the handling of matches and cigarettes—not only by children but also by adults. Multitudes are also caused by smoking in bed at home and in hotels and motels. To prevent these fires:

■ Dispose of cigarettes and matches safely. Never assume they are out when they might not be.
■ Keep matches and lighters out of the reach of children.
■ Do not smoke in bed. If you make a habit of smoking in bed, sooner or later (by the laws of chance) it is a virtual certainty that you will fall asleep while doing so.

The overuse of alcohol and other drugs is a particular hazard in combination with smoking—the person could lose consciousness before extinguishing the smoking materials.

Other fires are caused by cooking and heating equipment:

■ Keep cooking and heating equipment clean and in good repair, inspect it annually, and have experts service it.
■ Have heating systems and chimneys inspected every year; have experts make needed repairs.
■ If a gas pilot light or stove or oven burner goes out, ventilate the area thoroughly to dispel all fumes before relighting.

■ Turn pots on the stove so children cannot reach the handles. Keep the cords of electric cookware on the counter, not dangling.
■ Keep portable space heaters out of indoor traffic lanes, and turn them off before going to bed.
■ Keep cloth (curtains, pot holders, your own loose clothing) away from cooking surfaces and fires.

Still other fires are caused by flammable liquids:

■ Use such liquids only as directed.
■ Store them in safety containers that will not leak fumes into the air.
■ Store surplus quantities outside.

Related precautions:

■ Buy fireproof clothes for children. Be especially careful to buy fireproof pajamas, nightgowns, and robes.
■ Maintain your electrical wiring, and update it whenever you increase the load. Fuses (of the right size) and circuit breakers will keep wires from overheating to the fire point.
■ Maintain and repair tools, appliances, and electric cords when they show signs of wear. Have experts make repairs, especially on television sets.
■ Do not enclose television sets in tight spaces unless they are designed for such use.

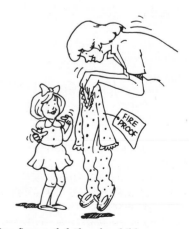

Buy fireproof clothes for children.

Three-hole wall receptacles mean the circuit is grounded. Three-prong plugs on appliances mean they *need* to be grounded to be safe. Plug them into three-hole plugs; and if you do not have such plugs, have your electrician install them.

What if a fire starts? It strikes me that planning what to do if a fire starts makes sense.

That is what the experts say. First of all, whenever you go into an unfamiliar building, imagine that it will start to go up in flames while you are in it, and plan your escape. Locate the exits, extinguishers, fire escapes, and stairways (never use an elevator in a fire). It is especially important to have an escape plan for your home. Figure out two ways to get outside from every room. Involve all your family members or roommates, including children. Make special plans to ensure that anyone who is handicapped can get out, too. Rehearse—even have a fire drill or two.

Picture the fire actually burning in your home or dwelling place—not for the sake of indulging in morbid imaginings but for further intelligent preventive work. By thinking through how a fire would spread from one place to another and how you would fight it, you can prepare the area in case such an emergency should arise. You will need a bucket here and another here. You will want to remove the trash from this area, so fire will not spread across it. You will need an outdoor faucet here and a hose nearby. Forethought is the only effective weapon; wishes are of no use in emergencies.

How about installing fire alarms in homes?

By all means do, and maintain them, too. Often, by the time people feel the heat or smell the smoke from a fire, it is too late to get out. Just a few minutes can be enough for poisonous fumes to accumulate—and most people die in fires because they

are unable to breathe, not because they are burned. Fire alarms, located in places where fires are likely to start, give people an early warning to make their escape. The fire alarms most recommended for homes are smoke detectors. Place them in locations that smoke would reach first—such as kitchens and peaks of ceilings—and within hearing range of the bedrooms.

Install fire extinguishers, too. But do not put them where the fire is most likely to be; put them where you can most likely get to them in case of fire. And learn how to use them. Using water on an electrical or chemical fire can cause more harm than good.

You mean if I use water, I can make a fire worse?

Yes, exactly. See Table S14–1.

OK, let's say a fire has started. Now what do I do?

First, grab a cloth (bedsheets work well), and wet it if possible. Cover your skin with it—most importantly, your nose and face. Put on hard shoes if you can get to them. Then, as you head for an exit, duck down. Do not run; crawl, because poisonous gases rise. If your clothes catch fire, roll on the ground, roll up in a rug, but *do not run*. Smother another person's flaming clothes with a coat or blanket.

Before you open a door, feel it; if it is hot, do not open it. (If there is no other way out, wait by a window; open it at the bottom for fresh air to breathe). When you do open a door, crouch behind it; expanding gas may explode into the room. Close doors behind you. And stay out of the elevator: elevators fail in fires. Use the stairs, or even jump from a window if necessary.

Put life before property. Do not try to save belongings unless you are sure you will have time. After everybody is out, call the fire department. See Appendix C for emergency measures to help the injured.

TABLE S14–1   Type of Fire Extinguishers and Fires

Type of Extinguisher	Class A (paper, wood, cloth, etc.)	Type of Fire Class B (chemical fire—burning gas, oil, paint, fat, etc.)	Class C (electrical fires involving live wires)
Carbon dioxide[a]	Yes, for small surface fires only	Yes	Yes
Dry chemical[b]	Yes, for small surface fires only	Yes	Yes
Foam[c]	Yes	Yes	Yes
Water[d]	Yes	No	No

NOTE: For a fire to burn, three components are necessary: fuel, oxygen, and heat. Removal of any of the three prevents or puts out fires.

[a]Carbon dioxide excludes oxygen. It leaves no residue, will not damage equipment or poison foods, and does not conduct electricity.

[b]Dry chemicals exclude oxygen. They leave a residue, produce a smothering gas that is effective on burning liquids, shield the operator from heat, and do not conduct electricity.

[c]Foam excludes oxygen and smothers fires. It does not dissipate; it stays on the material where it is sprayed, and it conducts electricity.

[d]Water saturates burning material and prevents rekindling of the fire—but will spread a burning liquid fire and, of course, conducts electricity.

SOURCE: Adapted from B. Q. Hafen and B. Peterson, *First Aid for Health Emergencies* (St. Paul, Minn.: West, 1977), Figure A–1, pp. 460–461.

Chapter 15

Infectious Diseases

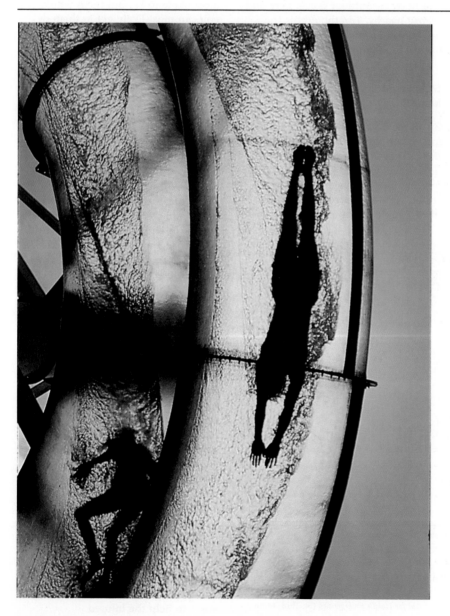

FOR OPENERS . . .

True or false? If false, say what is true.

1. It would be a great service to humankind if we could wipe out all microbes.
2. Antibiotics are among the few medicines effective against viruses.
3. Soap-and-water washing of the skin is useless against most infections.
4. Viruses have no way of eating.
5. Fevers are dangerous, especially when people have infections.
6. A hospital is a place where people can easily pick up infectious diseases.
7. Once a disease-causing microbe is in the body, it's too late to avoid the disease.
8. Sexually transmitted diseases (STDs) are rarely spread by anything except sexual activity.
9. Most cases of STD are known, treated, and reported.
10. To prevent STDs, a person can adopt a regimen of taking low doses of antibiotics daily.

(Answers on page 317.)

Advances in knowledge acquired in the last century account for a drastic difference between the causes of death that we face today and those faced by our ancestors. Medical research has bestowed on us techniques of both preventing and curing many of the **infectious diseases** that were killers in the past. Infectious diseases are no longer the leading cause of death in the developed nations. However, many infectious diseases still make people sick, and even with medical treatment, they can lead to consequences that last a lifetime. Also, there are still diseases for which no treatment exists.

RISKS OF INFECTION

You are surrounded. Microbes are all around you—on everything you touch, in the air you breathe, on the forkfuls of food that you lift to your mouth, and on your body. Most are harmless, but others can cause disease. This section describes the microbes and their world. The next section discusses two kinds of defense against disease-causing organisms: public health measures and your body's own remarkable devices to prevent infection.

A **microbe** is a living thing that is too small to be observed by the unaided human eye. Early scientists, using crude lenses, could see only the giants of the microbial world—molds, yeast, algae, and other creatures. With more powerful microscopes, smaller and smaller microbes have become visible, some so small that they contain only a few molecules.

In addition to being agents of disease, microbes have their good points. In the natural world, most microbes perform a service that is essential to life on earth: they break down life's wastes to their reusable nutrient components and other materials. They have far more impact than most people realize: in the top six inches of a square mile of soil, for example, there are 128 tons of **bacteria** at work; in one ton of soil, there are more than 900 trillion bacteria recycling waste materials back into useful forms. People have employed some microbes in the making of drugs, cheeses, breads, and alcoholic beverages. Through genetic engineering—splicing instructions for making a particular molecule into the microbial genetic material—microbes with no natural talents can be "taught" to make biological products needed by human beings.

Another service: the normal microbes of the intestines, the **endogenous bacteria**, manufacture vitamin K that the human body uses. For this reason, obtaining vitamin K is not a problem; you need not eat special foods to get enough.

Endogenous bacteria also protect against diseases by altering the body's internal chemistry. If they are reduced in numbers, infections become more likely, because disease-causing microbes, or **pathogens**, encounter less competition and find more nutrients available when they try to invade.

Some normally harmless endogenous bacteria can become pathogenic, however, given the opportunity. If a person's immune system becomes weakened, or if a wound occurs, these **opportunists** may invade and cause illness. All living things have evolved in harmony with microbial life forms, but each species has certain vexing microbes that can make it sick. Even the bacteria are attacked by smaller enemies—the viruses. The Miniglossary of Infectious Diseases names and defines a few of the diseases the pathogens produce.

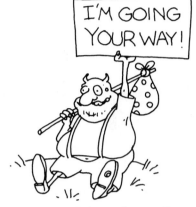

You are surrounded; microbes are all around you.

Microbe is a synonym for *microorganism*.

Vitamin K is essential for normal blood clotting.

PATH-oh-jen

Great fleas have little fleas upon their backs to bite 'em,
And little fleas have lesser fleas, and so *ad infinitum.*
And the great fleas themselves, in turn, have greater fleas to go on;
While these again have greater still, and greater still, and so on.
Augustus De Morgan (1806–1871), *A Budget of Paradoxes* (1872).

MINIGLOSSARY
of Infectious Diseases

acquired immune deficiency syndrome (AIDS): a fatal viral infection that is transmitted through mingling of body fluids, such as occurs during sexual intercourse or when drug users share needles. The words *immune deficiency* are often combined: *immunodeficiency*.

AIDS-related complex (ARC): a disease related to AIDS, thought to be a milder form or an early stage of AIDS. For other sexually transmitted diseases, see Table 15-1.

athlete's foot: a fungal infection of the feet, usually transmitted by wet floors; wearing rubber shower shoes will prevent its transmission.

bubonic plague: a bacterial infection causing swollen lymph glands and pneumonia, frequently fatal. Also called *black plague* or *black death*, it caused the near extinction of the population of Europe in the Middle Ages, and is still common in India today. It is transmitted by flea bites, so extermination of the rodent hosts aids in control of the disease; immunizations are also effective.

chicken pox: a usually mild, easily transmitted disease causing fever, weakness, and itchy blisters that, if scratched, may leave permanent scars on the skin. The herpes virus that causes chicken pox stays in the body for life and may later emerge as the painful skin condition called *shingles*. Once a person has been infected, immunity to chicken pox is lifelong.

cholera (KAH-ler-uh): a dangerous bacterial infection causing violent muscle cramps, severe vomiting and diarrhea, and severe water loss; without treatment, death is likely. People contract cholera by consuming infected water, milk, or foods (especially seafood harvested from contaminated water).

encephalitis: inflammation of the brain caused by viral infection. Mosquito control prevents transmission.

hepatitis: inflammation of the liver caused by one of several types of viruses that are transmitted mainly by infected hypodermic needles (drug use, tattoos, blood transfusions), by eating raw seafood harvested from contaminated water, and by any contact (including sexual) with body secretions from infected people. Sewage treatment and monitoring of commercial fisheries reduce these sources of infection.

Legionnaires' disease: a type of pneumonia caused by aquatic bacteria that can live in air-conditioning systems.

malaria: a parasite common to the tropics that resides within the red blood cells of the host, destroying the cells and causing high fever, anemia, and other symptoms. Mosquitoes transmit it to people who carry the parasite thereafter.

multiple sclerosis: a slowly developing disease of the central nervous system in which the nerve fiber coverings are destroyed. The cause is unknown, but a slow-acting virus is suspected.

mumps: a highly contagious viral disease that causes swelling of the salivary glands and, occasionally, of the testicles; preventable by immunization.

pneumonia: inflammation of the lungs with high fever, cough, and pain in the chest. A wide variety of bacteria, viruses, and some fungi cause pneumonia.

sexually transmitted disease (STD): formerly called *venereal disease (VD)*, one of the diseases caused by microbes that enter the body during sexual activity, especially intercourse. See Table 15-1 for specific diseases.

shingles: see *chicken pox*.

smallpox: a severe viral infection with skin eruptions similar to those of chicken pox but occurring all at once, about three or four days after the onset of the illness. Smallpox, once often fatal and permanently disfiguring to those who survived, is now under control worldwide, thanks to immunizations.

tetanus: a disease caused by a toxin produced by deep bacteria within a wound, which causes sustained contractions of body muscles and results in rigidity of the body and death from lack of oxygen or from exhaustion; preventable by immunization. Also called *lockjaw*.

traveler's diarrhea: sudden and severe diarrhea with general illness, caused by bacteria or parasites from the water supply; especially likely in countries with unsophisticated public health programs.

tuberculosis: a bacterial infection of the lungs.

Bacteria

The bacteria are one-celled organisms, similar to plant cells except that they lack chlorophyll. They alter their environment by way of their life processes, they use fuels in ways similar to human cells, and they sometimes produce toxins. Pathogenic bacteria grow and multiply best in conditions such as those found in the human body, which are:

- Warm.
- Dark.
- Moist.
- Nutrient rich.

Notice that oxygen is not listed as a requirement for bacteria. Some bacteria, the **aerobes**, require it, but others, the **anaerobes**, require environments that are devoid of oxygen. Anaerobes make puncture wounds dangerous, because they thrive in the interior of the wound, where medicines applied to the surface cannot reach. As first aid against them, the compound hydrogen peroxide is poured into the puncture, where it produces bubbles of oxygen that not only wash out the deep bacteria but also make conditions too airy for the anaerobes.

An infamous anaerobe is the one that causes **tetanus**, a disease that, once started, is fatal. Tetanus shots are important because they provide immunity against the bacterial toxin that causes the disease. Of course, any deep cut or puncture wound demands evaluation by a health professional. Appendix C offers a few basic wound treatment techniques. Much more can be learned in a first aid class.

A cut furnishes an opportunity for bacteria on the inhospitable skin to find themselves in warm, moist, nutrient-rich body fluid where they can grow and multiply. And multiply they do, not slowly, but geometrically— times 2 every hour or so (1 becomes 2, then 4, 8, 16, 32, 64, 128, and in just a few hours, millions).

As mentioned, microbiologists call these normally harmless resident bacteria opportunists, because they seize opportunities. If you fail to treat an infected cut, the bacteria may invade the bloodstream, causing a dangerous, generalized blood infection. Washing a wound and the surrounding skin with soap and water protects against opportunists. Soap does not kill bacteria but makes them slippery and allows the water to rinse them away. Also useful are **antiseptics,** chemicals that kill bacteria on the skin. Chemicals that kill bacteria on surfaces and elsewhere are **disinfectants** (household bleach is among the best).

Bacteria can invade uncut skin, too. One example is the endogenous skin bacteria that cause **acne** when the pores become clogged. Infection sets in when debris collects for the bacteria to feed on and they multiply. (Self-care tips for acne prevention are in the accompanying box.) Another example— people who use hot tubs often get bacterial skin rashes and ear infections from the bacteria that thrive in the infrequently changed warm water.[1*] (Hot tubs are harder to keep safe than regular swimming pools, because the heat and rapid water motion promote fast evaporation of the disinfectant chlorine.)

A bacterial infection of the lungs, **tuberculosis**, is the world's number one killer disease, affecting 1.5 billion people. In the United States, deaths from tuberculosis are rare, but the Public Health Service would like to reduce them further.

Viruses

The **viruses** are a unique life form. They depend entirely on the living tissue of other creatures; without it, they have no way of obtaining nutrients, purposefully moving about, managing energy, or reproducing themselves.

AIR-robe, AN-air-robe

Appendix C describes types of wounds and appropriate action to take when they occur.

✴ **STRATEGIES**
for Avoiding Infections

To avoid microbial illnesses:

✴ **Obtain medical treatment for deep wounds.**

✴ **Take measures to deter bacterial growth, both on your body and in your surroundings—maintain a cool, well-lit, dry, clean environment.**

✴ **Use soap and water to remove bacteria from skin; to kill bacteria, use antiseptics on skin and disinfectants on surfaces and elsewhere.**

*Reference notes are in Appendix D.

Acne

Most young people with acne are willing to go to considerable trouble and expense to find a remedy. But what is the remedy? To wash constantly? To sunbathe? To have the skin sanded? To take antibiotics? To spread vitamin A acid on the skin? To stop eating certain foods and drinking certain beverages? Or to try to find relief from stress? All of these approaches have been suggested, and each has helped some people in individual cases. But while advances are being made that give hope for the treatment of acne in the future, there is as yet no surefire way to get rid of it.

No one knows why some people get acne while others do not, but heredity plays a role—acne runs in families. The hormones of adolescence also play a role by increasing the activity of the glands in the skin. The skin's natural oil, **sebum**, is made in deep glands and is supposed to flow out through the tiny ducts around the hairs to the skin surface. In acne, the oily secretion is not brought to the surface of the skin.

Inside each of the ducts is a skin-like lining that regularly scales and flakes. The scales or flakes mix with the oil and then are pushed to the surface of the skin. At times, the scale sticks together and forms a plug, which may enlarge and weaken the duct, allowing oil and the skin-surface bacteria to leak into the surrounding skin. The oil and bacterial enzymes are irritating and cause redness, swelling, pus forma-

tion—and the beginning of a **whitehead**, or pimple. A **cyst** may be formed—a sort of enlarged, deep pimple. Or the skin may open above the plug, revealing an accumulation of dark skin pigments just below the surface—a **blackhead**.

Note that acne is not caused by the skin bacteria, although once the process has begun, they make it worse. Also note that the color of a blackhead is caused by skin pigments, not by dirt. Squeezing or picking at the lesions of acne in an attempt to remove their contents can cause more scars than the acne.

How, then, can acne be treated? Among the OTC acne treatments, preparations that contain benzoyl peroxide are safe and effective. The remedies mentioned at the start are sometimes helpful, too. Careful washing helps remove skin-surface bacteria and oil and keeps the oil ducts open; surface treatment with antibiotics also helps control the bacteria. A cream or gel containing retinoic acid (a member of the vitamin A family) can help: retinoic acid loosens the plugs that form in the ducts, allowing the oil to flow again so that the ducts will not burst. (This same medication may also smooth some wrinkling caused by sun.) But care is necessary in using it, because the acid may burn the skin and even cause pimples to form, making the acne look worse rather than better at first.

An internal medication, Accutane, is also related to vitamin A, and is reserved for the most severe cases

of acne. The drug has side effects, and can cause birth defects if taken during pregnancy. Women using it must take precautions against pregnancy.

At the end of adolescence, when the acne has subsided, a surgical procedure known as **dermabrasion**, or skin planing, can remove the scars—in some cases. (Be sure to request a second opinion beforehand, and select a dermatologist or plastic surgeon with a reputation for skill in this procedure.)

Prevention of acne has long been sought. Among foods charged with aggravating acne are chocolate, cola beverages, fatty or greasy foods, milk, nuts, sugar, and foods or salt containing iodine. None of these foods has been shown to worsen acne, and two have been shown not to worsen it—chocolate and sugar.

Stress, with its accompanying hormonal secretions, clearly worsens acne. Vacations from school pressures help to bring relief. The sun, the beach, and swimming also help, because they are relaxing, and also because the sun's rays kill bacteria and water cleanses the skin.

One remedy always works: time. While waiting for acne to clear up, keep the symptoms under control by using preparations with benzoyl peroxide or topical antibiotics available from a dermatogist. Even more important, prevent scarring by refraining from probing or picking at the skin. Also, keep a hopeful eye on the latest developments.

They do not eat, and they do not grow or mature. They have no metabolism. In fact, they may not really be alive at all. Furthermore, they can reassemble themselves after they have been taken apart—a characteristic living things do not share. Each virus has a unique body, made only of a protein coat that surrounds its genetic material.

Viruses cause diseases by invading cells. They usually attack cells that have soft, moist membranes, because such cells are easy to pierce and penetrate. Once inside, the invading viruses take over the cell's own genetic machinery and force it to serve their purposes—to reproduce viruses. The massive assembly line designed to replicate cell structures instead reproduces exact copies of the virus's genetic material and the parts that make up its outer coat, using up the cell's energy and raw materials in the process. From the pieces, new viruses assemble themselves. Then, typically, the cell bursts open, liberating multitudes of mature viruses to invade neighboring cells and restart the process. The one drawback to their system of survival is that, in order to reproduce, they must have access to the metabolic machinery of living cells.

When a person contracts a viral disease, treatment usually consists of minimizing damage and relieving symptoms while the disease runs its course. Antibiotics, effective against bacterial infections, are useless against viruses and can be dangerous in the long run.

Once the symptoms have subsided, the person may be free of the virus; however, some viruses can take up residence in the body to remain for life. In later years they can cause disease once again: an example is **shingles**, a painful skin condition in adults that is caused by the reemergence of the virus that brought them **chicken pox** as children. An adult with shingles can pass the virus to others, who will get chicken pox if they have not previously had the illness. Some of these lifetime viruses may act slowly over the years: one virus is suspected of eventually causing liver cancer, and another is suspected of causing the damage to nerve fibers seen in **multiple sclerosis**.

Parasites and Fungi

Literally, a **parasite** is an organism that lives at the expense of another; parasites depend on other organisms to produce the nutrients they need. The most familiar of the parasites are tiny animals that live on or in the body, and inflict bites on the victim to obtain blood. Worldwide, parasites cause many deaths from diarrhea, blood loss, and dehydration, especially among the very young or old, the malnourished, and those without access to medical treatment.

A class of plants that can cause disease, the **fungi**, do not capture the energy of sunlight to grow, as most plants do—they absorb and use nutrients manufactured by other organisms, living or dead. Microscopic, one-celled forms of fungi are **yeasts**; the multicellular types are **molds** and mushrooms. The yeasts can be pathogenic, and they cause an enormous variety of illnesses from **athlete's foot** to dangerous and incurable lung infections.

With so many microbes bombarding everyone every day, why aren't people ill from infection most of the time? Actually, it would be so, except that people have defenses. The public health system offers one, and people's immune systems provide another.

CONTROL OF INFECTIOUS DISEASE

For an infection to spread, several factors are required:

- A pathogen.
- A **reservoir** of infection—either water or a **host** (an animal or a person).
- A means of escaping from the reservoir (**portal of exit**).

MINIGLOSSARY
Acne

acne: chronic inflammation of the follicles and skin glands characterized by blackheads, cysts, whiteheads, and the accumulation of sebum (see below) inside the ducts around hairs.
blackheads: open lesions with an accumulation of dark skin pigment (not dirt) in their openings.
cysts: enlarged, deep pimples.
dermabrasion: a technique of planing the skin, used for the removal of certain kinds of acne scars.
sebum: the skin's natural oil, actually a mixture of oils and waxes, that helps keep skin and hair moist.
whitehead: a pimple caused by the plugging of an oil-gland duct with shed material from the duct lining.

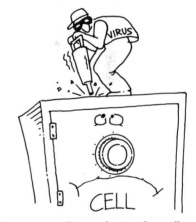

Viruses cause diseases by invading cells.

- A means of reaching the host, such as through the air, water, food, surfaces, sewage, and so on. A nonliving transmitter of infection such as a towel or drinking glass is a **fomite**; a living thing, such as an insect, that transmits an infection is a **vector**.
- A means of entering the host's body (**portal of entry**), such as the soft membranes of the mouth, nose, or eyes, or a break in the skin.
- Susceptibility to the infection in the new host.

To prevent the spread of infection, one of these factors must be eliminated. It may sound easy, but only a sophisticated public health system can succeed.

Public Health Defenses

The discoveries of the pathogens and of drugs to combat them are two reasons that death rates from infectious diseases have declined. Even more important are the public sanitation measures of developed countries that prevent **epidemics**. Chlorination of public water supplies and treatment of sewage destroy pathogens that could otherwise contaminate drinking water. Where sanitation is poor, sick people pass on such **endemic** diseases as **cholera** through sewage-contaminated water. When traveling to developing countries, you must take precautions against waterborne infections, which cause **traveler's diarrhea**: avoiding raw foods and salads and using the local water supply only after boiling it first.

Microbes are persistent and adaptable, despite public health measures. A disease new to this century that developed because microbes adapted successfully is **Legionnaires' disease**. In 1976, the American Legion held a convention at which many people became suddenly and violently ill with a mysterious onset of **pneumonia**. The new disease mystified scientists, who searched for a culprit in all the usual places—foods, water, and potential carriers—to no avail. Finally, they discovered that the hotel's air-conditioning coolant had become a habitat for aquatic bacteria never before identified as capable of causing disease. Tiny droplets of the bacteria-laden water were dispersed with the cooled air throughout the hotel and caused pneumonia in the lungs of those who inhaled them. Once the cause had been discovered, prevention was easily accomplished by disinfecting the water in the cooling system. That's how public health programs often work—by discovering the mode of transmission of disease and intervening. Another example: disinfectants applied to public showers and pool decks prevents transmission of the fungus that causes athlete's foot.

In contrast to bacteria and fungi, viruses cannot be so easily controlled, because they move directly from one living thing to another, where disinfectants cannot be applied. One method of prevention of both viral and bacterial diseases is vaccination. A **vaccination** or **immunization** is accomplished by injecting a drug made from destroyed and inactivated viruses, bacteria, or formerly toxic bacterial products. The drug trains the body's immune system to recognize the active viruses, bacteria, or toxins. Just as an airplane pilot in training practices on a flight simulator before trying out a real plane, the body practices on the vaccine as a sort of pathogen simulator. If the real invader arrives, the practiced reaction is so fast that disease never has a chance to develop. Thanks to aggressive vaccination efforts, not a single case of the devastating viral disease **smallpox** has been reported worldwide in over 10 years.

KAH-ler-uh

Pneumonia is really a group of diseases of the lungs, and it is a major threat to the lives of older people.

These examples have shown that understanding the mode of transmission of a pathogen provides a key to its control. A few more examples include **encephalitis, hepatitis, mumps**, and **bubonic plague**. If you are surprised that the ancient **pandemic** scourge bubonic plague is listed along with today's active diseases, keep in mind that the "controlled" diseases are simply that—they are under control. Their causes are alive and with us today, waiting in the wings for public health systems to break down, for catastrophes such as war to change things, or for drugs to lose their effectiveness. They could easily still cause disease should conditions become right once again.

Vigilance and effort are needed to keep up with the constantly changing status of infectious diseases. The diseases the U.S. Public Health Service is focusing on today are tuberculosis, hepatitis, pneumonia, Legionnaires' disease, AIDS (see later section), and hospital infections.[2] In hospitals, the high population density of people with infectious diseases favors the transmission of **nosocomial** (hospital-acquired) **infections**. It has been estimated that between 5 and 10 percent of people entering hospitals catch infections unrelated to their original condition, greatly extending hospital stays and expenses.[3]

The Body's Defenses

The skin and the membranous linings of the body's chambers are its first line of defense against invasion of microbes. The skin is a beautifully designed structure with salty, acidic sweat secretions (most pathogens don't like salt or acid) and one-way pores that let things out but won't let microbes in. However, the surfaces of the body chambers are lined with soft and moist membranes and are somewhat more susceptible to microbial attack than the tough outer skin. That is why most infectious diseases begin in the digestive, respiratory, reproductive, or urinary tracts. Still, the membranes fend off great numbers of microbes every day and are part of the body's first line of defense against diseases.

Should microbes penetrate into body tissues, the immune response provides a second line of defense. Usually, the immune system can intercept the invaders in time to prevent disease. Occasionally, though, the microbes multiply and produce illness. Not all diseases follow an orderly sequence of events, but many do, and five phases of the course of a typical disease have been identified (see Miniglossary: The Course of a Disease).

The prodrome, or general, symptoms listed in the Miniglossary are ones you might experience if you contracted one of a number of infections, many of them minor. One warning: if any of the symptoms listed in the box of Chapter 18 (When to Obtain Medical Help) are present, do not delay seeking help—they can mean the condition is serious.

Fevers have long been feared because they are associated with dangerous diseases, but the fever itself may actually assist the immune system. As mentioned in Chapter 7, fever stresses the body—it raises the heart rate and increases the tissues' demand for oxygen, and a weak heart could be damaged by the strain. Fever is not all bad, though. When fever is suppressed experimentally, sick animals are more likely to die from infection than when fever is allowed to run its course. Furthermore, animals kept continuously at fever temperatures resist viruses better than nonfeverish ones. Fever stimulates the immune system cells that fight infection.[4]

MINIGLOSSARY
The Course of a Disease

incubation: the period after initial invasion when microbes multiply in the body; the person may be unaware of the infection at this stage and may unwittingly infect others. The immune system may begin to detect the invaders; if the person was earlier vaccinated against the disease, the immune system will launch a full attack and stop the progression of the disease.

prodrome: the onset of general symptoms common to many diseases, such as fever, sneezing, and cough. Such symptoms are common to many diseases; in this stage, the disease is easily transmitted. The immune system is beginning to fight.

pro = before
drome = running

clinical period: the period of symptoms specific to the disease. The immune system is in full battle. (Medical intervention could possibly shorten this and succeeding stages.)

decline: the period when the immune system has almost won the fight against the infection, and symptoms are subsiding. Memory cells form.

convalescence: the period when the body repairs damage and returns to normal immune operations. The microbe may or may not remain in the body; if it does, the person may remain a carrier of the disease, able to infect others even if no symptoms are evident.

Oral temperatures over 104° F: Seek medical attention.
Oral temperatures over 100° F: Control with aspirin, acetaminophen, or ibuprofen.
Oral temperatures 100° F and less: Do not treat.
(If fever persists, see a health care provider.)

Public health and the body's defenses protect the population against many diseases, but these defenses can do only so much. At a certain point protection from infectious diseases becomes your own responsibility.

Sneezes contain millions of microbes.

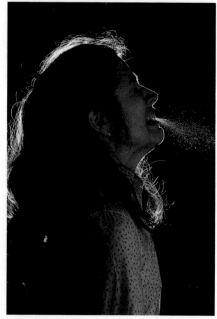

Strategies against Infectious Diseases

One of the most important steps a person can take to avoid infectious diseases is to keep immunizations up to date, especially against those diseases to which exposure is likely. This chapter's Life Choice Inventory lists immunizations recommended for children and adults, and it asks you to check your immunization records. If you don't know whether you've had the needed ones, call your health care provider to find out.

What can people do to prevent those diseases that have no vaccine? Some illnesses are so widespread and common that you need to be vigilant against them all the time—namely, colds.

The easiest way for viruses and bacteria to reach you is for you to pick them up and transfer them to your mouth, eyes, nose, or other portal of entry. One plan of defense is to avoid unnecessary contact with people who are ill or the objects that surround them. Don't touch what they touch, and wash your hands often with soap and water, especially before eating.

Millions of microbes are sprayed into the air by uncovered sneezes and coughs, so try to place yourself a good distance away from someone who is carelessly sneezing or coughing into the air. They probably have a cold, but it could be the prodrome of tuberculosis, pneumonia, or flu. Cover your own coughs and sneezes with disposable tissues to keep from spreading the infection.[5]

Keep up your resistance to infection by taking care of your immune system; it works best when given a balanced diet. For example, children in developing countries who show signs of vitamin A deficiency have a higher than normal rate of death and disease from infections. Vitamin A also plays a key role in maintenance of the skin and other barrier membranes; when the vitamin is lacking, the membranes break down, allowing microbes to enter. Vitamin A supplements are not what you need, though; the pills might become toxic with repeated use. Instead, choose vehicles of the non-toxic form of vitamin A: dark green, leafy vegetables and deep orange fruits and vegetables, in balance with the other foods you need. Related to diet is alcohol intake. Alcohol makes the body discard its supplies of many vitamins and minerals, to the detriment of the immune system.

Regular aerobic exercise supports the immune system, stimulating growth of its thymus gland and its infection-fighting cells.[6] Tobacco has the opposite effect. Chemicals in tobacco are thought to lower the number of immune cells. If you use tobacco, make plans to stop.

Stress management is a major part of your strategy against infectious disease. When the immune system is suppressed by sustained stress, lowered resistance can permit microbes to cause cold sores, acne flare-ups, and sore throats. You may have noticed that when you are worried or nervous about something, your throat tends to get sore. This is a warning that, before long, unless you manage the stress better, the microbes already present there will make you ill. Remember, it's not the events of your life that create stress; it's *how you perceive* them. To some extent, you can control your perceptions, and so you can modulate your stress response (see Chapter 2).

LIFE CHOICE INVENTORY

How well-protected are you against infectious diseases? Check *Yes* if you've been immunized for all that apply to you. If you check *No*, and you fit the description of who should be immunized, ask a health professional about it.

Your History

Age:	Vaccine:	Response:	
2 months	DPT (diphtheria, pertussis, tetanus), oral polio	Y	N
4 months	DPT	Y	N
6 months	DPT (Some physicians also recommend an additional dose of oral polio.)	Y	N
12 months	Tuberculin test	Y	N
15 months	Measles, rubella, mumps (combined vaccine MMR)	Y	N
18 months	DPT booster, oral polio	Y	N
5 to 6 years	DPT booster, polio booster	Y	N
14 to 16 years	Tetanus-diphtheria toxoid, adult type; booster every ten years or after a contaminated wound if more than five years have passed since the previous injection	Y	N

Your Present Status

Adults:	Vaccine:	Response:	
Never-vaccinated young men and women (nonpregnant)	Rubella, to decrease risks to fetuses	Y	N
Adults born after 1956 never vaccinated for the disease who have never had it	Live measles (People vaccinated between 1963 and 1967 with the killed measles vaccine should be revaccinated with the more effective live vaccine.)	Y	N
Anyone who has not had the disease or the vaccine	Mumps	Y	N
Nonimmunized adults over 65 years of age	Pneumococcal vaccine (One-time injection protects against the most common form of pneumonia.)	Y	N
All adults over 65 years of age and other adults with chronic ailments	Influenza (Vaccine changes yearly as the virus changes identity; given in anticipation of the varieties likely to attack.)	Y	N
People who hold high-risk jobs (health care workers); homosexuals; intravenous drug users	Hepatitis B series	Y	N
People who travel to high-risk areas, particularly to less-developed countries	Any of the above vaccines, plus polio, hepatitis A, plague, rabies, typhoid fever, cholera, and yellow fever	Y	N

SOURCES: C. Ballentine, Shots *adults* shouldn't do without, *FDA Consumer*, June 1986, pp.13-15; *Immunization—When and Why*, a 1981 leaflet available from Metropolitan Life Insurance Company; S. R. Preblud, Some current issues relating to rubella vaccine, *Journal of the American Medical Association* 254 (1985): 253-256.

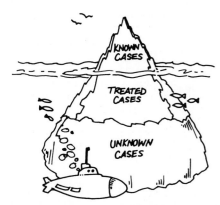

The known cases of STD: the tip of the iceberg.

Intelligent stress management can take you a long way toward the prevention of disease.

SEXUALLY TRANSMITTED DISEASE (STD)

Pathogens that cause the **sexually transmitted diseases** (STDs) make an easy living because they are transmitted directly from person to person by way of sexual contact. The delicate, vulnerable membranes of the reproductive tract make a perfect portal of entry for microbes. The moist, warm, dark environment encourages their growth, and the immune system develops no permanent defense against them. Some STDs, such as pubic lice, can be transmitted by any close body contact or by the sharing of towels or bedclothes, but most require genital, oral, or anal intercourse for transmission. None are transmitted through the air. Once in the body, STDs may threaten health, or they may be mere nuisances; some are treatable, and some are incurable. The known cases of STDs make up an epidemic of disease in the United States, and we are aware of only the tip of the iceberg. By far, most cases are unreported.

Common Sexually Transmitted Diseases

Until the discovery of antibiotics, contracting an STD led to severe, progressive, and inevitable consequences. In those days, the medical community had no power to stop the progression of symptoms and experienced the same helplessness as today's medical experts trying to help people who have contracted AIDS. Table 15–1 lists some of the most prevalent STDs and those that cause serious illness. AIDS is listed in the table, but the urgency of the problem and its grievous consequences demand fuller treatment, and we have devoted an entire later section to it. The margin notes some people who are believed to have suffered the progressive and devastating effects of syphilis.

Sometimes STDs can advance without giving any symptoms to warn that they are present; for example, gonorrhea infections, especially in women.

Famous and infamous people suspected of suffering from the brain damage and other symptoms of syphilis: Julius Caesar, Cleopatra, Napoleon Bonaparte, Catherine the Great, Peter the Great, Henry VIII, Mary Tudor, John Keats, Franz Schubert, Oscar Wilde, Vincent van Gogh, Friedrich Nietzsche, Ludwig van Beethoven, Thomas Mann, and Adolf Hitler.

TABLE 15-1 Sexually Transmitted Diseases

Name	Symptoms	Treatment	Potential Complications	Prevention
Acquired immune deficiency syndrome (AIDS)	Swollen lymph glands, diarrhea, pneumonia, weight loss, mental symptoms, rashes, infections	Symptom relief only; no cure	Severe illnesses leading to death in 6 months to 2 years	Use condoms, screen partners[a]
Bladder infection (bacterial)	Painful, burning urination; frequent urination; foul-smelling, cloudy urine; lower abdominal pain; blood in urine	Antibiotics	Recurrence	Urinate often, drink ample water, wear cotton underpants, urinate after sex[b]
Chlamydia infection	Burning on urination; vaginal discharge; symptoms of PID (see below); in males, infection of urethra	Antibiotics	Pneumonia of newborn, possible cervical cancer risk	Avoid multiple partners, use condoms
Genital bacterial infections	Yellow, green, or chalky white discharge; pain on urination; vaginal itching; painful intercourse; foul odor of discharge	Antibiotics	Infection of reproductive glands and organs, PID (see below)	Avoid multiple partners, use condoms
Genital herpes	Many blisterlike sores on genital organs, itching, pain	No effective known cure, but prescription cream may lessen the severity and duration of attacks	Recurrence of lesions, eye infection, generalized infection of newborn during birth	Avoid oral-genital contact or intercourse when sores are present, use condoms even if sores are not present, do not deliver a baby vaginally if sores are present
Genital warts	Dry, wartlike growths on penis, labia, cervix, vagina; constant discharge; itching	Removal	Recurrence of warts, cervical cancer risk	Avoid multiple partners; use condoms, do not deliver a baby vaginally if warts are present
Gonorrhea	Possibly no symptoms; vaginal/penile discharge; in males, painful urination, tender lymph nodes, testicular/abdominal pain, fever; in females, painful menstruation or urination, bleeding after intercourse	Antibiotics	Sterility, eye infections, blindness, PID (see below), arthritis, infection of heart lining, infection of eyes of newborns	Avoid multiple partners, use spermicides for some protection, use condoms
Pelvic inflammatory disease (PID)	Pain in abdomen, back, pelvic area, legs; fever; chills; vomiting; excessive menstrual bleeding; painful urination; painful sexual intercourse with bleeding afterward	Antibiotics	Sterility, chronic pain, chronic infections, abscess of ovaries or fallopian tubes	Avoid multiple partners, use condoms, avoid IUDs and douches

[a]See full description of AIDS beginning on page 313.

[b]Drinking cranberry juice is not effective for prevention or treatment.

(Continued on next page)

TABLE 15–1 Continued

Name	Symptoms	Treatment	Potential Complications	Prevention
Pubic lice	Itching, lice in pubic hair, eggs possibly visible clinging to strands	Medicated shampoo (prescription)	None	Avoid multiple partners and sharing of towels or bedclothes
Syphilis	*Primary* (3 weeks after exposure): Chancre on penis, vagina, rectum, anus, cervix *Secondary* (6 weeks after primary): Rash on feet and hands; flulike symptoms including anorexia, fever, sore throat, nausea; flat-topped growths; headaches *Tertiary* (10 to 20 years later): See "Potential Complications"	Antibiotics	Brain damage; heart disease; spinal cord damage; blindness; infection of fetus, causing death or severe retardation and the above complications	Avoid multiple partners, use condoms
Trichomoniasis	Possibly no symptoms in men; frothy, thin, greenish discharge; genital itching and pain; frequent urination	Antibiotics	None	Avoid multiple partners, use condoms
Yeast infection (*Candida*)	Thick, curdled discharge; itching and redness of external genitalia	Antibiotics	Recurrence	Medically prescribed douches, lose weight if obese, control diabetes

SOURCE: Adapted primarily from R. A. Hatcher and coauthors, *Contraceptive Technology 1984–1985* (New York: Irvington, 1984), pp. 270–278.

Another silent infection is pelvic inflammatory disease (PID), a dangerous infection of the uterus and associated organs that afflicts almost a million women each year. PID may be responsible for 30 to 40 percent of all cases of infertility among women and for about half of all ectopic pregnancies.[7] It is a good idea for every sexually active, healthy person to have an STD exam once a year or so, especially if the person has had more than one, or has changed, sex partners.

Another STD, genital herpes, is caused by a virus related to the one that takes up residence in the nerve fibers of the face and is responsible for fever blisters (cold sores) on the lips. In fact, the two viruses are so closely related that they can take each other's places—the genital type shows up in cold sores and the facial type, in genital infections. This means that a person with a cold sore or a genital herpes outbreak should not engage in oral sex or intercourse. Condoms can prevent genital transmission.

The two types share another aspect: both are incurable. This is so because once the virus has established residence in the nerve fibers, it is completely safe from any attempts at wiping it out. We have long known that the virus is transmitted from active sores to sexual partners; a more recent study found the virus in semen even when the men studied had no symptoms, causing suspicion that the disease might be transmissible even without lesions.[8]

Genital herpes is of minor medical importance; of greater concern is that its diagnosis causes some people excessive emotional turmoil, including episodes of depression, loss of self-esteem, and a sense of isolation. Some people avoid intimacy and sexual intercourse altogether when they learn they've been infected. Joining a local or national support group can help a person get over negative feelings.*

A virus also causes genital warts—warty, sometimes painful growths that are transmitted through sexual intercourse. Experts believe that the wart-causing virus is responsible for a fast-spreading cancer of the cervix that is occurring with increasing frequency among young women.[9] The warts themselves may be removed surgically, but the virus may be transmissible through the semen of infected men, with or without the presence of warty growths.[10]

Many STDs can reach a fetus and damage it in the uterus or attack it as it passes through the birth canal. To protect a baby against blindness from gonorrhea, drops of an antimicrobial drug are placed in the infant's eyes within minutes after birth. Science is working to perfect a vaccine against gonorrhea so that infant infections, as well as others, can be prevented. Genital herpes has also been known to infect infants during the birth process, causing blindness and severe mental retardation. A woman who has active herpes lesions when labor begins may require a surgical delivery to bypass the infected area of the birth canal. In a woman who has syphilis, the fetus is certain to become infected with the disease unless the mother receives treatment in early pregnancy. Syphilis may kill the fetus or cause birth defects, including severe mental retardation that may manifest itself in later childhood even if the infant appears normal. Curing syphilis after birth does not restore full potential for a normal life. Many a mentally retarded person in institutions today could have enjoyed a normal life had the mother's disease been diagnosed and treated.

Chlamydia infections, estimated to occur at ten times the rate of gonorrhea, cause minor irritations or no symptoms in men. In women and infants, though, the effects are severe. A woman with a *Chlamydia* infection may experience ectopic pregnancy; even if the location of the pregnancy is normal, the microbe may invade the uterus, causing PID. The infant, too, may be invaded during birth and suffer pneumonia or eye infection.

Strategies against STDs

Clearly, people must use strategies against STDs to protect themselves, each other, and future generations. This chapter's Strategies box is divided into two parts. The first offers guidelines for protecting yourself against the common STDs and actions to take if you suspect you may have been infected. Later, Part II of the box spells out what rules exist to protect against AIDS.

Many times STDs occur in pairs. Syphilis is a particularly dangerous second infection—its characteristic early symptom is a painless sore, easily disguised in, say, a cluster of herpes blisters. The herpes may or may not occur again, but the syphilis will spread throughout the body. The only external signs of advancing syphilis might be symptoms that resemble flu; meanwhile, the disease can progress to damage irreversibly such organs as the brain and heart. The second-infection threat holds true for all STDs listed in Table 15–1, even pubic lice. That is why medical treatment should be sought for even a simple problem: syphilis or gonorrhea may be lurking along with the symptomatic disease.

*An agency of the United Way is HELP, P.O. Box 100, Palo Alto, CA 94302.

STRATEGIES: PART I Rules for Avoiding Common Sexually Transmitted Diseases

To avoid contracting an STD:
1. Abstain from sexual activity. This is the only way to guarantee safety from STDs.
2. If you are considering a sexual relationship, choose your partner with extreme care. Know his or her sexual history for the past five years. If *any* of the person's past partners had an STD, then the disease may be passed on to you. Take your time in getting to know your potential partner and remember that many people are reluctant to disclose every past relationship.
3. Use condoms and spermicide (see Chapter 11 for details).
4. Observe your partner for rashes or sores before you have contact. If you find them, avoid contact until your partner has obtained medical treatment. (Remember, though, that not all diseases will be visible to the eye, so observation of no sores does not mean that no disease is present.)
5. Do not participate in casual sex or have sex with prostitutes.
6. Urinate immediately after sexual activity; this may help to expel infectious organisms from the urinary tract. Also, wash the genital organs.
7. If sexually active, get regular checkups and request an STD exam.
If you suspect you may already have an infection:
1. See a health professional. Treatment is reported, but confidentially—no one you know will find out.
2. Follow the prescribed treatment carefully.
3. Notify your sexual partner(s), and make sure they've been treated before you resume sexual activity.

If you care enough to hesitate, you care enough to tell your partner.

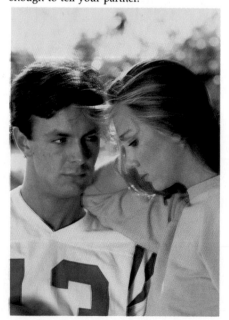

People who are sexually intimate have rights and responsibilities—the right to be informed if a dangerous disease is a possibility and the responsibility to inform all sex partners that treatment is needed, if a positive diagnosis has been made. After all, if you value someone enough to worry about losing his or her affection, then a way to prove you care is to warn the person of physical danger. Besides, simultaneous treatment of sexual partners is essential to keep them from reinfecting each other. The thought of telling a partner of a diagnosis of STD can be psychologically threatening to people who think that only people of low character get these diseases, but in reality, STDs are simply infections, just as colds are. Nice people who are careful can get them; having one is not a reflection on a person's character, only on the resourcefulness of microbes in attacking people.

The best way to tell someone is simply to do it as directly as possible—in person or on the phone, when you are sure only that person is listening. If telling someone this way is impossible—for example, if you are out of the country when the diagnosis is made—you should send the person a letter. A danger of this method is that letters have a way of getting opened by other people or lost in the mail. If a letter is the only option, include these elements:

- That you have been diagnosed with an STD and that your partner (or former partner) may therefore have it too, even if no symptoms have appeared.
- That the person should see a health care provider or go to a clinic at once.
- That the person should immediately inform anyone else who might have it.

Above all, it is essential to inform.

◼ ACQUIRED IMMUNE DEFICIENCY SYNDROME (AIDS)

A disease of enormous concern worldwide is **acquired immune deficiency syndrome (AIDS)**. It was first described in 1978 and was named in 1979. Since then, it has become pandemic, emerging in country after country, and the reaction of the mass-communication media has bordered on panic. In one way, the publicity is helpful—it focuses world effort on stopping AIDS from becoming a bigger problem. But it has a negative side, too; it presents a distorted view of a real threat and encourages hysteria rather than effective action.

Some degree of fear is rational. At present, tens of thousands of cases of AIDS have been reported in the United States alone, and no recoveries have occurred.[11] Most victims die within two years of developing symptoms. Public health strategies are failing to stop the general spread of AIDS, for several reasons. First, its carriers are human beings, so we cannot eliminate the vectors; second, its primary means of transmission, sexual activity, is beyond the reach of public health control; and third, a vaccine is slow in coming because the AIDS virus alters its identity, effectively hiding from even a prepared immune system.* A massive research effort on this last front is under way, because, as with other viral diseases, prevention may be the most effective means of controlling AIDS. The fruits of research are changing the established body of AIDS information almost daily. This section attempts to furnish a basic understanding of the AIDS virus, so that you can evaluate new information as it becomes available.

AIDS Infection

The disease's name describes it: acquired (people contract it; it is not genetic) immune deficiency (the immune system becomes unable to defend against invading disease) syndrome (the disease is characterized by a group of symptoms). Infection with the AIDS virus does not immediately lead to a full-blown case of the disease, although victims may experience a general body illness with tiredness and a run-down feeling within a few months of exposure. Afterward, victims usually remain in good health for many years (remain asymptomatic) or develop a milder illness called **AIDS-related complex (ARC)**. It is thought that people with ARC progress to the more lethal form of the disease and that asymptomatic infections later become AIDS or ARC. Over a hundred thousand people in the United States were suffering from ARC by the late 1980s.[12]

What *has* happened:

1979	AIDS-like symptoms observed
1981	AIDS identified
1986	25,000 total cases of AIDS, and up to 125,000 cases of ARC (see text), reported in the United States

What *might* happen:

1991	Predicted 270,000 reported cases and 179,000 total deaths; one of the top killers of adults

SOURCE: U.S. Department of Health and Human Services, *Acquired Immune Deficiency Syndrome*, Surgeon General's Report, HHS publication no. 86-888, 1986.

---

*The virus has been called *human T-lymphotropic virus, type III (HTLV-III)* or *lymphadenopathy-associated virus (LAV)*, or a combination of the two. As of 1986, the name *human immunodeficiency virus (HIV-1)* is official. Human immunodeficiency viruses, *Science* 232 (1986): 697. Researchers believe that a second, related virus (so-called HIV-2) may also be pathogenic and spreading.

AIDS begins when the virus selectively uses the immune system cells for replication, specifically, the immune cells called *T cells*. The virus acts as any other virus does, by invading the cell, taking over the replication machinery, and reproducing, using the cell's resources. The AIDS virus replicates faster than any other known virus and hides within the immune system's own cells to avoid detection.[13] The virus is transmitted from one person to another whenever body fluids containing infected cells pass from one to another—either through blood products or through contact with secretions of the reproductive organs, as explained later. As T cells are destroyed by replicating viruses, their number dwindles, disabling their essential function of triggering the production of antibodies. With the immune system thus crippled, other opportunistic infections thrive unchecked.

Shortly after the discovery of the AIDS virus, scientists developed a blood test to detect it. A positive test means that the person has been exposed to the virus. The test is most useful for screening blood products intended for medical use to prevent infection from transfusions. The diagnosis of AIDS is based on the presence of certain opportunistic diseases plus a positive result for the blood test.

The AIDS disease usually starts with swollen lymph nodes, skin rashes, fever, and diarrhea, although it has been known to start with mental symptoms.[14] It progresses to fungal infections of the mouth, rare types of pneumonia and cancer, a brain disorder of a type seen only in people with compromised, or damaged, immunity, and a long list of other opportunistic diseases. In children, the soft tissues, including the brain, calcify. The victims do not die of AIDS itself; they die of other diseases against which they have been rendered defenseless.

Physicians use drugs, radiation, and surgery to control the conditions suffered by AIDS victims, but with virus-damaged immune systems, the victims cannot be permanently cured. New drug testing is on a rush schedule, bypassing or shortcutting some of the safety controls normally applied before drugs or treatments can be used on people. Even toxic or experimental drugs are valuable to victims, if they can forestall the advancement of the disease and prolong life while research aims for treatments that will restore immunity.

In the United States, AIDS strikes people of certain population subgroups most often, with male homosexuals, intravenous drug users, blacks and Hispanics, and immigrants from AIDS-endemic countries being most significant. A few people were infected through blood products before screening of such products became routine; others are infected through heterosexual relations with AIDS victims; and a few others, infants, are infected at birth. Women contract AIDS less frequently than do men.

As time passes, more and more diagnoses of AIDS are made in people who do not belong to these subgroups. Both men and women can transmit AIDS, and some fear that AIDS could become one of the ten most frequent causes of death in both men and women in the United States by the early 1990s.[15]

It is as important to know how AIDS is *not* transmitted as to know how it is transmitted. Not one case of AIDS has occurred through casual contact (including kissing) with AIDS victims or carriers. No cases have been found in which AIDS has been transmitted by everyday household contact among family members.[16] Although the AIDS virus has been found in saliva and tears, exposure to either has never been shown to result in transmission.

Ambulance drivers, police, and fire fighters who have assisted AIDS sufferers have not become ill, although they are advised to minimize contact with injured people's blood. AIDS is also not transmitted by mosquitos, vaccinations, saunas, pools, or food handled by AIDS-positive persons.

People who work in hospitals that treat AIDS also seem, for the most part, to be safe from infection. There have been only a very few reports of health care workers who have tested positive for AIDS after being accidentally stuck by used hypodermic needles; a very few others tested positive after being splashed with infected blood. The latter few had skin abnormalities that offered a portal of entry for the virus, and they were not wearing the protective gear (such as rubber gloves) recommended for health care providers who are exposed to infectious diseases.

The risk of getting AIDS is increased by having multiple sexual partners, either homosexual or heterosexual. It is not enough to know the person for a few weeks or months; a history of multiple sex partners or intravenous drug use within the last five years signifies risk. People who appear perfectly healthy and who feel well may be in the symptomless incubation stage—a period of six months to five years, or even up to 14 years in some cases.[17] A person in the incubation stage is as contagious as someone with full-blown AIDS because, during incubation, the person has virus-infected T cells in the blood.[18] Public health measures such as blood donor screening are preventing some cases of AIDS, but evidence is strong that we need massive education to promote individual protection.[19]

Strategies against AIDS

Today, many cases of AIDS are being prevented. Blood products used in medical treatments are now considered safe because donors are screened for AIDS antibodies and carriers' blood is not used. As a backup, blood products are treated by methods that deactivate viruses. Still, a person who is planning to have surgery may choose to donate blood to be stored for use during the operation, should a transfusion be needed. Some people may fear (irrationally) that a danger is associated with medical uses of blood or even with *donating* blood. Blood banks and other blood collection centers use sterile equipment and disposable needles, so the risk in such settings is absolutely zero.

AIDS is not just a health problem. It is also a social, political, economic, and ethical one. Countries are blaming each other or denying the existence of AIDS to maintain the illusion that homosexuality and drugs are not their problems. In ignorance, some hospitals turn away AIDS victims; certain funeral parlors will not accept them. Some AIDS victims who have no easily transmissible diseases are barred from school or work. Known homosexuals are fired from their jobs for fear they might be carriers. These are hysterical, irrational reactions not based on science.[20] AIDS is frightening, but it is not easily transmitted: its transmission requires sexual activity, blood sharing, or infection at or before birth. Thus, you can protect yourself (see Strategies box, Part II).

Abstinence from sexual activity is a choice more and more people are making to protect themselves from AIDS and other STDs. Casual, unprotected sexual activity is no longer acceptable. Condoms are taking on double duty—contraception and prevention of disease and Chapter 11 describes their use.

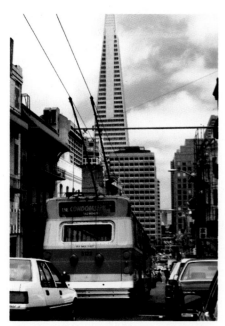

The condom is one defense against AIDS.

⊛ STRATEGIES: PART II   Rules to Prevent AIDS

If you are sexually active, the following strategies are recommended by the surgeon general:

1. Always use a condom and spermicidal cream, jelly, or foam during sexual activity, both homosexual and heterosexual, unless you have been in only one relationship for five years or more and neither partner has used intravenous drugs in the past five years.

2. If you suspect that your partner is at high risk for AIDS, or if he or she has a positive blood test, always use a condom during intercourse. Avoid mouth contact with the penis, vagina, or rectum.

3. Do not have sexual intercourse with prostitutes.

4. If you are addicted to an injected drug, seek help for the addiction; meanwhile, use only clean, unused syringes.

And you must protect your partner:

1. If you have had multiple sex partners, homosexual or heterosexual, or if you have injected drugs in the last five years, you should have a blood test to determine if you have been exposed to the AIDS virus.

2. If your test is positive, or if you are at risk and choose not to have a test, tell your sex partner. If you decide, and your partner agrees, to have sex, always use a condom (and spermicide) to protect your partner.

SOURCE: U.S. Department of Health and Human Services, *Acquired Immune Deficiency Syndrome*, Surgeon General's Report, HHS publication no. 86-888, 1986.

Adolescents should be warned emphatically about the AIDS threat. Unprotected sexual experimentation during the teen years is common and can put young people at high risk. They should understand, through explicit teachings, how AIDS is spread and how to prevent it.

It is tempting to sit back and trust that technology will soon solve AIDS as it has so many other medical puzzles. Drugs are being tested, and many look promising, but so far, none offers a cure. It is also comforting to feel a world apart from people at high risk for AIDS. Far from being safe, however, the population at large is at risk, and many who are lulled into feeling exempt or protected by technology could become part of the predicted epidemic ahead. *It is urgent* that every person not yet infected with AIDS adopt an aggressive, effective personal strategy to prevent it from occurring.

▮ STUDY AIDS

1. List the major beneficial roles microbes play in technology, the environment, and the body.
2. Compare and contrast bacteria, viruses, parasites, and fungi in terms of their requirements for life.
3. Describe how acne develops and what measures are effective against it.
4. Name the factors required for infection to spread.
5. Describe the importance of public health systems in preventing the spread of the most prevalent infectious diseases.
6. Explain how immunizations work to prevent diseases.
7. Describe the body's lines of defense against microbes and the order in which it uses them when pathogens attack.
8. List several personal strategies that strengthen defense against infectious diseases.
9. Give examples of some sexually transmitted diseases (STDs), and describe their detrimental effects on the body when they are allowed to progress untreated.

10. Describe some effects of STDs on fetuses and infants.
11. List some strategies useful to avoid contracting STDs.
12. List the characteristics of people who are at most risk for developing AIDS.
13. Describe ways in which transmission of AIDS occurs and how it can be prevented.

GLOSSARY

(See also separate Miniglossaries of Infectious Diseases, Acne, and the Course of a Disease on pages 300, 303, and 305. Table 15–1 defines the common sexually transmitted diseases.)

aerobe (AIR-robe): a microbe that requires oxygen to grow.

anaerobe (AN-air-robe): a microbe that requires an oxygen-free environment to grow.

antiseptic: agents that prevent the growth of microorganisms on the body surfaces and on wounds.

bacteria (singular, **bacterium**): microscopic, single-celled organisms of varying shapes and sizes, some capable of causing disease.

communicable disease: see *infectious disease.*

contagious disease: see *infectious disease.*

disinfectant: a chemical that kills microbes on surfaces, in surroundings, and in water.

endemic: a term used to describe a disease that is always present in at least a few people in a population.

endogenous bacteria: the normally harmless bacterial residents of the human body, which live on the skin, in the digestive tract, and elsewhere.

epidemic: a disease that appears suddenly in many people in the same geographical location.

fomite: a nonliving thing that transmits infection, such as a blanket, a dish, or a hypodermic needle.

fungi: plants and plantlike organisms of varying shapes and sizes. They include molds and mushrooms (visible), and yeasts (microscopic and one-celled, some causing diseases).

host: see *parasite.*

immunization: see *vaccination.*

infectious disease: disease caused by infection with microorganisms or their toxins; also called *communicable* or *contagious disease.* A separate Miniglossary of Infectious Diseases appears on page 00.

microbe (microorganism): minute organism, too small to be seen with the naked eye; bacteria, yeasts, and viruses.

mold: see *fungi.*

nosocomial (no-soh-COH-me-ul) **infection:** infection acquired in the hospital.
nosos = disease
comi = to care for

opportunist: in general, a creature that takes advantage of opportunities that come its way. Of microbes, one that can infect when an altered physiological state of the host provides an opportunity, although it ordinarily causes no harm.

pandemic: an epidemic that occurs around the globe.

parasite: an organism that lives within or on, and at the expense of, another organism (the *host* organism). An *internal parasite* lives in the internal chambers of the body; an example is intestinal worms. *External parasites* live on external surfaces, such as skin and hair; an example is lice.

pathogen: a disease-causing microbe.

portal of entry: a site in the body that allows microbes to enter.

portal of exit: a site in the body that allows microbes to exit.

reservoir (of infection): the source of an infectious disease agent, including people, animals, or water.

vaccination: injection with a suspension of modified infectious agents (vaccine) to induce an immune response and establish long-term resistance to a specific infectious disease. Also called *immunization.*

vector: a living thing that carries and transmits a disease-causing organism.

virus: an organism that consists of only DNA and a protein coat. Viruses draw on the contents of cells they invade for reproduction.

yeast: see *fungi.*

QUIZ ANSWERS

1. *False.* The great majority of microbes are valuable scavengers that break down refuse and rarely do any harm.
2. *False.* Antibiotics are useful against bacteria but useless against viruses.
3. *False.* Although soaps do not kill most microbes, they do make them slippery, so the water can rinse them away.
4. *True.* Viruses have no way of eating.
5. *False.* Low fevers are usually not harmful and are part of the body's defense against infection.
6. *True.* A hospital is a place where people can easily pick up infectious diseases.
7. *False.* Most often, disease-causing organisms that get into the body are intercepted by the immune system and never get the chance to cause disease.
8. *True.* Sexually transmitted diseases (STDs) are rarely spread by anything except sexual activity.
9. *False.* At any one time, more people have STDs without knowing or reporting it than the number who are being treated.
10. *False.* Antibiotics taken regularly do not prevent STDs.

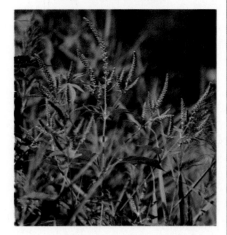

Allergy— Vandal of the Immune System

A man was stung by a wasp while he was out gardening. He had been stung once before, but this time he felt strangely light-headed, his breathing became difficult, his skin turned red, and he was almost unconscious by the time his friend got him to the hospital. A bank employee was presenting a report when a bout of uncontrollable sniffling and sneezing suddenly interrupted. A toddler, visiting his grandparents' country house, had been chasing chipmunks through the woods. Soon, a painful, itchy rash had covered his chubby legs and seemed to be spreading up his back. The boy's grandmother had her own problem: a case of hives she believed was brought on because she had eaten some strawberries.

No doubt you have guessed the plight of each of these people: **allergy**. Allergy is a reaction of the immune system, but unlike the development of immunity, the reaction occurs in response to normally harmless agents. It is an overreaction brought on by excessive release of **histamine**, the immune substance that causes inflammation.

How can such diverse problems all have a common cause?

Allergy can be caused by many different substances. The people in the stories are suffering from the four major types of allergies: those caused when allergens are injected, when they are airborne, when they are acquired by skin contact, or when they are eaten (food allergies). Allergy to an injected substance can occur as the result of an insect sting or animal bite, an injection of medicine that the person is allergic to, or an accidental transfusion of the wrong blood type. In these cases the **allergen**, the substance to which the body reacts, is injected directly into the blood, causing the severe blood disturbance **anaphylactic shock**. If left untreated, it can be fatal.

The gardener had been stung once before—why didn't he suffer the reaction then?

In most allergies more than one exposure to an allergen is needed to bring on the allergic reaction. Remember the workings of the immune system. The first time the body is exposed to an allergen, the immune system stores a memory of the encounter. Thereafter, the body is sensitized to it. The word *hypersensitivity* is often used to describe the condition, because the cells (and the person) are excessively sensitive to the normally nonthreatening material. When the sensitized cells again meet and recognize the allergen, the hypersensitivity reaction produces common allergy symptoms.

I guess the banker has the airborne type of allergy. Is this hay fever?

Yes. Hay fever is common and is usually harmless, because the reaction is confined to the membranes of the respiratory system—the allergen does not penetrate into the body. Hay fever causes millions of lost work days each year, and its symptoms are well known: itchy nasal membranes, irritated throat, watery eyes and nose, sneezing, and sinus swelling. Pollen of plants in spring and summer, spores of mushrooms and molds in fall, and dust or animal dander anytime may travel on the air and be inhaled, causing the symptoms.

You say that hay fever is not serious, but I've known people who couldn't breathe normally during pollen season.

Simple hay fever can progress to the more serious disease **asthma**. Asthma can also result from allergies other than the airborne variety. For example, a food allergy could easily express itself as asthma in susceptible people. In an asthma attack, the smaller air tubes of the lungs close up, making it hard to breathe and producing the characteristic wheezing sound. Asthma can also be brought on by infection or drugs and is worsened by mental or physical fatigue and by stress.

About the toddler—it sounds as if he had a poison ivy rash, but what does that have to do with allergy?

The toddler did have poison ivy rash, and it is a type of allergy that can result from skin contact with an allergen. When the poison ivy oil contacts sensitized skin cells—those that have antibodies attached to them—the cells are destroyed in the allergen-antibody reaction, and they release histamine. One of the immune functions of histamine is to open up the surrounding blood vessels to bring on fresh supplies in the battle against an invader. The large quantity of histamine released in allergy causes fluid to leak through the blood vessel walls into the surrounding tissue; the result is swelling. In

the case of poison ivy, the result is an itchy, bumpy rash; in the case of hay fever, swollen, itchy nasal membranes; in asthma, swollen lung tissues. In food allergies, the antigen is absorbed from the digestive tract and travels to many locations, so it can cause a wide variety of symptoms.

Why is it that some people develop allergies and others don't?

Although all the reasons why some people develop allergies are not known, a strong factor is heredity. The tendency to allergies usually runs in families.

When someone is diagnosed with an allergy, what can be done about it? Is there a cure?

First, it must be determined what exactly is causing the symptoms; then, steps can be taken to avoid contacting the cause. This may be easier said than done, because the allergen may be in the dust of air conditioning and heating systems, in bedding, or on the family pet. To find the cause, a physician (an allergist) introduces tiny amounts of probable allergens under the skin and watches for the characteristic histamine reaction. If the allergy is to an airborne substance, the vents and filters of heating and cooling systems can be cleaned regularly; offending weeds can be removed from the yard; bedding can be replaced with the nonallergenic types; and some relief is probable.

OK, so the person tries to avoid the allergen. But can't drugs help?

Medical treatment of allergy can be aimed at either relief of the symptoms or at curing the body of the allergy altogether. For symptom relief, antihistamines might help (see Chapter 7). Antihistamines oppose the action of histamine, reducing swelling and fluid buildup. Antihistamines also make people sleepy and hence make driving unsafe. Actually, many people choose to suffer the symp-

toms of allergy rather than suffer the side effects of the drugs.

What about a real cure for the underlying problem?

Those who hope for permanent relief can receive a series of injections of the allergen given over a long period of time and in increasing amounts. The shots desensitize the immune system. This approach is most effective for people who suffer from severe allergic reactions, such as the potentially fatal anaphylactic reactions to injected antigens. For these people, even a reduction in the severity of the reaction can buy time to obtain medical help in the event of a sting or bite. For others, the best bet may be to endure the allergy symptoms; at least some evidence indicates that allergic reactions may reduce the person's risks of developing cancer.[1*]

I read in a magazine that people can now be tested for allergy by mail. What do you make of that?

Be extra careful when you evaluate claims for allergy testing or cure. To a quack selling snake oil, allergies are the perfect ailment. People want relief because allergies are so uncomfortable, but legitimate testing and treatments are long and expensive procedures with uncertain outcomes.

Some recent allergy ripoffs tout sophisticated-sounding laboratory work. Cytotoxic testing, for example, is done to see what foods your blood cells "react" to. Some blood cells are mixed with pureed foods and observed for "changes." As you might guess, this is not a valid test for allergy, because the isolated blood cells are cut off from the immune system that produces the allergic response. Other terms that should alert you to allergy quackery are *brain allergy*, *metabolic rejectivity syndrome (MRS)*, and the term *ecology* when applied to body function.

*Reference notes are in Appendix D.

Heart and Artery Disease

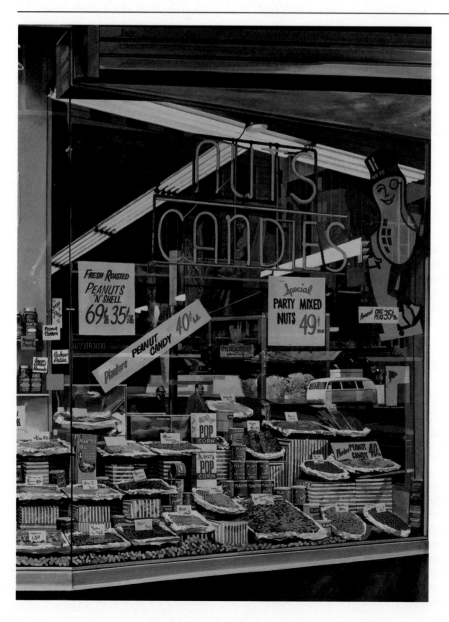

FOR OPENERS . . .

True or false? If false, say what is true.

1. Thanks to the constant presence of blood in its chambers, the heart needs no arteries to provide it with nutrients and oxygen.
2. Veins appear blue under the skin because the blood within them is blue.
3. Most people who have suffered heart attacks can be helped by heart surgery.
4. Chelation therapy cleans out arteries by stripping the cholesterol from their walls.
5. A person with hypertension has high blood pressure.
6. Everyone is developing atherosclerosis.
7. You can tell whether your blood pressure is high by the way you feel.
8. Once atherosclerosis has begun to clog the arteries, it cannot be reversed.
9. A primary dietary measure to avoid heart disease is to eat more margarine and less butter.
10. To avoid salt, fat, and cholesterol, you should shop in the dietetic foods section of the grocery store.

(Answers on page 339.)

"That's the lifeblood of the operation." "Let's go to the heart of the matter." *Lifeblood, heart*—the words are used to mean that something is absolutely essential, vital to survival. This chapter is about the heartbeat and lifeblood of the body and what this system needs to support its health.

■ THE CIRCULATORY SYSTEM

The tissues of the body require a constant supply of nutrients and oxygen, removal of wastes, and communication between their parts. These tasks are assigned to the **circulatory system**—the heart and its associated blood vessels. Also called the **cardiovascular system**, it pumps around the body the equivalent of 4,000 gallons of blood each day, propelled by over 85,000 heartbeats.

The heart, at the center of the system, is almost all muscle, with hollow chambers inside that collect blood and then squirt it out again into tough, elastic arteries. The heart has four chambers: two that function as receiving areas and two, as shipping areas. The receiving chambers, the **atria**, pool the blood as it arrives from the body, and the shipping chambers, the **ventricles**, contract powerfully to send the blood on its way again. One atrium and ventricle, on the right side of the heart, collect used blood—blood that has visited the tissues—and send it to the lungs to pick up fresh oxygen supplies. The other atrium and ventricle, on the left side of the heart, collect blood that is returning from the lungs freshly oxygenated and force it out to the body tissues again.

The heart derives no direct benefit from the blood inside of its own chambers. It relies for nourishment on its a network of arteries that lie on its surface—the **coronary arteries**—and on **capillaries** embedded in its muscle tissue (see Figure 16–1). This fact becomes important to understanding how the heart is affected by artery disease.

You have probably listened to your own or someone else's heartbeat and noticed its two-step rhythm, sometimes called *lub-dub*. The first beat (lub) is the sound made when the atria contract to send the blood they have pooled to the ventricles below; the second beat (dub) is the sound made when the ventricles contract to send the blood on its way to the body (the atria relax and pool more blood during the dub). You may be wondering why the contraction of the heart muscles should make any sound at all, and in reality it does not. The sound comes from the slapping shut of the heart's valves, flaps of tissue located at the entrances and exits of the chambers. Normally, the valves allow blood to flow in only one direction on its way through the heart, but if the valves are damaged or unusually shaped, some blood will flow backward, changing the sound (a **heart murmur**). Heart murmurs are usually no cause for alarm, but occasionally they reflect conditions that require medical attention.

The job of the ventricles is to maintain the correct pressure of the blood in the **arteries** and to keep the blood moving at the rate that best maintains the tissues. The arteries are built to withstand the pressure of the blood pulsing from the ventricles. The arteries branch out, the branches become smaller in diameter and more numerous, and they end in networks of capillaries—webs of tiny vessels too small to see. The artery walls are thick and keep substances from escaping, but the thin capillaries allow nutrients, oxygen, and chemical messengers such as hormones to be forced through their walls from the blood into the tissues. Also, the blood in the capillaries

■■■■■■■■■

FIGURE 16–1 The Heart's Major Arteries

The coronary arteries feed the heart muscle itself; the heart obtains no nourishment from the blood inside its chambers

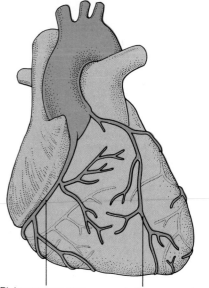

Right coronary artery   Left coronary artery

receives wastes from the tissues. The capillaries that carry waste-laden blood then merge with others to form greater vessels, the **veins**, and these transport this used blood to the lungs for renewal. Blood in the veins appears to be blue under the skin; the bluish cast occurs when blood has been stripped of its oxygen by the tissues. Figure 16–2 diagrams the cardiovascular system.

A certain blood pressure is vital to the trading of materials between tissues and the bloodstream. The pressure of the blood against capillary walls is what pushes fluids, with their cargo of nutrients and oxygen, out into the tissues. As the blood moves through a capillary net, much of its fluid is strained out, leaving a high concentration of blood cells and dissolved materials inside the capillaries. This attracts fluids carrying wastes from the tissues, and these fluids seep back into the bloodstream. Thus the tissues

FIGURE 16–2   An Overview of the Cardiovascular System

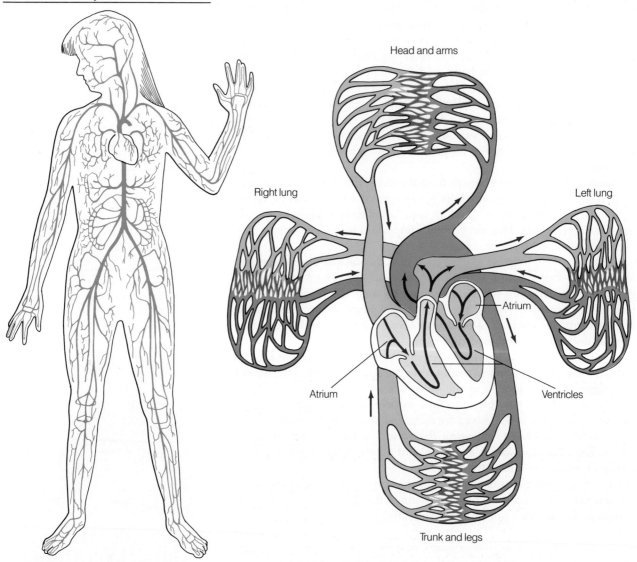

A. Arteries conduct blood away from the heart toward the tissues. Veins are not shown, but they form a similar network conducting blood back to the heart.

B. This is a simplified diagram that depicts the blood flow through the heart, out into arteries, through capillaries, and back to the heart by way of veins.

are nourished and cleansed. A similar exchange in specialized capillary networks within the kidneys removes certain wastes from the blood and disposes of them into the urine.

Blood in the veins is under comparatively little pressure. It must travel uphill against gravity on the return trip from the lower parts of the body such as the legs to the heart. The veins' walls are thinner and weaker than those of the arteries, and they are equipped with valves at intervals along their length to hold blood against the downward pull of gravity. These valves can become too weak to hold the heavy blood, which then pools inside the delicate veins, causing them to bulge out visibly under the skin, a condition called **varicose veins**. People who stand for long periods are especially vulnerable. Elevating the legs for short periods each day may help prevent the condition, and during exercise, contraction of the muscles that surround the veins helps keep the venous blood moving. Thus musclular fitness promotes vascular health.

Disease in any part of the circulatory system affects the tissues that depend on the blood supply for nutrients and waste removal. **Heart disease** is any disease that affects the heart muscle or other working parts of the heart. The term **cardiovascular disease (CVD)** covers diseases of all parts of the cardiovascular system, including the heart. The most prevalent form of CVD is **atherosclerosis**, which can lead to heart attack and stroke (see pages 325–327). These are discussed in the following sections, with attention to the question of how people can minimize their risks.

CARDIOVASCULAR DISEASE

Cardiovascular disease is the number one killer of adults in the United States. Nothing else kills even half as many adults each year; many of these deaths occur long before retirement. One in every four people suffers from some form of this disease, and many more are developing it.[1]* Everyone is susceptible to heart and artery disease, but fortunately, everyone can take measures to reduce the risks of developing it.[2]

Atherosclerosis and Blood Clotting

Atherosclerosis, a type of hardening of the arteries, begins with an accumulation of mounds of soft fat along the inner walls of all the arteries of the body. Such mounds gradually enlarge and harden with mineral deposits to form **plaques**, which make the artery walls lose their elasticity and narrow the passage through them (see Figure 16–3 on page 324). As mentioned, the heart muscle depends on blood flow through its own arteries for nourishment and oxygen—the blood it pumps through its chambers cannot meet its needs. The end result of atherosclerosis, then, may be disease of both the heart and the arteries (CVD).

Normally, as blood surges through the arteries, they expand to allow blood to pass, and they contract with each beat of the heart to push it along. Arteries hardened and narrowed by plaques cannot expand or contract, and so the blood must squeeze through. The pressure inside the arteries increases beyond normal, because the blood backs up at the restricted areas while the heart works ever harder to push it through. This high blood pressure, or **hypertension**, is a major contributor to cardiovascular disease.

*Reference notes are in Appendix D.

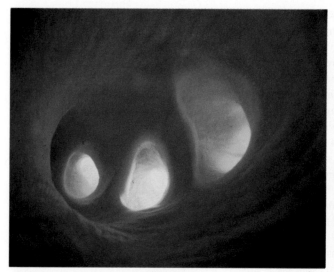

The aorta of an infant, illuminated from behind.

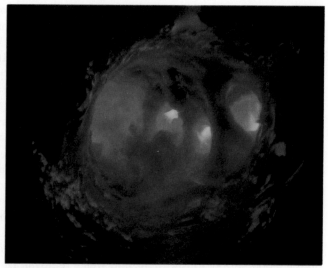

The aorta of a middle-aged man, almost totally occluded by plaques.

FIGURE 16–3   Plaques in Arteries

AN-your-ism

Hypertension damages the artery walls further and can even cause them to go into spasms, blocking blood flow. The heart, pumping blood against this back pressure, is also under a strain. As pressure builds up in an artery, the arterial wall may become weakened and balloon out, forming an **aneurysm**. An aneurysm can burst, and when this happens in a major artery such as the aorta, it leads to massive bleeding and death.

324

Abnormal blood clotting is another factor that contributes to life-threatening events. Under normal conditions, clots form and dissolve in the blood all the time. Small, cell-like bodies in the blood, known as **platelets**, cause clots to form whenever they encounter injuries—a protective function that prevents blood loss from minor wounds. Clots also form inside the blood vessels when the platelets encounter rough spots such as plaques, but they soon dissolve again unless they are needed to plug a leak. In atherosclerosis, the balance between clot formation and dissolution is disturbed. The platelets are triggered to begin the clotting process more often than normal.

Prostaglandins control the action of the platelets, and an imbalance among those regulators may contribute to the formation of clots. Particles released when platelets break down also may worsen atherosclerosis by adding to the growth of plaques. A person who has suffered a minor stroke may feel that the problem is being dismissed lightly when the health care provider orders daily aspirin as preventive therapy. Aspirin, though, modifies the prostaglandins and so can suppress the platelet clotting action (see Chapter 7).

Atherosclerosis can cause blockage of an artery in any of three ways:

- The plaques can grow large enough to completely block the blood flow.
- A blood clot may form on a plaque and gradually grow (a **thrombus**), eventually cutting off the blood supply. In the arteries of the heart, such a blockage is called a **coronary thrombosis** (a type of **heart attack**). In a vessel that feeds the brain, such a blockage is a **cerebral thrombosis** (a type of **stroke**).
- A clot can also break loose, becoming a traveling clot (an **embolus**), and circulate until it reaches an artery too small to allow its passage. The sudden blockage of the vessel is called an **embolism**.

When an artery is blocked, the tissue normally supplied by the blocked vessel may suddenly die. If blockage occurs gradually, tissue death can occur gradually, too, resulting in organ damage. Figure 16–4 shows a thrombus and an embolus.

No one is free of atherosclerosis. Autopsies on soldiers as young as 18 have shown that their arteries were already clogged with plaques. The condition advances with age. The question, then, is not whether you have atherosclerosis, but how far advanced it is. The development of atherosclerosis reaches a **critical phase** at which more than 60 percent of the surfaces of the arteries are covered with plaques. Once in the critical phase, a person faces substantial risk for a CVD event, such as heart attack or stroke.

Heart Attack

Heart attack is the most common of the life-threatening conditions brought on by atherosclerosis. It is especially likely in men in later midlife, but a significant number of heart attacks occur earlier, and some even before age 30. Before menopause, women are less susceptible to heart attacks than men are; female hormones possibly delay the onset of CVD in women. Women who take oral contraceptives, however, and especially those who also smoke, are at extra risk for CVD development and for heart attack.

A heart attack occurs when the arterial blood supply to the heart becomes so restricted that some of its muscle tissue dies. When muscle tissue dies, it is replaced by nonfunctional scar tissue, and the remaining heart muscle then must work harder to compensate.

Another problem, caused by reduced blood flow and restriction of oxygen to the heart, is pain. When the oxygen supply to the heart is reduced but

EM-boh-luss

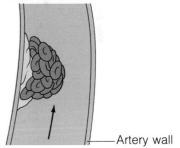

FIGURE 16–4   A Thrombus and an Embolus

A thrombus grows in size until the blood flow in an artery is cut off. An embolus breaks away, travels in the bloodstream, and plugs the first vessel it encounters that is too small to allow its passage.

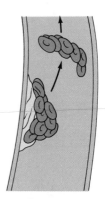

Thrombus

Artery wall

Embolus

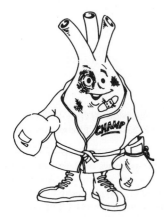

Even if damaged the heart keeps pumping.

is still sufficient for sedentary life, a sudden exertion or emotional upset can bring on a pain in the chest, **angina**. Angina is not always a symptom of heart attack, but it can be. Some heart disease victims do not have angina and so may not be forewarned of an impending heart attack. Others may deny that a heart attack is occurring and blame the symptoms on "indigestion." Many heart attack victims could have been saved if they had told someone of their symptoms.

When blood flow to an area of the heart is reduced, alternate vessels begin to deliver the needed blood. These smaller **collateral blood vessels** detour around the blockages, and can prevent tissue death. Some evidence from studies using animals suggests that exercise, especially in the young, stimulates the heart to form new collateral vessels.[3] In human beings, the development of such vessels may be a factor in the excellent post-heart attack recovery seen in those who exercise.[4]

A person who has suffered a heart attack or infection that has damaged the valves may develop **congestive heart failure**. The name does not mean that the heart has stopped pumping altogether, but it certainly is pumping less well. The disabled heart cannot fully empty its chambers of blood at each beat, and blood backs up in the veins that are trying to return it to the heart. As blood collects in the veins, fluid is forced out of the capillaries into the tissues, especially into the feet and legs, causing swelling—**edema**. Fluid also can collect around the lungs, making breathing difficult.

Heart attacks do not always end in permanent disability. Many times a person who experiences a minor heart attack can recover fully through treatment and be motivated to adopt habits that could help prevent another. Drugs such as **digitalis** may be used to strengthen and stabilize the heartbeat; drugs that correct fluid imbalances or that dissolve clots quickly are also useful. A **pacemaker** is an implanted device that electrically stimulates a failing heartbeat. The latest models even automatically adjust the heartbeat to exercise levels. Sometimes, though, surgery is needed.

Heart transplants are infrequent and the use of artificial hearts is controversial; more common is **coronary artery bypass surgery**, in which the surgeon replaces the blocked coronary arteries with sections of the person's own veins or with synthetic tubing. In **angioplasty**, a tiny tube is inserted into the artery and expanded to widen the passageway. Although these and other techniques are promising, nothing has been found that will cure atherosclerosis. Medicine can probably prolong life, but blockages recur, and people may require repeated surgery or treatments.

An exercise trend does seem to be emerging, though. Not only is moderate exercise helpful in reducing hypertension and correcting blood cholesterol levels, but if heart and artery disease has already set in, a monitored exercise program may actually help to reverse it.[5] Medical advances are exciting, but in the end, health habits may well turn out to be more reliable in preventing, and even permanently reversing, heart disease.

Stroke

Strokes are not as common as heart attacks, but they still claim a substantial portion of the lives that are lost to CVD each year. Sometimes a person will suffer a small stroke, called a **transient ischemic attack (TIA)**—a warning that a blockage is forming. Like a minor heart attack, a TIA may have no lasting effect except to startle a person into taking action to reverse damaging habits.

When a major stroke occurs, a part of the brain is starved for blood and dies. This dead tissue interferes with the person's mental and physical functioning, depending on the location of the damage, as shown in Figure 16–5.

Stroke victims may be robbed of their former abilities, requiring that they start from scratch to learn such elementary functions as personal hygiene or walking. Most stroke victims can recover basic functioning, but it requires dedication from all participants—the victim, family and friends, and the medical team—to support them while they do so.

Stroke can occur in the same ways that heart attack does: as a result of occlusive plaques, thrombus formation, or embolism. Strokes also occur in one other way—**hemorrhage**. Hemorrhage occurs when an artery that feeds the brain becomes weak and the blood pressure causes it to burst. As with heart attacks, strokes require immediate medical attention. Figure 16–6 illustrates a hemorrhage and an aneurysm.

To prevent further strokes, medical treatment, such as anticlotting medication, is sometimes required. If the exact location of a blockage has been discovered by **arteriogram**, a type of X-ray designed especially for locating such blockages, surgery to remove the plaques may be required.

■ RISK FACTORS

Most of the diseases we face today are not primarily those caused by the microbes discussed in Chapter 15, but the lifestyle diseases that develop over years. CVD is just such a disease; cancer is another. When people are diagnosed with CVD, they may be as surprised as if they had just come down with the measles, but many of their own personal choices, made day after day, year after year, may have made the disease practically inevitable.

Preventive strategies against heart disease are based on analyzing **risk factors**. The risk factors for a disease are those factors (hereditary, environmental, and behavioral) that research has revealed to be associated with the occurrence of the disease—that is, factors that show a **correlation** with the disease. They are candidates for causes of the disease, not yet voted in or out. We can say with confidence that the cause of influenza is a virus that attacks a vulnerable system. We cannot, on the other hand, name "the" cause of heart disease with such confidence, but we can name risk factors, some of which are strongly implicated as causal.

An analogy may help to clarify the difference between correlation and cause. Suppose that there is an outbreak of crime in a certain city—arson,

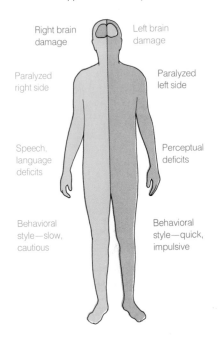

FIGURE 16–5   The Effect of Stroke Location

Brain damage affects opposite side of body.

Right brain damage

Left brain damage

Paralyzed right side

Paralyzed left side

Speech, language deficits

Perceptual deficits

Behavioral style—slow, cautious

Behavioral style—quick, impulsive

The warning signs of stroke:
Report to a physician immediately any of the following:

1. Sudden, temporary weakness or numbness in any part of one side of the body.
2. Temporary loss of speech or understanding of speech.
3. Dizziness, unsteadiness, or unexplained falls.
4. Temporary dimness or loss of vision, particularly in one eye.

FIGURE 16–6   A Hemorrhage and an Aneurysm

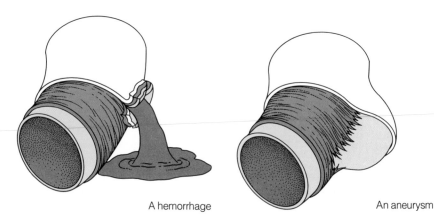

A hemorrhage

An aneurysm

CHAPTER 16 ■ HEART AND ARTERY DISEASE

for example. Someone is setting fires, and the police are on the trail. They discover that a certain person, Mr. Tagalong, is always seen in the neighborhoods when the fires start, and they suspect him of setting them. It may be, however, that a very sneaky individual, Ms. Match, is the real culprit and that Mr. Tagalong is only following her around. Mr. Tagalong, then, is associated with, but not a causal agent in, the setting of the fires. The evidence against him is only circumstantial (correlational). If the police could show that whenever he was locked up no fires occurred and that whenever he was let out the fires started again, then the evidence against him would be stronger, but still only circumstantial. The police could be sure Mr. Tagalong was the culprit only if they caught him pouring the gasoline and lighting the match. (This is equivalent to finding the mechanism by which a disease is caused.) Risk factors have not yet been caught in the act of causing disease (the mechanism is still unknown). Still, the identification of risk factors is a start toward the identification of causes.

To determine whether a risk factor is a cause of disease, scientists must perform **intervention studies**. The theory is simple: intervene in a group of people's lives by removing a risk factor, and prove that the disease then does not develop; next, compare this group with a similar group of people who experienced no intervention, and show that the second group did develop the disease. Studies of this kind indicate that lifestyle choices are indeed linked to CVD.

Among the many risk factors linked to CVD are age, heredity, smoking, sex (being male), race, hypertension, diabetes, lack of exercise, obesity, stress, abnormal heartbeat, high blood cholesterol levels, many nutrient excesses and deficiencies, personality characteristics, and more. Some of the risk factors are powerful predictors of CVD. If you are young and have none of them, the statistical likelihood of your developing cardiovascular disease in the next six years may be less than 1 in 100. If you are older and have all the major ones, the chance may rise to close to 1 in 2.[6] The Life Choice Inventory shows one way of calculating your risk score. The correlation isn't perfect; a few people with many risk factors live long lives without disease, and a few people with only a few or none die young of CVD. On the average, though, the more risk factors in a person's life, the greater that person's risk of disease.

The major factors that respond to lifestyle changes and that have emerged as the most powerful predictors of risk of CVD are:

- Smoking.
- Hypertension.
- High blood cholesterol.
- Diabetes.

The chances of having a healthy heart and arteries are much greater if you do not smoke, if your blood pressure and blood cholesterol are normal, and if you keep any symptoms of diabetes under control. (This chapter's Spotlight is devoted to diabetes.)

Heredity

A health care provider may ask, "Do you have any relatives with heart disease? What did your grandparents die of?" Susceptibility to CVD runs

To reduce your CVD risk:

⊗ **Learn the major risk factors, and evaluate your own degree of risk.**

LIFE CHOICE INVENTORY

How healthy is your heart? Every disease has risk factors; those for heart disease are among the best known. The better you know the nature of the risks you face, the better you can decide what prevention measures may be appropriate. To determine your risk of heart disease, add up the numbers in each category that most nearly describe you:

	H	E	A	R	T
Heredity[a]	**1** No known history of heart disease	**2** One relative with heart disease over 60 years	**3** Two relatives with heart disease over 60 years	**4** One relative with heart disease under 60 years	**6** Two relatives with heart disease under 60 years
Exercise	**1** Intensive exercise, work, and recreation	**2** Moderate exercise, work, and recreation	**3** Sedentary work and intensive recreational exercise	**5** Sedentary work and moderate recreational exercise	**6** Sedentary work and light recreational exercise
Age	**1** 10 to 20	**2** 21 to 30	**3** 31 to 40	**4** 41 to 50	**6** 51 to 65
Lb	**0** More than 5 lb below standard weight	**1** ± 5 lb of standard weight	**2** 6 to 20 lb overweight	**4** 21 to 35 lb overweight	**6** 36 to 50 lb overweight
Tobacco	**0** Nonuser	**1** Cigar or pipe	**2** 10 cigarettes or fewer per day	**4** 20 cigarettes or more per day	**6** 30 cigarettes or more per day
Habits of eating fat[b]	**1** No animal or solid fat	**2** Very little animal or solid fat	**3** Little animal or solid fat	**4** Much animal or solid fat	**6** Equal to the typical meat-eater's diet

Your risk of heart attack:

4 to 9: Very remote.   16 to 20: Average.   26 to 30: Dangerous.
10 to 15: Below average.   21 to 25: Moderate.   31 to 35: Urgent danger—reduce score!

Other conditions—such as stress, high blood pressure, and increased blood cholesterol—detract from heart health and should be evaluated by your physician.

[a]Diabetes and hypertension in the family are also predictors.

[b]If you know your blood cholesterol, use it instead. Below 180 = 0 points, 181 to 200 = 1,201 to 235 = 2,236 to 260 = 4,261 to 300 = 5, and over 300 = 6.

SOURCE: Courtesy of Loma Linda University.

in families. If your parents have it, chances are good that you will develop it, too.

Note that to be born with a hereditary *disease* is different from being born with a genetic *tendency* to develop a disease later in life. Hereditary diseases inevitably cause abnormalities in function; they are present at birth; they must be managed throughout life. In contrast, genetic tendencies may or

⊕ Learn about your heredity and use the information: control the lifestyle factors that may affect you.

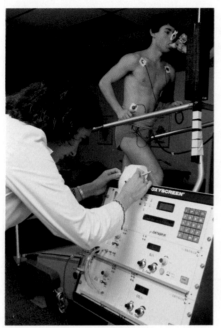

If you have a hereditary tendency toward CVD, consider taking a stress test.

⊕ Make use of screening tests to learn the status of your heart and arteries.

⊕ Don't smoke, or plan to cut down or stop.

may not result in disease states themselves, depending on lifestyle choices and environmental factors.

You cannot change your heredity, but you can be aware of it and pay attention to its significance for you. If several close relatives have CVD, then you should probably adopt additional preventive measures, even if you have no symptoms.

If you have a hereditary tendency toward CVD, or if you want to be screened as a preventive measure, two tests may be worth considering: an **electrocardiograph** (**ECG** or **EKG**) and an exercise stress test. The first of these, the ECG, records the heart's own electrical impulses at rest and produces a graph of the heart's beat pattern. An abnormal heartbeat pattern may indicate damage in the heart muscle. Sometimes an abnormality makes itself known only in times of physical activity. An exercise stress test (described in Chapter 6) consists of an ECG taken while exercising on a stationary bicycle or treadmill. The tester gradually increases the work load until the person reaches a level of exertion close to maximal or until a heart abnormality shows up on the monitor. The stress test is often used to determine whether a person can safely start exercising after years of sedentary life. If you learn that CVD is developing, then you have the opportunity to begin taking appropriate preventive measures.

Smoking

When tobacco smoke enters the lungs, it delivers to the ,blood a load of nicotine, a stimulant that triggers the stress response. This raises the blood pressure and increases the heart rate, and it greatly increases the heart's need for oxygen. At the same time, carbon monoxide from the smoke is mistakenly picked up by the blood, because it closely resembles the chemical structure of oxygen—but instead of providing oxygen to the tissues, the carbon monoxide continues to ride in the blood, starving the tissues. To the extent that carbon monoxide occupies the blood, oxygen cannot be picked up from the lungs. The results of smoking are an increased demand for heart activity and a reduced supply of oxygen to support its work. Not only that, but nicotine directly damages platelets, making clot formation more likely. (Chapter 9 lists more of the effects of nicotine and smoking on health.) In short, smoking:

- Elevates blood pressure.
- Increases heart rate.
- Increases the heart muscle's oxygen requirement.
- Deprives the heart and other tissues of oxygen.
- Increases the likelihood of clot formation.

The action needed to reduce the risk of CVD from smoking is straightforward. Don't smoke, or if you do, make plans to cut down or stop. Even people who have smoked for years can reduce their risks by quitting.

Hypertension

The term *hypertension* refers to excess pressure in the arteries. To understand how the blood pressure can rise too high, consider how the body works to raise it when it falls too low.

Next to lack of air, no condition threatens life so direly as dehydration, which diminishes the supply of blood and causes the blood pressure to fall too low to deliver fluid to the tissues. The kidneys control what products leave the body as urine (wastes) and what products are returned to the blood. The kidneys respond to dehydration by setting in motion two mechanisms to raise the pressure again. First, they send out a message to constrict the blood vessels, because the squeezing action will raise blood pressure. Second, they instruct their own adrenal glands to send out a hormone that will conserve fluid and increase the blood supply. This hormone works by preventing sodium excretion so as to raise the blood sodium level: because water stays with sodium, the blood volume increases. (Most tissues get their water this way—they gather up sodium, and water accompanies it.)

Normally, this response of the kidneys is protective: their conservation of water helps prevent the dire consequences of dehydration and ensures that blood pressure is maintained until more water can be drunk. In atherosclerosis, though, the kidneys can actually create problems rather than help to solve them, by bringing on hypertension.

When atherosclerosis has narrowed the kidneys' arteries, they experience this condition in the same way as dehydration, because the flow of blood through them is diminished. This time, however, the cause of the problem is different—the reduced blood flow is due to a reduced *delivery* of blood rather than a reduced supply. Still, the kidneys set in motion the sequence of events that leads to water retention—only now, it raises the blood pressure above normal. When the blood pressure has finally risen high enough to deliver sufficient blood to the kidneys, they stop calling for water retention, but now the whole body's blood pressure is too high. The heart now has to pump harder to push the extra fluid around against constricted arteries. Thus atherosclerosis contributes to hypertension, and the person then suffers from two degenerative conditions instead of one. Hypertension worsens kidney damage, makes strokes and heart attacks more likely, and damages artery walls, increasing the likelihood of plaque formation.

Hypertension produces its harmful effects without a single symptom. You can't rely on your body to warn you; you must actively seek information about your own blood pressure to find out whether you have hypertension. Hypertension has a hereditary component; it runs in families. Learn your own family's blood pressure pattern. People who are middle aged or elderly, black, obese, heavy drinkers, users of oral contraceptives, or suffering from kidney disease or diabetes are especially prone to hypertension.[7]

The most effective single step you can take to protect yourself from CVD is to know your blood pressure, or at least to know whether it is above normal or not. At checkup time, you should see a professional to get an accurate blood pressure reading (self-test machines do not give accurate readings). If your blood pressure is above normal, the reading should be double checked. Depending on how high it is, and on your age, physical state, and family history, different treatments are appropriate.

⊕ **Know your blood pressure—or at least know whether it is high or not.**

When blood pressure is measured, two numbers are important: the pressure during contraction of the ventricles of the heart and the pressure during relaxation of the ventricles. The first number is the pressure in the arteries during **systole** (dub); the second number is the pressure during **diastole** (lub). Normal systolic blood pressure is between 100 and 140;* normal di-

---

*Blood pressure is read in millimeters of mercury. The silver column that rises on a blood pressure instrument is a column of mercury; the height to which it is pushed is marked off in millimeters.

astolic pressure is between 60 and 90. Figure 16–7 shows how to interpret your blood pressure reading.

A word of caution about interpreting blood pressure readings: many factors can affect them. Blood pressure rises when you speak, so it is important to remain silent as the reading is being taken. Body position, too, is important for accuracy: your blood pressure is lowest when you are lying down, higher when you are sitting up, and higher still when you are standing. And the cuff should be of the right size. People with excess body fat may sometimes get a falsely high blood pressure reading simply because the cuff is too small.

Hypertension can be controlled, especially if the cause is known. Medication can control some people's blood pressure. Other people can control it by means of lifestyle strategies: eating high-fiber and low-fat foods, reducing their intakes of salty foods while increasing their intakes of nutrient-rich whole foods, losing weight, exercising aerobically, and applying stress management techniques. You have seen these recommendations before, for many other ills besides atherosclerosis and hypertension are preventable by the same chosen habits.

There is some controversy about how to treat moderate hypertension (see Figure 16–7). Some authorities feel that, since any degree of hypertension can cause some damage to the heart, arteries, and kidneys, even moderate hypertension should be aggressively treated with drugs to bring it down. Others, though, prefer to avoid drug use if possible: they think that lifestyle factors should be modified first. They recommend trying weight reduction, exercise, and dietary measures before using drugs.[8] That way, not only is the condition alleviated but a boost is given to health in other ways as well.

Body fatness aggravates hypertension. A single pound of extra body fat requires miles of extra capillaries to feed it; and the heart has to pump the blood around those extra miles. Distribution of body fat seems important, too. Fat around the abdomen seems to correlate most closely with CVD,

✳ To reduce CVD risk, prevent or control hypertension:
    Control weight.
    Do not add salt to foods.
    Reduce fat and increase fiber in the diet.
    Exercise regularly.
    Take prescribed drugs faithfully.
    Practice relaxation techniques.

Regular aerobic exercise helps keep blood pressure normal.

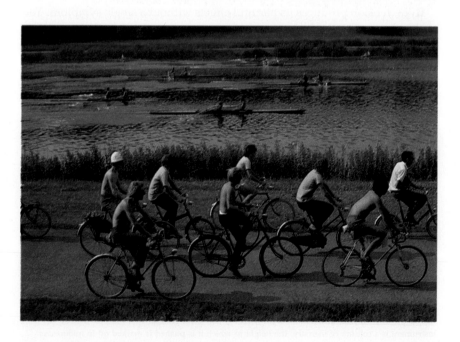

FIGURE 16–7   How to Interpret Your Blood Pressure

When the blood pressure is taken, two measures are recorded: the systole first, the diastole second (example: 120/80). High blood pressure is defined differently for different purposes, but generally, a systolic reading over 140 or a diastolic reading over 90 indicates a too-high blood pressure.

120 { This is the systolic pressure. If this number is above 140, you may have hypertension.

80 { This is the diastolic pressure, the most sensitive indicator of hypertension. Interpret this number as follows:

Less than 85	Normal blood pressure
85 to 89	High normal blood pressure
90 to 104	Mild hypertension
105 to 114	Moderate hypertension
115 or more	Severe hypertension

especially in men, so a rule of thumb has been developed: if your abdomen protrudes when you lie flat on your back, you may have more body fat than is consistent with good health. (Ideally, if you place a ruler across your hipbones while lying on your back, relaxed, it should touch both bones.)

Some evidence indicates that restricting dietary sodium will produce a drop in blood pressure.[9] But the relationship of sodium to blood pressure is not simple. It may not be just any form of sodium, but only sodium as part of salt (sodium choloride) that is the culprit, and then not for everybody. Many people can tolerate large amounts of salt without a rise in blood pressure. In addition, diets high in sodium and chloride are often deficient in other minerals such as potassium and calcium. Some researchers think that increasing dietary calcium intake is the real key to lowering blood pressure.[10] In any case, the use of highly salted foods certainly contributes to hypertension in people with a genetic tendency to develop it.

It takes time for people to get used to the flavors of food without salt, but eventually the taste buds adjust, and the lower levels become the preferred taste. This chapter's Strategies box gives tips on cutting down the amounts of salt and sodium in the diet. The margin lists some high-salt foods, so that you can limit your intake of them.

When lifestyle factors fail to control hypertension and drugs are prescribed, a lifelong dependency on drugs begins. Hypertension drugs do not cure the underlying problems, but they keep the blood pressure under control as long as they are in the system. The drugs may have side effects, such as dizziness, nausea, muscle cramps, and sexual dysfunction; predictably, many people simply stop taking them. A wiser move is to consult the prescribing physician—a change in prescription that could alleviate the side effects may be possible.

Elevated Blood Cholesterol

Another silent, symptomless risk factor for cardiovascular disease is much talked about but little understood: elevated blood cholesterol levels. Cholesterol is a type of fat, one of the lipids (see Chapter 4); it is found in foods and is also made and destroyed in the body.

Foods that are high in sodium:
   Those prepared in brine, such as pickles, olives, and sauerkraut.
   Salty or smoked meat, such as bologna, corned or chipped beef, frankfurters, ham, luncheon meats, salt pork, sausage, and smoked tongue.
   Salty or smoked fish, such as anchovies, caviar, salted and dried cod, herring, sardines, and smoked salmon.
   Snack items such as potato chips, pretzels, salted popcorn, and salted nuts and crackers.
   Bouillon cubes; seasoned salts (including sea salt); soy, Worcestershire, and barbecue sauces.
   Cheeses, especially processed types.
   Canned and instant soups.
   Prepared horseradish, catsup, and mustard.

These foods are low in fat, cholesterol, and sodium, and high in fiber and nutrients.

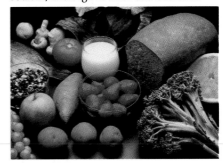

STRATEGIES: Cutting Down on Sodium

To avoid too much sodium, follow these suggestions from the U.S. Department of Agriculture:
1. Learn to enjoy the unsalted flavors of foods.
2. Cook with only small amounts of added salt.
3. Add little or no salt to food at the table.
4. Cut down on the foods listed in the margin.
5. Read labels. Look for the word *soda* or *sodium* or the symbol Na on labels, but watch out particularly for salt.
6. Eat whole foods instead of processed ones. (It isn't necessary to buy expensive, specially prepared "dietetic" foods.)
7. Use only cold, unsoftened water for cooking and drinking. (Softened water contains extra sodium and hot or softened water tends to dissolve toxic metals from pipes.)

Blood cholesterol may be high for any of a number of reasons. Some people seem to inherit tendencies to make too much or to fail to destroy it on schedule. Others have high blood cholesterol for lifestyle reasons: they eat too much fat or too much saturated fat, undergo too much stress, exercise too little, are obese, possibly even drink too much coffee,[11] or all of these. A blood test to determine high blood cholesterol levels, the **blood lipid profile**, can give you an idea of your standing as to this risk factor. Table 16–1 shows how to interpret your blood cholesterol level. Note that acceptable cholesterol levels go up as a person ages.

Cholesterol does not travel freely in the blood; it travels in particles called **lipoproteins**. The two kinds of lipoproteins that transport cholesterol are **low-density lipoproteins (LDL)** and **high- density lipoproteins (HDL)**. The first type (LDL) carries cholesterol from the liver, where it is made, to the tissues, where it is used for making hormones, building cell membranes, and making vitamin D. LDL also tend to deposit cholesterol along the artery linings when the tissues have all they need. HDL, on the other hand, work to gather up excess cholesterol from the tissues and the arteries and carry it back to the liver to be dismantled.

TABLE 16–1 Blood Cholesterol Readings and Risk of CVD

Age	Moderate Risk	High Risk
2 to 19	Over 170[a]	Over 185[a]
20 to 29	Over 200	Over 220
30 to 39	Over 220	Over 240
40 and up	Over 240	Over 260

[a]Blood cholesterol is measured in milligrams per deciliter of blood.

SOURCE: Consensus conference statement: Lowering blood cholesterol to prevent heart disease, *Journal of the American Medical Association* 253 (1985): 2080–2090.

A raised LDL concentration in the blood is a sign of high risk of CVD. (When the overall cholesterol level in the blood is high, it usually reflects raised LDL.) In contrast, raised HDL concentrations are associated with a lowered risk for CVD. (In this case, the overall cholesterol reading would still be low.) In fact, numerous studies now agree that for men over 50, the most potent single indicator of heart attack risk may be the HDL level—the higher the better.

Several factors affect blood cholesterol level. Some of them you can control and some you can't. First, being female is an asset; women have higher HDL levels than men. Second, nonsmokers have uniformly higher HDL levels than smokers. Maintaining appropriate weight for height is helpful (see Chapter 5). Diet and exercise also affect blood cholesterol. Evidence suggests that regular aerobic exercise lowers LDL and raises HDL in the blood.[12] The role of diet is complex, but the complexities are worth learning.

The public has been confused about the relationship of diet to high blood cholesterol, often thinking that cholesterol in foods contributes to high levels of cholesterol in the blood. It does, but ordinary dietary fat, especially saturated fat, contributes much more. The most important key to lowering blood cholesterol seems to be to eat less total fat. The fat you do eat should be the unsaturated type.

Fish oils apparently offer a protective effect beyond merely substituting for saturated fat. Fish oils contain a type of fatty acid that lowers blood cholesterol.* In addition, they alter the prostaglandin balance to favor the dissolving of blood clots over the making of them.[13] One or two fish dishes a week are all it takes to exert a significant effect,[14] and the fattiest cold-water fish are the most effective: mackerel, herring, sardines, bluefish, salmon, tuna, oysters, anchovies, squid, and others.

Dietary fiber may also confer benefits. People on high-fiber diets have been shown to excrete more cholesterol and fat than those on low-fiber diets. One reason is that the high-fiber diet shortens food's transit time through the digestive tract, and so allows less time for cholesterol to be absorbed. When cholesterol from the diet is thus reduced, the body must turn to its own supply to make necessary body compounds. Diets high in fiber are typically low in fat and cholesterol anyway—another advantage to emphasizing fiber. Some cases of elevated blood cholesterol do not respond to changes in lifestyle, and control may be achievable only with cholesterol-lowering drugs.

Emotions and the Heart

Up to this point, the risk factors discussed have been powerfully associated with the development of CVD and are considered by some to be proved causes. Emotional health may be equally important in CVD risk, but so far the findings are less clearly correlational, and certainly not proven to be causal. Still, they are intriguing. For example, people with many social ties develop less heart disease than people with few or none. Married men have less heart disease than single men, and owners of pets (even pet fish) have lower blood pressure than other people.

People (at least some people) can learn to lower their blood cholesterol by practicing meditation, prayer, or whatever relaxation techniques work

⊛ To reduce CVD risk, control blood cholesterol levels:
Do not smoke.
Control weight.
Reduce fat intake, especially saturated fats.
Exercise regularly.

Saturated fats are:
  Solid at room temperature.
  Found in and around cuts of red meat.
  Found in animal products such as butter, whole milk, cheese, and lard.
  Found in a few plant products, such as cocoa butter, coconut oil, and palm oil.
  Found in hydrogenated (hardened) vegetable oils, including margarine (the hardened, stick variety), processed peanut butter, and shortening.

Unsaturated fats are:
  Liquid at room temperature.
  Found in plant products such as grains, seeds, and nuts.
  Found in a few meats, such as fowl and fish.
  Found in liquid cooking oils, liquid and soft margarines, and unprocessed peanut butter.

The heart prefers fiber to saturated fat.

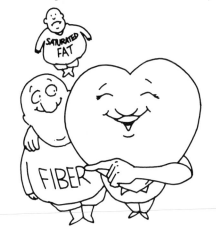

*The fatty acid is eicosapentaenoic acid (EPA), one of the omega fatty acids.

for them. Similarly, plain old affection and love affect the heart and arteries. Rabbits that are petted deposit only a third as much cholesterol in plaques as rabbits that receive no affection. Clearly the mystery of CVD, like all the great human mysteries, involves the mind and spirit as well as the body.[15]

A striking example of the link between CVD and personality type is the study of **type A** and **type B** personalities (see Table 16–2). The type A person finds it hard to cope with leisure time and must feel constantly busy accomplishing things. The type B person accomplishes things, too, but is able to rest when tired and rarely becomes upset. Studies have identified people as As or Bs and then followed them over a period of years; these studies found the type As to have more than twice the rate of CVD as the type Bs. The A versus B difference showed up even when other risk factors were taken into account.[16]

Another study identified three personality types. The alphas were steady and self-reliant. The betas were lively and lighthearted. The gammas were moody and insecure. After classifying students into these three types, the researchers followed their health history for some 30 years beyond graduation. They found that the gammas experienced a much higher rate of heart attacks and cancer than either the alphas or the betas.[17] When people say that someone "takes everything to heart," meaning the person's emotional rections to life are often exaggerated, their description may be literally correct.

The research just described has been criticized. Its detractors point out that the relationship may be correlational rather than causal. Still, if you identify yourself as a type A (or gamma) personality, stress control might help you. Stress causes water retention, increases the blood volume, and

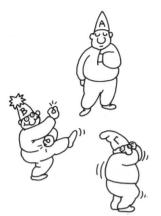

Personality types correlate with heart disease susceptibility.

TABLE 16–2   Type A and B Personality Traits

Characteristics of Type A	Characteristics of Type B
Cynical, mistrustful	Trusting
Aggressive, hurried	Easygoing, relaxed
Ambitious, dominant	Patient, slow
Energetic, quick	Leisurely, quiet
Determined, forceful	Retiring, silent
Excitable, extroverted	Cautious, introverted
Greater reported life satisfaction	Less reported life satisfaction
More often married (men)	Less often married (men)
More often self-employed (men)	Less often self-employed (men)
Change residences more often (men)	Change residences less often (men)
Have higher incomes (men)	Have lower incomes (men)
Drink more alcohol and smoke more cigarettes	Drink less alcohol and smoke fewer cigarettes
Spend less time on physical leisure activity	Spend more time in physical leisure activity
Have high blood cholesterol	Have normal blood cholesterol
Have high diastolic blood pressure	Have normal diastolic blood pressure

SOURCE: Compiled from S. Herman and coauthors, Self-ratings of Type A (coronary prone) adults: Do type A's know they are type A's? *Psychosomatic Medicine* 43 (1981): 405–413; M. Koskenvuo and coauthors, Psychosocial and environmental correlates of coronary-prone behavior in Finland, *Journal of Chronic Disease* 34 (1981): 331–340.

**CHAPTER 16 ■■ HEART AND ARTERY
DISEASE**

raises blood pressure. Some people think that the key to prevention lies in control of the stress response.

Many type A people, having learned of the connection between their personality type and CVD, feel guilty about being type A. But type A behavior is nothing to be ashamed of. After all, competitive, achievement-oriented people get things done. They keep their promises, meet their deadlines, honor their commitments. If you recognize yourself as a type A person, you can take pride in those characteristics. But type A people need to learn to minimize the destructive aspects of their behavior. They need to learn to be sensitive to their feelings of fatigue, and they need to learn to stop and relax totally at frequent enough intervals to avoid paying the price later.

Why is it that making healthful choices is so difficult? Part of the reason is that a person must go against the grain of society: pass up the fried, heavily salted (and heavily advertised) fast foods and the cigarettes that promise to make people more manly or womanly and, instead, search the grocery shelves to pick out the low-fat products.

Does this mean that to remain healthy, you must live a Spartan life and bid a final farewell to ice cream and pizza? No, it does not. The effects of life choices are cumulative. If, *most of the time*, you choose low-fat, high-fiber meals and if on most days you exercise; then on occasion you can relax and indulge in the most outrageous dessert without noticeably adding to your risks. In fact, "moderation in all things" can be interpreted to mean that you *should* indulge, but only once in a while. It is the majority that weights the average, so make most of your choices healthful ones, and savor your occasional treats.

Throughout this chapter, you learned about CVD and about personal choice making as the number one strategy against it. The next chapter shows that remarkably similar choices can affect the development of cancer.

⊛ **To reduce CVD risk, learn to relax and control stress.**

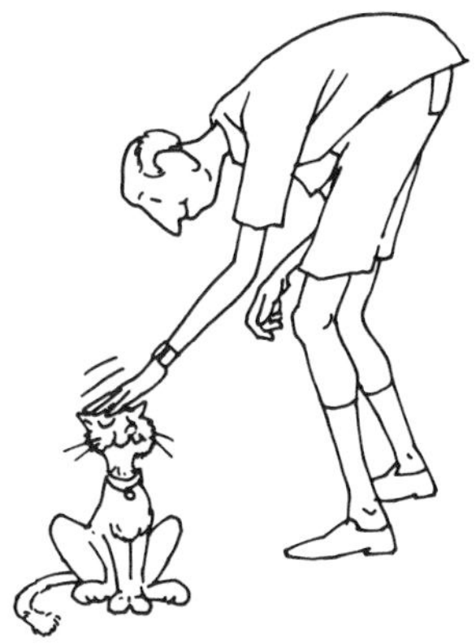

Stop and relax totally at intervals.

STUDY AIDS

1. Describe the circulatory system, and explain how blood moves from place to place in the body.
2. Explain the role of the capillaries.
3. Describe the development of atherosclerosis.
4. Describe the event called heart attack and its effects on the heart.
5. Define *congestive heart failure.*
6. Describe the event called stroke and its effects on the brain.
7. Identify the principal risk factors for coronary heart disease and stroke.
8. Explain ways in which smoking strains the heart, precipitating or worsening heart disease.
9. Explain the relationship of hypertension to CVD.
10. Describe the kidneys' role in raising blood pressure.
11. Describe how blood pressure readings are taken, what factors can affect the reading, and how to determine whether the reading is normal.
12. State your blood pressure, or at least whether it is high or not.
13. Identify methods of controlling high blood pressure.
14. List and describe some ways people can influence their own blood lipid levels.
15. Discuss the relationship of personality type and stress management to chronic diseases.

GLOSSARY

aneurysm (AN-your-ism): the ballooning out of an artery wall at a point where it has been weakened by deterioration.

angina (an-JYE-nuh or ANN-juh-nuh): pain in the heart region caused by lack of oxygen. The complete term is *angina pectoris* (peck-TORE-iss or PECK-tore-iss).

angina = to strangle
pectus = chest

angioplasty: a procedure to reduce the size of plaques in arteries by inserting a tube into the artery to put pressure on and flatten the plaques.

arteries: blood vessels that carry blood from the heart to the tissues.

arteriogram: an Xray used to locate blockages in arteries, such as those that occur in atherosclerosis.

arteriosclerosis (ar-TEER-ee-oh-scler-OH-sis): hardening of the arteries.

atherosclerosis (ATH-uh-roh-scler-OH-sis): the most common form of arteriosclerosis, a disease characterized by plaques along the inner walls of the arteries.

   athero = porridge or soft
   scleros = hard
   osis = too much

atria (singular, **atrium**): the two upper chambers of the heart.

blood lipid profile: a test that reveals the amounts of various lipids in the blood.

capillaries: minute weblike blood vessels that permit transfer of blood and tissue materials.

cardiovascular disease (CVD): a general term for all diseases of the heart and blood vessels.

cardiovascular system: see *circulatory system*.

cerebral thrombosis: see *thrombus*.

chelation therapy: an unproved therapy for heart disease.

cholesterol: see Chapter 4 Glossary.

circulatory system: the system of structures that circulates blood and lymph throughout the body. Also called the *cardiovascular system*.

   cardio = heart
   vascula = blood vessels

collateral blood vessels: small, alternate blood vessels in the heart that form a detour around blocked or narrowed larger arteries, permitting the heart to deliver blood and thus preventing tissue death.

congestive heart failure: an insufficiency of heart action, causing blood backup in the veins, edema, and breathing difficulties.

coronary arteries: the two arteries that supply blood to the heart muscle.

coronary artery bypass surgery: surgery to provide an alternate route for blood to reach heart tissue, bypassing a blocked coronary artery.

coronary artery disease (coronary heart disease): disease of the coronary arteries, a major contributor to CVD.

coronary thrombosis (coronary occlusion): see *thrombus*.

correlation: an association of two variables, such that when one increases, the other increases (or decreases). A *variable* is anything that varies, such as age, height, or heart attack risk.

critical phase: in atherosclerosis, when plaques cover more than 60 percent of the interior surfaces of the arteries making a CVD event likely.

diastole (die-ASS-toh-lee): the part of the heartbeat in which the heart ventricles relax. Diastolic (die-uh-STAHL-ick) blood pressure is the lowest pressure in the veins and arteries and is represented by the second number in a blood pressure reading. See also *systole*.

   diastellein = to expand, dilate

digitalis: a drug derived from the foxglove plant that increases the force of the heart's muscle contractions.

edema: the accumulation of fluids in parts of the body, resulting from a backup of blood in veins.

electrocardiograph (ECG or EKG): a record of the electrical activity of the heart that, if abnormal, may indicate heart disease.

embolism: see *embolus*.

embolus (EM-boh-luss): a clot that breaks loose and travels through the bloodstream. When it causes sudden closure of a blood vessel, the event is an *embolism*.

   embol = to insert

HDL: see *lipoproteins*.

heart attack: the event in which vessels that feed the heart muscle become blocked, causing tissue death. Also called *myocardial infarction*.

   myo = muscle
   cardial = of the heart
   infarct = tissue death

heart disease: any disease of heart muscle or other working parts of the heart.

heart murmur: a heart sound that reflects abnormal or damaged heart valves.

hemorrage: bursting of a blood vessel with resultant bleeding.

high-density lipoprotein (HDL): see *lipoproteins*.

hypertension: high blood pressure—a systolic reading higher than 140 or a diastolic reading higher than 90.

intervention studies: research studies designed to determine whether certain risk factors are causes of a disease by comparing two similar groups. If a risk factor is reduced in one population and the incidence of the disease also decreases, and if the risk factor is not reduced in the other population and the incidence of the disease does not decrease, this is taken as evidence that the risk factor is causal.

LDL: see *lipoproteins*.

lipoproteins: clusters of protein and fat molecules that transport lipids in the blood and lymph. *Low-density lipoproteins (LDL)* carry large amounts of fat and cholesterol from the liver, where the fat and cholesterol are made, to the tissues and also deposit excess cholesterol in arteries, forming plaques. *High-density lipoproteins (HDL)* carry smaller amounts of fat and cholesterol away from the tissues (and from plaques) back to the liver for breakdown and, ultimately, excretion from the body.

low-density lipoprotein (LDL): see *lipoproteins*.

myocardial infarction: see *heart attack*.

pacemaker: a device that delivers electrical impulses to the heart to regulate the heartbeat.

plaques (placks): mounds of lipid material, mixed with smooth muscle cells and calcium, that lodge in arterial walls and contribute to atherosclerosis. (The same word is used to describe a different kind of accumulation of material on teeth, which promotes dental caries.)

   placken = patch

platelets: tiny, disk-shaped bodies in the blood, important in blood clot formation.

   platelet = little plate

risk factor: a factor that is associated with a disease by correlation but that is not proved to be causal.

stroke: the shutting off of the blood flow to the brain by a thrombus or embolus, or by hemorrhage.

systole (SIS-toe-lee): the part of the heartbeat in which the heart ventricles are in contraction, during which the blood is pushed out into the arteries. Systolic blood pressure is the maximum blood pressure in the vascular system and is represented by the first number in a blood pressure reading. See also *diastole*.

   sustellein = to contract

thrombus: a stationary clot. When it has grown enough to close off a blood vessel, the event is a *thrombosis*. A *coronary thrombosis* (coronary occlusion) is the closing off of a vessel that feeds the heart muscle. A *cerebral thrombosis* is the closing off of a vessel that feeds the brain.

   coronary = crowning (the heart)
   thrombo = clot
   cerebrum = part of the brain

transient ischemic (iss-KEE-mic)

attack (TIA): a small, usually mild, reversible stroke; a warning signal that a major stroke is threatening.

type A: a personality style associated with increased incidence of CVD, characterized by impatience, hostility, and aggression.

type B: a personality style associated with decreased incidence of CVD, characterized by patient, easygoing behavior.

variable: see *correlation*.

varicose veins: visible bulging out of the veins, especially in the legs, sometimes accompanied by pain and ulcers. Treatment may include elevating the feet each day, wearing supportive stockings, or undergoing surgical removal of the largest veins. Tiny, spidery purple marks on the skin are normal and are not related to varicose veins.

veins: blood vessels that carry used blood from the tissues back to the heart.
ventricles: the two lower chambers of the heart.

QUIZ ANSWERS

1. *False*. The blood that passes through the heart's chambers donates no nourishment to the heart tissues; the heart depends on its own network of arteries, just as other tissues do.

2. *True*. Veins appear blue under the skin because the blood within them is blue.

3. *False*. Heart surgery, although highly publicized, usually is not required for recovery from a heart attack.

4. *False*. Chelation therapy is useful for heavy metal poisoning but useless in treating atherosclerosis.

5. *True*. A person with hypertension has high blood pressure.

6. *True*. Everyone is developing atherosclerosis.

7. *False*. High blood pressure gives no warning signs.

8. *False*. Efforts at reversing atherosclerosis are beginning to prove successful; still, prevention is better than attempting reversal.

9. *False*. The primary dietary measure to avoid heart disease is to eat *less total fat*; a secondary measure is to replace some saturated fats such as butter with polyunsaturated fats such as soft or liquid margarine.

10. *False*. To avoid salt, fat, and cholesterol, choose whole foods and limit fats (especially animal fats); special foods or expensive products are not needed.

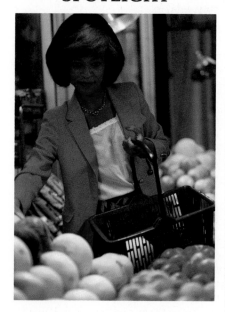

Diabetes

In **diabetes**, the blood sugar (glucose) builds up and is not cleared away normally. One out of every four people in the United States has diabetes in the family, and it is a risk factor for CVD.

Why doesn't the body handle glucose normally in diabetes?

The answer centers around the hormone insulin, which enables the body tissues to remove glucose from the blood. Two conditions can interfere with the normal use of glucose: either a person's body makes too little insulin, or the tissues lose their sensitivity to the insulin the body does make. Without insulin or the sensitivity needed to use it, glucose does not enter the tissues, where it is needed to furnish vital energy. The kidneys normally allow no glucose to escape into the urine. But in diabetes, the concentration of glucose in the blood exceeds the kidneys' capacity to conserve it, and some of the excess is lost in the urine.

Why is that a problem to the body?

The problem lies in the resulting imbalance in the chemistry of the blood. The composition of the blood is normally tightly controlled, with many centers throughout the body providing checks and balances. In diabetes, the blood contains its normal amount of water, but has too high a concentration of glucose. The body experiences the condition as a lack of water in the blood, so it sends fluid from the tissues into the bloodstream to dilute the glucose to its normal concentration. The kidneys then detect the excess water in the blood and excrete it, but excrete with it many of the other vital blood components as well. Frequent urination causes dehydration. Two of the warning signs of diabetes, excessive thirst and urination, are caused by the movement of water out of the tissues and into the urine. Table S16–1 lists the warning signs of diabetes.

TABLE S16–1 The Warning Signs of Diabetes

1. Excessive urination and thirst.
2. Weight loss with nausea, easy tiring, weakness, or irritability.
3. Craving for sweets or other food.
4. Frequent infections of the skin, gums, or urinary tract.
5. Vision disturbances.
6. Pain in the legs, feet, or fingers.
7. Slow healing of cuts and bruises.
8. Itching.
9. Drowsiness.

SOURCE: J. M. Couric, Diabetes is a controllable disease with a growth factor, *FDA Consumer*, November 1982, pp. 21–23.

Without glucose for energy, how do tissues stay alive?

Most cells of the body are equipped to handle long periods of carbohydrate depletion, as would occur during fasting or starvation. When glucose is not available, the tissues resort to using their other energy fuels—protein and fat—and produce **ketones**. Ketones are the acidic byproducts of fat breakdown; they can change the acid-base balance of the blood, and they can disturb brain function if they reach too-high levels. In diabetes, the ketones can overwhelm the brain, producing coma.

I've heard that diabetes affects people's feet, and that they can go blind. Why would sugar in the blood cause trouble for the feet or eyes?

The effects of untreated diabetes on the body seem unlikely, at first glance: disease of the feet and legs, sometimes requiring amputation; kidney disease, sometimes requiring intensive hospital care or kidney transplant; cataracts in the eye, leading to blindness; and nerve damage. The root cause of all these conditions is the same. Diabetes causes destruction and blockage of the small arteries that feed the tissues—with effects like those of atherosclerosis.[1]* The tissues of the feet, kidneys, cornea, and other parts of the body die from lack of nourishment when the arteries that feed them become diseased. That is why uncontrolled diabetes is a powerful risk factor for heart disease or stroke. Hypertension and elevated blood cholesterol are much more common in people with elevated blood glucose than in others.[2]

Is is possible for people with diabetes to avoid developing these conditions?

Yes. Many people with diabetes live long, healthy lives provided they obtain and follow medical treatment to control their diabetes. In some cases the person with diabetes may attain higher levels of health than a person without the condition because the person with diabetes is inspired to adopt healthy behaviors. Treatment of diabetes focuses on controlling blood glucose in these ways:

- Obtaining insulin or oral medication, if required.
- Daily monitoring of blood glucose.
- Following a dietary regime to match insulin and control blood glucose.
- Achieving and maintaining appropriate body weight.
- Exercising regularly.

The person with diabetes is advised to have regular physician visits and to obtain an individualized meal plan from a registered dietitian. Controlling blood glucose increases the chance of avoiding complications.

Can people prevent diabetes from occurring?

Yes, sometimes they can. Diabetes has its own risk factors, some of which can be controlled and others that cannot. One that cannot be controlled is inheritance; people from families with diabetes stand a greater chance of developing it than do oth-

*Reference notes are in Appendix D.

MINIGLOSSARY

adult-onset diabetes: see *type II diabetes.*

diabetes: a condition of abnormal carbohydrate metabolism, resulting in too much glucose in the blood and the presence of glucose in the urine. Diabetes is caused by inadequate production of insulin or the failure to use the insulin produced. The common form, *diabetes mellitus,* is a major risk factor in the onset of heart disease and stroke and causes many organ diseases.

gestational diabetes: a type of diabetes mellitus that develops during pregnancy and is associated with birth defects in offspring; often a forerunner of type II diabetes.

ketones: acidic by-products of fat metabolism produced during a time of carbohydrate deficit in the tissues. Buildup of these chemicals causes diabetic ketosis (see page 92) and coma.

type I diabetes: a type of diabetes mellitus that begins in childhood and is characterized by a lack of insulin in the blood, thinness, and failure to grow. Also called *juvenile-onset diabetes.*

type II diabetes: a type of diabetes mellitus that sets in during adulthood and is characterized by the presence of adequate insulin in the blood, a lack of tissue response to the insulin, and obesity. Also called *adult-onset diabetes* or *maturity-onset diabetes.*

---

ers.[3] Among those risk factors that can be controlled is obesity. Susceptible people who are overweight develop the major form of diabetes as they get older (**type II**, or **maturity-onset, diabetes**). Type II diabetes accounts for over 90 percent of all diabetes in the United States. Inactivity also can contribute to this type of diabetes, and exercise can be preventive. In addition, women who develop diabetes during their pregnancies (**gestational diabetes**) face a greater risk than normal of developing the disease outright, as well as a higher risk of birth defects in their infants. Gestational diabetes is often preventable by gaining appropriate weight for pregnancy, without excess.

Is there a type of diabetes that is not preventable?

Yes. About 10 percent of people develop diabetes in childhood (**type I diabetes**). The cause is unknown, but it is suspected that a virus may cause or worsen the condition. In type I diabetes, the immune system attacks and destroys the cells of the pancreas that make insulin, creating an insulin deficiency. A child with the disease usually becomes thin and fails to grow.

Why do some people require insulin shots whereas others do not?

People with type I diabetes do not make insulin at all. It has to be supplied through injections or other means such as implanted pumps that deliver the drug automatically. In contrast, people with type II diabetes may produce plenty of insulin but fail to respond to it. Sometimes a person with type II diabetes benefits from insulin shots or insulin-producing drugs. Some people with type II diabetes can manage the disease by diet and exercise alone.

Is it true that people with diabetes have to avoid eating sweets and ice cream?

In most cases, yes. Especially for an overweight person, a diet low in fat and sugar, high in unrefined whole foods provides the needed starch, fiber, vitamins, and minerals while helping with weight loss and maintenance of normal blood glucose levels. Such a diet also helps lower blood cholesterol for control of CVD.

However, each case of diabetes is as unique as each human being. The goal of the diet is to maintain normal blood glucose levels and a healthy body weight. For this reason, it's essential to obtain an individual plan developed by three people working together: the physician, the registered dietitian, and most important, the person with diabetes who must live with it every day.

Cancer

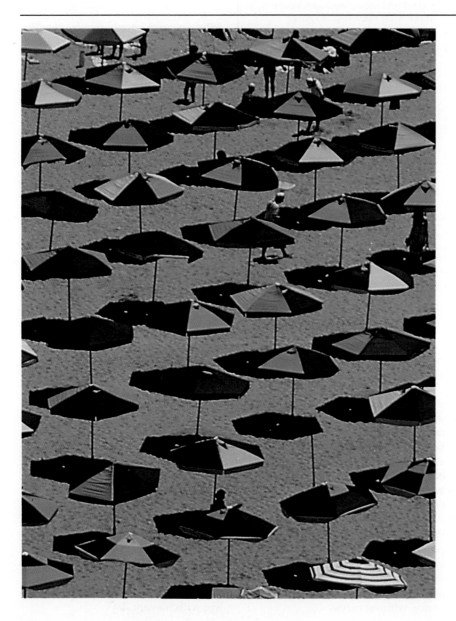

FOR OPENERS . . .

True or false? If false, say what is true.

1. Once cancer has started in a person's body, it can be eliminated only by surgery, chemotherapy, or radiation treatment.

2. The majority of cancers may be preventable by changes in lifestyle factors.

3. In addition to lung cancer risk, smoking is linked to an increased incidence of cancers throughout the body.

4. People with darkly pigmented skin do not need to use sunscreen to prevent skin cancer.

5. People who would like to tan while avoiding the risk of skin cancer can do so in tanning booths or with lamps.

6. People can help ward off certain cancers by choosing the right diet.

7. If you work hard at it, you can prevent cancer.

8. A person who notices a suspicious body change should observe it for a month, and if it persists, have it checked.

9. To cure cancer, a treatment must destroy or remove every cancer cell from the body.

10. Some of the most effective cancer drugs have been discovered in wild plants and animals.

(Answers on page 359.)

At the turn of the century, the forecast for most people diagnosed as having **cancer** was bleak, but today, millions of people have fought and won battles with cancer and are living normal lives. Although the numbers vary with the type of cancer and how early it is detected, the average rate of complete and permanent recovery from cancers of all types is approaching 50 percent and 80–90 percent for some individual types. Recent news concerns cancer prevention. Researchers estimate that 80 percent of all cancer cases result from the circumstances of people's lives, many of which they can control themselves.[1]* For example, the number one cancer in both men and women is now lung cancer, which is seen only rarely in people who don't smoke. It has been estimated that 30 percent of all cancers could be eliminated if people stopped using tobacco.

Cancer affects one out of every four people in the United States today. Over a hundred diseases are called cancer, and each has its own name and characteristic progression of symptoms, depending on its type and location in the body. Some cancers are given names that reflect the location of the tissue from which they arise, with the suffix *-oma*, meaning tumor, added on. For example, cancer of the pigmented cells of the skin, the melanocytes, is called **melanoma**. A tumor of the bone marrow is a **myeloma**—*myelos* means marrow. The names of cancers are numerous and this chapter will keep naming to a minimum.

WHAT IS CANCER?

Generally, all cancers can be assigned to one of four classes, depending on tissue type:

- Cancers of the immune system organs are **lymphomas** (limf-OH-mahz).
- Cancers of blood-forming organs are **leukemias** (loo-KEE-me-ahz).
- Cancers of the glands and body linings such as the skin, lining of the digestive tract or lungs, or other linings are **carcinomas** (car-sin-OH-mahz).
- Cancers of connective tissue, including bones, ligaments, and muscles, are **sarcomas** (sar-KOH-mahz).

The word *cancer* refers to a type of tissue, a **tumor**, that is growing out of control in the body. The tumor has needs, just as other tissues do. The body provides for those needs as though the tumor were normal body tissue, building arteries and veins to supply nutrients and oxygen to it and to remove wastes from it. Thus a tumor may grow rapidly, with full support of the body's systems.

Initially, the cancer begins when a normal cell changes into a cancer cell with altered metabolism and uncontrolled reproduction. The steps in the development of cancer are thought to be:

1. Exposure to a type of **carcinogen** called an **initiator**. One environmental agent may work alone to initiate cancer, or two or more such factors may work together as **co-carcinogens**.
2. Entry of the initiator into a cell.
3. Alteration by the initiator of the molecules responsible for cell division.
4. Possible acceleration of cancerous alterations by a **promoter**.
5. Out-of-control multiplication of the cells.
6. Tumor formation.

*Reference notes are in Appendix D.

CHAPTER 17 ■ CANCER

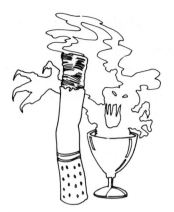

Two factors that work together as carcinogens: tobacco and alcohol.

be-NINE

ON-co-jean

meh-TASS-tuh-sized

An example of how initiators and promoters work together (see Figure 17–1) is the interaction between alcohol and tobacco in the development of cancers of the mouth, throat, and esophagus. Normally, these cancers are rare. In a person who smokes two packs of cigarettes a day, the risk of developing a cancer is one and a half times greater than for the nonsmoker, but should that person also drink two alcoholic drinks each day, the risk becomes 15 times greater. Alcohol alone does not increase the risk for these particular cancers, so it is thought likely to be acting as a cancer promoter, not as an initiator. The chemicals in cigarette smoke probably act in both ways: they initiate the cancer and promote it, too, to some degree.[2]

All of the changes that lead to cancer happen inside an individual's cells, so cancer itself is not contagious. Once it has started, though, it can attack any tissue inside the body, from the solid bone to the fluid blood.

Normally, cells can discriminate when and whether to divide to produce new cells. For example, if some of the tissue of your liver were to become damaged, the remaining healthy cells of the liver would multiply to replace the damaged part and then stop. A cancerous cell, though, appears to have lost responsiveness to the signal that says "stop dividing," and so it and all its progeny divide continuously. The result is a lump of nonfunctional tissue, a tumor. Sometimes the tumor is a harmless bump—a **benign** tumor—that does not spread, forming a well-defined, solid mass that is contained in an external membrane. A cancerous, spreading tumor that has less-defined boundaries and invades surrounding tissues is called **malignant**.

The processes that transform normal cells into malignant ones are unknown, but the cells' genetic material is believed to be involved. Researchers suspect that an **oncogene**, a portion of a cancer cell's genetic material, plays a key role in the transformation process. Oncogenes probably undergo **mutation**—that is, they change. Alternatively, they could originate from the genetic material of a virus left behind from an infection. In either case, an oncogene changes the cell's protein products. These changed products influence the cell's reproduction and metabolism, giving it the malignant characteristic. Because the oncogene is part of the genetic material of the cell, it is passed on to each of the cell's offspring, so that they also are malignant.[3]

As a malignant tumor gains in size, it competes with normal tissues around it for nutrients and space, and it eventually interrupts the normal function of the tissue or organ in which it has grown. In cancer of the large intestine, for example, the tumor may block the passage of the intestinal contents; in cancer of the brain, the growing tumor threatens the mind's function and body control.

In addition to invading surrounding tissues, cancer cells break loose from the original site and ride the rivers of body fluids to colonize new locations. When the tumor is just beginning, it sheds only a few cells. As it enlarges, however, more and more of these wild cells escape and start new growths in other body parts, and the cancer is said to have **metastasized**. Cancer causes death of the person when it interrupts the functioning of vital organs such as the lungs, digestive system, or brain.

The immune system is on the watch for escaped cancer cells and works to stop these dangerous travelers before they lodge in body tissue. But the immune system is limited in the number of cancer cells it can eliminate at any one time. The success of treatment often depends on whether a cancer has metastasized before it is detected.

After the initiating event, some cancers take as long as 20 years to develop. It is impossible to look back and discover which initiator or which promoters facilitated the long chain of events that ultimately led to cancer. However, research has uncovered some factors that are known, or strongly suspected, to be causal. Genetic susceptibility, suppression or defect of the immune system, geographic location, environmental chemicals and radiation, life-style choices, age, sex, and personality are all risk factors. Separating their effects is a problem.

RISK FACTORS THAT PEOPLE CAN CONTROL

The incidence of many cancers in the United States has not declined over the last 20 years, and researchers are trying to pinpoint the environmental factors that may cause or contribute to them.[4] Environmental factors that can affect cancer include not only air, water, food, and surroundings, but also disease agents (microbes), stress, exercise—in short, every aspect of existence except heredity. This chapter's Life Choice Inventory can help you evaluate the known controllable factors in your life.

Tobacco

Smoking is probably the most familiar of the cancer risk factors, and with good reason—the evidence against it is overwhelming. Hospital studies show consistently that 80 percent of lung cancer victims are smokers; population studies show that an increase in smoking precedes a jump in incidence of lung cancer; and animal studies show that direct application to the skin of condensed chemicals from tobacco smoke causes cancer.

In addition to the connection with lung cancer, smoking is linked to an increased incidence of cancers throughout the body, and it is related to about a third of all cancer deaths. Cancer of the larynx (voice box), mouth, esophagus, urinary bladder, kidney, and pancreas all have been attributed to smoking. Second-hand smoking also increases risks.

Painless, whitish patches (**leukoplakia**) form in the mouths of people who turn to smokeless tobacco; these are a warning sign of changes that may lead to lethal cancers of the mouth and throat—cancers most frequently seen in tobacco users. Other times, red patches may appear. Both of these warnings should be evaluated by a health care practitioner. Using alcohol as well as tobacco, even at different times, is dangerous: they work together to increase the cancer odds enormously.

Radiation

The sun's ultraviolet rays are a carcinogenic form of radiation, and too much exposure to them is the leading cause of skin cancer. Skin color can help predict susceptibility—the darker the skin, the more resistant to cancer.

Concentrated doses of the sun's radiation, such as the amount received with sunburn, are most likely to promote cancerous changes. Melanoma is the most lethal form of skin cancer; formerly one of the less common skin cancers, it is now on the rise.[5] According to one study, a single blistering sunburn in the teen years can double a person's risk of melanoma in later

FIGURE 17–1 Cancer Initiators and Promoters

In cancer research, initiators and promoters are found to work together to produce many more tumors than initiators alone.

Experiment 1

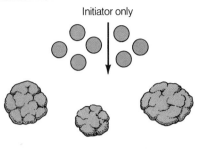

Initiator only

A few tumors result.

Experiment 2

Promoter only

No tumors result.

Experiment 3

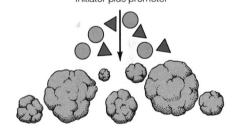

Initiator plus promoter

Many tumors develop.

⊕ STRATEGIES to Minimize Cancer Risks

To cut your risks of cancer:

⊕ **Do not smoke; do not use tobacco in any form.**

⊕ **Encourage people around you to stop smoking; choose nonsmoking areas whenever possible.**

How well do you protect yourself against cancer? You cannot eliminate all cancer risk from your life, but you can take steps to reduce your risk of developing the disease. Questions answered no indicate opportunities for improvement.

1. Are you a nonsmoker?
2. Are you careful not to sunburn?
3. Do you question the necessity of X-ray examinations?
4. Do you read and follow instructions on the labels of chemicals that you use in the home, in the garden, or on the job?
5. Do you choose foods in a balanced diet that supply adequate fiber, vitamin A, and vitamin C, without too much fat? Do you eat cabbage and related vegetables often?
6. Is your weight within the normal range for your height?
7. Do you limit your intake of cured and smoked meats?
8. Do you limit your alcohol intake?
9. Do you exercise regularly?
10. Do you practice breast or testicular self-examination regularly?

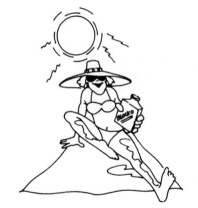

Use sunscreen and take along a big hat.

✳ Take care to avoid burning when sunbathing; take along some sunscreen and a big hat.

✳ Question "routine" X-ray procedures; if they are not essential, ask that they be omitted.

life.[6] People who receive small, daily doses of sunlight tend to develop the more common, easily diagnosed and cured forms of skin cancer.*

All types of sunlamps and tanning booths, including the ultraviolet-A type, bombard the skin with radiation and provide no health benefits. A recent twist is a high-intensity quick-tan lamp used in tanning booths. According to the FDA, unless these lamps are properly filtered, they can not only cause cancer but also damage blood vessels and cloud the lens of the eye (**cataracts**).[7]

People are exposed to a great deal of background radiation from the cosmos, from the soil, and from the air and water. Artifical radiation bombards us from medical and dental X-rays and from above-ground nuclear weapons testing.[8] Researchers believe that throughout life, a person living in the United States normally receives about one-third the minimum radiation required to cause the cancer leukemia.[9]

People cannot escape radiation entirely, nor is such a goal in keeping with good health. In the case of ultraviolet radiation from the sun, small doses are essential to make vitamin D and other compounds, so moderate exposure is the goal. But you should take certain precautions to avoid dangerous overexposure. Be aware that ultraviolet rays penetrate clouds, so that even on cool, cloudy days, you can get burned. Use a sunscreen product that will block ultraviolet radiation and prevent burning. The higher a product's sun protection factor (SPF), the more protection it gives. When choosing a sunscreen for your skin color, start with a high SPF, say 25, to avoid the possibility of being caught out in the sun without adequate protection. To receive the intended level of protection, a person in a bathing suit should apply a full ounce of product with each application. Plan to enjoy the sun for short times on many occasions rather than on an all-day trip, and take along a big hat.

Another strategy for avoiding unnecessary radiation exposure is to tell your dentist and health care practitioner that you wish to avoid X-rays whenever possible. When they are unavoidable, be sure that the technician

*The most common skin cancer is basal cell carcinoma; second is squamous cell carcinoma.

takes precautions to protect the parts of your body that are not being X-rayed, especially the abdomen and genitals.

Diet and Exercise

Evidence about the cancer effects of food and diet is piling up. Food brings with it into the body materials from the external environment, and food constituents become a part of the body, thus influencing cancer's development. Further, food substances moving through the digestive tract affects these organs directly, even if the substances themselves pass through intact, without being absorbed. This chapter's Spotlight describes ways that the constituents of food are suspected to promote or inhibit the development of cancer.

Exercise may also be important in cancer prevention. Some evidence indicates that people who are sedentary contract cancer of the large intestine more often than people who exercise regularly.[10] More research in this area is needed.

■ RISK FACTORS BEYOND PEOPLE'S CONTROL

Even if a risk factor cannot be controlled directly, it may still be one you can take steps to minimize. Generally, wherever a risk factor is outside of your own control, many other controllable ones can work to oppose it.

Environment

Chemical carcinogens, both natural and artifical, surround us, and taken together, they create a cancer risk. City dwellers are exposed to engine exhaust and factory chemicals, while people in the country run a risk from using pesticides and other agricultural chemicals. Certain occupations also entail greater cancer risks than others. Chapter 19 delves further into environmental chemicals that cause cancer and other ills.

Cancers are sometimes specific to geographic locations. It may be that people are exposed to different risk factors in different places. In India and China, for example, cancers of the uterus and penis are common; liver cancer is prevalent in Africa and Indochina. Inadequate hygiene practices probably contribute to cancer of the penis; for liver cancer, it is suspected that a virus common to the area is the root cause. When people change locations, especially if they are young, their cancer risks change to those of the new locality. Diet change is a prime suspect, and the anticancer diet strategies are probably effective no matter where they are practiced.

Stomach cancer is becoming rare in most developed nations, yet in a northern geographic belt extending from Iceland to Japan, stomach cancer shows up frequently. It is thought that in those countries, absence of chemical preservatives and poor refrigeration allows carcinogens to develop in the food supply more often than in developed countries. Of course, this does not mean that you should search out foods with preservatives to reduce your cancer risk; it does mean that you should eat only unspoiled food.

Sex, Age, and Personality

Whether you are a man or a woman partially determines your likelihood of developing cancer of all types. Overall, women are slightly more likely to develop it than men are, but in men, cancer is more likely to be fatal.

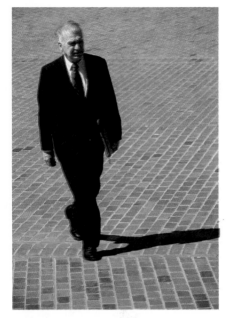

Exercise daily, all your life.

✳ **Exercise regularly.**

✳ **Select employment carefully; some jobs are associated with higher cancer incidence. If your job carries a hazard, take all the recommended precautions at all times.**

✳ **Throw away any food on the verge of spoilage.**

Age plays an important role in a person's chances of developing cancer. Young people rarely contract and die of cancer; older people frequently do. The relationship is linear: the older the person, the more likely he or she is to contract cancer. Age is outside the control of the individual. But a shift in emphasis from prevention alone to prevention and early detection through screening tests will help a person to exert maximum contol over the disease. Screening tests are described in a later section.

Cancer may have a connection with personality type. The theory of the cancer-prone personality states that such people, **type C** individuals, demonstrate helplessness, passivity, and a desire to appease others.[11] It is unknown whether severe cancer itself may bring such traits on or whether such a coping style is a risk factor for cancer.[12] Unsatisfactory interpersonal relationships may also be linked with subsequent cancer development.[13] Learning to handle stress and grief and improving relationships bring many benefits, and they just may turn out to be important in cancer prevention.

Heredity

The genetics of cancer is complex. It is relatively certain that cancer itself, with rare exception, is not inherited. Normal cells are thought to change into cancerous ones during a person's lifetime.

Oncogenes are one focus of interest. Scientists are striving to identify products that oncogenes produce; blood tests to detect those products could then identify people who are at risk for cancer development. The goal is to screen families of people with a particular form of cancer and be on the lookout for the disease in the earliest, most curable stages.

Viruses are connected with the genetics of cancer. Remember from Chapter 15 that a virus's genetic material uses the host cell's manufacturing equipment to reproduce copies of the virus. Scientists think that cancer-causing viruses may also trick the cells into dividing. It may be that the viral oncogenes fool the cells into producing the very molecule that gives the go-ahead signal for cell division. Normally, the cells would be triggered to produce this molecule only when cell replacement was required for health, but under the influence of the virus, replication could go on unchecked, forming a tumor. An alternative idea is that people's genetic material carries viruslike sections that can be induced by an initiator to pop out of place and start the multiplication.

The virus that causes the genital warts (a sexually transmitted disease described in Chapter 15) is believed to cause cancer of the cervix in women. Early research found that women most likely to get such cancer began sexual activity at an early age and had multiple partners. More recently it was discovered that a woman stands a three to five times greater chance of getting the disease by pairing with a man whose former partner contracted cervical cancer. Finally, researchers determined that men with genital warts were likely to have partners with cervical cancer and that the virus from the cancer was the same as the one in the warts.[14] The virus is suspected of causing cancer by altering the genetic material in cervical tissues. This sexually transmitted form of cervical cancer is especially likely to attack young women who began intercourse in their early teen years. It is thought that the cells of the cervix are most susceptible to mutations during the final stages of maturing.

Although cancers usually are not inherited, the tendency to develop certain cancers can run in families. People with a family history of cancers should alert their health care providers so that they may obtain tests for them.

SCREENING AND EARLY DETECTION

The treatment of cancer makes use of sophisticated equipment, powerful drugs, and specialized medical staff, but the detection of common cancers requires mostly routine tests and self-examinations. The sooner a cancer is detected, the better the chances for a complete cure. Table 17–1 lists the cancers that most often cause deaths among young people and the symp-

TABLE 17–1   Cancers Causing Death in People Ages 15 to 34

Disease	Early Symptoms	Survival with Early Diagnosis and Prompt Treatment[a]
Leukemia	Mimics infection, with fever, lethargy, and other flulike symptoms; may also include bone pain, tendency to bruise or bleed easily, and enlargement of lymph nodes	Poor to good (up to 50%), depending on the type of disease
Brain and nervous system cancer	Personality changes, bizarre behavior, headaches, dizziness, balance and walking disturbances, vision changes, nausea, vomiting, or seizures	Poor to good
Hodgkin's disease	Swelling of lymph nodes in neck, armpits, or groin; susceptibility to infection	Good (54%)
Breast cancer	Unusual lump, thickening, change in contour, dimple, or discharge from the nipple	Good (about 50%)
Testicular cancer	Small, hard, painless lump; sudden accumulation of fluid in the scrotum; pain or discomfort in the region between the scrotum and anus	Good to excellent (66 to 86%)
Uterine cervical cancer	Abnormal Pap test results; later symptoms include urinary abnormalities, unusual bleeding or vaginal discharge between menstrual periods or following intercourse	Excellent (80%)
Skin cancer	Unusual discoloration, swellings, sores, or lumps; change in color or appearance of a wart or mole; tenderness, itching, or bleeding from a lump or mole	Excellent (up to 90%)

[a]The survival rates are estimates based on five years of disease-free survival. For all cancers, survival rates drop dramatically after metastasis.

toms associated with each. Any of the symptoms listed should be checked by a health care provider immediately.

Often, cancer gives some warning to the person who is developing it. Cancer can develop without symptoms, but it is wise to heed all the messages your body sends you, particularly those the American Cancer Society points to as warnings of cancer:

FIGURE 17–2   Breast Self-Examination

The next two steps are designed to emphasize any changes in the shape or contour of your breasts. As you do them, you should be able to feel your chest muscles tighten.

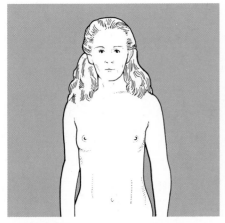

1. Stand before a mirror. Inspect both breasts for anything unusual, such as any discharge from the nipples or puckering, dimpling or scaling of the skin.

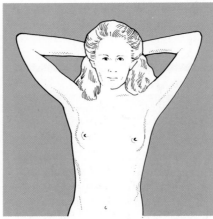

2. Watch closely in the mirror, clasp hands behind your head, and press hands forward.

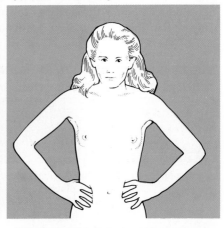

3. Next, press hands firmly on hips and bow slightly toward the mirror as you pull your shoulders and elbows forward.

Some women do the next part of the exam in the shower. Fingers glide over soapy skin, making it easy to concentrate on the texture underneath.

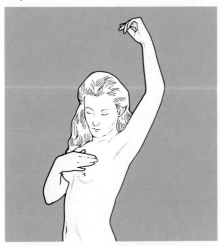

4. Raise your left arm. Use three or four fingers of your right hand to explore your left breast firmly, carefully, and thoroughly. Beginning at the outer edge, press the flat part of your fingers in small circles, moving the circles slowly around the breast. Gradually work toward the nipple. Be sure to cover the entire breast. Pay special

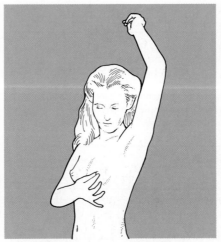

attention to the area between the breast and the armpit, including the armpit itself. Feel for any unusual lump or mass under the skin.

5. Gently squeeze the nipple and look for a discharge. Repeat the exam on your right breast.

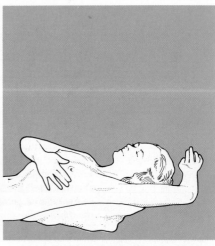

6. Repeat steps 4 and 5 lying down. Lie flat on your back with your left arm over your head and a pillow or folded towel under your left shoulder. This positions flattens the breast and makes it easier to examine. Use the same circular motion described earlier. Repeat on your right breast.

- Change in bowel or bladder habits, such as diarrhea or constipation.
- A sore that does not heal.
- Unusual bleeding or discharge.
- Thickening or lump that suddenly appears anywhere in the body.
- Indigestion or difficulty swallowing.
- Obvious change in a wart or mole.
- Nagging cough or hoarseness.

To help remember this list, recall that the first letters in the warning signs spell the word *caution*. Having one of these symptoms does not necessarily mean that you have cancer. A cold or eating too much might bring about some of them, for example. Just remember that when signals last for more than a week, or when they recur, they require the attention of a health care provider.

Self-examinations are particularly useful for early detection of cancer. If you are a woman, you can check your breasts; the test is easy (see Figure 17–2). In young women, lumps are most often not cancerous, but they should be checked by a health care provider nonetheless.

If you are a man, you can help protect yourself from cancer of the testicles through self-examination (see Figure 17–3). Although it occurs less frequently than breast cancer, testicular cancer is dangerous because it advances rapidly. Once-a-month testing of either breasts or testicles is usually sufficient. Try to test at the same time each month (women should time the test to follow the menstrual period, because the breasts can be lumpy beforehand.) Many people find the tests easy to remember and perform in the shower or bath.

Self-examinations have proved valuable in early cancer detection. A person who often examines his or her body becomes familiar with it and may be more likely to detect an abnormality than a medical professional who examines the person only once a year or so. (Of course, a professional can detect a lump in places not easily examined at home.) Other forms of self-examination are catching on, too; for example, a person who wants a test for colon abnormalities can buy an inexpensive home test that detects hidden blood in the stools, a primary indicator of developing cancer.* The person

*The name of one such home test is Hemoccult.

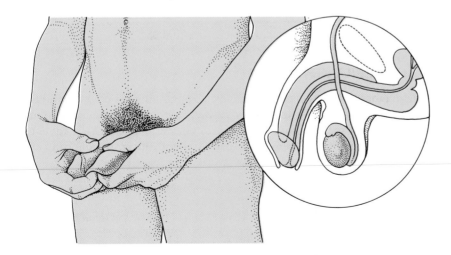

FIGURE 17–3 Testicular Self-Examination

Roll each testicle between the thumb and fingers; the testicles should feel smooth, except for the normal raised organ located on the back of each. Report any hard lump, enlargement, or contour changes to your health care provider.

CHAPTER 17 ■ CANCER

collects a small sample at home and sends it to a laboratory for checking. Such tests should not be used as substitutes for periodic screening, however.

Laboratory tests are important, too, and enormous strides have been made in the development of new cancer detection methods. The most accurate detection method for breast cancer is the **mammogram** (X-ray examination). The procedure does carry some risks, including the slight risk of inducing cancer, but the risks are lessening as the technique is improved. Mammograms are used sparingly; Table 17–2 instructs women to have one done at age 35 to use for a baseline comparison, repeating the test in later life. All women with increased breast cancer risk should be examined by mammography. Table 17–2 lists other medical tests to detect cancer and the appropriate ages at which to seek them.

One standard test is the **biopsy**, which is the surgical removal of a small amount of tissue for microscopic and chemical study. In the case of small, local tumors, a biopsy can be the cure as well as the test. In other cases, it will reveal information vital to the treatment of the disease, such as the tissue in which the cancer originated. Imaging tests are used to discover the size of the mass and the extent of invasion. Physicians often use X-ray examination, including the **CT (computerized tomography) scan**, a computerized organization of X-ray information into a visual image of the tumor. Another method is **thermography**, the detection of heat produced by a tumor in contrast to the cooler normal tissue around it.

People should be tested routinely for the most likely cancers—those of the lungs, skin, cervix, prostate, uterine lining, breasts, large intestine, and rectum. Within these few common locations, the disease can take a great number of forms, and a specific test is needed to detect each one. Specific tests are performed on people with a family history of cancers or with other known risk factors. A health care provider can judge which may be necessary for you. In the future, it may be possible to detect the presence of cancer in the body simply by performing a blood test that detects molecules associated with cancer.[15]

Even though the earliest possible detection is crucial to successful treatment, new detection tests may not be the first priority in cancer research. A better use of resources would be to discover how to prevent cancer's occurrence. No disease has ever been cured out of existence. As is now the case with smallpox and polio, we can claim success only when the disease is prevented from occurring. The rate of cure, although better than in the past, has been relatively stable for many years, while the number of cases remains high, and for some cancers is rising higher.

▓▓▓ CANCER TREATMENT

Being diagnosed as having cancer can be a frightening experience, and fear can impair the body's healing response. But cancer has a tremendous number of treatment success stories, and it is important to know about advances in cancer treatment. For more information about cancer, people can call a cancer hotline number.*

---

*The National Cancer Institute's information service number is (1-800) 4CANCER. In Alaska, it is (1-800) 638-6070; in Washington, D.C., and suburbs, 636-5700 (local number); and in Hawaii, 524-1234 (local number). Spanish-speaking staff are available in some areas.

TABLE 17-2 Medical Tests for the Early Detection of Cancer in Asymptomatic Persons

Test	Sex	20	35	Age 40	50	60
Pap	F	Every year; then, after 2 negatives 1 year apart, every 3 years[a]	At least every 3 years	At least every 3 years	At least every 3 years	—
Pelvic examination	F	Every 3 years	Every 3 years	Every year	Every year	Every year
Breast examination (by physician)	F	Every 3 years	Every 3 years	Every year	Every year	Every year
Testis and prostate examination	M	Every 3 years	Every 3 years	Every year	Every year	Every year
Thyroid, lymph nodes, oral region, and skin examination	M, F	Every 3 years	Every 3 years	Every year	Every year	Every year
Mammography	F	—	Once at 35, to establish baseline[b]	—	Every year	Every year
Digital rectal examination	M, F	—	—	Every year	Every year	Every year
Uterine lining tissue sample	F	—	—	—	Once, at menopause	—
Stool slide test	M, F	—	—	—	Every year	Every year
Colon examination	M, F	—	—	—	Every year; then, after 2 negatives 1 year apart, every 3 to 5 years	At least every 3 years

[a]Start younger if sexually active.

[b]Have additional mammograms on health care provider's recommendation.

SOURCE: Adapted from American Cancer Society recommendations.

Cancer cells move freely in the body, and surgical removal or destruction of a tumor does not necessarily eliminate all of them. Cancer *cure* comes when every cancer cell is either removed from the body or destroyed by treatments.

Surgery is the primary mode of treatment for many cancers. Removal of the tumor stops the cancer growth at the site, especially if the cancer is still small. Figure 17-4 shows cure rates for many types of cancer *by surgery alone*; notice how the cure rate drops off as the tumor invades surrounding tissues and metastasizes. For example, the large intestine may contain growths called **polyps**, which may become cancerous; removal of polyps protects against cancer. If a cancerous polyp begins to invade just a few millimeters into the tissue, however, its surgical removal no longer guarantees complete freedom from cancer at that site.

A small tumor on the skin or another external membrane sometimes can be destroyed by freezing with liquid nitrogen. Such a procedure is often performed in the physician's office and causes little inconvenience or pain.

FIGURE 17–4 **Cancer Progression and Cure Rate by Surgery Alone**

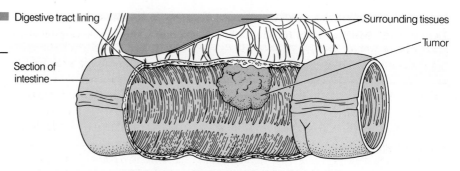

Digestive tract lining

Section of intestine

Surrounding tissues

Tumor

(a) When the tumor is local, surgery alone can cure it 80% of the time.

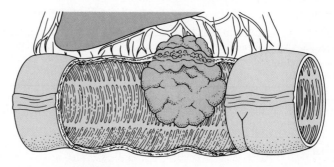

(b) When the tumor has advanced into the surrounding tissues, the cure rate by surgery drops to 40%.

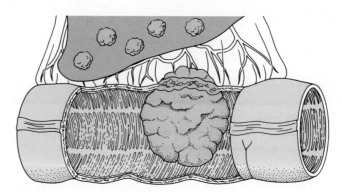

(c) A tumor that has widely invaded the surrounding tissue and has metastasized can be cured by surgery alone only 20% of the time.

You have probably heard the name of one type of surgery for breast cancer—the **radical mastectomy**. In medicine, the word *radical* means curative; **mastectomy** means removal of the breast. The mastectomy was originally developed only to make clients with advanced cancer comfortable—**palliative therapy**—but even some of these advanced cases were cured by the procedure. Still the best choice for some cases, the radical mastectomy removes muscle, bone, and glands as well as the breast, and it cures the disease about half the time. In other cases, it is possible to remove less tissue, because the surgery is usually accompanied by other treatments aimed at wiping out cancer cells not removed by surgery. These treatments have been shown, at least by some research, to be as effective as radical mastectomy.[16]

Another treatment for cancer, **radiation therapy**, is similar to surgery in that both are local forms of treatment and both must remove normal tissue to kill cancer tissue. In some cases, as in cancer of the head or neck, radiation is chosen over surgery because surrounding structures may be too delicate to permit surgery. To kill a tumor with radiation, a beam is focused on the area known to be cancerous. Alternatively, radioactive materials are injected into the bloodstream and selectively absorbed by the tumor, or the materials may be implanted. Under bombardment from the radioactivity, the fast-growing cells of the cancer become disrupted and die off.

People who receive such treatments may suffer from skin irritation, nausea, diarrhea, hair loss, and fatigue. Developments in technology have helped to minimize these effects by minimizing the damage to healthy tissues.

Chemical treatment of cancer, called **chemotherapy**, has a major advantage—the drugs are taken orally or by injection and are distributed throughout the body to seek out and destroy the escaped cancer cells and any new tumors that may be just starting. More than 40 drugs are now used against cancer in some way, to cure, to inhibit cancer growth, to relieve pain, and to allow the person to lead a more normal life.

A typical anticancer drug works by blocking cell division—for example, by interfering with the action of the vitamin folacin. Cancer cells need more folacin than other dividing cells, because they are dividing more rapidly, and the anticancer drug is chemically similar enough to folacin to fool cancer cells into accepting it instead of the vitamin. When the drug settles into the spot normally occupied by folacin, the cancer cells' attempts at division are unsuccessful, and they die. Other drugs work in different ways to accomplish the same thing—blockage of cell division and death of the cancerous tissue. Several of the most effective anticancer drugs are chemicals that occur in nature: an extract of the periwinkle plant and a substance made by ocean sponges. Scientists are scanning other wild species for anticancer chemicals yet unknown.

Anticancer drugs also kill normal tissues, although more slowly than they kill cancerous ones. In the digestive tract, for example, the normal, rapid cell division is disturbed; diarrhea, nausea, and vomiting result. Blood cells are also a rapidly dividing tissue, so their production is impaired in people being treated with anticancer drugs.

New developments in packaging and delivery of the drugs may help prevent such side effects. Microscopic time-release capsules now can be injected directly into the cancer site. That way, the drug stays in the immediate vicinity of the cancer and causes fewer side effects. All anticancer drugs have narrow margins of safety.

A dramatic improvement over any one of these methods alone is attained by the combination of surgery or radiation with chemotherapy, **adjuvant therapy**. Clients are given drug treatments soon after, or sometimes even before, surgery or radiation to prevent the possibility of a tumor's showing up in another location.

A new treatment with great promise, although still experimental and currently only about 50 percent effective, is immunotherapy. Immunotherapy consists of activating a person's own powerful immune system against the cancer. Currently, researchers at the National Cancer Institute are testing a drug (Interleukin 2) that works to activate the immune system's killer cells against cancer. So far, the results look promising—even some advanced cases of inoperable cancer have been improved by the therapy. Another approach

Not all cancer treatments called cures are effective. Frauds in health are always cruel, but those aimed at cancer victims are especially so—they prey on people who are already suffering. Laetrile (also called amygdalin or vitamin B_{17}) is a cancer-cure hoax, not a vitamin by any stretch of the imagination. Another such hoax is called immuno-augmentative therapy, or IAT; this one sends people with cancer to foreign countries for dangerous blood transfusions that not only do not fight cancer but spread AIDS and hepatitis to the already sick victims. Any number of nutrient, vitamin, or mineral "therapies" can also be found.

Sometimes people will report that a phony cancer cure worked. A famous quack-buster, Victor Herbert, has identified five possible scenarios to account for this: the person never had cancer; the cancer was cured by conventional therapy, but the quack took the credit; the cancer is silently progressing, the person only *thinks* that cure has taken place; the person has died of cancer, but is represented as cured; the person's cancer went away by itself, and the quack took the credit.

The proponents of bogus treatments capitalize on people's fear of cancer and scare them into believing that the medical establishment frowns on their methods for dishonest reasons. "The doctors don't care if you die," they say, "so long as you pay huge sums for their services." Loving life, wanting to trust someone, wanting to hope that a cure is possible, victims of cancer easily fall prey to this sort of deception, as do relatives and friends who are willing to try anything to help their loved ones get well.

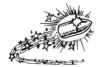

Quacks will stop at nothing to cheat people of their money.

is to use the person's own cancer cells to make a vaccine to activate the immune system against the cancer.[17]

Listed here are only a few avenues of approach in the treatment of cancer. A person who gets cancer has reason to be hopeful about possibilities for a cure.

LIVING WITH CANCER

For cancer treatment, the focus is necessarily on machines, drugs, and techniques that battle an abnormally growing tissue. That the tissue is within a living, feeling human being and that the treatments often invade the person's life in intimate ways goes unappreciated. People diagnosed with cancer have fears to cope with, and their emotions may need to move through the stages of grief before they can take part in their own treatments and recovery.

Some people, of course, face the crisis with courage; they take an active part in treatment and recovery. They are spurred into action, not despair; they cultivate a sense of humor in the midst of fear. Such people maintain strong family bonds and bonds of friendship throughout the illness, and they have that indefinable asset to recovery—the will to live.

A form of positive self-talk, known as **positive imaging,** or **guided imaging,** is useful for people struggling with the pain of cancer. A therapist who teaches positive imaging may tell the person to image the pain as a mad dog. Then the therapist tells the person to approach the dog, try to coax it into stopping its snarling and growling, and gradually tame it to the point where it begins to wag its tail and respond in a friendly fashion. The pain then becomes less of an enemy. Cancer clients who use positive imaging have been shown in some experiments to survive longer than those who do not.[18]

The family and friends of a person with cancer are all affected by the illness. There exists a mutual need for support and love. Family and friends can help by taking over chores, filling out insurance forms, and the like. But even more important, they can acknowledge that the person is the same as before—loved as before, accepted with the diagnosis as much as without. Friends who listen, talk about fears, and continue their friendships can assist the person who has many difficult feelings to work through. The disease should be discussed freely, but other topics should be brought in, too; everyday conversation can help lessen the focus on the disease.

People who have been cured of cancer may live in fear of its recurrence. The stress of this fear can be enormous. Self-help groups can assist people to live with cancer or cope with the fear of its return. The American Cancer Society can direct you to groups in your area.

Sometimes the cancer is not curable. In that case, the person must accept that death will occur from the disease and meanwhile, live the remainder of life with cancer. Chapter 13 discusses death and grief.

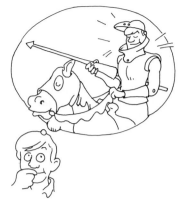
Imagine yourself able to conquer dragons.

THE THINGS THAT MATTER

A young book salesman approached an old farmer who was out plowing in his field to show him a marvelous new book about how to farm with modern technology. After inspecting the book, the farmer handed it back to the young man and said, "Son, this is a fine book, but I don't farm half as well as I already know how." We can make an analogous point: we do not need more new technologies to enjoy better health; we simply must do what we already know how to do.

Sensational reporting may lead people to worry about and try to control such generally harmless factors as food additives (see this chapter's Spotlight). Those same people may choose to ignore real dangers such as tobacco use, alcohol abuse, overeating, and lack of exercise. When you ask the question "How many deaths each year are related to food additives?" the answer would be "almost none"; compare that with the effects of the second group, which are the risk factors and causes of the great majority of deaths each year. Choose carefully where you spend your health care energy and money. Some things truly matter—concentrate on them.

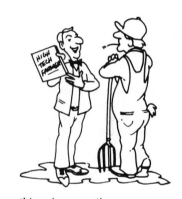
Keep things in proportion.

STUDY AIDS

1. Describe the characteristic course of cancer development and the factors that affect it.
2. Explain the terms *carcinogen* and *promoter*, and name one of each.
3. Delineate the differences between malignant tumors and benign tumors.
4. Describe how cancer spreads.
5. Identify and describe the major risk factors for cancer.
6. List some steps to take to reduce your cancer risks.
7. Describe the possible role of viruses in cancer development.
8. List cancer's warning signals.
9. Identify and state the usefulness of several home screening tests for cancer.
10. Describe screening and early detection for cancer.
11. Name and describe several types of cancer treatments.

GLOSSARY

adjuvant therapy: cancer treatment through a combination of surgery or radiation and chemotherapy.

benign: see *tumor.*

biopsy: surgical removal of a piece of tissue for examination by microscope or other means.

cancer: a malignant tumor that spreads into surrounding tissues and into other body parts by way of the circulatory and lymphatic systems.

carcinogen (CAR-sin-oh-jen or car-SIN-oh-jen): a substance that causes normal genetic material to mutate into cancer-causing oncogenes (an initiator). *Co-carcinogens* are two or more factors that may be harmless when alone in the body, but induce cancer when they occur together. See also *mutagen, oncogene, initiator,* and *promoter.*

    carcin = cancer
    genesis = beginning

carcinoma (car-sin-OH-mah): a class of cancers that arisees in the skin, body chamber linings, or glands.

cataract: clouding of the lens of the eye that diminishes and endangers sight.

chemotherapy: the administration of drugs that have a specific harmful effect on the disease-causing entity but that do not harm the client, or at least usually do not harm the client as much as the disease does.

co-carcinogen: see *carcinogen.*

CT scan: computerized tomography scan (formerly called CAT scan), computer-processed X-ray pictures; the X-ray beam is rotated to cover the body area in question, and the computer organizes the individual images into a whole picture of a thin section of the body tissue, including any tumors that might be present. It is especially useful for areas not easily accessible, such as the brain.

guided imaging: see *positive imaging.*

initiator: a carcinogen, an agent required to start the formation of cancer.

leukemia (loo-KEE-me-ah): a class of cancers that arises in the blood cell-making tissues, characterized by an abnormally high number of white cells in the blood. There are several classes and types of leukemia.

leukoplakia (loo-koh-PLAY-kee-ah): white patches on the lining of the tongue, lips, or cheek that are smooth, irregular in shape, hard, and occasionally sore. Leukoplakia often become malignant.

lumpectomy: see *mastectomy.*

lymphoma (limf-OH-mah): a cancer that arises in an organ of the immune system. See Chapter 2's Miniglossary of Immune System Terms.

malignant: see *tumor.*

mammogram: X-ray examination of the breast, a screening test for cancer.

mastectomy: surgical removal of the breast and varying amounts of surrounding tissue as the primary treatment for breast cancer. The most extreme form is the *radical mastectomy,* in which the breast, underlying muscle tissue, and lymph glands are removed; a *modified radical mastectomy* is removal of the breast and lymph glands, but not the underlying muscle; a *simple mastectomy* is removal of the breast only; a *lumpectomy* is the removal of the tumor with a minimal amount of the surrounding tissue, usually leaving the skin and nipple intact.

melanoma: cancer of the pigmented cells of the skin, related to sun exposure in people with light-colored skin.

metastasize (meh-TASS-tuh-size):migration of cancer cells from one part of the body to another, starting new growths with characteristics of the original tumor.

modified radical mastectomy: see *mastectomy.*

mutagen: see *mutation.*

mutation (myoo-TAY-shun): a change in a cell's genetic material. Once the genetic material has changed, the change is inherited in the offspring of that cell. A *mutagen* (MYOO-tah-gen) is a substance or event (such as radiation) that causes such changes in genetic material.

myeloma: a cancer originating in the cells of the bone marrow.

oncogene (ON-co-jean): genetic material that has been modified and produces irregular cell products that characterize malignant tumors.

palliative therapy: measures given to relieve discomfort or alleviate symptoms, without producing a cure.

polyp: a tumor that grows on a stem, similar in appearance to a mushroom. Polyps bleed easily and some have the tendency to become malignant.

positive imaging: a technique used to help achieve the relaxation response; the person imagines achieving positive outcomes to present experiences. Also called *guided imaging.*

promoter: a substance that assists in the development of malignant tumors, but does not initiate them on its own.

radiation therapy: the application of cell-destroying radiation to kill cancerous tissues.

radical mastectomy: see *mastectomy.*

sarcoma (sar-KOH-mah): a class of cancers that arises in the connective tissue cells including bones, ligaments, and muscles.

simple mastectomy: see *mastectomy.*

thermography: a method of detecting tissues of high metabolice, such as tumors, by the heat they release.

tumor: an abnormal mass of tissue that has metabolism and replication, but performs no physiologic service to the body. A *malignant* tumor, or cancer, is a fast-growing disease that endangers the victim by shedding cells into body fluids, in which they are carried to new locations to start new cancer colonies. (The general term *malignant* means "growing worse.") A *benign* (be-NINE) tumor lacks the characteristics of a malignant tumor and does not metastasize.

    malignen = to attack
    benignus = gentle, mild

type C: a designation given to people with personality characteristics suggesting cancer- proneness—helplessness, passivity, and a desire to appease others. (For type A and type B, with reference to heart disease, see Chapter 16.)

QUIZ ANSWERS

1. *False*. Cancer develops in several steps, and the healthy body's immune system can bring defenses to bear at every step.

2. *True*. The majority of cancers may be preventable by changes in lifestyle factors.

3. *True*. In addition to lung cancer risk, smoking is linked to an increased incidence of cancers throughout the body.

4. *True*. People with darkly pigmented skin do not need to use sunscreen to prevent skin cancer.

5. *False*. Tanning booths or sunlamps are not safer than sunbathing as far as cancer risks are concerned.

6. *True*. People can help ward off certain cancers by choosing the right diet.

7. *False*. You can reduce your likelihood of getting cancer, but some cancers attack even people who have taken all known precautions.

8. *False*. A month is too long to wait. Symptoms that suggest cancer and that persist for more than a week should be checked.

9. *True*. To cure cancer, a treatment must destroy or remove every cancer cell from the body.

10. *True*. Some of the most effective cancer drugs have been discovered in wild plants and animals.

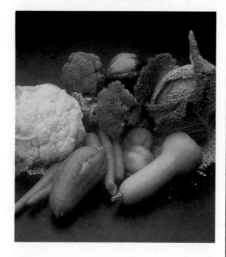

SPOTLIGHT

Nutrition and Cancer Prevention

Among the links of environmental factors with cancer, the diet connections are tenuous. Science tantalizes us with glimpses of promising avenues of research, but it has not, at least so far, mapped for us a certain path to cancer prevention. To draw conclusions about what people should eat would be premature. Popular books and magazines that do so are responding to popular demand—people will buy promises of control over cancer. Still, connections exist between diet and cancer. Food constituents may speed cancer's development, or they may protect against it.

What do you mean by food constituents?

Chapter 4 stated that foods are made of chemicals—the nutrients, of course, chemicals—the nutrients, of course (protein, carbohydrate, fat, and the vitamins and minerals), and also a wide variety of nonnutrients such as the deep red pigment of beets, the aromatic substances in bananas, and the pungent principles of hot peppers that confer on them their characteristic color, aroma, and "bite." Many thousands of nonnutrient chemicals occur in foods; some benefit the plant or animal in some way and so occur naturally, and some form when the food is cooked. Table S17–1 shows the chemicals in three familiar breakfast foods. Each chemical in every food could potentially affect cancer development, but the effects of just a few are known.

So even natural foods have chemicals in them. What about the additives in processed foods? Do they have more potential to cause cancer than the natural chemicals?

For prevention of cancer, "natural" is not better. Food additives have little to do with the causation of cancer—the law forbids the addition to food of any substance that has ever been shown to cause cancer in experimental animals. This is not to say that foods do not contain chemicals that

are capable of initiating cancer—they do contain naturally occuring carcinogens, but in amounts so dilute as to have no effect. As just one example, wholesome roasted turkey contains a proven carcinogen, but to receive enough of it to initiate cancer you'd have to eat two tons of turkey. The body easily detoxifies the amount of the carcinogen in your Thanksgiving dinner. Almost every meal contains such chemicals, so the body has evolved with the ability to handle them.

You said that chemicals that cause cancer can't be added to foods, but I've seen soft drink and food labels warning that saccharin causes cancer in laboratory animals. Are you certain that additives are safe?

Companies that produce food are restricted as to which chemicals they may add to it. Conditions of use and amounts are monitored. All of today's additives have been extensively studied and proved safe when used within federal guidelines.

As for saccharin, it has been in use for over 100 years as a sweetener, but was almost banned in 1977 when evidence showed that extremely high doses caused bladder tumors in the offspring of rats. (The law requires that an additive must have absolutely no connection to cancer for it to remain in use.) The public outcry in favor of retaining saccharin was so loud, however, that this one exception was made—Congress placed a moratorium on any action, with the condition that saccharin-containing food bear the warning label you mentioned. That moratorium is still in effect. Recently, researchers reviewed saccharin-cancer experiments and concluded that high doses of saccharin probably can cause cancer in rats. They could not conclude that saccharin is associated with increased cancer risk in people.[1]*

People worry about what might be present in their food, and that con-

*Reference notes are in Appendix D.

TABLE S17–1 Ingredients in Your Breakfast of Foods *without Additives*

Coffee	Toast and Coffee Cake	Scrambled Eggs
Caffeine	Gluten	Ovolbumin
Methanol	Amino acids	Conalbumin
Ethanol	Amylose	Ovomucoid
Butanol	Starches	Mucin
Methylbutanol	Dextrins	Globulins
Acetaldehyde	Sucrose	Amino acids
Methyl formate	Pentosans	Lipovitellin
Dimethyl sulfide	Hexosans	Livetin
Propionaldehyde	Triglycerides	Cholesterol
Pyridine	Monoglycerides and	Lecithin
Acetic acid	diglycerides	Choline
Furfural	Sodium chloride	Lipids (fats)
Furfuryl alcohol	Phosphorus	Fatty acids
Acetone	Calcium	Lutein
Methylfuran	Iron	Zeaxanthine
Diacetyl	Thiamin (vitamin B_1)	Vitamin A
Isoprene	Riboflavin (vitamin B_2)	Biotin
Guaiacol	Niacin	Pantothenic acid
Hydrogen sulfide	Pantothenic acid	Riboflavin (vitamin B_2)
	Vitamin D	Thiamin (vitamin B_1)
	Methyl ethyl ketone	Niacin
	Acetic acid	Pyridoxine (vitamin B_6)
	Propionic acid	Folic acid (folacin)
	Butyric acid	Cyanocobalamin
	Valeric acid	(vitamin B_{12})
	Caproic acid	Sodium chloride
	Acetone	Iron
	Diacetyl	Calcium
	Maltol	Phosphorus
	Ethyl acetate	

SOURCE: The Manufacturing Chemists' Association.

cern is well-placed, but not with additives. Environmental pollutants, such as pesticides, industrial by-products, and the metals lead, cadmium, and mercury pose extreme hazards when they break through controlling safeguards and enter the food and water chain. Pollution is beyond the scope of this discussion, but is the topic of Chapter 19. Here, it stands as an example of a real hazard to compare with the highly controlled food additives.

I feel better about additives, but isn't it still best to choose fresh foods?

Yes, fresh foods contribute to dietary adequacy (most processed foods have lost nutrients) but do scrub fruits and vegetables to remove pesticide residues before eating them. Fresh foods may even protect against cancer, to the degree that they are low in dietary fat (many processed foods are high in fat). Scientists have strong suspicions that dietary fat and excess food energy play a role in promoting cancer. For example, it is well known that the number of mammary tumors in rats increases with increased dietary fat. Fat is just one among many naturally occurring substances that promote tumor growth, after the cancer has been initiated by some other environmental influence. (Alcohol is another.)

Many theories exist as to exactly how fat may promote cancer. A high-fat diet may change the way body tissues respond to hormones, causing rapid cell division (and thus tumor formation). Or fat may interfere with chemical signals that control cell division (prostaglandins). Or perhaps fat is culpable only in its contribution to obesity, a known cancer risk factor. Still another lead—excess dietary fat may inhibit the body's immune response and allow cancers to start that would otherwise be wiped out.

Would cutting down on fat lessen people's chances of developing cancer?

First, keep in mind that the associations are not proven and that the theories mentioned have been developed on the basis of work with experimental animals, not people. Scientifically, findings about rats cannot be assumed true about people. Studies are progressing to determine if people with cancer or at risk of developing it can benefit from the same kind of diet that benefits experimental rats—one low in fat.[2] There would appear to be no harm in reducing the fat intakes of adults by about half, and in bringing energy intakes into line with energy needs. (In the United States, children's fat intakes, on the average, are about right—lowering them could retard growth.) For the average adult, this would mean choosing low-fat foods, drastically reducing fat used in food preparation, and refraining from adding fats such as butter, margarine, salad dressings, and gravies at the table.

Aside from fat, what other food components are thought to promote cancer?

One suspect for promoting cancer of the stomach is a group of chemicals, **nitrosamines**, produced in the stomach from **nitrites**. Natural sources of nitrites include the water supply and vegetables. They are added to most processed meats, such as bacon and lunch meats, to prevent the growth of microbes that cause **botulism**, a deadly kind of food poisoning . The human body makes large quantities of nitrites, and processed meats add only small quantities of them. Anyone wishing to control the conversion of nitrites to the cancer-promoting form nitrosamines would do well to eat plenty of fresh fruits and vegetables. Vegetables contain nitrites, but they also contain vitamin C which inhibits the conversion of nitrites to nitrosamines.

One other concern about meats: carcinogens form whenever meat or fat is burned, charred, or smoked. A person who wishes to minimize cancer risks should limit intake of smoked or charbroiled meats to one or two servings a week.

Are certain breakfast cereals protective against cancer, as some advertisers claim?

Nothing is absolute in the food-cancer connection, and advertisers often imply an absolute causal relationship when scientists would not do so, to speed sales. Cereals and

other high-fiber foods have at least some evidence in their favor, although it is not as strong as the evidence implicating fat. In general, research shows that wherever the diet is high in fat, it is simultaneously low in vegetable fiber. It is difficult to single out the effects of either one. Still, fiber may independently help to protect against some cancers at the same time as fat promotes them. One theory has it that since fiber speeds the transit of materials through the large intestine, it helps minimize contact of body tissues with harmful constituents. Another suggests that fiber attracts digestive secretions and removes them from the intestine.

Evidence from Finland suggests that fiber exerts a protective effect even when the diet is high in fat. The Finns eat an unusual diet—one high in both fat and fiber. Their colon cancer rate is low, suggesting that fiber is protective even in a high-fat diet.[3] Other evidence for fiber's protective effect: vegetarians such as the Seventh-Day Adventist religious group and others have lower rates of breast cancer than those of meat eaters. Since meat is high in fat, and vegetables are high in fiber, the fat-fiber connection may be working here. On the other hand, it could be something other than fiber in the vegetables that is protective.

Do researchers know what that "something" in vegetables might be?

They have some ideas. Some vitamins are likely candidates, as are other components of vegetables. Careful comparisons of stomach cancer victims' diets with those of case controls show less use of vegetables in the cancer group—less volume of vegetables, fewer fresh vegetables, fewer green vegetables, and fewer that contain vitamin C.[4] People with colon cancer have been found to have eaten fewer vegetables throughout life, and specifically, less of the **cruciferous vegetables**—cabbage,

broccoli, brussels sprouts, and others. Another group of cancers (those of the skin, head, and neck) are related to smoking and alcohol consumption primarily, but are also related to a low intake of fruits and vegetables, particularly those that are rich in vitamin A.[5] The vegetable form of Vitamin A, **carotene**, may interfere with the earliest cancerous changes in cells. Abundant evidence makes clear that anyone at risk for cancer should obtain vegetables rich in carotene—yellow, orange, or dark green leafy ones.

Can I just take a supplement to be sure I get enough vitamins? Preparing fresh vegetables is a bother.

More will be known about the efficacy of supplements against cancer at the conclusion of a study now under way: a group of doctors agreed to take a supplement of carotene for the rest of their lives to see if it protects against cancer. If all goes well, in about 30 years we will have one piece of evidence about how one vitamin in supplement form affects cancer. Right now, however, no evidence supports the idea that a supplement can do what vegetables do. For one thing, vegetables have fiber as well as vitamins, and they supply other nutrients known to be important to immune function—vitamin B_6, folacin, vitamin E, iron, zinc, and many others not found in supplements. For another thing, vegetables contain many nonnutrients, such as the chemical that gives cruciferous vegetables their cabbage-like taste. These nonnutrients may turn out to be important in preventing some kinds of cancer. It is admittedly trouble to prepare fresh vegetables and other protective foods, but there are benefits—those of an adequate diet described in Chapter 4.

The best way to get all the nutrients and nonnutrients that may be protective against cancer is to eat a wide variety of fresh foods, limit fats, choose foods with fiber, and choose fresh vegetables often, especially the ones listed in Table S17–2. One other suggestion: Vary your choices. Don't let your diet become monotonous. Whenever you switch from food to food, you are diluting whatever is in one food with what is in the others. For example, if you eat a ham sandwich for lunch today, choose rice and beans tomorrow, and something entirely different the next day. If you take these steps, you have every reason to feel confident that you are providing your body with the best nutrition at the lowest possible risk for cancer. Some fringe benefits: you will be boosting your immune power and probably helping protect yourself against heart disease, diabetes, and many other diseases as well.

TABLE S17–2 Cruciferous Vegetables and Vitamin A-Rich Fruits and Vegetables

Cruciferous Vegetable	Vitamin A-Rich Fruits and Vegetables
Broccoli	Apricots
Brussels sprouts	Asparagus
Cabbage (all varieties)	Broccoli
Cauliflower	Cantaloupe
Greens (collards, mustards, turnips)	Carrots
Kale	Green onions
Kohlrabi	Greens (all varieties)
Rutabaga	Lettuce (dark green)
Turnip roots	Mango
	Oriental cabbages
	Papaya
	Parsley
	Spinach
	Squash (hard, winter)
	Sweet potato

Chapter 18

The Consumer and the Health Care System

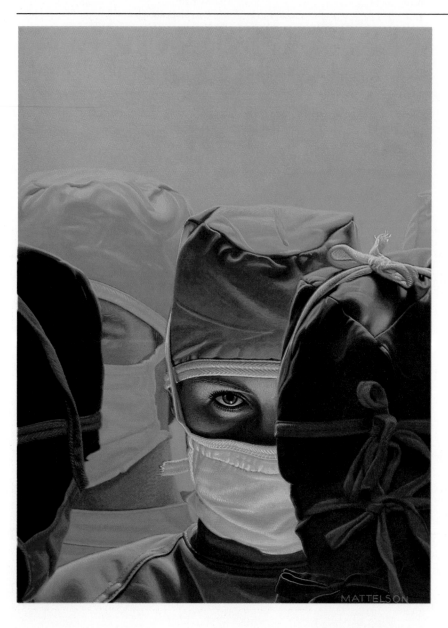

MATTELSON

FOR OPENERS . . .

True or false? If false, say what is true.

1. If you have medical and surgical insurance, you are probably covered for most medical expenses you might incur.

2. When someone successfully sues a physician for malpractice, the physician's insurance company absorbs the cost.

3. If you have a severe sore throat, you should go to the hospital emergency room.

4. If you can show the physician or hospital that your insurance covers a medical treatment, you will not have to pay in advance for it.

5. If a person arrives at the hospital bleeding to death, the hospital has to provide emergency treatment.

6. A certificate of accreditation indicates that a hospital has met certain standards for health care.

7. HMO stands for home medical operation—minor surgery that people can perform for themselves.

8. An osteopath (D.O.) is just as well qualified to perform most medical services as a physician is and is legally permitted to do so.

9. Chiropractors (D.C.s) are called "doctor," but they don't have nearly as much medical education as medical doctors (M.D.s).

10. Anyone can adopt the title "doctor," but there are penalties for claiming to be a medical doctor (M.D.).

(Answers on page 380.)

The health care system is a big system, consisting of big businesses and big suppliers. It can serve you well, but it can also serve you ill, for many of its transactions are governed by the motives of profit, power, and prestige. This chapter offers the information you need to use the health care system to best support your health. Its Life Choice Inventory can help you discover how much you already know about the system and how skilled you are in using it.

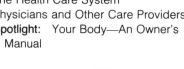
THE HEALTH CARE SYSTEM

Let us suppose you are going to have three problems this year, all currently unknown to you. For one thing, you are developing a heart condition (even though you may be as young as 18), although you will not have any noticeable symptoms for 15 years. For a second thing, you are going to get a severe sore throat, which, unless promptly treated, will develop into a major, whole-body infection. Third, you are going to break your arm.

Now consider several different scenarios. The first is the simplest: you have no insurance, no physician, and no health care plan. The developing heart condition therefore advances silently for the entire year, without your awareness. When the sore throat strikes, you attempt to soothe it with cough drops until you have become extremely ill; then a friend takes you to the

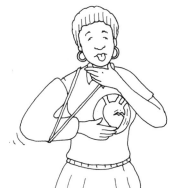

Suppose you are going to have three things happen to you this year.

LIFE CHOICE INVENTORY

How well do you know and use the health care system? For each yes answer, give yourself 1 point:

1. Do you take responsibility for your own health insurance? (Someone else may pay for it, but did you obtain your own policies, and are you acquainted with their contents?)
2. Are you familiar with the five types of health insurance you may need? (Can you name them?)
3. Do you know what breaks you can obtain on health/medical insurance, based on your lifestyle choices?
4. Have you ever compared a health maintenance organization (HMO) with the traditional medical care system? (Could you explain to someone else what an HMO is?)
5. Given the choice, when you need prompt medical treatment, do you work out a way to go to a clinic or health care practitioner's office, rather than to the hospital emergency room?
6. Before paying a bill for medical care, do you (or would you) check it to make sure that you received all the services it lists?
7. Should you move to a new location, would you know how to go about selecting a health care practitioner (personal physician or other)? (Can you name several steps you would take to find the appropriate one?)

8. Do you know what is reasonable to expect during a general physical checkup? (Can you identify the steps the health practitioner should take in examining you?)
9. If you meet a "doctor," do you keep in mind that the person may not be an M.D.? (Can you name several other possibilities?)
10. Can you spot a quack? (Extra credit: give yourself an extra point if you have ever reported quackery to a regulating agency.)

Scoring:

9 or more: You are a skilled consumer of health care services.

7 or 8: You know the system fairly well, but have a little more to learn.

5 or 6: There is room for improvement in your skill at using the health care system.

4 or less: You are unlikely to benefit from the available services to any significant extent, and in fact, you may be losing out in significant ways.

hospital emergency room. You are required to pay in advance, given a prescription for antibiotics, and dismissed; the visit and the medicine cost you close to $100. Because you became so sick before seeking treatment, you lose a week of classes or work. When you break your arm, you are rushed to the hospital again, and you find, to your amazement, that they will not even treat you until you have again paid your bill in advance. They charge you $500. Then they set your arm in a cast, and you return to the hospital's outpatient clinic for periodic checkups and finally to have the cast removed. Total cost of treatment for the year: about $600 and a week of missed classes or work.

With insurance, the scenario would be slightly different. You might pay, say, $50 a month for coverage as an individual. Still, no one would discover the need for preventive measures against your heart condition, but when you went to the hospital on your two trips, you would be admitted without question and without agonizing delays. Afterward, you would receive bills for your treatment, but either you or the hospital would apply for reimbursement from your insurance company. If you had to pay the bills at first, you would soon receive reimbursement. Alternatively, you might simply receive notice that the bills had been paid for you. Total cost to you: still $600 for the year, but in 12 equal installments of $50 rather than in two surprise lump sums, and still a week of missed classes or work.

To create still another scenario, suppose you have your own personal physician, Dr. A, who sees it as a physician's responsibility not only to treat but also prevent illness. Dr. A gives you a routine physical examination this year, and instructs you to lose a few pounds and to alter your diet. The effect, if you follow Dr. A's recommendation, is to postpone the onset and reduce the severity of your heart condition, years later. When your sore throat develops, you telephone Dr. A's office, and the nurse tells you to come in immediately for a throat culture. The condition is thus caught early, and prompt antibiotic treatment spares you the loss of a week's classes or work days. When you break your arm, you still go to the hospital emergency room, and your experience is essentially the same as before. With insurance coverage as before, your expenses add up only a little differently. Your insurance does not cover your general physical examination, so you are out $100 for that—but with benefits to come in the distant future that outweigh the price paid now. Insurance does pay for the sore throat treatment and for the arm. Cost: $600 for insurance, $100 for the general physical exam, and no loss of a productive week.

As a student, you may have an option similar to this but less expensive: the student health center. For nonstudents, another less-expensive option, at least for the sore throat, is the community public health center.

Yet another variation on this theme is as follows. You belong to a health maintenance organization (HMO). These organizations vary, but let's say the particular one you have chosen offers the most comprehensive services possible. The fee for membership, payable monthly, is a fixed fee and entitles you to many services "free." At your physical examination, your physician, who is a disease-prevention advocate, explains the specific risk factors for heart disease and not only recommends diet changes but also refers you to a dietitian down the hall who can advise you on how to implement them in your particular situation. The physician also sends you to an exercise specialist for a personalized exercise prescription, and you are entitled to use the HMO's gym and track if you like. You are encouraged to return for periodic checkups on your weight, blood pressure, and blood lipid profile, and for further advice on diet and exercise as needed.

As a member of the HMO, you do not hesitate to go in when you have a sore throat, because it does not cost anything extra. Therefore, although you do not see your regular HMO physician on this occasion, you receive prompt treatment, and you do not lose a week to illness. (Your prescription for an antibiotic costs extra, but you fill it at the HMO pharmacy at a discount.) And when you break your arm, although you go to the hospital for treatment, the HMO pays the fees.

Another possibility, not a true alternative but potentially a powerful adjunct to the traditional and modern hospital/physician-based systems just described, is a strengthened system of self-care. Health education could teach people to do much more for themselves than they now know how to do. By studying your family history, you might detect that heart disease was a likely problem for you—and institute the lifestyle changes that would lower your risk. You might prevent your sore throat—both by guarding against precipitating factors and by avoiding exposure to infective agents. You might even be able to prevent that broken arm, if you were aware of the principles of accident prevention and willing to apply them. This chapter's Spotlight suggests some ways in which you can be your own physician. The accompanying Strategies box itemizes the elements of care you might want to learn to provide for yourself. The box, "When to Obtain Medical Help," tells you when you should seek professional care, and Table 18–1 describes a schedule of physical examinations for a lifetime.

There are many other variations on the preceding health care scenarios. What will work best for you is a combination unique to your situation, and

 STRATEGIES: Elements of Self-Care

You can provide these elements of health care for yourself:

1. Learn to practice truly effective preventive dental hygiene.

2. Learn and practice good posture habits.

3. Do a preventive breast or testicular examination every month.

4. Learn when to go and when not to go to a health care provider.

5. Doctor your own mild, temporary conditions.

6. Learn to take your own temperature and pulse.

7. For women: conduct regular vaginal self-examinations.

||| When to Obtain Medical Help

You need to see your health care provider if you have or have had:

■ An oral temperature above 104 degrees Fahrenheit. (Between 102 and 104°F, call and ask whether you should be seen, or control with aspirin, acetaminophen, or ibuprofen.)

■ Any serious accident or injury, including animal bites, puncture wounds, wounds with much blood loss, severe burns, suspected breaks or fractures, or possible poisoning.

■ Falls with possible injury to the head or spine, followed by headache; vision abnormality; vomiting; bleeding from the ears, nose, or mouth; unusual behavior or drowsiness; paralysis; or convulsions.

■ Sudden, severe pain or cramps in the abdomen.

■ Breathing difficulty.

■ Loss of consciousness, even if brief.

■ Persistent severe headache.

■ Intense itch.

■ Sudden high fever.

■ Bleeding or loss of any fluid from any body opening with unknown cause. (Blood in vomit or stools may appear black or brown, like coffee grounds; blood in urine may make it appear pink, red, or smoky.)

■ Possible internal bleeding, as indicated by faintness, dizziness, weak or rapid pulse, shallow or irregular breathing, cold or clammy skin, or a bluish cast to the lips or fingernails.

■ Possible cardiovascular abnormality, as indicated by a noticeable increase or decrease in heart rate.

■ Possible nervous system damage, as indicated by impaired thought processes, vision (especially a halo effect), hearing, sense of touch, or ability to move.

■ Any adverse drug reaction.

■ Continuous diarrhea or vomiting.

TABLE 18–1   Lifetime Health Monitoring Program

Young Adulthood (18 to 24 years)

Health Goals	Professional Services
1. To facilitate the transition from dependent adolescence to mature independent adulthood with maximum physical, mental, and emotional resources. 2. To achieve useful employment and maximum capacity for a healthy marriage, parenthood, and social relations.	1. One professional visit with the healthy adult, including a complete physical examination; tetanus booster if not received within 10 years; tests for syphilis, gonorrhea, malnutrition, cholesterol, and hypertension; and medical and behavioral history. This visit may be provided upon entrance into college, the armed forces, or the first full-time job, but it should occur before marriage. 2. Health education and individual counseling, as needed, for nutrition, exercise, study, career, job, occupational hazards and problems, sex, contraception, marriage and family relations, alcohol, drugs, smoking, and driving. 3. Dental examination and prophylaxis every two years.

Young Middle Age (25 to 39 years)

Health Goals	Professional Services
1. To prolong the period of maximum physical energy and to develop full mental, emotional, and social potential. 2. To anticipate and guard against the onset of chronic diseases through positive health habits and early detection and treatment where effective.	1. Two professional visits with the healthy person—at about ages 30 and 35—including tests for syphilis and gonorrhea (if not monogamous), hypertension, anemia, cholesterol, cervical cancer, and breast cancer, as well as instruction in self-examination of breasts, skin, testes, neck, and mouth. 2. Professional counseling regarding nutrition; exercise; smoking; alcohol use; and marital, parental, and other aspects of health-related behavior and lifestyle. 3. Dental examination and prophylaxis every two years.

Older Middle Age (40 to 59 years)

Health Goals	Professional Services
1. To prolong the period of maximum physical energy and optimum mental and social activity, including menopausal adjustment. 2. To detect as early as possible any of the major chronic diseases, including hypertension, heart disease, diabetes, and cancer, as well as vision, hearing, and dental impairments.	1. Four professional visits with the healthy person, once every five years—at about ages 40, 45, 50, and 55—with a complete physical examination and medical history; tests for syphilis and gonorrhea (if not monogamous) and specific chronic conditions; and appropriate immunizations. Counseling should help with changing nutritional needs and physical activities; occupational, sex, marital, and parental problems; and use of cigarettes, alcohol, and drugs. 2. For those over 50, annual tests for hypertension, obesity, and certain cancers. 3. Annual dental prophylaxis.

you will have to discover it for yourself. To do so requires working out answers to the following questions:

1. What kind(s) of insurance do I need, if any?
2. What hospitals are available near me? Which will be best for me?
3. Should I consider joining an HMO? Are other alternatives available?
4. Should I have a personal physician? What are the alternatives?

The sections that follow contain information to help you assess your own needs.

TABLE 18–1   Continued

The Elderly (60 to 74 years)	
Health Goals	*Professional Services*
1. To prolong the period of optimum physical/mental/social activity. 2. To minimize handicapping and discomfort from the onset of chronic conditions. 3. To prepare in advance for retirement.	1. Professional visits with the healthy adult at 60 years of age and every two years thereafter, including the same tests for chronic conditions as in older middle age, and professional counseling regarding lifestyle changes related to retirement, nutritional requirements, absence of children, possible loss of spouse, and probable reduction in income, as well as reduced physical resources. 2. Annual immunization against influenza (unless the person is allergic to the vaccine). 3. Annual dental prophylaxais. 4. Periodic podiatry treatments as needed.
Old Age (75 years and over)	
Health Goals	*Professional Services*
1. To prolong the period of effective activity and ability to live independently, and to avoid institutionalization so far as possible. 2. To minimize inactivity and discomfort from chronic conditions. 3. When illness is terminal, to ensure as little physical and mental distress as possible and to provide emotional support to both the client and the family.	1. Professional visit at least once a year, including complete physical examination; medical and behavioral history; and professional counseling regarding changing nutritional requirements as well as changes in activity, mobility, and living arrangements. 2. Annual immunization against influenza (unless the person is allergic to the vaccine). 3. Periodic dental and podiatry treatments as needed. 4. For low-income and other persons not sick enough to be institutionalized but not well enough to cope entirely alone, counseling regarding sheltered housing, health care visitors, home help, day-care and recreational centers, meals-on-wheels, and other measures designed to help them remain in their own homes and as nearly independent as possible. 5. Professional assistance with family relations and preparations for death, if needed.

NOTE: This health monitoring program was developed from two separate traditions—public health and medical practice. The two differ, but they are similar in important ways. They focus on personal health service; they identify specific preventive measures for specific age groups; they call for examinations to be spaced appropriately according to age rather than an annual ritual; they rely heavily on scientific proof of effectiveness but venture to apply prudent interpretation of available evidence where proof is not yet available; and they include educational and counseling procedures aimed at prevention, as well as specific tests aimed at the detection of risk factors and early disease onset.

SOURCE: Adapted with permission from L. Breslow and A. R. Somers, The lifetime health-monitoring program: A practical approach to preventive medicine, *New England Journal of Medicine* 296 (1977): 601–608.

Insurance

Health insurance is one way to reduce the risk of incurring medical expenses you can't afford. Shopping for health insurance requires considerable know-how.

There are several kinds of health insurance to consider—**accident insurance, hospitalization insurance, surgical insurance, medical insurance, major medical insurance**, and **disability insurance** (see Miniglossary of Health Insurance Types page 370). The first three of these may be combined into single policies, but when you shop for insurance, be sure your policies cover them all, or that you have *intentionally* left out one or more. In each area,

✴ **STRATEGIES**
for Purchasing Insurance

Before signing on insurance:

✴ **Be sure to cover these five areas:**
Hospitalization.
Surgical.
Medical.
Major medical.
Disability.

369

✳ Read each policy to be sure it meets your needs. What is the deductible? Does it cover:
  In-hospital and outpatient costs?
  Diagnostic tests?
  Second opinions?
  Medicines?
  Prevention?
  Education?
  Ambulance service?
  Psychological counseling?

✳ Use your healthful lifestyle habits to obtain breaks on insurance rates.

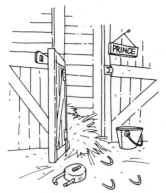

This is not the time to discover that you do not have insurance.

policies differ; read them with attention to your particular needs. For example, if you are planning to start a family soon, be sure your insurance covers the cost of prenatal care, delivery, and newborn care—and be aware that if you are already pregnant when you buy the policy, the costs of your current pregnancy will not be covered.

If your lifestyle compares favorably with that of other buyers, you may be able to obtain breaks on insurance rates. Some policies offer reduced rates for nonsmokers (or people who can prove they have quit), some favor people of normal weight, some consider nonuse of alcohol to be worth a reduction in rates, and some even offer discounts to people who exercise regularly.

Other types of health insurance that apply to special groups are **Medicare** and **Medicaid**. Medicare provides hospital expense and medical insurance coverage for senior citizens who are entitled to Social Security benefits. Medicaid is a program of medical insurance designed for those who receive public assistance (welfare) and for others who are identified as medically needy.

Insurance has saved the financial skins of millions of individuals who have faced unexpected medical costs, but no matter how much insurance you have, you cannot be sure of covering every eventuality, particularly in the later years, when long-term care may be needed. Increasing numbers of families today are finding themselves in a nightmare of limited options when they discover that extended care facilities are not covered by Medicare or conventional health insurance policies. Many people think Medicare includes nursing home care, but it does not. Costs for nursing homes can exceed $24,000 a year and range up to $60,000 and higher. Medicare pays less than half; it may not pay at all, unless the person is receiving specific types of medical care. Clients and their families pay most of the costs.[1*] Insurance is not a substitute for careful financial planning.

Insurance is imperfect in another way: It can be abused. The chief insurance abuse contributing to the high cost of medical care today is the abuse of **malpractice insurance**. Malpractice insurance serves an important purpose; it repays people for the cost to them of physician negligence, ignorance, or error. Unfortunately, however, it is possible for unscrupulous people and their attorneys to exploit it. Although only a few physicians are unethical or incompetent, all feel compelled to protect themselves with insurance against lawsuits.

Malpractice awards can be extraordinarily high. Some exceed a million dollars. Such awards tempt clients to sue for malpractice more often and for larger amounts. Each time a client wins a suit, the client's lawyer draws a third to half of the award as the fee—so attorneys are also powerfully motivated to encourage clients to sue.[2] To be prepared to pay such high damages, the insurance companies have to charge fees as high as a third of a physician's annual income. This forces the physician and the hospital to raise fees, and the person who ends up paying is you, the consumer.

Not all nations' health care systems operate as the United States system does, with a massive, complex, and competitive insurance industry as its main financial provider. For example, Canada has a national program of hospital and medical care insurance that is standardized and covers more than 99 percent of its citizens. Such a system has been proposed for the

*Reference notes are in Appendix D.

United States as well, but the medical, insurance, and attorneys' lobbies have opposed it.

Hospitals and Other Facilities

Each hospital has its own strengths and weaknesses, including specialties in emergency treatment. The better you know them ahead of time, the better you can choose which one to go to in time of need. The Miniglossary of Hospitals and Related Facilities on page 373 defines the major types.

Several strategies can help you save money and needless struggles. If at all possible, do not go to a hospital emergency room. Make an appointment to see a health care practitioner during office hours. If you need special tests or surgery, you may be able to schedule them in the health care practitioner's office. Before submitting to extensive tests or surgery, though, get a second opinion. Some operations, especially **tonsillectomies** and **hysterectomies**, are overperformed—that is, often recommended when they are not necessary. Insurance covers the price of obtaining second opinions for some operations; if the two opinions differ, consider getting a third.

If you have to go to the emergency room, here are a few hints to make your visit easier:

- Have only one person go with you, not the whole family.
- Have identification and your insurance card with you.
- Tell the person at the admissions desk if you have been there before; if you have, they can retrieve your file and will not have to ask you as many questions.
- Always wear your ID bracelet or carry a card to alert health professionals to any chronic condition you may have, such as diabetes.
- Know your own medical history and what medicines you are taking. Carry a short record with you, if your memory is not reliable.

If you need special tests or surgery, you still have choices to make. For simple surgery, you can use a walk-in center rather than the large, general hospital; that way, you will not have to pay for an overnight stay. For surgery requiring hospitalization, ask to have tests performed before you go in. Plan to check into the hospital on a weekday and check out before the weekend, if possible: the weekdays are when the work gets done. If you need a vacation, you can go to a fine hotel for less than the cost of a hospital room.

Many hospitals must give some care to people who cannot afford to pay. Look for the sign "Notice—Medical Care for Those Who Cannot Afford to Pay" in the admissions area.* Hospitals that serve as teaching facilities where medical and nursing school students can learn their professions often are required to take all comers in return for the federal money that supports their programs.

As a hospital client, you have certain rights. You are entitled to considerate care, privacy, confidentiality, accurate information on your diagnosis and treatment, and continuity of care; furthermore, you have the right to refuse treatment. You are also entitled to an explanation of your bill.

STRATEGIES for Selecting and Using Medical Care Facilities

To get the best from medical facilities:

- **Know what facilities are available and what their specialties are.**
- **Avoid emergencyroom visits.**
- **Get a second opinion.**
- **Consider alternatives to hospital tests and surgery.**
- **Use the hospital on weekdays in preference to weekends.**
- **Discover each facility's policy on payment.**

*Ask for an application and for a copy of the "Individual Notice." After you have turned in the application, the hospital must inform you, within two working days, if you are eligible for free care. If you can't get a copy of your determination of eligibility, complain to your Department of Health and Human Services (DHHS) regional office. U.S. Department of Health and Human Services, Public Health Service, *Free Hospital Care* (leaflet), HHS publication no. (HRA) 80-14520, August 1980.

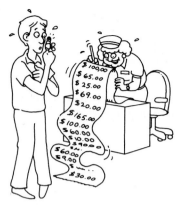

The cost of medical care can be high.

✳ **Find out the physician's and hospital's ways of handling insurance claims. Get help filing for insurance, if available.**

✳ **Protest if the bill is in error.**

✳ **When choosing a place to live, consider the availability of hospital care.**

✳ **Be sure the hospital you choose will take you as a client.**

✳ **Be willing to go out of state, if necessary, for specialized medical care.**

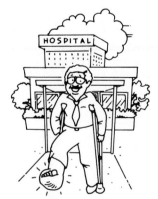

Some medical dramas have happy endings.

About payment: the time when you receive your bill is not the time to discover that you do not have adequate insurance coverage. *Before* the need arises, check your insurance policies—today, for example. When you are scheduling an operation or other treatment, ask in the physician's office whether your insurance will cover it and what help will be available in filing your claim. Many hospitals and physicians' offices expect you to pay the bill immediately, then file a claim to get your insurance company to reimburse you. Some will help you file the claim; some will do it for you. Other hospitals and physicians' offices will *not* require you to pay, but will collect directly from your insurance company and then bill you (sometimes weeks or months later) for the portion not covered.

As many as 90 percent of most hospital bills contain errors.[3] Read through your bills to verify that you did receive all the services for which you are being asked to pay. If you question the accuracy of a bill, ask for an itemized list of services rendered, and send it to your insurance company with an *unsigned* claim form. If the insurance company agrees that the charges are too high, it may be possible to get them reduced. As a last resort, try obtaining access to the peer review committee or grievance committee of the local medical society.

The hospital system can be highly successful in treating illness. No drama surpasses the swift sequence of events of a medical emergency beginning with rushed transit in an ambulance and ending with cure and dismissal. Such dramas are played out daily in the world's great medical centers, but they don't always end so happily. At every step are obstacles to the client's receiving the needed care.

The problems are many. One is supply: there are not enough care facilities or health professionals to serve the population. Another is distribution: especially in rural areas, people may find themselves far from needed services. Other problems are those of coordination and referral: it is hard to find the exact services needed, and it is possible to be turned away for lack of funds, even in an emergency (people have died after being turned away from a hospital emergency room because they could not pay for their care). Still another is quality control: although the medical profession attempts to police itself, mistakes, incompetence, and even dishonesty are not excluded.

Another problem is cost—which is high and rapidly growing higher, not only because of inflation. Among factors that contribute to the spiraling cost of health care is malpractice insurance, already mentioned. Others are the high cost of hospital technology; the self-serving decisions of some medical providers; and the **fee-for-service system** which rewards health care practitioners for each service they perform, tempting them to perform unneeded services.

The problems, then, are many: supply, distribution, coordination, referral, quality control, and cost. Solutions to them are of two kinds—those that work within the system and those that involve alternative systems.

The problems of supply and distribution of health care practitioners and health services may respond best to alternative approaches: institutions other than hospitals, personnel other than physicians. An example is the community clinic, staffed by people trained in particular aspects of health care—such as nurse practitioners trained to deliver women's health care and well-baby care or nurse midwives trained to supervise normal births. Another example is the health maintenance organization (HMO), described in the following section.

Coordination and referral problems are largely the concern of you, the consumer. It is up to you to learn what health services and providers are available in your community and which ones you may need for what.

As for quality control, some elements of the system are intended to deal with that, and they do so with some success. The American Hospital Association has an **accreditation** board that evaluates a hospital's delivery of services on request and furnishes a certificate of accreditation to hospitals that qualify. Accreditation is a seal of approval that indicates to you, the consumer, that a hospital has met certain standards for health care. Think twice before choosing one that has not.

Until recently, it has been typical of the health care system that people have spent enormous amounts of money consulting medical professionals after they were in trouble, but seldom before. But why wait until you are sick to get needed health care? If you have just had a heart attack at the age of 40, what good will it do you to be told all the things you should have done to prevent it? Wouldn't it have been better to have been encouraged to start taking preventive measures at age 19? The **health maintenance organizations (HMOs)** are set up to emphasize preventive measures more strongly than traditional hospitals do.

Health Maintenance Organizations (HMOs)

The HMO consists of a group of health care providers (physicians and associated staff) who are still associated with a hospital, but with a difference. The HMO offers comprehensive health care, including out-of-hospital, in-hospital, and preventive health services. It charges a flat monthly fee to its members, regardless of what services they require (a **prepayment system**, in contrast to the fee-for-service system mentioned earlier). This enables people to budget for their medical costs. It reduces the need for some kinds of insurance, although major medical coverage is sometimes still necessary. It also encourages people to come in for preventive health services—such as checkups and advice—because they don't have to pay extra for them. Table 18–2 on page 374 compares the HMO system with the traditional medical system.

HMOs are one form of response to consumer needs that have not been satisfactorily met by the traditional hospital system. Many variations on the types described here exist; others will doubtless evolve in the future.

▉ PHYSICIANS AND OTHER CARE PROVIDERS

Among professional health providers, important distinctions exist. A person who gets sick usually will think in terms of "going to the doctor"—but what is a doctor? Anyone can adopt the title doctor, but not all are trained the same way, and not all offer beneficial services. The next few sections are devoted to medical professionals.

The Health Care Provider

The health care provider most people think of when they think of medical care is the **medical doctor**, or **M.D.** (this book refers to such a person as the *doctor* or *physician*). This is as it should be, for medical school training equips the M.D. to handle many kinds of medical problems.

MINIGLOSSARY
of Hospitals and Related Facilities

birthing center: a center where people can give birth in a homelike atmosphere with the family in attendance (see Chapter 12).

convalescent home: a center where people can recover from illness or surgery, similar to a hospital but without intensive care, surgical, and emergency treatment facilities.

extended care center: a center for the care of the chronically ill, similar to a convalescent home, but with more medical and nursing services.

government hospital: a hospital run by the federal government, for example, a Veterans Administration—that is, VA—hospital.

health center: a center to serve the routine health care needs of a special group.

nursing home: a center for the care of the elderly who can no longer live independently. Essentially a residential, not a medical, facility. See also *extended care center*.

private (also called **proprietary**) **hospital:** a hospital run by individuals for profit.

teaching hospital: a hospital that serves a medical and/or nursing school as a place where students can learn their professions.

trauma center: see *walk-in emergency center*.

voluntary hospital: a nonprofit hospital run by a community for the benefit of its own citizens.

walk-in emergency center (also called a **trauma center)**: a center for emergency care, similar to the emergency room of a hospital, but operated as a separate institution.

walk-in surgery center (also called **one-day surgery center)**: a facility that performs surgery that doesn't require overnight care.

women's health center: a health center that focuses on the routine health care of women and, sometimes, their infants and children.

TABLE 18–2 Comparison of HMO and Traditional Medical Care

Characteristic	HMO Care	Traditional Care
Philosophic emphasis	Preventive care	Sickness care
Mode of payment	Partial or complete prepayment by group insurance; occasional small fees per visit[a]	Fee for service (can be reimbursed by individual's insurance if applicable)
Provision for out-of-town care	Visit to an out-of-town physician or facility as approved by HMO; reimbursement by HMO	Visit to an out-of-town physician or facility at consumer's discretion; reimbursement by insurance
Needs covered	"One stop": emergency, out-of-hospital care, preventive services,[b] home visits,[c] lab, pharmacy	Many stops: each service provided by a different supplier or facility
Client referral	Initial visit between client and intake specialist; referral to appropriate physician; alternatively, same as in traditional care system	Management of client care by one personal physician; referral to others only for special treatment as needed

[a]Alternatively, in some instances, services are paid by members' insurance companies.

[b]Preventive services include regular checkups; screening and immunization programs; counseling and classes to help people control their blood pressure and weight, develop personalized exercise and diet regimens, plan their families, stop smoking, and learn first aid and safety; and others.

[c]Some HMOs also offer a limited number of mental health visits; service in intermediate and long-term care facilities; service in vision, dental, and more extensive mental health facilities; fertility and family planning services; and rehabilitation therapy.

SOURCE: *HMO—Is It for You?*, a booklet available from Metropolitan Life Insurance Company.

A nurse practitioner is an autonomous health professional.

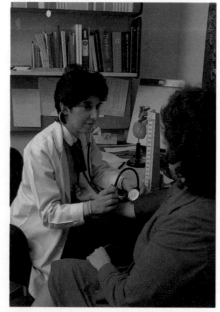

A physician pursues a long course of education to obtain the M.D. degree and the license to practice medicine. Another type of health care provider, the **osteopath (D.O.)**, takes the same course of training as an M.D., but in a school of osteopathy, which specializes in disorders of the musculoskeletal system. People with D.O. degrees can take the same examination given to medical doctors and, on passing it, receive a license to practice medicine and surgery in all states. They may be granted staff privileges, internships, and residencies in accredited hospitals, and so in many ways they are equivalent to physicians.

Following four years of college, the person seeking to become a physician attends medical school, a three-year program. This is followed by a two-year internship and a one-year residency. Then the person is required to pass a state examination to receive a license to practice. Additional schooling is necessary to become a specialist.

A physician is an **autonomous health professional**—that is, a person who is licensed to provide medical care under his or her own authority. Other such professionals are the **nurse practitioner (N.P. or R.N.P.)** and the **physician's assistant (P.A.)**. These people have received considerable medical school training and are equipped to handle all routine medical problems—but they consult physicians when necessary. The Miniglossary of Autonomous Health Professionals lists these and other health care providers and what they are qualified and empowered to do.

How do you go about choosing a health care provider? For ordinary health concerns, it may be sufficient to see the staff at a health center. For continuity of care, though, you may want to have a personal health care provider. This person will get to know your medical history, and will be able to refer you to others whom you may need to see—for example, a gynecologist for women's special problems, an obstetrician for care through pregnancy and childbirth, a pediatrician for the medical care of children. For some periods in your life, you may visit only the one person periodically; for other periods, you may be in frequent contact with specialists.

A reasonable first step in selecting a health care provider is simply to ask friends whom they recommend or to call the county medical society. Then, check the recommended providers' credentials: look for the degrees listed by their titles in this chapter's glossaries, and find out what you can about the reputations of the institutions where they obtained their degrees.* For physicians, look in the *AMA Directory* or *Directory of Medical Specialists* in the local public library.

*If you are especially concerned with finding a physician who has strong credentials and experience, then after you have some names, make sure the person is a member of the American College of Physicians (or American College of Surgeons, if a surgeon). Also, ask the hospital to provide you with a list of staff physicians and their ranks and privileges; this will give you some sense of the extent to which the person has earned the respect of fellow physicians.

STRATEGIES
for Choosing a Health Care Provider

To choose among health care providers:

- **Ask for recommendations.**
- **Check the provider's credentials.**

MINIGLOSSARY
of Autonomous Health Professionals

autonomous health professional: a person authorized to offer a health service without supervision.
dietitian: a person trained in diet planning. A *registered dietitian (R.D.)* is a dietitian who has graduated from a state-approved program of dietetics, has passed the professional American Dietetic Association registration examination, and has served in an internship program to practice the necessary skills. Some states require licensing for dietitians; others do not.
medical doctor (M.D.): a *physician*; a person trained to provide medical care and licensed by the state to practice.
nurse: a general term for any person who provides health care. A *registered nurse (R.N.)* is a nurse who has graduated from a state-approved school of nursing, has passed the professional nursing state board examination, and has been granted a license to practice within a given state.
nurse practitioner (N.P.): a registered nurse (R.N.) who has received additional medical training to assess the physical and psychosocial status of individuals and families and can manage some of the common illnesses of people in a colleague relationship with a physician. Some are registered as nurse practitioners (R.N.P.).
osteopath (D.O.): a health care provider who takes the same course of training as a physician, but in a school of osteopathy, which specializes in disorders of the musculoskeletal system.
physician: see *medical doctor (M.D.)*; also *osteopath (D.O.)*.
physician's assistant (P.A.): a person with medical training, authorized to perform medical services under the supervision of a physician (and therefore, strictly speaking, a semiautonomous health professional). Training includes two to four years of college and two years of specialized training. In some states, physician supervision can be by telephone, and in some, P.A.s can prescribe certain drugs.
registered dietitian: see *dietitian*.
registered nurse: see *nurse*.

Most degrees listed next to health care practitioners' names are strong degrees that equip people to practice their specialties competently. However, **bogus** degrees complicate the picture. Not everyone who posts a doctor's diploma on the office wall has spent all those years studying and passed all those examinations. Some organizations simply sell official-looking diplomas for $50 or $75 by mail. Some unscrupulous people working in strategic positions within a university can manipulate computer files to bestow a degree on someone who has not completed the required course of study. The price may be in the thousands of dollars, but the degree is still fraudulent for qualifying someone to practice.

To find out whether an institution is a genuine graduate school, do some research. The university should have an address, some buildings, and a faculty consisting of people with bona fide degrees. If you ask to speak to the dean of graduate studies, such a person should exist. A post office box number without a street address is practically a guarantee that the degree-granting institution is a fraud. Also, the university should be accredited by a professional accediting association, (for example, the AMA for physicians, the APA for psychologists). But watch out. There are bogus associations, too. And bogus accrediting agencies and bogus licenses to practice also abound. The rule seems to be that for every valid symbol of legitimacy, there is a counterfeit that copies it. If you can apply to an institution for a degree, a diploma, or a license to practice in the name of your pet poodle—and get it—then you have uncovered a fraud.

For every valid symbol of legitimacy, there is a counterfeit that copies it.

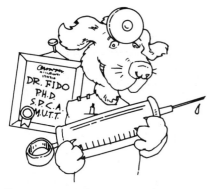

If you can apply for a degree in the name of your pet poodle—and get it—then you have uncovered a fraud.

A key to understanding just who is legitimate and who is not is the **license to practice**. Each state has a health licensing agency, which regulates the practice of health occupations within its borders. Do not visit a health professional who has no license to practice.

Besides licensing, other controls on quality of practitioners exist: **certification** and **registration**. Each health care profession has a society with defined qualifications and fees for membership, and each society scrutinizes candidates for registration (for example, course work and experience) and administers an examination. Those candidates who pass are then listed on a register with the other approved practitioners within the profession. Many societies have requirements for periodic updating of registration; for example, a practitioner may have to keep taking approved course work every year and reapply for registration every five years or lose the status. When you see the term **registered dietitian (R.D.)**, for example, that is what it means. Of course, in every health care profession you may find fake certifications, registrations, and licenses, so the buyer must still beware, but the legitimate titles are workable controls on quality.

Once you have found a qualified health care provider, call the person's office and ask the questions listed in the margin. Then, on your first appointment, you can gather your own impressions of the person and staff. Most people want someone they can talk to. If the health care provider and staff willingly furnish all of the information you are requesting, the match may be a good one. It is a good idea, especially if you are intimidated or hurried, to:

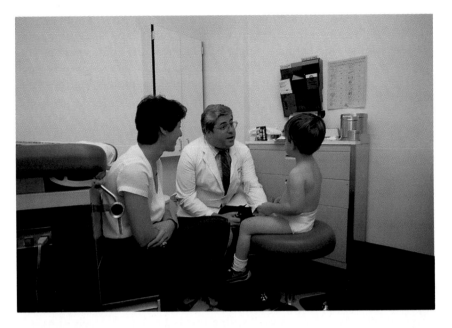

When visiting a health care provider, expect to be listened to and to have your questions answered.

⊕ **Ask these questions:**
What are the fees for office visits? Other visits? What are the office hours?
Can I obtain advice by phone? At what times?
Does the person recommend that I have periodic checkups? How often?
If I am sick, will the person visit me at home? What is the fee for this service?
Who handles the calls when the person is not around?
Notice how your first appointment goes.

⊕ **Expect to be listened to.**

⊕ **Expect a thorough history.**

⊕ **Expect a thorough physical examination.**

⊕ **Expect to have your diagnosis and instructions clearly explained.**

■ Write out your observations and thoughts on your condition beforehand, and give them to the person at examination time.
■ Write out your questions for your own reference, and write down the answers you receive as the interview takes place.

Expect a thorough **history**—that is, a question-and-answer session about your past medical history. How well you communicate with the person in this session is of great importance. The history provides about 70 percent of the information needed for an accurate diagnosis; time spent communicating will likely save money on medical costs later.[4] A truly well-informed health care provider will ask you about your exposure to occupational and environmental threats to health, use of safety belts, eating and exercise habits, sexual history, and stress management and coping skills, as well as many other questions.

Also expect a thorough **physical examination**, head to toe. The person who gives you a once-over-lightly is not starting by getting to know your physical condition very well. Expect certain tests as aids to diagnosis—for example, a blood and urine analysis, a chest X-ray procedure if you have been having trouble breathing; or an EKG if any heart trouble is indicated.

Expect to be told the diagnosis and to have it explained. When a treatment is prescribed:

■ Write down the directions you are given. Follow them.
■ If in doubt, ask about alternative treatments.

By the time you leave the office, you should feel satisfied that you have been well received, understood, and instructed. The person has spent adequate time with you, has focused attention on listening to you, has learned everything important about your previous medical history, has examined you carefully, has made an expert diagnosis (or taken the first necessary steps in that direction), and has answered all your questions. If this description does not apply to your interaction, you may want to find another health care provider.

The physical examination should be thorough.

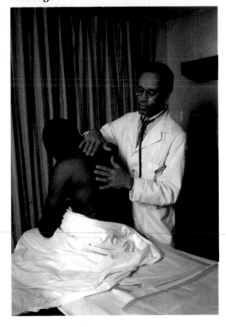

Once your choice is made, periodic contact over the years should help to establish a mutually respecting and trusting relationship. Your health care provider can become an increasingly valuable resource. On occasion, you can obtain advice efficiently just by telephoning. (Do not abuse this privilege, though. If you have more than a simple, routine question, go to the office and pay the fee.)

Other Professionals—Including Some Not So Professional

Besides those already mentioned, many other people practice as autonomous health professionals singly or in **group practice**, in private offices or clinics. Some of these people may be well qualified to help you with what ails you or even to help you improve and prolong your already good health. Some have skills within limited realms that are useful. Some may be out-and-out frauds waiting to ambush anyone with full pockets and an unsuspecting nature.

An assortment of unorthodox health practitioners of varying quality is listed in the Miniglossary of Other Health Practitioners. Some offer useful services; some are essentially harmless; some are unscrupulous and dangerous quacks. New "specialties" spring up all the time to deceive unwary victims. Anyone can claim the title doctor; there are penalties only for falsely claiming to have an M.D. degree from a particular medical school. Thus where credentialing and licensing are not standardized, the guarantee that a health care provider will give you useful service is not secure. Medical doctors are of different stripes, too; not all are the fine, upstanding, ethical persons we wish them to be. Some are dishonest, incompetent, or impaired—

MINIGLOSSARY
of Other Health Practitioners

acupuncturist: a health practitioner who punctures the body with needles to relieve pain and achieve other physiological effects. Needles inserted at nerve synapses can alter the transmission of pain sensations. Acupuncture is an ancient art in China; depending on the practitioner, it has been found to be of some usefulness in the United States for pain management.

allopath: see *naturopath*.

chiropractor: a person who is trained to treat people with pain said to be caused by misalignment of the skeleton. Chiropractic treatments use "adjustments"—that is, manipulations of the joints that can, at best, relieve pressure on nerves, and at worst, cause permanent disability.

clinical ecologist: a practitioner who claims to be able to cure people's illnesses by diagnosing and treating allergies to substances and materials in the environment.

homeopath: the practitioner of a scientifically unproven practice of using small doses of poisons to prevent or relieve harm caused by those poisons.
    homeo = same

iridologist: a person who claims to be able to diagnose illnesses by studying the patterns of color in the iris of the eye. "Training" consists of payment of $400 to purchase a chart of the iris and a list of diseases indicated by various color patterns.

lay midwife: a birth attendant who may or may not be an R.N. and may be educated in any number of ways, from informal observation of births to three-year lay midwifery programs. There are no licensing boards for lay midwives.

naprapath: a person who treats connective tissue and ligament disorders by manipulation and massage.
    napra = connective (tissue)

naturopath: a person who uses "natural" products such as foods and herbs to treat people's illnesses. Naturopaths distinguish themselves from traditional medical practitioners, whom they call *allopaths*—people who use medicine, surgery, X-ray examinations, and other "unnatural" tools to treat illnesses.
    allo = other (than natural)

nutritionist: a person who specializes in the study of nutrition. Some nutritionists are registered dietitians, some have considerable course work in nutrition, and some are self-described experts whose training may be minimal or nonexistent.

orthomolecular psychiatrist: a psychiatrist who uses "natural" treatments, especially vitamins and minerals, to rectify mental illnesses, assuming they are caused by wrong amounts of nutrient molecules in the system.
    ortho = right (amount)

but the chance that this is so is less than it used to be, because the safeguards are greater. Chapter 1 offered strategies for sorting fiction from fact in the world of health claims.

One specialist many people use as a health care provider is the **chiropractor** (doctor of chiropractic, or D.C.). Not everyone realizes that this person, although called "doctor," has been through a much shorter course of training than the M.D.—only two years of college and two years of chiropractic school before beginning to practice. (Compare the M.D. or D.O. schooling described on page 374.) A chiropractor's training makes it possible to set up an office that resembles a physician's office, and some of the services offered there can relieve pain (especially from pressure on nerves), but others cause more severe health problems than they solve.[5]

The wise consumer uses all the strategies, resources, and services mentioned in this chapter, and more. The person who knows how the health care system works and how to avoid health fraud is way ahead of the game when it comes to self-care.

STUDY AIDS

1. List alternative choices for treating medical problems and the payment systems likely to accompany them.
2. Describe various kinds of health insurance.
3. List strategies for purchasing an appropriate insurance package.
4. Describe insurance abuses and their effects on health care providers, medical care facilities, and consumers.
5. Compare a traditional hospital with a health maintenance organization.
6. List strategies for selecting and using medical care facilities.
7. List elements important in choosing a health care provider.
8. List criteria that help the consumer distinguish between various health care providers, both professional and unprofessional.
9. Describe how to determine whether a health care provider's credentials are fraudulent.
10. Describe what to look for during an initial visit to a health care provider.
11. Describe a variety of health care practitioners whose qualifications to practice are limited or nonexistent.

GLOSSARY

(This chapter has several Miniglossaries. For health insurance types, see page 370; for hospitals and related facilities, page 373; and for types of health professionals, pages 375, and 378.)

accreditation: approval; in the case of hospitals or university departments, approval by a professional organization qualified to judge the quality of the service or educational program offered. See also *bogus.*

bogus: fake. There are bogus doctors, bogus professional organizations, bogus accrediting agencies, bogus licenses to practice, bogus certifications, bogus registrations, and probably bogus refereed journals, too (see Chapter 1).

certification: approval granted by an organization, signifying that an individual is qualified to perform a service according to a certain standard. See also *bogus.*

fee-for-service system: the system of payments for medical care that charges a fee for each service.

group practice: an organization of physicians who practice medicine together; an example is the HMO.

health maintenance organization (HMO): a group practice organization based on a prepayment system.

history (medical): an interview in which a health care professional obtains information from a client relating to past medical experience.

hysterectomy: removal of the uterus, an operation performed more often than necessary.

license to practice: permission under state or federal law to use a certain title (such as medical doctor, osteopath, attorney, etc.) and to offer certain services, obtained by passing a state-administered examination.

malpractice insurance: a type of insurance that can be carried by any person offering a service or selling a product. If the person is sued by someone claiming to have been harmed by the service or product, it pays all or part of the fines awarded by the court.

physical examination: an examination performed as part of a general checkup or to achieve a diagnosis.

prepayment system: the system of payments for medical care that charges a fixed monthly fee regardless of the services provided in a given month.

registration: with respect to health professionals, a listing signifying that the professional has met requirements such as course work, experience, and the passing of an examination, and so may use the title and practice the profession.

tonsillectomy: removal of the tonsils (in the throat), an operation sometimes performed unnecessarily.

QUIZ ANSWERS

1. *False.* You may need as many as five different kinds of insurance to be adequately covered against medical expenses; even then, long-term care might well not be covered.

2. *False.* Although the physician's insurance company pays the fee, the physician pays the premium, and the client indirectly absorbs the cost.

3. *False.* The place to go to get a sore throat treated is your health care provider's office or the health clinic—during regular office hours.

4. *False.* You may have to pay in advance for treatment, then get reimbursed by your insurance company.

5. *False.* Hospitals can turn away people who can't afford to pay, even if they need emergency treatment.

6. *True.* A certificate of accreditation indicates that a hospital has met certain standards for health care.

7. *False.* HMO stands for health maintenance organization. People should not perform surgery on themselves!

8. *True.* An osteopath (D.O.) is just as well qualified to perform most medical services as a physician is and is legally permitted to do so.

9. *True.* Chiropractors (D.C.) are called "doctor," but they don't have nearly as much medical education as medical doctors (M.D.).

10. *True.* Anyone can adopt the title "doctor," but there are penalties for claiming to be a medical doctor (M.D.)

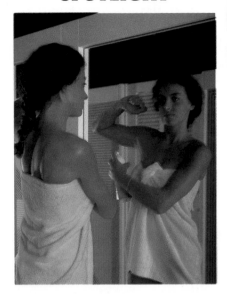

Your Body— An Owner's Manual

This chapter talked a lot about hospitals and physicians—whom to see, how to pay. But an important aspect of health care—in fact, the most important, most of the time—is *self*-care. Doing a few simple things for your body can enable you to maintain it at least as lovingly as you would maintain a fine car.

That sounds like a worthwhile objective. How much do I have to do?

Surprisingly little—just the basics. Some things you need to do daily, others only once a month or once a year. Tooth care is a daily chore, but there is not much to it.

I know what's involved in tooth care—and why it's important. Tooth decay can lead to major illness of the whole body.

True. And what are the steps to take?

Brush and floss the teeth after each meal to remove all food particles. There's nothing more to it than that.

Actually, there is something more. It is important to brush at the gum line, as well as to brush your teeth. Dental plaque takes hold at the gum line and beneath it, and the gums themselves deteriorate if plaque gets out of hand. Gum disease causes most people's mouth odor and contributes more to tooth loss than tooth decay does. Ninety percent of all adults will develop gum disease; the early symptom is gums that bleed easily. No one need ever develop it.

I didn't know that. Ninety percent of all adults get gum disease? OK, I'll start brushing my gums. Any other pointers?

Yes, that is the purpose of flossing, too. Use the floss to pull the plaque up from below the gum line, *between* the teeth. Use the brush or a toothpick to dislodge plaque from below the gum line *along* the teeth (see Figure S18–1). If you do this only once a day, you will be doing more to protect your teeth than any amount of brushing of tooth surfaces can.

If you do all that, do you still have to visit the dentist?

Yes, you certainly do. A professional cleaning about once every six months and a full examination about once a year can go a long way toward helping you keep your teeth for life. Your dentist can advise you what intervals are appropriate for you. And, of course, you should obtain adequate fluoride and avoid sugary snacks.

What else should a body owner do by way of daily maintenance?

Some things, such as bathing, are too elementary to discuss, but others may not be learned during the growing years and are important. For example, the way you walk, sit, and sleep affects your skeleton profoundly over the years. The bones and disks of your spine are of particular interest, and if you have had even a twinge of back pain, you will know why. Think of your spine as a set of 26 delicate hollow bones (**vertebrae**) stacked up on one another like doughnuts with pads between them (the disks). Think of your spinal cord running right up through the holes in the doughnuts.* (A difference from doughnuts is that the holes in the vertebrae are near their edges, not at the center; see Figure S18–2). Major nerves exit and enter at every level between the vertebrae—and if the bones or disks are damaged, they can pinch those nerves. The result: stabbing pain, like an electric shock, torturing the muscles of the neck, shoulders, back, or legs. The odds are that it can happen to you. During their adult lives, eight out of ten people have back pain

---

*Counting the "tailbones," there are 33 vertebrae in most people's spines; some have 34.

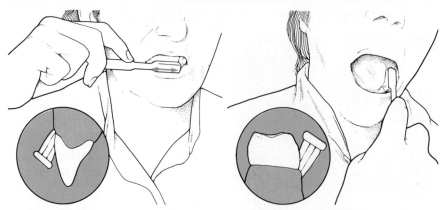

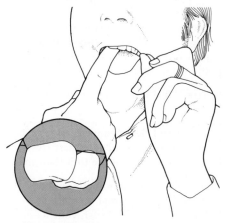

Brush tooth surfaces back and forth, not up and down, so as not to push food particles below the gum line.

Brush the gums, especially inside at the gumline (gently), to dislodge plaque there.

Use floss to pull plaque up from below the gum line between the teeth.

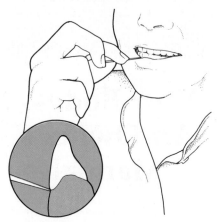

Use a toothpick or brush to dislodge plaque from below the gum line along the teeth.

severe enough to warrant a visit to the doctor.[1]*

That's still not likely to happen to me. I don't do strenuous work using my back.

You might be surprised to learn that people in the sedentary (sitting) occupations are most susceptible. If they don't exercise, their back and abdominal muscles become weak, and their spines tend to become less and less well supported. Poor posture combined with weakened muscles is a virtual guarantee of major back trouble.

What do the abdominal muscles have to do with it? Are you telling me I should do sit-ups to protect my back?

Yes. Overly strong back muscles can bend your spine backward unless you have strong abdominal muscles to work against them.[2] Sit-ups and leg lifts are therefore important. And how you sit, stand, and walk also matter a lot. The image to keep in mind is of that stack of doughnuts. Keep it in its normal S curve so that it will not topple; so that it will hold your heavy head up by balancing, not by straining; and so that the nerves run straight through it unimpeded.

You mentioned how I sleep as being important, too.

Yes. You spend a third of your life sleeping, remember. By the time you have lived 75 years, you will have spent a quarter of a century lying down. Whatever position you choose to lie in for 25 years is bound to af-

*Reference notes are in Appendix D.

fect the shape of your skeleton permanently.

I never saw it quite like that. I hope you're not going to tell me to change the position I sleep in. I doubt I could learn to sleep in any other position.

No one position is right for sleeping, but there are some to avoid. Figure S18–3 shows the principles. In general, the idea is to keep your spine in its normal curve while sleeping, just as you would try to do while awake. If you sleep on your back, support your knees, so as not to develop a swayback, and do not use too high a pillow under your head. If you sleep on your side, use a pillow just high

enough to keep your neck straight. Do not sleep on your stomach. Figure S18–3 shows how to sit, stand, and walk, too.

That sounds like good advice. Any other habits I should be conscious of?

None we haven't covered elsewhere. We have stressed nutrition, fitness, and alcohol, drug, and tobacco use enough already.

You certainly have. You mentioned monthly chores, though. What did you have in mind?

Breast and testicular self-examinations fall into that category. Chapter 17 showed how to do them,

FIGURE S18–2 The Spinal Column

The spinal cord runs through the hollow part of the bones of the spine. Branches of nerves leave the main trunk at each level to carry messages to and from the body parts. Disks provide padding between the bones. Disk A is normal and protects the nearby nerves from being pinched. Disk B has bulged out of shape and is pinching the nearby nerves. Depending on how high in the spine this defect is, the result will be pain in the neck, shoulder, lower back, or legs. Other common back damage causing pain includes flattened disks, bone spurs, worn-cut vertebral joints, or degeneration of the vertebrae themselves (osteoporosis).

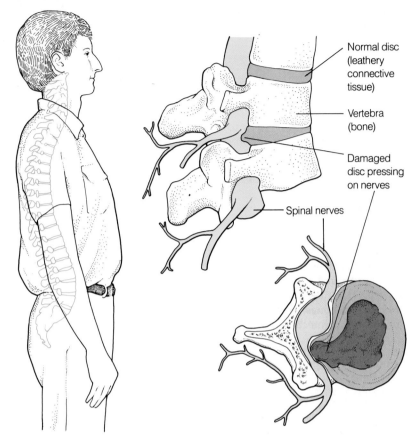

Normal curve of the spine. When the bones are stacked this way, the discs bear the weight evenly, and the nerves feel least pressure.

Labels on figure:
Normal disc (leathery connective tissue)
Vertebra (bone)
Damaged disc pressing on nerves
Spinal nerves

MINIGLOSSARY

glaucoma (gla-oh-CO-ma): a disease of the eye, caused by high pressure of the fluid inside the eyeball, that causes blindness. An early symptom is that lights appear to have halos around them.

speculum: an instrument used to spread the vaginal opening so that the cervix can be viewed.

vertebrae (singular, **vertebra**): the bones of the spine—26 above the point of attachment to the pelvis, 7 or 8 below it.

but knowing how is not enough. You also have to *remember* to do the examinations every month. Some people keep a reminder with the monthly bills.

Women can also examine their own internal sex organs monthly, if they wish. Medical personnel have traditionally performed these examinations, but women can learn to examine themselves, using a **speculum**, a mirror, and a flashlight (see Figure S18–4). In some ways, women can do this better than someone else might do, because they can learn from frequent inspections just how their own tissues change in color and texture at different times of the month. A health care provider would

be less likely to recognize what appearances are normal for a particular woman.

A woman does need to go to a health care provider for an annual Pap smear, though. The early changes characteristic of cancer are not visible to the naked eye.

That would be part of an annual physical examination, right?

Actually, although a woman needs a Pap smear every year, she doesn't necessarily need a complete physical examination every time. The most effective strategy seems to be for everybody to adopt some broad preventive measures, and then for individuals with specific risk factors to adopt some additional measures tailored especially for them. That about

takes care of all the maintenance activities you need to engage in to keep your body in smooth running order—other than to seek medical help when necessary, of course.

To be thorough about it, shouldn't you also visit the eye doctor and get your hearing checked every now and then?

Vision and hearing are mentioned specifically for the over-40 age group in Table 18–1. It is assumed that your regular checkup will include the screening necessary to detect problems before that time. But after age 40 your vision is expected to deteriorate, and correction is likely to be necessary. Hearing deteriorates after age 40, too, and people can gradually

FIGURE S18–3 Care of the Spine

become deaf without being aware of it.

I don't want my vision and hearing to deteriorate. What can I do to prevent that?

For vision—watch television from six feet or more away and with lights on in the room. Don't stare into the television from up close, especially in a dark room. Don't expose your eyes to any kind of radiation other than ordinary light; never stare at the sun or at an ultraviolet light. For hearing—don't listen to loud music through earphones, and if you use guns, use earprotecting muffs along with them.

You didn't say "don't read without good light."

No, contrary to popular belief, reading in the dark will not hurt your eyes. The reason you are advised not to do it is that it will make you tired.

If I'm sure that my vision and hearing are fine, do I still have to have them checked after age 40?

You can't know that your eyes are all right, and it is extremely important to have them checked periodically after age 40. A condition known as **glaucoma** (rhymes with *cow coma*), in which the fluid inside the eyeball exerts too-high pressure, can progress rapidly to blindness before you are aware of it. (A warning sign is that lights appear to have halos around them; if you ever have this symptom, see a physician right away.) Glaucoma typically sets in after age 40, and that is the main condition the eye check is intended to catch.

As for your hearing, that is up to you. Prevention of damage is the key to both hearing and sight acuity in the later years, because both the ears and the eyes work by way of nerve

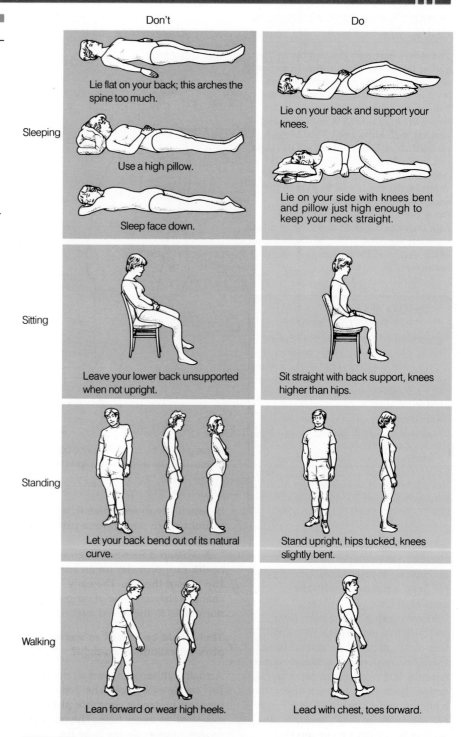

Don't

Do

Sleeping

Lie flat on your back; this arches the spine too much.

Use a high pillow.

Sleep face down.

Lie on your back and support your knees.

Lie on your side with knees bent and pillow just high enough to keep your neck straight.

Sitting

Leave your lower back unsupported when not upright.

Sit straight with back support, knees higher than hips.

Standing

Let your back bend out of its natural curve.

Stand upright, hips tucked, knees slightly bent.

Walking

Lean forward or wear high heels.

Lead with chest, toes forward.

FIGURE S18–4 Medical Self-Care Techniques

These are observations you can make, yourself, before visiting a health care professional. The keener your self-awareness, the better you can take care of yourself, and the better you can cooperate with medical personnel when necessary. ➡

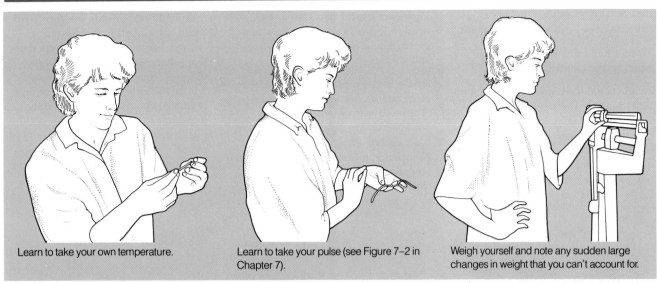

Learn to take your own temperature.

Learn to take your pulse (see Figure 7–2 in Chapter 7).

Weigh yourself and note any sudden large changes in weight that you can't account for.

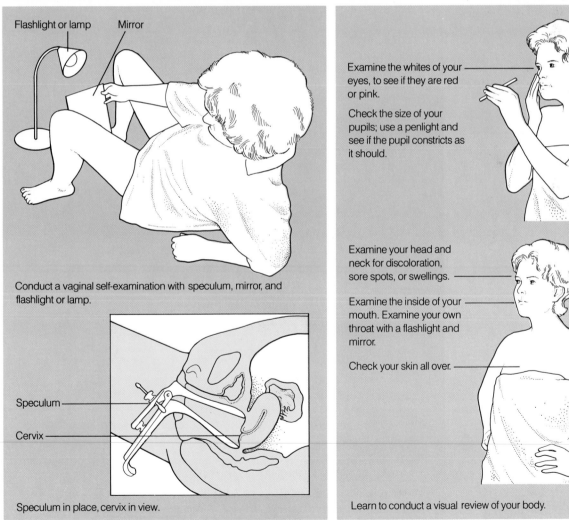

Flashlight or lamp   Mirror

Conduct a vaginal self-examination with speculum, mirror, and flashlight or lamp.

Speculum

Cervix

Speculum in place, cervix in view.

Examine the whites of your eyes, to see if they are red or pink.

Check the size of your pupils; use a penlight and see if the pupil constricts as it should.

Examine your head and neck for discoloration, sore spots, or swellings.

Examine the inside of your mouth. Examine your own throat with a flashlight and mirror.

Check your skin all over.

Learn to conduct a visual review of your body.

tissues, and these do not recover from damage beyond a certain point.

What other signs should send me running for medical care?

People could save themselves a lot of time, money, and needless worry if they knew when *not* to visit a health care provider, as well as when *to* see one. One time not to go is when you have an ordinary cold. You also need not go if you have:

■ A mild rash without other symptoms.
■ A single episode of vomiting or diarrhea without abdominal pain.
■ A fever of less than 102 degrees Fahrenheit (39 degrees centigrade).

Those are useful lists. Now, all I need to know is how to take a temperature and how to take a pulse, and I'll be all set.

Figure S18–4 offers these and a few other techniques everyone can learn to use. To learn more of the same, you may want to purchase a self-care book such as the American Medical Association's *Family Medical Guide*. You should also learn and practice the basics of accident prevention, and take a course in first aid, to be

maximally responsible for your own health care. And if you have a chronic condition (such as hypertension, diabetes, arthritis, or kidney disease), there are many ways in which you can learn to monitor and regulate it yourself. Self-care initiatives do not replace professional health care, but they certainly complement it nicely, and they give you the sense, which is appropriate, that your health care is your own responsibility.

The Environment and Personal Health

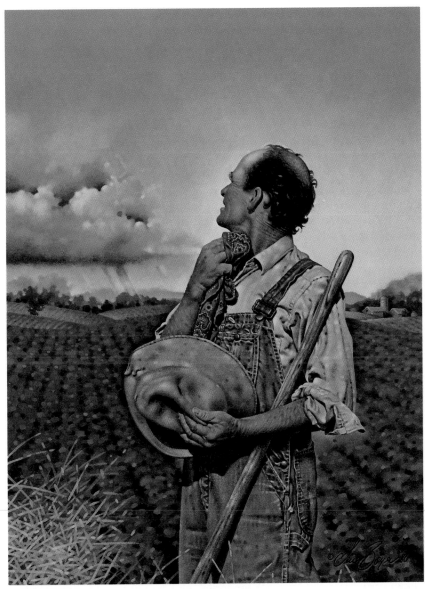

© Gene Boyer '86.

FOR OPENERS . . .

True or false? If false, say what is true.

1. There is no clear boundary between a person and the environment.

2. Air pollution has existed on earth since before the dawn of human history.

3. The greenhouse effect is beneficial to the earth, because it promotes the growth of plants.

4. As long as the ozone hole stays at the South Pole, it won't hurt the people on the major continents.

5. Pure water can pollute the environment if it is of the wrong temperature.

6. To minimize environmental impact, human sewage should be returned to the earth after treatment, not to the water.

7. Radioactive wastes can't be detoxified; they can only be moved from place to place.

8. Radioactivity alters the genetic material in living cells, including ova and sperm cells, creating mutations that can persist for generations.

9. When birds can't survive in an environment, that is a sign that people's health is likely to suffer there, too.

10. The most promising way to approach the world's environmental problems is for all nations to work equally hard on all of them.

(Answers on page 417.)

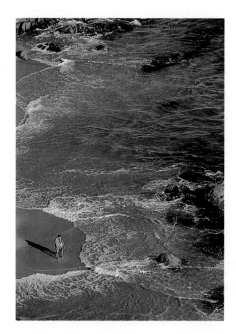

Technically, an **environment** might be defined as all things that exist or originate outside of an individual. Several environments might be described that way—the home environment, the cultural environment, the biological environment, and so forth. But to define an environment as *outside* implies a separateness that is not real. When you are breathing, is the air outside of you, or inside? When you are conversing with a teacher, where do the thoughts you are sharing come from—inside or outside of you or the teacher? Materials, energy, and information constantly flow into and out of us. We and our environments are not only interdependent but also continuous, part of the same whole. Our biological environment, for example, supplies the materials our bodies are made of and the forms of energy (light, heat, sound) that make our lives possible. Conversely, we alter and interfere with the environment in many ways.

Healthy environments support personal health; damaged environments detract from it. Consider your needs. Ideally, wherever you lived and worked—inner city, farm, or wilderness—the air would be clean, the water pure, the food nourishing and safe, the surrounding scenery and sounds enjoyable, the space sufficient for play, the people nearby stimulating and loving, the events interesting, and all other elements, both seen and unseen, in harmony together. It is unrealistic, of course, to think that everyone in today's world can enjoy such a life, and it is also untrue that such perfect conditions are indispensable to health. It is true, however, that we will survive or thrive only so long as we maintain our environments sufficiently so that they can sustain us. This chapter focuses on our biological environment—the planet Earth.

You may wonder why a book about personal health should have a chapter on such a seemingly impersonal subject. The book's philosophy, stated on the first page of Chapter 1, is that you control your health, and its mission is to help you do a good job of it. The emphasis throughout is on your choices. But in what sense do you make choices that affect your "environmental health"?

You make such choices all the time. You do not leave the earth the same from one day to the next. Each day of your life, you breathe its air, eat its food, leave your wastes on it—and you either restore more of its resources than you consume, or you do not. To make your choices consciously, you have to be informed about the impact you are having on the earth as you interact with it. This chapter is intended to raise your consciousness, partly so that you can make many little choices every day with that awareness.

The environment also has an impact on you. If its air is clean, your lungs can be healthy. If its water is pure, you can drink it without fear. If its soil is free of toxins, it will bring forth food that will sustain your life. Because you are a biological creature, you depend on the environment for the physical necessities of your life—air, water, soil, climate, and living plants and animals. You may be unaware of the vast changes taking place in your environment today, but once your eyes are open you can see these changes all around you and recognize their effects. We want you to become aware, because your awareness can lead to action.

You have the right to a healthy environment. You have the right to demand of your fellow human beings that they maintain it so as to support you and your children and grandchildren. You have the right to clean air, pure water, uncontaminated food. So this chapter has a second mission—to increase your awareness of the ways other people's choices impinge on you. Together with your neighbors you can demand that other people respect your rights. As large as the world's environmental problems may be, they are all caused by people's choices. They can also only be solved by people's choices, and you can influence those choices. Every time you drop a word of awareness into someone else's consciousness, you start a ripple that may grow into a wave.

Some of the choices are small—for example, that of the motorist who keeps the car running while it sits for ten minutes in a traffic jam: turned off, it would pollute the air a little less. (The mere sharing of that thought might be all it would take to solve that problem.) Some are big—for example, that of the hospital administrator who chooses for profit's sake to have disease-carrying refuse dumped into the nearest river rather than disposing of it properly. (Effective legislation backed by vigilant police work and stringent punishments for violations might be needed here.) In any case, all such choices begin with consciousness of what the problems and their causes are, so that is where this chapter begins.

The chapter is divided, somewhat artificially, into realms: the air and green plants first, then the water, then the land—but of course, these realms are interconnected, and anything that affects one of them affects them all (see Figure 19–1 on pages 390–391). The Life Choice Inventory allows you to assess the present state of your earth awareness, and the Spotlight ends the chapter with an emphasis on personal choices that affect the environment.

LIFE CHOICE INVENTORY

How closely attuned to your natural environment are you? To find out, try answering the following questions (2 points each):

1. Trace the route of the water you drink from rainfall to your drinking glass.
2. How many days is it until the next full moon (within two days)?
3. How many inches of rain fall every year where you live (within 1 inch for every 20 inches)?
4. What kind of soil lies beneath your homesite?
5. Which way is north? (Point without hesitating.)
6. Where does your kitchen garbage go?
7. Where does your waste water go?
8. Name five birds that reside in your region and five that migrate through it.
9. What primary geological event or process formed the land on which you live?
10. From what direction do rainstorms generally come in your region?

Extra credit (1 point each):

11. What species, now extinct, roamed the land where you live?

12. What spring wildflower is consistently among the first to bloom where you live?
13. How long is the growing season where you live?
14. Name five native edible plants in your region and the seasons in which they are available.
15. At what time of year do the deer mate in your region, and when are the young born?

Scoring: With respect to the natural world that surrounds you:

19 to 20   Your awareness is keen. The earth needs you.*
16 to 18   Your awareness is commendable.
11 to 15   You are paying attention.
8 to 10   You have a fair grasp of its obvious features.
4 to 7   You are unaware.
0 to 3   You are woefully unaware.

*In the words of the original writers of this quiz, "You not only know where you're at, you know where it's at."

SOURCE: Excerpted with permission from a quiz by Leonard Charles, Jim Dodge, Lynn Milliman, and Victoria Stockley, in *CoEvolution Quarterly*, Winter 1981, now known as *Whole Earth Review* (subscriptions: $18/year, 4 issues, from WER, 27 Gate Five Rd., Sausalito, CA 94965. Back issues: $3.50 from same address).

**FIGURE 19–1 All Things Are
Connected**

The Earth *before* Human Impact

THE AIR

Animals and people take up oxygen (○) and release carbon dioxide (◉).

The sun's rays, passing through clear air, provide energy for plants and algae to free oxygen (○) from carbon dioxide (◉).

Green plants on land and algae in the ocean take up carbon dioxide (◉) and return oxygen (○) to the atmosphere.

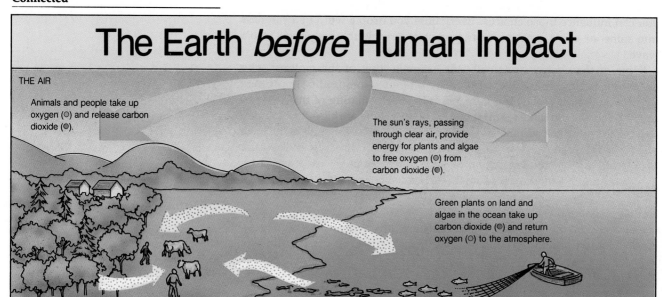

THE WATER

Water evaporates from waterways to form clouds.

Rain falls from the clouds, supports the plant life, and replenishes the water in the waterways.

Abundant plant life transpires water from beneath the ground to the air.

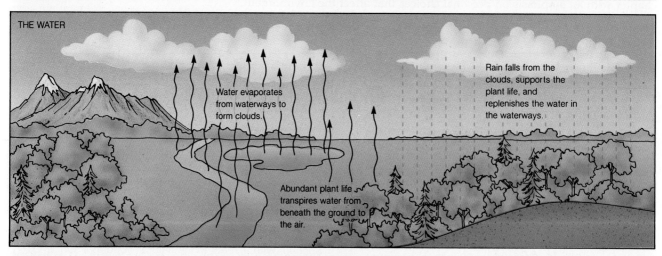

SOLID WASTE

Plants use the animal waste as natural fertilizer to support their own growth.

Cleansed by the plants and by filtration through the earth, pure water returns to the waterways.

Animals use plants to support their growth.

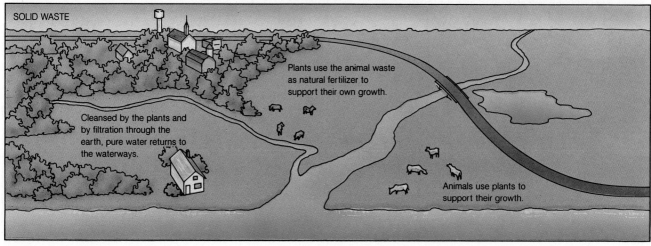

The Earth *with* Human Impact

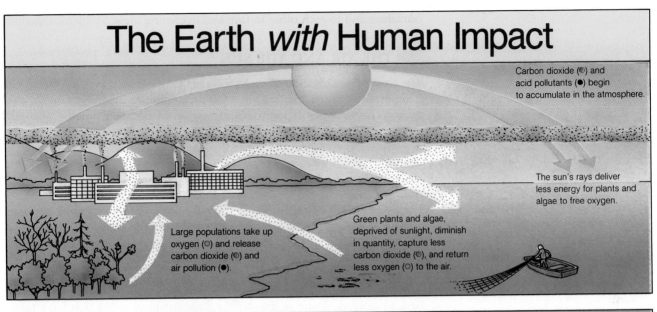

Carbon dioxide (◎) and acid pollutants (●) begin to accumulate in the atmosphere.

The sun's rays deliver less energy for plants and algae to free oxygen.

Large populations take up oxygen (○) and release carbon dioxide (◎) and air pollution (●).

Green plants and algae, deprived of sunlight, diminish in quantity, capture less carbon dioxide (◎), and return less oxygen (○) to the air.

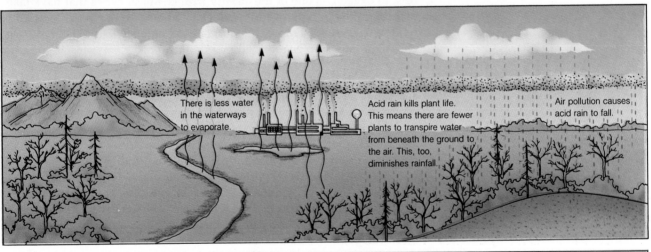

There is less water in the waterways to evaporate.

Acid rain kills plant life. This means there are fewer plants to transpire water from beneath the ground to the air. This, too, diminishes rainfall.

Air pollution causes acid rain to fall.

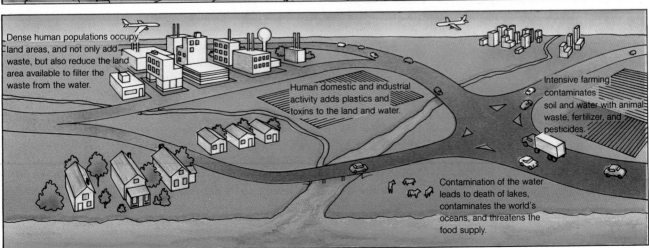

Dense human populations occupy land areas, and not only add waste, but also reduce the land area available to filter the waste from the water.

Human domestic and industrial activity adds plastics and toxins to the land and water.

Intensive farming contaminates soil and water with animal waste, fertilizer, and pesticides.

Contamination of the water leads to death of lakes, contaminates the world's oceans, and threatens the food supply.

A warning: this chapter describes some monumental environmental problems. Do not be disheartened: work your way through them to the end, where solutions are proposed to which you can contribute. We all owe it to ourselves and to each other to face and overcome these problems together.

■ THE AIR AND THE SUN

The air supports life in such obvious ways that we tend to take it for granted. It offers the oxygen you breathe in from minute to minute, to burn your body's energy fuels. It receives the carbon dioxide you breathe out with every breath. It conveys the energy of sunlight to green plants, and they use that energy to consume the carbon dioxide and restore the air's oxygen as they grow. In brief, the air, the sun, and green things are indispensable to life. To support life best, the air must be reasonably fresh (oxygen rich), clear (so that sunlight can penetrate it), and pure (carrying few harmful gases or particles). It must be of the right temperature to support life. And to receive the energy of sunlight and return oxygen to the air, there must be green plants. The more carbon dioxide in the air, the more green plants there must be to convert it back to oxygen.

The **oxygen cycle**, in which oxygen moves through animals and people to become carbon dioxide and the carbon dioxide is then processed by plants back to oxygen, is one of the earth's great chemical cycles that have taken place since the beginning of life on earth. All of the resources life depends on, like oxygen, are limited; all must be continuously recycled for life to go on. Water must also be returned pure to the earth; plants must continue to grow.

Next to the earth's surface, normal clean air consists of about 1/5 oxygen and 4/5 nitrogen, with trace amounts of inert gases mixed in. Natural processes add variable amounts of water vapor (from evaporation), carbon dioxide (from forest fires, volcanoes, and the life processes of living plants and animals), and small quantities of a few other gases contributed by the decomposition of protein matter. Any components other than these that get into air are **contaminants**—forms of **pollution**.

The air has never been perfectly fresh, clear, and pure. The natural processes just described have always released temporary bursts of contamination into the air, but these have always dispersed, leaving the atmosphere as before. However, polluted air surrounds the earth today. The reason is that the earth now sustains vast numbers of human beings who use fuel intensively for both domestic and industrial processes. Natural **air pollution** is, in general, intermittent and diffuse, whereas people-generated pollution is continuous, concentrated, and in many cases growing more intense from year to year.

People-generated pollutants come from four main sources: fuel burned to run cars and other forms of transportation, fuel burned to heat and cool homes and run their appliances, wastes from manufacturing, and solid wastes being burned for disposal. These add large amounts of carbon dioxide to the air— a natural substance, but unnatural in the quantities in which it now occurs in the atmosphere. In addition, they add pollutants, including carbon monoxide (already mentioned in Chapter 9), compounds of nitrogen and sulfur, and gases and particles containing many other substances. The effects of these chemicals on earth's climate, plants, animals, and people are often harmful and potentially catastrophic.

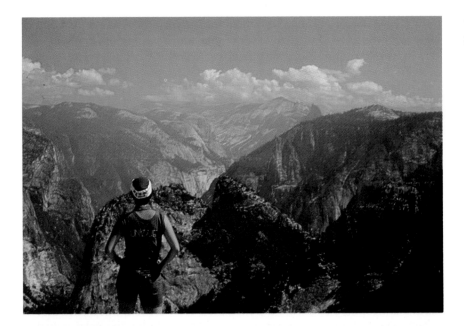

The Earth is better off where there are fewer people on it.

Warming of the Climate

Take carbon dioxide, for example. In its normal quantity, which until 30 years ago had remained about the same for billions of years, it blocks the escape of heat into the outer atmosphere and helps to keep the earth warm. Without it, the earth would have been 54 degrees colder for all those years, and life as we know it would have been impossible. In the thirty years between 1958 and 1988, however, the concentration of carbon dioxide in the earth's air has increased by 25 percent, mostly as the result of increased burning of oil and coal by people all over the world. The result is that the earth is warming up—the so-called **greenhouse effect**.[1]*

The greenhouse effect is expected to raise the earth's average temperature by 3 to 8 degrees in the next half-century (before 2050)—an amount that may not sound like much, but that is expected to have major effects. Most scientists believe that these effects are already occurring. Worldwide, summer heat is setting new high temperature records. Rainfall is declining across the corn and wheat belts in the United States, Europe, Russia, and Asia, resulting in drought and loss of crops. The water level below the ground is falling. Inland, the rivers are shrinking, creating hardship for areas that depend on their water. Along the coastlines salt water is invading areas where fresh water formerly kept it out, depriving both vegetation and people of needed water. In the oceans, the water is expanding as it warms while the polar ice caps are melting, so the sea level is rising. Governments are faced with the choice of seeing coastal cities and shores going under water or building dikes and levees to hold the water back. Forests and agricultural crops, adapted for thousands of years to a certain climate, are being stressed by rising temperatures and becoming increasingly vulnerable to disease. Whole species of animals and plants, including agricultural crops that human beings depend on, are becoming extinct as the earth's climate changes by

*Reference notes are in Appendix D.

only a few degrees. Having studied the problem, observers have commented, "We have tended to assume that the earth and its complex machinery would continue into the indefinite future as they have for the billions of years leading up to this moment. We forgot the one force capable of upsetting the balance that it took those billions of years to create. Ourselves."[2]

Thinning of the Ozone Layer

Another atmospheric effect of air pollution is taking place far out, in the outer atmosphere. Where intense sunlight strikes the outer atmosphere, a layer of gas known as the **ozone layer** continuously forms and breaks down from oxygen. The ozone layer has for billions of years screened out 99 percent of the ultraviolet rays of the sun, allowing just enough through to support plant growth. Life probably did not begin until after the earth's protective ozone layer was formed.[3]

Now, air pollution from all over the earth is eating a hole in that layer at the South Pole—the so-called **ozone hole**—and each antarctic summer, the hole grows larger. Diffusion of the remaining ozone from the rest of the earth's atmosphere re-covers the hole after each season, but at the cost of thinning the layer over the rest of the earth. As a result, ultraviolet radiation of higher and higher intensities is reaching the earth's surface each year. This radiation causes cancers and mutations in animals and people, and damages plants and crops.

Chief among the pollutants that destroy ozone are compounds known as **chlorofluorocarbons** (trade name **Freon**). The chlorofluorocarbons that destroy ozone are used to cool refrigerators, freezers, and air-conditioning systems; to create foams (including some styrofoams); and to expel liquids under pressure from aerosol cans (such as deodorant sprays).

CLOR-oh-FLOR-oh-car-bons, FREE-on

People and nations have been taking action to reduce chlorofluorocarbon output. Since 1978, aerosol deodorant sprays, window-cleaning sprays, and other sprays used by individual consumers have been largely replaced by roll-ons and pump devices. Industrial use of chlorofluorocarbons has continued to rise, however, and as of this writing it is still rising at the rate of 2 to 5 percent a year. Since it takes these molecules up to 40 years to reach the outer ozone layers, the destruction of ozone may continue long after their production has ceased.[4] At the current rate of increase, according to several independent predictions, the ozone layer will be seriously depleted within 100 years. Skin cancer rates, already on the increase, are expected to rise proportionately—to 1 in 90 by the year 2000 and 1 in 3 by the year 2075.[5] But individual cases of cancer do not constitute the biggest threat. Ultraviolet rays in excess of the norm disrupt the genetic material in all living tissues, damaging all future generations, not only of human beings, but also of forests, agricultural crops, grasslands, gardens, and animal life on land and in the seas.

In response to the destruction of the ozone layer, for the first time in history, an international conference on an environmental problem has led to *preventive* action. In the Montreal Protocol of 1986, 30 nations agreed to reduce their output of chlorofluorocarbons by 50 percent within the following decade. (The United States, unfortunately, agreed only to reduce the *rate of increase* of its chlorofluorocarbon production.) This historic event reflects a new and hopeful trend in history—the world is now united as never before by instantaneous mass-media communications, and governments can respond more quickly than ever before to global problems.

Health Effects of Local Air

When people are close to the sources of air pollution, they feel its effects more directly than they may feel such distant events as the change in the ozone layer. For example, wherever traffic and industrial processes are intense, **smog** forms, a type of air pollution familiar to everyone who lives in cities. Smog arises when sunlight strikes certain pollutants in the air, and one of its components is **ozone**—the very compound that provides protection from intense rays of the sun in the outer atmosphere. This nearby ozone breaks down before it reaches the outer atmosphere, so it cannot help to fill the ozone hole, but before breaking down it can damage people's lungs and reduce their ability to perform work or exercise.

Another air pollutant always surrounds automobile traffic: carbon monoxide from tailpipe exhaust. Electrocardiograms of people with heart disease reveal changes after time spent in heavy freeway traffic, where the concentration of carbon monoxide is high. People with heart disease, lung disease, or anemia (reduced oxygen-carrying capacity of the blood) can be severely disabled or even killed by carbon monoxide levels that merely impair function in healthy people. Even at relatively low concentrations, carbon monoxide also impairs mental and visual function and alertness.[6]

Another form of air pollution is **thermal pollution**, which occurs locally, particularly in cities and on cleared land where trees are absent and reflecting surfaces concentrate the heat. Thermal pollution adds significantly to the stress people in such environments face, and contributes to global climate warming.

Acid in the Air

As mentioned, air pollution cannot help but affect the water and soil as well. One problem arising from air pollution is **acid rain**. Each time it rains, the air is scrubbed of its pollutants; they fall to the earth. Many of them, when combined with water, form acids, which affect living things profoundly. It doesn't matter what compound forms the acid—it can be a compound of carbon, sulfur, nitrogen, or any other element. The effects are similar, because the acid part is always the same: a tiny, charged particle of hydrogen. This chemical busybody disrupts cell membranes, distorts the proteins that do the work of living cells, and changes the characteristics of fluids so that they cannot support normal life processes.

Just as there has always been air pollution, so too there has always been acid rain. But in the last 100 years, the world has become increasingly industrialized, and the air's acid burden has grown greater, primarily because of the burning of coal and petroleum.

The pH (see margin) of rainfall is normally slightly acidic, because falling rain always captures some carbon monoxide on its way to the earth, but

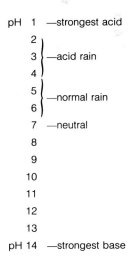

pH 1 —strongest acid

2

3 —acid rain

4

5 —normal rain

6

7 —neutral

8

9

10

11

12

13

pH 14 —strongest base

Acid is measured in pH units.* Each increment presents a ten-fold increase in concentration of hydrogen particles.

---

*The pH is the negative logarithm of the hydrogen ion concentration. It is a convenient unit, because it captures the 10,000,000-fold variation in hydrogen ion concentration within a seven-point scale—one point for each zero.

measurements taken today in some places show pHs in the 2 to 4 range—strongly acidic. Of particular concern to North Americans is the rain in the Northeast, made acid by pollution that drifts northeastward from the industrial Ohio Valley. Thousands of lakes in New England and Canada, once filled with fish and waterfowl, now stand clear and lifeless.

Snow and ice hold acid, just as rain does. When they melt, they suddenly dump high concentrations of acid into the waterways. The time of melting often coincides with the critical time in the spring when fish eggs and other eggs are just developing into young animals—a time when they are particularly vulnerable to environmental water conditions. Acid snowmelt causes massive kills of young fish and other fry and deforms those that survive.

Acid is neutralized by compounds (bases) in the soil. Where soils are thin and lie on top of rocks (on mountaintops and ocean islands, for example), this neutralizing capacity is limited, and ultimately the soil itself turns acid, killing the plants and trees that grow in it or weakening their resistance to diseases and insect pests. Millions of acres in many areas of the world, including U.S. mountain ranges, the Black Forest in West Germany, many parts of China, and elsewhere have been deforested by acid rain. Acid particles in the air are also directly harmful to human lungs, second only to cigarette smoking as a cause of lung disease.[7]

These forms of pollution are a people problem. The more people there are in an area, the more deforestation (removal of air-cleansing forests) there will be, the more burning of fuels and waste materials, the more cars and other traffic, and the more industry. This chapter returns to the population problem at the end.

THE WATER SUPPLY

When you draw water from the tap into a glass and drink it, it is not only water that you are drinking. Chlorine may have been added to it, to kill microorganisms that might otherwise convey disease. Fluoride may be present in it naturally, or it may have been added. In addition, it contains other naturally occurring minerals, live microorganisms, and a variety of toxic compounds. The minerals in water often make significant contributions to people's nutrition. A case in point is fluoride, which combines with the crystals of teeth and bones, hardening them and making them resistant to mineral loss. Other examples are calcium and magnesium, which are found in **hard water**, and which seem to help protect people against hypertension (see Chapter 16), and sodium, found in **soft water**, which has the opposite effect.

The microorganisms in water are mostly from human sewage and animal waste (agricultural animals and fertilizers). Many are harmless, but some are disease organisms. Sewage treatment plants must reduce the microbial count enough so that when the treated water is released into the water supply, the resulting dilution will make the water safe for human use. (The treatment of sewage, because it yields sludge that is deposited on the land, is described further in the next section, "The Land.")

High standards for sewage treatment in the developed countries ensure that most people have drinking water safe from microbial disease, but for the rest of the world, microbial contamination remains the primary cause of human diseases and epidemics. Two of the most basic public health needs of the world's people are safe drinking water and effective waste disposal.

Even in developed countries such as the United States and Canada, a major epidemic of disease would occur should we allow the public health system to go unsupported.

Among the harmful compounds in water are many contributed by agricultural fertilizers, pesticides, and industry. In the wilderness, waterborne contamination either falls on the ground and then is filtered by the soil before arriving in underground waterways, or, if it falls in a river, its contaminants quickly disappear back into the earth as the river flows along its course, leaving the water pure again. But neither the earth nor its rivers can purify completely the water polluted by today's intensive agricultural and industrial processes. Water leaving a factory may contain concentrations of contaminants so high that some are still present in the water after treatment, the water that reaches consumers. When the factory uses some of this water again, the concentrations of pollutants grow higher. The law requires polluting industries and water-processing plants to adhere to set standards, but enforcement often fails. Both government and consumer groups must be vigilant in detecting, reporting, and preventing dangerous levels of contamination, because our water is a vital resource.

⊛ **Study your own water supply to assure yourself of its purity.**

Some forms of water pollution first affect living things other than ourselves. When chemicals such as nitrates and phosphates (usually from sewage or fertilizer) are released into lakes and ponds, microorganisms in the water use them as nutrients to grow on. Life in waterways declines by a process known as **eutrophication**. First, the nutrients support the growth of large quantities of algae—so large that some are shaded out, die, and sink, filling the lake or pond with dead plant material. Bacteria thrive on this dead matter, and as they break it down, they use up the water's oxygen. The ultimate result is death of all life forms in the lake, including fish.

YOU-troh-fih-CAY-shun

Thermal pollution of lakes and streams also takes its toll on living things. Consider a factory that discharges hot water into a trout stream. The discharge may be pure H_2O, but it still kills the fish, because it is too hot for them to live in.

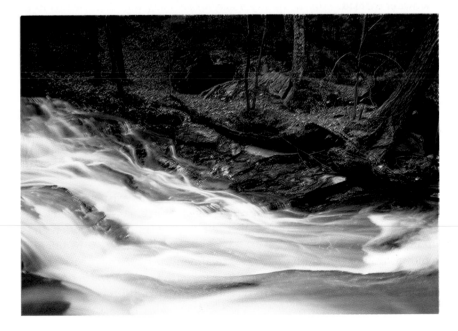

An abundant supply of fresh water is vital to all life forms on Earth.

The discussion of water to this point has focused on water *quality*. Water *quantity* is also of concern, as already mentioned. Not only droughts and encroachment of salt water but also the agricultural and industrial use of water strain the supply. Used by agriculture for irrigating and by industry for transporting, dissolving, washing, rinsing, cooling, flushing away waste, and many other purposes, water in huge quantities is diverted from its original, natural uses. In the future, it may be the water supply that first limits human activities.

▨ THE LAND: SOLID AND TOXIC WASTE

Like the air and the water, the land has a job to do in supporting human life, and all life, on earth. Today, when large masses of land lie under highways, parking lots, and city sidewalks, we no longer ask that *all* the soil be uncontaminated, but it remains essential that *some* of it be so, because it is on the soil that our food supply grows, and it is the soil that filters and purifies water after human, agricultural, or industrial use.

Two classes of contaminants are deposited directly in the ground as the result of human life and activity. One is **solid wastes** (nontoxic wastes such as ordinary sewage, garbage, and trash); the other is **toxic wastes** (mostly pesticides and industrial waste products).

Solid Waste

People and animals have always excreted solid wastes onto the earth. Bacteria break the waste material down and return its constituents to the soil. Plants then use those compounds as fertilizers—that is, building materials. Later, the plants either die or are eaten and are themselves similarly recycled. Everyone knows that manure makes excellent fertilizer. Human manure is no exception—provided that it is first treated to remove pathogens. However, today's large populations generate more sewage than can practically be used on the land areas that they occupy, and much of it is dumped into the water instead.

In nature, one ten-member wolf pack occupies a 25-acre territory; they and the other animals on that territory excrete a burden of waste that the land can easily handle. The waste is within the land's **carrying capacity**. By contrast, human beings live in densities of up to hundreds per acre in some cities, the cities are paved with tar and concrete, and the land is not able to recycle the waste. Cities burden the land far beyond its carrying capacity. The people in a single city the size of Philadelphia excrete fecal matter amounting to millions of gallons of sewage a day; after its water is removed, 100 tons of solid waste have to be disposed of each day. The mass of a typical city's sludge would, within a year, cover the whole city to a depth of 17 feet.

Where does it all go? Most people are unaware of its existence after they flush their toilets and see it disappear. But of course, sewage doesn't disappear. It often flows into the nearest river or bay untreated; it often ends up in the ocean. Ideally, however, it undergoes three steps of treatment—removal of the solid matter (**sludge**), treatment of the remaining water to kill pathogenic microorganisms, and release of the treated water onto land (not into waterways) to deposit its dissolved nutrient fertilizers where plants

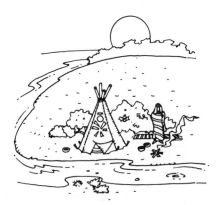

Live within the earth's capacity to carry the burden you place on it.

can use them, rather than where aquatic weeds will grow and strangle waterways. After this treatment, the water returns to the waterways free of contamination. The solid matter can be treated to purge toxic contaminants and kill microorganisms and then can also be returned to the land as fertilizer. Few cities treat even part of their sewage this way.

⊛ Know how the sewage in your area is treated. Support responsible sewage treatment.

Another form of solid waste is what people throw away—their garbage and trash. In so-called advanced civilizations, many people enjoy immediate removal of their throwaways and never have to wonder what becomes of them. Of course garbage and trash do not just disappear; they must be burned (polluting the air), buried (polluting the soil), or released into rivers or the ocean (polluting the water). Nothing ever really goes away.

It is hard to comprehend how massive the problem of solid waste is, but you can get some idea of it by simply becoming conscious of the amount of trash you throw away in a day. Multiply that by 200 million people (the population of the United States alone), try visualizing all that trash piling up *each day* just from personal consumption in one nation—and ask where it all *does* go.

⊛ Be aware of the effect of the overpopulation of an area on the land.

At best, items discarded by people undergo **recycling**; that is, they are transformed into materials that can be used again. Food garbage, for example, once rotted in the soil, makes excellent fertilizer (**compost**) for the next crop of plants; but if put down the sink, it fertilizes water weeds to choke waterways instead. Materials that don't occur naturally, such as glass, paper, and metal, can be reused if communities organize themselves to recycle them. In the simplest case, everything that is **biodegradable** would be allowed to recycle naturally, while everything that is **persistent** would either be banished from use or recycled. The case is oversimplified, however; human communities are overwhelmed with excess items and materials that cannot be treated either way.

A case in point is plastics, most of which are nonbiodegradable. Hundreds of tons of plastic debris litter landscapes all over the world, and vast quantities have found their way into the ocean. Each year, thousands of seabirds and sea mammals get caught in them or swallow them, and die.

In summary, human waste materials can cycle through the natural world in ways that benefit life on earth or at least do no harm—but when there are too many of them, and when they are dumped in the wrong places, they can spread disease among people, pollute the water, and threaten all life forms.

Another form of waste that people throw away is toxic wastes—poisons and other chemicals used in homes, pesticides used in agriculture, and wastes from industrial processes. Toxic wastes are the opposite of biodegradable; they are persistent—that is, they accumulate in the organs of living things and therefore become concentrated at the top of the **food chain**, in big fish, birds, carnivorous animals, and human beings, as shown in Figure 19–2.

What can be done with toxic waste? The earth, large as it is, is a limited place, and wherever we dump our wastes, they have a way of coming back to haunt us. Unfortunately, they often don't come back quite in time to haunt those who dumped them; rather, they affect innocent bystanders who happen to settle unknowingly on the land near the dump site, where waste-containing drums leak poisons into the environment. The toxic waste problem is so severe that it deserves a section of its own.

FIGURE 19–2 How a Food Chain Works

A person whose principal animal protein source is fish may consume about 100 pounds of fish in a year. These fish will, in turn, have consumed a few tons of plant-eating fish in the course of their lifetimes. The plant eaters, in their lifetimes, will have consumed several tons of photosynthetic producer organisms. If the producer organisms have become contaminated with toxic chemicals, these chemicals become more concentrated in the bodies of the fish that consume them. If none of the chemicals are lost along the way, *one person* ultimately eats the same amount of the contaminant as was present in the original *several tons* of producer organisms.

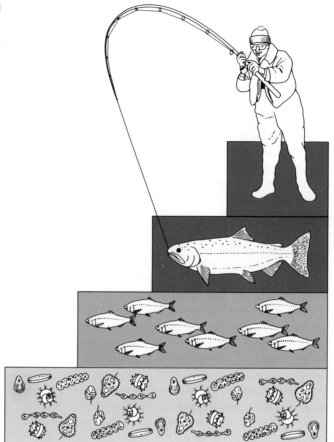

Level 4
A 150-pound person

Level 3
A hundred pounds
of fish

Level 2
A few tons of
plant-eating fish

Level 1
Several tons of
producer organisms

✳ Scrub all fresh fruits and vegetables before eating or cooking them.

Toxic Waste

Of great concern because of their toxicity are agricultural pesticides that find their way into foods. Pesticides have to be poisonous to living things, of course, but ideally, after exerting their effects against the pests they are aimed at, they will disappear so that no residues remain in foods to harm the user. In reality, pesticide use can seldom be so well controlled, and there is reason for concern that hazardous pesticide residues drift onto other crops, pollute the water, contaminate the soil, and accumulate in the tissues of animals and people. The largest contributor of pesticides to the environment is commercial agriculture, but individual homeowners and gardeners add significantly to the total. The consumer's chief defense against ingesting pesticide residues that may remain on food is to make a habit of washing all fresh fruits and vegetables before eating or cooking them.

When pesticides were first used, the persistent ones were chosen, because they would not get washed away or chemically altered. These were considered most desirable because they would control pests the longest. One of the most satisfactory pesticides from this point of view was DDT. Then it became apparent that DDT's persistence created problems. It began to show up in high concentrations in the fatty tissues of animals. Scientists showed that it was a threat to the survival of the American eagle, whose eggs became too fragile to protect new chicks. DDT also turned up in big fish, in carnivorous animals, and in human breast milk. Finally, its widescale agricultural use in the United States was banned, but it is still used in other countries.

National and international agencies do monitor pesticide levels in the environment, and often report that they appear to be within established limits. The agencies assume, though, that people do not overconsume any one food and so ingest a harmful pesticide dose. Also, the tests used do not necessarily detect all the pesticides currently in use. Furthermore, toxicity to nerves is sometimes slow to show up and is not detected. Pesticide use worldwide is increasing; the hazards may be considerable; and many of them are unknown.

On occasion, accidents occur with pesticides, such as spills, mixing of the poisons into animal or human feed, or illegal overuse. Then these chemicals, no longer a gradually growing threat to life, precipitate a sudden crisis. They become deadly contaminants of air, water, and food. For example, in Arkansas, the milk of both cows and human beings became contaminated with heptachlor, a powerful, illegal pesticide that causes cancer. A gasohol dealer used heptachlor-treated grain in his distillation process and then sold the grain residue to farmers at cut-rate prices. Not knowing it was toxic, the farmers fed it to their cattle, whence it found its way into milk, ice cream, and meat products in eight states. Mothers who had been been breastfeeding their infants were advised to stop, thousands of gallons of milk had to be dumped, and dairy farmers had to cease selling their products for periods from several months to close to two years, losing their chief source of income.[8] Such episodes are rare, but when they occur, they are devastating.

Pesticides are only one of many classes of toxic compounds people release into the environment today. Most of the others are the by-products of fuel use and industrial processes, and these have been accumulating in the environment at an accelerating rate, especially in the last few decades. For many people, however, awareness of the problem of toxics in the environment dates only from 1980, when the U.S. surgeon general declared it an environmental emergency. In that year, Congress created the Superfund, a $1.6 billion, five-year crash program intended to clean up the worst of many leaking dump sites. Little was accomplished by the Superfund program in the allotted five years, and it is now estimated that to clean up the nation's worst hazardous waste sites will cost more than $1,000 per U.S. household.[9]

In the crush of other environmental emergencies, the toxics problem may seem to be just one more, but it is one of the most pressing problems. Scientists are alarmed by the growing use of toxic chemicals: over 65,000 chemicals are in commercial use in the United States, and only a few have been tested for their health effects.[10] Screening, regulation, and monitoring of their use and disposal are urgently needed.

More subtle, but no less lethal, are gradual releases of poisons into the soil and water supply. These threaten everyone's ability to produce safe food or to obtain pure drinking water.

The chemicals most likely to enter the food chain, and so of greatest concern, fall into three major categories—heavy metals, halogenated compounds, and a third group that is diverse. An example from each group illustrates the kinds of problems that environmental contaminants create.

The most serious heavy metal pollutant in our domestic environment today is lead. Symptoms of mild lead poisoning include reduced ability of the blood to carry oxygen, intestinal cramps, fatigue, and kidney abnormalities; these symptoms may be reversible if exposure stops soon enough.

⊛ Keep alert to news of contamination episodes in your area. Take recommended measures in individual instances.

⊛ Be aware of the toxic waste issue.

More severe lead poisoning, however, causes irreversible nerve damage, paralysis, mental retardation in children, abortions, and death.[11]

Lead is readily transferred across the placenta and its most severe effects on the fetus are on the developing nervous system. Absorption of lead is five to eight times greater in children than it is in adults, and it tends to stay in their bodies.[12] Only one year of exposure can cause irreversible effects on the brain, nervous system, and psychological functioning.[13] Furthermore, recent experiments have shown that the effects occur with lower doses than has been thought in the past. Even children who have only moderately elevated blood lead levels and who have never had high exposures show deficits in school performance—in speed, dexterity, verbal memory, language functions, concentration, and reasoning. Based on these experiments, one million children in the United States may now be at risk of showing permanent damage caused by lead.[14] Three trends are occurring simultaneously. Scientists are discovering that lead poisoning has more *subtle* effects than had heretofore been appreciated; these effects are more *permanent* than had been known earlier, and they are being found at *lower levels of exposure* than before. At least 1 out of every 50 children in rural areas and more than 1 out of every 10 inner-city children are afflicted with lead poisoning—an average of about 4 percent of all children.[15]

Lead appears in all foods, and is also the nation's most significant contaminant in drinking water.[16] Whether some of it is naturally present is not known, but much of it is known to come from industrial pollution. People use lead in gasoline, paint, batteries, pesticides, and in industrial processes that release it into the air and water. Exposures are higher in urban and industrial areas, near highways, and in slums where children may accidentally ingest leaded paint by teething on old furniture, toys, and the railings of old buildings. Old plumbing is made of lead and it dissolves into water—especially soft water. A major source of lead is canned food, including evaporated milk, because many cans are sealed with lead solder. Food is also contaminated in the fields by the air pollution from leaded gasoline, by way of rainfall and soil. Scientists have recommended a standard for weekly acceptable intakes of lead,[17] but there is no monitoring system to keep track of the amounts to which people are actually exposed.

The reduction of the use of leaded gasoline for automobiles and the application of new technology and material to the canning process are helping to limit the amounts of lead in the environment and in food. Children's blood levels of lead have declined, but preschool children's lead levels are still of concern in 4 to 6 percent of cases. More leaded gas is still being sold than anticipated, so considerable lead is appearing newly in the soil. Consumers would be wise to take ultraconservative measures to protect themselves and especially their small and unborn children from lead poisoning. Practical implications of these findings are itemized in this chapter's Strategies Box.

Lead is only one of many heavy metal pollutants in the environment. Another is mercury. In the United States today, certain seafood cannot be commercially harvested because of excess mercury contamination.

An example of the next class of pollutants, the halogenated compounds, is the polychlorinated biphenyls, or PCBs. For years, industry produced PCBs as an insulating material, only to realize recently that this practically indestructible toxin is now appearing in the food supply through unanticipated channels.[18] Animal studies have shown that PCBs can be breathed in, absorbed through the skin, or swallowed, and suggest that they can

STRATEGIES: Minimizing Lead Exposure

To minimize exposure to lead:

1. In contaminated environments, prevent hand-to-mouth ingestion (keep small children from putting dirty or old painted objects in their mouths).

2. Make no baby formula from canned, evaporated milk.

3. Once you have opened canned food, immediately remove it from the can, and always store it in a regular storage container to minimize lead migration into the food.

4. Have the water in your home tested by a competent laboratory.

5. Use only cold water for drinking, cooking, and making baby formula (cold water absorbs less lead).

6. When water has been standing in pipes, flush the cold water pipes by running water through them until it is as cold as it can get (this may take as long as two minutes).

7. If lead contamination of your water supply seems probable, obtain additional information and advice from EPA and your local public health agency.

SOURCE: *Lead and Your Drinking Water*, U.S. Environmental Protection Agency, Office of Water, April 1987 (OPA 87-006).

cause or promote liver disease, cancer, reproductive abnormalities, acne, hair loss, and eye damage. Offspring of animals exposed to PCBs suffer behavioral and learning disabilities.

Toxins such as PCBs are stored in every county of every state across the United States. There is no out-of-the-way place to put them. They cannot be made to disappear; they can only be moved from one place to another.

Within the third category—miscellaneous compounds, dioxin is one of the most deadly. In the mid-1970s, the town of Times Beach, Missouri, hired a man to spread oil on ten miles of unpaved streets to keep the dust down. The man spread more than oil; he spread oily waste material from a chemical factory that contained dioxin, a poison so powerful that one drop in 10,000 gallons is considered dangerous. Birds died all over town, dogs and cats bore stillborn litters, several horses died, and two children developed skin lesions caused by the poison. The town had to be abandoned; no one lives there now. Twelve years later, the long-term effects on people had not been evaluated, the area had not been cleaned up, and no one yet knows how to dispose of the wastes.[19]

These three examples serve to illustrate the intensity of individual toxic waste cases, but not the magnitude of the problem as a whole. Multiply the worst cases by 10,000, spread them all across the United States, and you will have some idea of the problem's extent and seriousness (see Figure 19–3).

Toxic wastes can sometimes be disposed of, but disposal is profoundly difficult and expensive. Sometimes it fails. One such episode took place beginning in 1979 on the Susquehanna River in Pennsylvania, where a small company illegally dumped toxic wastes into some mine shafts many times over a several months' period. The company was fined $750,000; the EPA supervised the cleanup, and in 1982 it took the site off its priority list. Then came Hurricane Gloria, which stirred up the river, and 100,000 gallons of toxic waste came boiling to the surface. In effect, nothing had been accomplished by the cleanup.

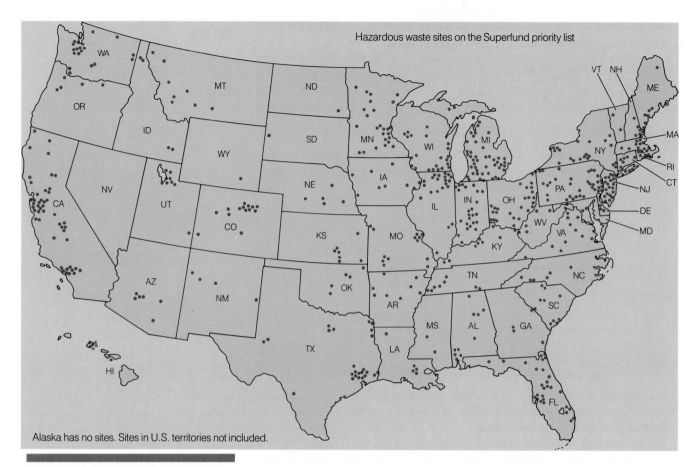

Hazardous waste sites on the Superfund priority list

Alaska has no sites. Sites in U.S. territories not included.

FIGURE 19–3 Hazardous Wastes in the United States

What is a cleanup, anyway? How do you set about cleaning up hundreds of thousands of gallons of oily sludge out of a river, a bay, or an underground watercourse? The task is horrendous, requiring massive earth-moving equipment and labor. Then, once the material has been collected, what can be done with it? Often it will have leaked from old drums stored at the site. Should it be stored in new drums, which will become old? Should it be moved "somewhere else"? Where? In whose backyard should it be placed to leak again?

Ideally, toxic waste should be disposed of as natural waste is—by being converted chemically to harmless, inert, or useful compounds. Sometimes, that is possible. Meanwhile, let no one believe it is ever excusable or permissible to pollute the earth as people do now. The only enlightened way to deal with the toxins produced by industry is to stop them at the source, before they have entered the air, soil, and water.[20]

The U.S. Public Health Service has worked out many objectives for monitoring the health effects of toxic wastes, but some citizens' groups think that the proposed measures are insufficient to protect our rights to pure air, water, and food. They believe that the law should have teeth in it—that is, should punish polluters severely. "Someone else" will not control runaway technologies, they say, nor will they voluntarily control themselves. "Indeed, much of the chemical industry is actively fighting *against* government curbs on toxic exposures."[21] Citizens must band together to make their demands heard— marshalling the scientific evidence, lobbying Congress, litigating in court, alerting the press—to force industry, the government, and their neighbors to curb the hazards.

To be most effective as an activist, one has to understand the members of the opposition—if possible, even better than they understand themselves. Whenever an industrial process is found dangerous, those who stand to lose the most financially are most opposed to controls. This seems so obvious as to be hardly worth saying, but it is worth a moment's thought. The next two paragraphs offer some clues into the motivation behind such actions.

What is it in human nature that makes people willing to poison others? It is not just that there is profit in it. Consider being in that position yourself. Something you produce, or a service you perform—something in which you have an immense personal investment in money and pride—suddenly is accused of killing people. You had no idea that this would ever happen. Your first reaction is disbelief: it can't be. Then you feel threatened: what if they take this way of life away from me? I'll be ruined. And, often enough, it is true that the unwitting producers of the poisons are themselves victims of the situation—they intended no wrong; at worst, they failed to think through the consequences of their actions. When they are caught and brought to account, they will not be compensated for their losses or given back the time and money they invested in their enterprises. Looked at from this point of view, it is easy to see why the perpetrators of environmental crimes are often the last to see the harm they may be doing and the most persuasive in arguing in their own defense.

The point of seeing the problem from the opposing point of view is not to argue that they be let off, of course—but to show what must be done to stop them. It is necessary to educate producers of toxic waste in advance about the possible consequences of their actions, and to set up the situation to minimize the chance that they can get away with crimes against the environment. "Do not dump unknown chemicals down abandoned mine shafts," they will then tell themselves. "The chemicals may end up poisoning people's drinking water—and besides, there's no way we can get away with this. We will pay such a high price that it's obviously not worth taking the chance."

Radioactive Waste

Outranking the worst of the other toxic wastes in the hazard it presents is radioactive waste. The term **radioactivity** refers to the kind of radiation that alters molecules chemically, including the genetic material in living cells. A material that is radioactive gradually loses this ability over time, becoming completely inactive after a period of days, weeks, months, years, or centuries. The most hazardous radioactive materials produced by human activity have extremely long lives, numbering in thousands of years. Since radioactivity passes through most barriers as if they were not there, it is difficult to store radioactive materials in such a way that they will not damage nearby life unalterably for all future generations.

Some radioactive materials are present in the earth naturally—for example, radon, already mentioned in Chapter 14. Another example is uranium, which is collected from mines for use in nuclear power plants and nuclear weapons. Nuclear power plants are intended to improve the quality of life by providing inexpensive energy for human use, but whether they are succeeding is questionable. Nuclear weapons are supposed to stabilize world peace, but

⊛ Learn; be prepared with a viewpoint; take action with other citizens when concerned.

U.S. cities with nuclear power plants with Chernobyl-type containment systems:
Decatur, AL
Waterford, CT
Baxley, GA
Palo, IA
Clinton, IL
Cordova, IL
Morris, IL
Seneca, IL
St. Francesville, LA
Plymouth, MA
Newport, MI
Monticello, MN
Port Gibson, MS
Southport, NC
Brownsville, NE
Salem, NJ
Toms River, NJ
Brookhaven, NY
Scriba, NY
North Perry, OH
Berwick, PA
Peach Bottom, PA
Pottstown, PA
Vernon, VT
Richland, WA

Plants with other failure-prone containment systems are in:
Cornelius, NC
Bridgman, MI
Clover, SC
Daisy, TN
Spring City, TN

SOURCE: Adapted from N. Maxwell, Chernobyl's message: Look again at containments in the United States, *Nucleus* (a quarterly report from the Union of Concerned Scientists), Summer 1986, pp. 3, 7.

there are those who question their success, also. In any case, both enterprises produce radioactive wastes, and the threat of accidents grows. One of the best-known recent accidents occurred in 1986 at Chernobyl in the western Soviet Union and spewed radioactive waste over the whole world. But there have been many other accidents. A chronology of the worst of them is shown in Table 19–1.

With such a record behind them, it seems unlikely that nuclear plants will have an accident-free record ahead. As evidence that other accidents similar to that of Chernobyl can be expected domestically in the future, the Union of Concerned Scientists reports that 39 nuclear plants in the United States employ containment systems similar to the one that failed in the Chernobyl plant, allowing the escape of radioactive waste, and that ten others have a different type of system, but one that is also susceptible to failure.[22]

Even without such accidents, with 100 nuclear plants in operation, an immense amount of dangerous radioactive waste is accumulating, and a place must be found to dispose of it. It will not decay fast enough to become less of a threat in the next 10,000 years. Disposal is a national problem, and the Department of Energy has undertaken the task of selecting sites for nuclear dumps. Among the locations under consideration in the late 1980s were sites in Texas, Washington State, Nevada, Georgia, Maine, Minnesota, New Hampshire, North Carolina, Virginia, and Wisconsin; dumping at the first site chosen was to begin within 20 years.[23]

Radioactive waste spills are the most serious known. No human sense can detect radioactivity, and so it can do immeasurable harm before people are even aware of it. From Chernobyl alone, evidence indicates that all the animals over a wide area, including all the reindeer of Lapland, picked up enough radioactivity to alter their genetic material; presumably the people did, too.

Clearly, the spilling of radioactivity over a large area of the earth's surface is incompatible with human well-being. Such accidents can be prevented in only two ways—either by eliminating the sources so that accidents can't happen or by making the nuclear power plants and arsenals totally safe from accidents or vandalism. Many believe that only the first alternative will work.

▬ NATURAL ENVIRONMENTS

The earth's natural environments renew themselves and the resources we need to sustain our lives. Forests renew clean air and soil; wetlands restore clean water and serve as breeding grounds for each season's new generations of animal life. Today, however, the world's rapidly growing human population is displacing the natural environments on which life depends. The earth is like an aquarium in which the plants and fish are interdependent: it is large, but it is still limited in capacity. With too many fish in it, an aquarium fills with too many wastes and its plants fail to regenerate sufficient food and oxygen. Then both the plants and the fish die.

People and Land

Even without industrialization, a large enough mass of human beings upsets the life-sustaining balance in an area. The migration of human beings down

TABLE 19–1   A Chronology of the World's Worst Nuclear Accidents

When	Where	What
December 2, 1952	Chalk River, Canada	Employee error leads to 1 million gallons of radioactive water leaking inside an experimental nuclear reactor, forcing a six-month cleanup.
October 7–10, 1957	Windscale Pile, Liverpool, England	A fire in a plutonium-production reactor leads to the largest then known accidental release of radioactive material. Government later attributes 39 cancer deaths to it.
Month unknown, 1957	Ural Mountains, Soviet Union	A nuclear accident occurs, probably at a weapons facility. From available information, it is believed that hundreds of square miles had to be evacuated.
May 23, 1958	Chalk River, Canada	A second accident, sparked by an overheated fuel rod, leads to another long cleanup.
January 3, 1961	Idaho Falls, Idaho	A steam explosion at a military experimental reactor kills three servicemen.
October 5, 1966	Enrico Fermi plant, Detroit, Michigan	In an experimental breeder reactor, part of the fuel core melts, producing high radiation levels within the plant.
October 17, 1969	Saint-Laurent, France	A fuel-loading error leads to partial meltdown.
November 19, 1971	Monticello, Minnesota	A power company's reactor's waste storage space overflows, releasing 50,000 gallons of radioactive water into the Mississippi River.
March 22, 1975	Browns Ferry reactor, Decatur, Illinois	A worker using a candle to check for air leaks starts a $150 million fire that lowers cooling water to dangerous levels.
March 28, 1979	Three Mile Island, Middletown, Pennsylvania	A partial meltdown occurs, and some radioactivity is released into the atmosphere in what some consider the worst U.S. commercial nuclear mishap. Plant still being decontaminated in 1988.
August 7, 1979	Top secret fuel plant, Erwin, Tennessee	Accidental release of enriched uranium exposes 1,000 people to above-normal doses of radiation.
February 11, 1981	Sequoyah 1, Tennessee Valley	More than 100,000 gallons of radioactive coolant leak into the containment building; eight workers are exposed to radiation.
April 19, 1984	Sequoyah 1, Tennessee Valley	A second accident occurs when superheated radioactive water erupts during a maintenance procedure.
April 26, 1986	Chernobyl, Soviet Union	A fire starts, meltdown occurs, and a cloud of radioactive fallout spreads worldwide. 2,000 people near the plant are affected, 11 die, many receive bone marrow transplants, many more are expected to contract cancer and other illnesses and to pass on genetic defects to their unborn children.

SOURCE: Adapted from A chronology of notable nuclear accidents worldwide, *Tallahassee Democrat*, 30 April 1986.

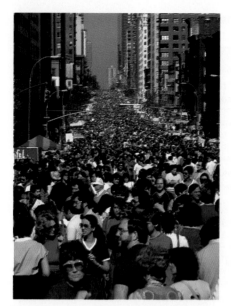

Every person in an industrialized society taxes the earth's resources more heavily than a person in a primitive society.

the western coast of North America is blamed for the extinction, by hunting, of all the species of large animals that used to live in that area. The mountains of China are now bare over thousands of square miles because people of earlier times, living in primitive conditions, burned all the trees for firewood. Now, erosion has worn the mountains to bare rock, and the land has become an uninhabitable moonscape. The cedars of Lebanon were wiped out in the same way, beginning in biblical times, and even the Sahara Desert is a desert partly because of human misuse of once-fertile land.[24] All over the world, deserts are growing. Dust blown from the ever-growing Sahara Desert now darkens the air all the way to Florida; dust from China is detectable in Hawaii.

The vast wastelands of China, Lebanon, the Sahara, and many others like them were created by people living *primitively*—cutting trees for firewood and to clear the land for agriculture. People living in modern industrialized societies use many times the fuel and generate many times the waste, and faster, so they use up the land faster. Witness the fact that the United States produces 3,000 pounds of toxic wastes for every man, woman, and child, every year.[25] When you put the two factors together (the sheer numbers of people we add up to and the increasing industrialization that makes each of us a tremendous polluter), then you may be able to imagine how seriously the earth is threatened. No place on earth is now pollution-free—no mountaintop, no river, no icecap, no valley.

Where there is human habitation, there is also light and noise—and **light** and **noise pollution**. Pure darkness is needed for the renewal of many kinds of wildlife. (Baby turtles hatch on the beach on moonless nights and instinctively crawl toward the reflections of stars on the water; but when a highway is built too near the beach, they crawl instead toward the highway lights and are killed by passing cars.) Silence also is needed. (When the noise of cars and radios is audible within half a mile of the nests of water birds, they become unable to raise their young and abandon the nesting site.) Periods of darkness and silence are also human needs, and excessive light and sound are forms of stress. The effects of various intensities of sound on the ears of living creatures are shown in Figure 19–4.

The Rainforests: A Case in Point

The disappearance of wild lands through human intervention today is nearing is final stages. A case in point is the rapid loss of the world's tropical rainforests (see Figure 19–5). These forests are fast disappearing all over the globe; in the Amazon River valley alone they are being destroyed at the rate of an area the size of Massachusetts every month. Because the tropical rainforests contain more than half of all the species that remain on earth, the loss of those forests is now bringing about the greatest destruction of life forms that has ever occurred on earth.

The rainforests have existed for millions of years. They are vast—three-dimensional—miles wide, miles long, and over a hundred feet deep. Millions on millions of species of animals and plants not yet known to science thrive in their honeycomb of multitudinous spaces. Within one acre of these forests dwell 800,000 pounds of living things.[26]

The forests are destroyed for many purposes people call "development." One such purpose is to grow beef cattle. If an acre of rainforest is cleared to plant grass and grow beef, it is useful for that purpose for only about eight years. Within the eight years it takes for a million-year-old acre of

Sound Intensity (decibels)	Your Experience	Characteristics of Conversation with Others	Common Examples
150 —			
—			
140 —			
—	Painful loudness		Aircraft carrier deck jet
130 —	Limitation of		takeoff
—	amplified speech		
120 —			
—	Need for		Rock music club
110 —	maximum		Car horn, 3 ft
—	vocalization		Jet takeoff, 2,000 ft
100 —		Shouting in ear	
—	Annoyance		Busy subway station
90 —	Damage to	Shouting, 2 ft apart	Heavy truck, 50 ft
—	hearing after 8 hr		Pneumatic drill, 50 ft
80 —	Irritation	Speaking very	Alarm clock
—		loudly, 2 ft. apart	Train, 50 ft
70 —	Difficult phone use	Speaking loudly, 2 ft	Interstate traffic, 50 ft
—	Distraction	apart	
60 —		Speaking loudly, 4 ft	Air-conditioning unit, 20 ft
—		apart	
50 —	Quiet	Conversing normally,	Light auto traffic, 100 ft
—		12 ft apart	Living room
40 —			Bedroom
—			Library
30 —			Quiet whisper, 15 ft
—			
20 —			Sound studio
—			
10 —	Sound barely		
—	audible		
0 —	Hearing threshold		

FIGURE 19–4 Sound Intensities and their Effects

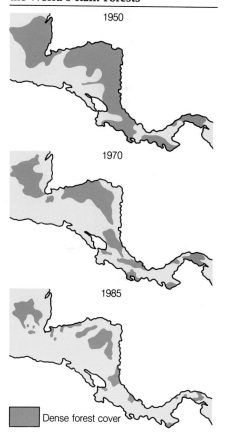

FIGURE 19–5 The Rate of Loss of the World's Rain Forests

1950

1970

1985

☐ Dense forest cover

forest to die, the acre will produce 50 pounds of cattle per year—400 pounds in all. Of that, 200 pounds is usable meat, enough to yield 800 4-ounce hamburgers. The trade-off: 55 square feet of forest, representing half a ton of forest life, lost permanently for each hamburger.[27]

At the end of eight years of such use of the land, the soil's fertility is depleted. It then requires large applications of fertilizer, pesticides, and irrigation to make the land "useful" for any purpose whatever. When the whole region's forest is gone, the land becomes uninhabitable, not only for cattle but also for all other life, including human beings. The last of the soil washes away, leaving bare clay, and ultimately, rain ceases to fall. This is one of many ways in which natural environments are turning to deserts all over the world.

Loss of soil, worldwide, is one of the greatest threats facing the human race. It is increasing every year. At present, it amounts to 25 billion tons a year, enough to fill Yankee Stadium 175,000 times.[28] Nature (where there are trees) creates new soil at the rate of a centimeter every 80 to 280 years, but soil loss due to human misuse of the land today is taking place at a much greater rate.

The reasons why deforestation and soil loss are occurring are complex, but they often have to do with land ownership and greed. In Central America, for example, the poor own little land, and as they multiply, they are forced onto "undeveloped" government land (wild land) to attempt to support their families. They make roads into the rainforest, and start the process by which "development" can take place. They make a little money by clearing the land; speculators then follow them, exploit the land, reap their profits, and move on. By way of this process, between 1950 and 1980, nearly two-thirds of Central America's lowland and mountainside rainforests was cleared or severely degraded.[29] Within 20 more years, the process will be over, for no more forest will be left. In El Salvador, the end has come already.

Left alone, rainforests are more valuable than when "developed" in this way—but valuable by a measure other than dollars gained in the year of their destruction. The forests can, for example, support human agriculture indefinitely if handled in the age-old way developed by the forests' original people. The natives in such an area, living on small, cleared patches beneath the undisturbed forest canopy, were able to grow 5,000 pounds of shelled corn *and* 4,000 pounds of root and vegetable crops each year on each acre of plots for five to seven years. Then they would allow the plots to return to forest and clear others. They rotated their crops of citrus, rubber, cacao, avocado, and papaya in a system known as **agroforestry**, which could be continued indefinitely. If the government of the country wants to solve its people's hunger problem and produce crops for export, it can do no better than to encourage an agricultural method like this one. "Food production systems practiced by traditional rainforest Indians are, without exception, more productive than the pasturelands that are replacing these systems."[30]

Even though we consumers may not personally be clearing rainforest land, our demands for products are driving the process. U.S. companies annually purchase more than 330 million pounds of beef from Central American countries alone—an amount that represents 90 percent of that region's beef exports.[31] The demand comes largely from our innumerable fast-food hamburger establishments. Consumers buy the beef, and the trees continue to fall.

The money to convert Central America's rainforests to grasslands comes largely from international banks, which have supplied billions of dollars to finance cattle ranching in Central and South American since 1970. The banks claim that they are helping to close Central America's "nutrition gap," but in reality, they are doing nothing of the kind. They prefer to finance the production of a resource that will be paid for by the U.S. market for imported beef than to finance an effort to improve the native people's malnutrition problems with no sure return in sight.

Some argue that the process benefits the country as a whole. It is, after all, a form of economic development. It brings money in; it encourages international trade. So it does, but this ignores the question to whom, within the country, the money is going. It goes to wealthy speculators, not to the people who live or work on the land. As beef production in Central America has increased, the people there have eaten less and less beef, for two reasons. First, foreign companies are willing to pay higher prices than the people can afford to pay. Second, the population has increased, so more people are competing for the beef that remains within the country. Even an American house cat eats more beef than the average Central American.[32]

People concerned with the destruction of tropical rainforests to grow beef ask, "Why can't we produce our own beef?" or "Why can't we import beef from elsewhere?" In fact, we do both. Only 2 percent of the beef we consume, or about two pounds per person (220 square feet of rainforest per person per year), comes from rainforest land, but this beef is not labeled as such. We cannot avoid using it, except by foregoing beef altogether. Even the fast-food establishments that buy beef do not know which packages are from the rainforest, because by the time they see them, they are all labeled "domestic."

The problem is solvable. It has been called *simple*. To solve it with maximum speed and effectiveness requires the participation of several sets of people: knowledgeable biologists and others in a position to influence policy; U.S. legislators; officials in international banks; and American consumers.*

Development as traditionally practiced—by destroying natural environments—cannot permanently achieve solutions to any of the world's problems. To make clear what development is really doing, we need ways of expressing the value of the land other than by assigning dollar values to the products it brings forth. What is rainfall worth? Soil? Forest vegetation? Animal life? The clean air and water that they generate?

The traditional concept of development by exploitation must be replaced by that of **sustainable development**. This kind of development is:

- Stable—it does not disrupt the ecology or way of life of the country in which it takes place.
- Nonexploitative—it involves the rational use of renewable resources; it does not plunder and leave desolation behind.
- Resilient—it is adaptable to changes, whether in the weather or in governments.
- User-friendly—its methods are easy for the local people to understand.
- Productive—it creates surpluses above people's minimum needs for survival.
- Self-reliant—it helps people become free of dependence on handouts and assistance from outside.
- Complicated and challenging—it requires much more intimate knowledge of individual locales and situations than does, say, one massive technology (such as beef production) applied to an entire area.[33]

The Value of Species Diversity

The preservation of natural environments matters, not only in terms of air, water, and land for people, but also for wild species that otherwise will become extinct. So far, scientists have studied, for medicinal use, only about 2 percent of all the likely plants and animals on earth, yet every single day several plant and wildlife species become extinct because people destroy their habitats. By the end of this century, if extinction continues at the present rate, we shall have lost one million of the five to ten million species we now still possess. This may mean hundreds of thousands of lifesaving drugs, for more than 50 percent of such drugs prescribed today trace their origins to such species. A dramatic example is penicillin, a lifesaving drug from a wild mold. Also, drugs prepared from a tropical forest plant, the rosy periwinkle, are used to treat young people with leukemia, and have improved their chances for remission from 1 in 5 to 4 in 5. Commercial sales of drugs from this one plant alone now total around $100 million per year. The total spent on all drugs of plant origin is around $20 billion a year.

More examples are these: some types of birth control pills from the Mexican yam; digitalis (a heartbeat strengthener) from the purple foxglove; re-

Wild species possess many still-undiscovered treasures.

*One way to help is to join and work with the Rainforest Action Network, 300 Broadway #28, San Francisco, CA 94133.

serpine (a tranquilizer) from the root of a small Asian shrub; and quinine (an antimalaria drug) from the bark of the cinchona tree. The octopus yields an extract that relieves hypertension; a sea snake produces an anticoagulant; and a Caribbean sponge manufactures a compound that acts against viruses, much as penicillin does against bacteria.

Not only do wild species supply materials for our direct use but they also furnish models for scientists to imitate when they devise strategies against diseases. For example, in the expectation of helping human beings, scientists are currently trying to discover why certain snails and bison never get cancer. Experts might look forward to many more discoveries as important to health as penicillin, if only the species still exist to be studied.

There is another reason we should attempt to preserve the quality of our environment: the needs of all living things are similar. If the trees, grasses, birds, and flowers in our surroundings are not flourishing, then whether we perceive it or not, the conditions that we need to survive are deteriorating. Biologists know that "birds are indicators of the environment, a sort of litmus paper. Because of their furious pace of living and high rate of metabolism, they reflect subtle changes in the environment rather quickly; they warn us of things out of balance."[34] In fact, the biological quality of a region can be measured by the abundance and variety of its bird life. Miners know this, too; the practice of taking a canary into the mine is the miner's way of self-protection. If the canary sickens and dies, it's time for the miner to hurry out of the mine, for the air is becoming too foul to support human life.

To some people, the extinction of species matters simply for its own sake, as well. We affiliate with other organisms; we need them deeply.[35] The preservation of other species is a moral and ethical responsibility; it concerns us in a deep, spiritual way. Our native American predecessors, the Indians, have always known:

This we know. The Earth does not belong to man; man belongs to the Earth. This we know. All things are connected like the blood which unites one family. All things are connected. Whatever befalls the Earth befalls the sons of the Earth. Man did not weave the web of life, he is merely a strand in it. Whatever he does to the web, he does to himself.

—Chief Seattle, 1854

THE POPULATION PROBLEM

At the beginning of this chapter, we promised that if you would work your way through the huge problems described in these sections, we would present some solutions at the end. There is hope—because the world's nations are able to act as a unit, and to act quickly, for the first time in history. What makes this possible is two current trends: the explosion of scientific knowledge about environmental problems and the world's increasing use of fast communications to make that knowledge available to all governments simultaneously. Information is a form of stored energy, and energy can do work. Information and awareness shared among people can bring about rapid decision making and action. The new global awareness of our shared problems is the source of our hope.

Every expert agrees that all the other problems described up to this point are tied to the greatest problem of all—the world's exploding population. This second-last section therefore focuses on that problem. If we are aware

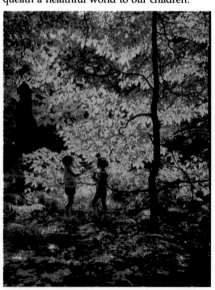

Population growth must stop if we are to bequeath a healthful world to our children.

412

of it and face it as a single species working together, we can solve it. The chapter ends with "global strategies" to which you can contribute with your own personal awareness and sense of urgency.

These three trends are occurring simultaneously, threatening life on this earth:

1. The spread of industrialization.
2. The destruction of natural environments.
3. The multiplication of people.

The effects of each trend compound those of the others, because, as emphasized earlier, every person in an industrialized society devours the earth's resources and pollutes the environment much more heavily than a person in a primitive society.

Our present dilemma has been developing throughout human history. It took us a million years to arrive at a population size of a billion in the mid-1800s. A mere 80 years later, we numbered two billion; in the 50 years following, we more than doubled again. As this book goes to press, we number five billion, and each year, the number of people added to the population is greater than the number added the year before.[36] If the growth rate remains steady, in less than 50 years, the number of people on earth will reach the maximum that the earth can support—close to 10 billion people.[37] At that level, life for most people will barely be possible, and conditions will be much worse than they are today. Already millions are starving; agricultural and grazing lands are eroding and others are being irreversibly paved over; soils are becoming more salty; petroleum and other fuel supplies are dwindling; water shortages are increasing; rainfall is diminishing as the world's forests shrink; ocean pollution and overfishing are leading to smaller catches and less variety; and widespread extinctions of plants and animals are occurring.[38] As shortages develop, people and nations become aggressive in an attempt to meet their needs; as people grow needy, they become irrational, and the threat of global destruction through nuclear war looms ever greater.

Even the richest and most protected people on earth are now feeling the effects of the population's growth. This growth is taking place even in the United States and Canada, where people have been acting responsibly and limiting family size. Immigrants escaping from overcrowding in their own countries account for at least half of the growth of our population. People feel the impact of population growth as stress from lack of space, more noise, more cars, more toxins, more crime, more illness, and simultaneously less peace, less quiet, less greenery, less oxygen, less clean air and water. They also experience the effects of population growth indirectly, in the scarcity of resources that once were common. The more people crowd into cities, the more land outside the cities is needed to produce food for those people, but as the suburbs advance, *less* land is available—hence the rising costs of food, water, fuel, and other resources.

People in industrial societies often fear that to stop population growth would be to stop progress. This view assumes that growth and progress are the same thing, but they are not. Growth means only greater numbers; progress is intentional movement toward a goal. Further increases in population will drain the economy, not foster its growth, because rising numbers of people mean more people living in poverty. Progress toward meeting the basic needs of our present population could take place better without growth.

People who must scramble for food and water have no energy to strive for higher purposes. In fact, growth must stop for real progress to continue; people must limit their numbers.

It used to be thought that the growth rate would slow as industrial development proceeded. This has proved true only when industrial development actually improved the economic lot of the people. More often, industrial development has increased crowding and intensified poverty. The Central American development of rainforest land is one example; the growth of Mexico City is another. As Mexico's capital city has developed industrially, it has failed to stem population growth, and its crowds, pollution, and rampant poverty are notorious. Leaders of less-developed countries no longer question whether a need for population control exists, but only how best to deliver birth control to the people who need it.

Two factors hinder success in population control. One is that people who want to use birth control methods often can't get them; their other is that many people resist using them. They want too many children.[39] In India, for example, there are 600 million sexually active adults and each couple wants on the average, 9 children.

Of the two problems, that of birth control availability is easier to solve, but it is no small task. It requires materials, experts, transport, planning, money—and political support. Not only are the resources hard to obtain but also the political support is unpredictable.

It is even harder to change people's desires for large families, but political decisions can override them. The leaders of China, for example, have tried to limit the offspring of each family to one child by offering tax incentives and other motivators. The first hints of such initiatives in the United States are now appearing as well.

In the name of public health, precedents already exist for regulations that limit individual rights. Mandatory vaccinations and safety belt laws are two familiar cases in this country. With an issue as urgent as population control, each society must look at needs both within and beyond its borders and meet those needs with programs that are socially and politically right for them—and for the earth.

■ A WAY TO THE FUTURE

An encouraging development in work toward the world's future is that some of the best minds are bringing their powers to bear on these problems. For example, much powerful, positive thinking is coming from the Worldwatch Institute—an independent, nonprofit research institution created to analyze and focus attention on global problems.* Worldwatch is funded by private foundations and by the United Nations, and its papers are written for a worldwide audience of decision makers, scholars, and students. Its *State of the World* report, which comes out annually, not only keeps track of trends in all areas such as deforestation and fuel use but also goes beyond the mere presentation of facts on environmental emergencies to analyze and compare possible solutions. *State of the World* is used as a text in more and more college courses, and is helping to make tomorrow's leaders aware of the areas on which they need to focus their attention.

*Worldwatch Institute, 1776 Massachusetts Avenue NW, Washington, DC 20036.

An ingenious suggestion appears in *State of the World 1987*. Nations that have the greatest power to affect each problem should focus on that problem. For example, of the 83 million people added to the world's population last year, China and India accounted for a third of the total. Those two countries should emphasize population control the most heavily, and be encouraged to do so by the others. Similarly, of all the world's increases in carbon dioxide and global warming, caused by the burning of fossil fuels, half appears to be caused by only three nations— the United States, the Soviet Union, and China. Similarly, three nations contain more than half of the remaining tropical rainforests—Brazil, Indonesia, and Zaire—so efforts at conservation should focus on them. Substantial changes can be brought about if the right efforts are made by the right groups.[40]

One of those groups is American consumers. Earlier, this chapter named four main sources of people-generated pollutants (page 392). The first two were fuel burned to run cars and other forms of transportation and fuel burned to heat and cool homes and run home appliances. These reflect personal individual choices—our own lifestyle choices. The days when we could blame major industrial polluters for most of our problems are over— they still do their share, but small consumers are now the major contributors to the pollution of our environment. When asked at a major conference on the rainforest what we as individuals could do to help reverse the growing deforestation tragedy, several world experts said, "Convince U.S. consumers to change their own lifestyles." Many avenues are open to us—we can demand that our cars be designed to get 200 miles to the gallon—already a feasible possibility. Or we can demand that they be fueled in the future with hydrogen, whose waste product is pure, nonpolluting water. We can also eat less beef.

Such choices require that citizens learn to live by a less materialistic value system than in the past. To do so will help considerably to reduce the burden we human beings place on the earth's carrying capacity. It can also bring each of us great personal satisfaction, as this chapter's Spotlight reveals.

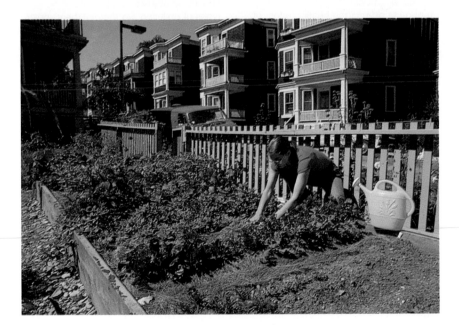

A spot of shared earth enables city dwellers to grow their own vegetables, promoting both mental and physical health.

CHAPTER 19 ▪ THE ENVIRONMENT AND PERSONAL HEALTH

415

STUDY AIDS

1. Define the term *environment*, and describe the relationship that exists between human beings and their external environment.
2. Describe how air, water, and soil support human life and how human beings can in turn support them.
3. Explain what the greenhouse effect is, why it is occurring, and what its effects are expected to be.
4. Explain why the ozone hole is forming in the antarctic atmosphere, and why this is of concern to human health.
5. List the main sources of human-made air pollutants, their effects on human health, and their impact on the physical environment.
6. Describe the four classes of compounds found in water and their impacts on human health.
7. Explain why water quantity is as important as water quality.
8. Discuss two classes of contaminants deposited directly on the soil as the result of human life and activity, and describe measures to manage them.
9. Define the term *carrying capacity*.
10. Explain why toxic waste is a pressing environmental problem.
11. List examples of toxic waste that pose particular problems, and explain why they offer cause for special concern.
12. List personal strategies to deal with environmental hazards.
13. Explain why human beings are likely to suffer detrimental effects from the continuing extinction of plant and animal species.
14. Discuss the relationship between population size and industrialization and its impact both on human beings and on the environment.
15. Describe current trends in population growth, along with outcomes that are likely if those trends continue.
16. Describe measures designed to cope with the population problem.
17. List long-range objectives for worldwide environmental protection.

GLOSSARY

acid rain: rain that has picked up chemicals from the air that convert to acid when combined with water; a form of pollution.

agroforestry: agriculture within a tropical rainforest, as practiced by the indigenous people, notable for high productivity and for not destroying the forest.

air pollution: contamination of the air with any gases or particles not normally found there.

biodegradable: of chemical compounds, those that can be decomposed by living organisms to harmless waste products so that they do not persist in the environment. For contrast, see *persistent*.

carrying capacity: the total number of living organisms that a given environment can support without deteriorating in quality.

chlorofluorocarbons (CLOR-oh-FLOR-oh-car-bons; the trade name of one of these is **Freon**): chemical compounds containing chlorine, fluorine, and carbon. They are produced by industrial processes and, when released, react with ozone to destroy it; see *ozone*.

compost: rotted vegetable and animal matter, used as fertilizer.

contaminants: chemicals that ordinarily do not occur (and therefore do not "belong") in a given environment; especially toxic chemicals.

environment: everything "outside" the living organism—air, water, soil, other organisms, forms of radiation.

eutrophication (YOU-tro-fih-CAY-shun): death of waterways caused initially by nutrients, then algae and bacteria, and finally oxygen depletion.

  eu = well

  troph = to grow

food chain: the sequence in which living things serve as foods for one another—actually, a pyramid (see Figure 19-2).

Freon (FREE-on): the trade name for a propellant and refrigerant (see *chlorofluorocarbons*).

greenhouse effect: the heating effect of trapping carbon dioxide in a closed space that is warmed by sun. In a greenhouse, the trapped carbon dioxide keeps heat from escaping and facilitates plant growth. The same effect in the air surrounding the earth keeps the earth warm, but now is occurring to excess.

hard water: water containing high concentrations of calcium and magnesium.

light pollution: see *pollution*.

noise pollution: see *pollution*.

oxygen cycle: the cycle through which oxygen moves—from the air into living things which convert it to carbon dioxide, then back to the atmosphere, then into plants to be regenerated as oxygen.

ozone: a photochemical oxidant, toxic when in direct contact with lung tissue; an air pollutant. See also *ozone layer*.

ozone hole: a hole in the ozone layer at the South Pole, caused by air pollution.

ozone layer: a layer of ozone in the outer atmosphere that protects living things on earth from harmful ultraviolet radiation from the sun.

persistent: a term that refers to chemicals that cannot be broken down to harmless waste products and that therefore accumulate in the food chain (see Figure 19-2). For contrast, see *biodegradable*.

pollution: contamination of the environment with any substance or influence that impairs its ability to support life. Among types of pollution are *thermal* (heat) *pollution*, *noise pollution*, and *light pollution*. See also *air pollution*.

radioactivity: the release of radiation from the nuclei of atoms.

recycling: using materials over again in the same process as before.

sludge: the solid material that remains after fluid has been drawn off (as from sewage or industrial waste).

smog: the form of air pollution that arises when sunlight strikes certain compounds in the air.

soft water: water containing a high concentration of sodium.

solid wastes: a term used primarily to refer to sewage and animal waste; secondarily to nonpoisonous artificial materials such as paper, glass, plastic, and metal. See also *toxic wastes*.

sustainable development: development that betters people's economic well-being, not only in the short term, but also in the long term.

thermal pollution: see *pollution*.

toxic wastes: waste materials, primarily from industrial processes, that are toxic to plants, animals, and people.

QUIZ ANSWERS

1. *True*. There is no clear boundary between a person and the environment.

2. *True*. Air pollution has existed on earth since before the dawn of human history.

3. *False*. The greenhouse effect is now harming the earth, because it is causing global warming.

4. *False*. Even though the ozone hole is developing only at the South Pole at present, it is leading to thinning of the ozone layer all over the earth's outer atmosphere and affecting people on the major continents.

5. *True*. Pure water can pollute the environment if it is the wrong temperature.

6. *True*. To minimize environmental impact, human sewage should be returned to the earth after treatment, not to the water.

7. *True*. Radioactive wastes can't be detoxified; they can only be moved from place to place.

8. *True*. Radioactivity alters the genetic material in living cells, including ova and sperm cells, creating mutations that can persist for generations.

9. *True*. When birds can't survive in an environment, that is a sign that people's health is likely to suffer there, too.

10. *False*. The most promising way to approach the world's environmental problems is for each nation to work hardest on the problems to which it contributes the most.

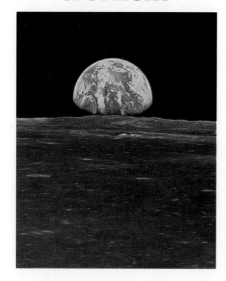

Personal Strategy— Voluntary Simplicity

The problems of the environment and the world's multiplying population may appear so great that they seem approachable only by way of worldwide political decisions. But consider this: you can change the world. To describe some ways in which an individual can accomplish this is, perhaps, the most fitting way to conclude a book about personal choices. After all, a society is the sum of its individuals; as we go, so goes our world.

I feel much too insignificant to have any effect on the way the world goes. In fact, when I think about what's happening around me, I feel overwhelmed, depressed, and pessimistic.

Every thoughtful person feels that way at times and is tempted to give up. Optimism can be cultivated, though, and many people are intentionally doing just that.[1]* They know that optimism gives them energy and makes their efforts to shape the world's future more effective.

How do I go about cultivating optimism?

By living your own life. Don't try to solve all the world's problems. Mentally draw a circle around yourself, and work as energetically as you can to better yourself through education, spiritual growth, and physical health. Work, too, to better the small world within the circle around yourself.

That sounds simple enough, but I don't see how it will help anything. In fact, it almost sounds selfish.

It will help, though. Every move you make leaves the world a better or worse place. Your actions have a ripple effect, often far beyond what you may think. Tending compassionately to the lives nearest you, including your own, is your first responsibility. Many great religious teachings express that value.

*Reference notes are in Appendix D.

Your second responsibility is to make sure you can answer yes to the question, If everyone lived as I do, would the children of today grow up in a better world? Those who study the future are convinced that the hope of the world lies in everyone's adopting a simple lifestyle. As one such person put it, "the widespread simplification of life is vital to the well-being of the entire human family."[2]

Are you implying that everybody needs to adopt a life of poverty? I can't envision how my being poor would help anyone. Besides, wealthy people would never agree.

No, the suggestion is not that everyone become poor. It is said that "poverty is repressive, simplicity is liberating. Poverty generates a sense of helplessness . . . simplicity fosters creativity. Poverty is mean and degrading . . . simplicity is enabling."[3] In other words, to become poor would solve nothing—poverty obstructs personal growth; simplicity opens the way to it. You are also right that few people would willingly give up their wealth, even if it did help. What *is* advocated has nothing to do with wealth. It is a lifestyle, a commitment to live more simply in view of the world's limited resources.[4]

What does living a life of voluntary simplicity involve?

A thousand small decisions—of which we will offer a hundred. Before reading them, be sure to understand that they are not "the" rules, but only a sampling deemed appropriate by one school of thought. *Voluntary* is a key word, just as *simplicity* is. Each individual must look within to discover a personal sense of what is appropriate. "Crucial to acting in a voluntary manner is being aware of ourselves as we move through life. This requires that we not only pay attention to the actions we take . . . but also that we pay attention to the person [ourselves]."[5] Each person needs to find a balance—a path, suitable for that individual, that leads between the extremes of poverty and self-indulgence.

That makes sense. Now tell me: what are the 100 ways?

Here are 99 of them, in Table S19–1. They were developed by a team of researchers who had been given the assignment of describing the elements of a simple lifestyle. They wrote 99 short chapters under ten headings: heating and cooling, other

TABLE S19–1 Ninety-nine Ways to a Simple Lifestyle

Heating and Cooling	Other Home Conserving	Food	Gardening	Solid Waste
Save heat and insulate	Light house efficiently	Consume less meat	Garden on available land	Avoid disposable paper products
Keep furnace operating properly	Save water	Select unprocessed foods	Grow vegetables	Refrain from purchasing plastic-wrapped items
Regulate humidity in heated homes	Avoid aerosol sprays	Avoid non-nutritious food	Plant fruit trees	Ban non-returnables
Conserve cooking energy	Use few cleaning products	Reduce intake of refined sugar	Fertilize wisely	Sort trash
Refrigerate wisely	Budget resources	Eat wild foods	Use natural pesticides	Use flush-less toilets
Design buildings with ecology in mind	Build a yurt	Learn to preserve food	Compost and mulch	
Cut hot-water costs	Make home repairs	Conserve nutritional value of food	Keep bees	
Economize with modular heating	Paint the home	Be aware of agribusiness		
Cool conservatively and ventilate	Make, repair, and reuse furniture	Organize a food co-op		
Dehumidify in summer	Eliminate unnecessary appliances	Bake bread		
Air condition minimally		Prepare various food products		
Convert to renewable fuel sources (organic, solar, wind)[a]		Drink homemade beverages		
		Advocate breast feeding		
		Question pets and pet food		

Clothing	Fulfillment	Health	Transportation	Community
Choose fabrics wisely	Have a hobby	Use simple personal products	Know bicycle benefits and servicing	Live communally
Pick quality clothing	Become artistic	Select safe cosmetics	Bike safely	Refurbish old homes
Make clothing	Decorate the home simply	Beware of hair dyes	Encourage mass transit	Provide pure drinking water
Mend and reuse garments	Create toys and games	Do not abuse drugs	Share the car	Join a craft co-operative
Do not wear fur from endangered species	Preserve a place for quiet	Stop smoking cigarettes	Avoid unnecessary auto travel	Care for the elderly and ill
Protect the feet	Camp and backpack	Curb alcohol abuse	Buy cars thriftily	Have simple funerals
	Enjoy recreational sports	Prepare for environmental extremes	Choose proper gas	Influence legislation
	Exercise without equipment	Guard against home hazards	Drive conservatively	Consumers beware
		Recognize signs of chronic disease	Seek proper maintenance and service	Battle utilities
		Care for teeth		Demand corporate responsibility
		Watch weight		Start recycling projects
		Learn to rest and relax		Fight environmental pollution
				Improve land use
				Create work and study opportunities

[a]The book from which this list was adapted devotes a chapter each to organic, solar, and wind fuel sources.

SOURCE: Center for Science in the Public Interest, Simple Lifestyle Team, *99 Ways to a Simple Lifestyle* (Garden City, N.Y.: Anchor Books, 1977).

methods of home conservation, food, gardening, solid waste, clothing, fulfillment, health, transportation, and community. The book from which the list was taken offers many more pointers under each heading, of course, but you can get a sense of what comprises a simple lifestyle just by reading the titles.*

But you said there were 100 ways. What's the last one?

To better yourself. Improving yourself is the first step toward improving the world—remember the ripple effect. Learn all you can; work on your emotional and spiritual growth. You will then be better equipped to participate fully and responsibly in the world community.

Do you really think that if everyone made choices like these, it would help the state of the world?

Yes. Every agency that has studied the future has reached the same conclusion: voluntary simplicity can work. It does not mean living primitively; most people prefer beauty and ease to ugliness and discomfort. It does mean seeking a life free of distractions, clutter, and pretense—a life that includes self-discipline. The words of an old poem speak to this idea, and they are a fitting close to this discussion:

Beyond a wholesome discipline, be gentle with yourself. You are a child of the universe, no less than the trees and the stars; you have a right to be here. And whether or not it is clear to you, no doubt the universe is unfolding as it should. Therefore be at peace with God, whatever you conceive him to be, and whatever your labors and aspirations . . . keep peace with your soul.

—*Desiderata*, found in Old St. Paul's Church, Baltimore, dated 1692, author unknown.

---

*Another book of excellent suggestions for meeting personal responsibilities to the world is one produced under the auspices of the American Friends Service Committee: J. Bodner, ed., *Taking Charge of Our Lives: Living Responsibly in a Troubled World* (San Francisco: Harper and Row, 1984).

Addresses

The following resources offer health information related to the chapters in this book as follows. Of interest in connection with many chapters are the resources listed under "Consumer Information" and "Handicapped People."

Chapter 1—see "Consumer Information."

Chapters 2, and 3—see "Mental Health," and "Self-Help Groups."

Chapters 4 and 5—see "Foods and Food Safety" and "Nutrition."

Chapter 7—see "Drugs and Drug Abuse."

Chapter 8—see "Alcohol and Alcohol Abuse."

Chapter 9—see "Smoking."

Chapter 11—see "Infertility" and "Pregnancy."

Chapter 12—see "Child Health."

Chapter 14—see "Accident Prevention."

Chapters 15–17—see "Diseases."

Chapter 18—see "Health Maintenance Organizations."

Chapter 19—see "Cosmetics," "Environmental Safety," "Foods and Food Safety," and "Occupational Safety."

ACCIDENT PREVENTION

American National Red Cross
National Headquarters
Washington, DC 20006

New York City Poison Control Project
Bellevue Hospital Center
27th Street and First Avenue
New York, NY 10016

ALCOHOL AND ALCOHOL ABUSE

National Clearinghouse for Alcohol Information
Box 2345
Rockville, MD 20850

National Council on Alcoholism (NCA)
733 Third Avenue
New York, NY 10017

Alcoholics Anonymous World Services
P.O. Box 459
Grand Central Station
New York, NY 10017

Al-Anon Family Group Headquarters
P.O. Box 182
Madison Square Station
New York, NY 10010

Toughlove
P.O. Box 70
Sellersville, PA 18960

▇ CHILD HEALTH

National Center for Education in Maternal and Child Health
P.O. Box 28612
Washington, DC 20005
(202) 842–7617

▇ CONSUMER INFORMATION

Consumer Information Center
Department 609K
Pueblo, CO 81009
(Ask for the *Consumer's Resource Handbook.*)

National Council Against Health Fraud (NCAHF)
P.O. Box 1276
Loma Linda, CA 92354

Center for Science in Public Interest (CSPI)
1755 S. Street, NW
Washington, DC 20009

Office of the Secretary
Federal Trade Commission (FTC)
Washington, DC 20580
(202) 523–3598

▇ COSMETICS

Food and Drug Administration (FDA)
5600 Fishers Lane
Rockville, MD 20852

▇ DISEASES

Arthritis Information Clearinghouse
P.O. Box 9752
Arlington, VA 22209

American Dental Association (ADA)
211 East Chicago Avenue
Chicago, IL 60611

American Diabetes Association (ADA)
2 Park Avenue
New York, NY 10016

American Heart Association (AHA)
7320 Greenville Avenue
Dallas, TX 75231

American Medical Association (AMA)
535 North Dearborn Street
Chicago, IL 60610

High Blood Pressure Information Center
120/80, National Institutes of Health (NIH)
Bethesda, MD 20205
(703) 558–4880

DRUGS AND DRUG ABUSE (SEE ALSO *ALCOHOL*)

Food and Drug Administration (FDA)
5600 Fishers Lane
Rockville, MD 20852

National Clearinghouse for Drug Abuse Information
5600 Fishers Lane, Room 10A-56
Rockville, MD 20857

ENVIRONMENTAL SAFETY (WATER, PESTICIDES, HAZARDS)

Public Information Center (PM-215)
Environmental Protection Agency (EPA)
Washington, DC 24060
(202) 755–0707

FOODS AND FOOD SAFETY

Food and Drug Administration (FDA)
5600 Fishers Lane
Rockville, MD 20852

Food Safety and Inspection Service (FSIS)
Consumer Inquiries
U.S. Department of Agriculture (USDA)
Washington, DC 20250
(202) 472–4485

HANDICAPPED PEOPLE

Clearinghouse on the Handicapped
330 C Street, SW
Washington, DC 20202
(202) 245–0080

National Information Center for Handicapped Children and Youth
1555 Wilson Boulevard
Suite 600
Rosslyn, VA 22209
(703) 522–0870

HEALTH MAINTENANCE ORGANIZATIONS (HMOs)

Office of Health Maintenance Organizations
Department of Health and Human Services (DHHS)
12420 Parklawn Drive
Rockville, MD 20857
(800) 638–6686

INFERTILITY

RESOLVE, Inc.
National Office
P.O. Box 474
Belmont, MA 02178

National Committee for Adoption
Suite 326
1346 Connecticut Avenue, NW
Washington, DC 20036

MENTAL HEATLH

National Clearinghouse for Mental Health Information
National Institute of Mental Health (NIMH)
5600 Fishers Lane, Room 11A-33
Rockville, MD 20857
(301) 443–4513

NUTRITION

Human Nutrition Information Service (HNIS)
U.S. Department of Agriculture (USDA)
Federal Center Building
Hyattsville, MD 20752

American Dietetic Association
430 North Michigan Avenue
Chicago, IL 60611

OCCUPATIONAL SAFETY

Office of Information and Consumer Affairs
Occupational Safety and Health Administration (OSHA)
Department of Labor
Room N3637
200 Constitution Avenue, NW
Washington, DC 20210
(202) 523–8151

PREGNANCY

National Center for Education in Maternal and Child Health
P.O. Box 28612
Washington, DC 20005
(202) 842–7617

SELF-HELP GROUPS

Self-Help Center
1600 Dodge Avenue
Evanston, IL 60201

The National Self-Help Clearinghouse
33 West 42nd Street
Room 1227
New York, NY 10036

SMOKING

Technical Information Center
Office on Smoking and Health
5600 Fishers Lane, Room 1–16
Rockville, MD 20857

American Cancer Society
(look up the local address in your phone book)

American Lung Association
(check your phone book)

Smokenders
(call 1–800–243–5614 east of the Mississippi, or 1–800–828–4357 west of the Mississippi.)

American Institute for Preventive Medicine
1911 West Ten Mile Road
Suite 101
Southfield, MI 48075

Nutrient and Food Standards

The consumer of nutrition information and products needs to know the standards against which to measure claims. Among the most important of the standards used in nutrition are the Recommended Dietary Allowances (RDA) and the **U.S. RDA.**

The RDA (shown in Table B–1), are daily recommended intakes of nutrients intended to provide for individual variations among most normal, healthy people in the United States under usual environmental stresses. RDA are set for energy, ten vitamins, and six minerals; similar recommendations known as "estimated safe and adequate intakes" (Table B–2) are set for three other vitamins and nine trace minerals. A third set of recommendations, the RDA for energy, appear as a set of ranges of energy intakes for individuals of different ages (Table B–3). No RDA is set for carbohydrate or fat. The assumption is that you will first use a certain minimum number of calories for the protein you specifically need, and then will use the remaining calories for carbohydrate, fat, and possibly alcohol (according to your personal preference) to meet your energy RDA. The Canadian recommendations for nutrients (RNI) and calories are given in Tables B–4 and B–5.

The RDA should not be confused with **MDR** (minimum daily requirements), a term used in the past on the labels of nutrient supplements. The MDR are not much used any more because they often misled the public into thinking of them as absolute minimum requirements. The RDA are also different from the U.S. RDA, used on labels (see the discussion that follows.).

The government-appointed committee that determines the RDA is composed of highly qualified scientists selected by the National Academy of Sciences. They are based on available scientific evidence to the greatest extent possible, and the committee reviews them about every five years in the light of new findings and revises them if necessary. The RDA are for healthy persons only. Medical problems alter nutrient needs.

Because the RDA are generous recommendations intended to cover even people with unusually high nutrient needs, they cannot be taken as literal, all-or-none recommendations for any individual. You can't know exactly what your own personal requirement may be. Moreover, the Committee on RDA makes several assumptions that do not apply to all real situations. It assumes, among other things, that you are eating a generally adequate diet including sources of complete protein and that you are consuming adequate calories and nutrients. It assumes that you store and cook your foods with reasonable care and that large amounts of nutrients aren't lost in these processes.

> **MINIGLOSSARY**
> **of Nutrient and Food**
> **Standard Terms**
>
> **Minimum Daily Requirements (MDR):** an obsolete standard of nutrient intake; supposedly the minimum amount of nutrients necessary to prevent deficiency diseases. Actually, because requirements vary, a single accurate minimum value can't be set for a population.
> **nutritional quality guidelines:** guidelines provided by the FDA for the nutrient contents of convenience foods such as TV dinners.
> **Recommended Dietary Allowances (RDA):** a standard for nutrient intakes developed by the Committee on RDA of the National Academy of Sciences. They are designed for the maintenance of good nutrition among most normal, healthy people in the United States under usual environmental stresses.
> **Recommended Nutrient Intakes for Canadians (RNI):** a standard for nutrient intakes developed by the governmental agency Health and Welfare Canada. They are designed to cover individual variation in essentially all of a healthy population subsisting on a variety of common foods available in Canada.
> **standard of identity:** the composition of a food product as designated by the Food and Drug Administration, spelling out the required ingredients and the percentages in which they must be present. For example, any frozen confection labeled *ice cream* must contain a certain percentage of milk fat. Products for which there exist standards of identity are not required to list ingredients on labels.
> **U.S. RDA:** "United States Recommended Dietary Allowance," a standard for the daily intake of nutrients designed for use on food labels.

TABLE B–1 Recommended Dietary Allowances (RDA), 1980

Age (years)	Weight (kg)	(lbs)	Height (cm)	(in)	Protein (g)	Vitamin A (RE)	Vitamin D (µg)	Vitamin E (mg)	Vitamin C (mg)	Thiamin (mg)	Riboflavin (mg)	Niacin (mg equiv.)	Vitamin B₆ (mg)	Folacin (µg)	Vitamin B₁₂ (µg)	Calcium (mg)	Phosphorus (mg)	Magnesium (mg)	Iron (mg)	Zinc (mg)	Iodine (µg)
Infants																					
0.0–0.5	6	13	60	24	kg × 2.2	420	10	3	35	0.3	0.4	6	0.3	30	0.5	360	240	50	10	3	40
0.5–1.0	9	20	71	28	kg × 2.0	400	10	4	35	0.5	0.6	8	0.6	45	1.5	540	360	70	15	5	50
Children																					
1–3	13	29	90	35	23	400	10	5	45	0.7	0.8	9	0.9	100	2.0	800	800	150	15	10	70
4–6	20	44	112	44	30	500	10	6	45	0.9	1.0	11	1.3	200	2.5	800	800	200	10	10	90
7–10	28	62	132	52	34	700	10	7	45	1.2	1.4	16	1.6	300	3.0	800	800	250	10	10	120
Males																					
11–14	45	99	157	62	45	1000	10	8	50	1.4	1.6	18	1.8	400	3.0	1200	1200	350	18	15	150
15–18	66	145	176	69	56	1000	10	10	60	1.4	1.7	18	2.0	400	3.0	1200	1200	400	18	15	150
19–22	70	154	177	70	56	1000	7.5	10	60	1.5	1.7	19	2.2	400	3.0	800	800	350	10	15	150
23–50	70	154	178	70	56	1000	5	10	60	1.4	1.6	18	2.2	400	3.0	800	800	350	10	15	150
51 +	70	154	178	70	56	1000	5	10	60	1.2	1.4	16	2.2	400	3.0	800	800	350	10	15	150
Females																					
11–14	46	101	157	62	46	800	10	8	50	1.1	1.3	15	1.8	400	3.0	1200	1200	300	18	15	150
15–18	55	120	163	64	46	800	10	8	60	1.1	1.3	14	2.0	400	3.0	1200	1200	300	18	15	150
19–22	55	120	163	64	44	800	7.5	8	60	1.1	1.3	14	2.0	400	3.0	800	800	300	18	15	150
23–50	55	120	163	64	44	800	5	8	60	1.0	1.2	13	2.0	400	3.0	800	800	300	18	15	150
51 +	55	120	163	64	44	800	5	8	60	1.0	1.2	13	2.0	400	3.0	800	800	300	10	15	150
Pregnant					+30	+200	+5	+2	+20	+0.4	+0.3	+2	+0.6	+400	+1.0	+400	+400	+150	a	+5	+25
Lactating					+20	+400	+5	+3	+40	+0.5	+0.5	+5	+0.5	+100	+1.0	+400	+400	+150	a	+10	+50

The allowances are intended to provide for individual variations among most normal, healthy people in the United States under usual environmental stresses. They were designed for the maintenance of good nutrition. Diets should be based on a variety of common foods in order to provide other nutrients for which human requirements have been less well defined.

The Committee on RDA has published a separate table showing energy allowances in ranges for each age-sex group and another table for vitamins and minerals not previously covered by the recommendations.

Reproduced from *Recommended Dietary Allowances*, 9th ed. (1980), with the permission of the National Academy of Sciences, Washington, D.C.

aSupplemental iron is recommended (30 to 60 mg).

When you use the RDA for yourself and compare your nutrient intakes with them, you should keep in mind that the RDA are not absolute requirements. *R* stands for *recommended*, not for *required*. They are allowances, and they are generous. Even so, they do not necessarily cover every individual for every nutrient. In planning your own diet, it is probably wise to aim at getting 100 percent or more of the RDA for every nutrient.

On the other hand, it is naive to think of the RDA as minimum amounts. A more accurate view is to see your nutrient needs as falling within a range, with danger zones both below and above it. The 1980 RDA reflect this consideration especially clearly in the tables that state the recommendations in ranges with an "adequate" intake at the bottom of the range and a "safe" intake at the top (Table B–2).

The U.S. RDA (Table B–6) are derived from the RDA for use on food labels. A food label is most meaningful if it expresses the food's nutrient contents as a percentage of your need. For example, it is useful to you to learn from the label of a cereal box that one serving of the cereal provides you with 25 percent of the iron you need for the day. Your RDA could be used to give you this information; but the trouble is, the makers of the label don't know who you are: a 10-year-old boy, a 70-year-old woman, or a pregnant teen-age girl. To standardize labels, four sets of U.S. RDA were developed for different groups of people. The most commonly used of these is the U.S. RDA for adults, and this is the one referred to here. The idea behind the U.S. RDA for adults was to develop a single set of standards for a sort of generalized adult human being whose nutrient needs are high— as high as people's needs generally go. If you read on a label that a serving of cereal provides 25 percent of the U.S. RDA of iron, you can be sure that it will also provide at least 25 percent of *your* iron RDA. Your nutrient needs, in other words, are covered by the U.S. RDA.

Another set of standards exist to regulate the quality of foods sold in the marketplace. You can evaluate the nutrition value of ordinary foods such as fish or beans by looking them up in a table of food composition. You can evaluate foods that present information panels like breakfast cereals, because their contents and nutrient composition are listed on their labels. But what about foods that simply say "TV dinner" or "macaroni and cheese"? The FDA has devised **nutritional quality guidelines** for the nutrient contents of many kinds of convenience foods: frozen dinners; breakfast cereals; meal replacements; fruit-type or vegetable-type beverages; and main dishes such as pizza or macaroni and cheese. If a product complies with the nutritional quality guidelines, it may carry on its label the statement that it "provides nutrients in amounts appropriate for this class of food as determined by the U.S. government." For example, frozen dinners must contain one or more sources of protein from meat, poultry, fish, cheese, or eggs, and these must make up at least 70 percent of the total protein; they must include one or more vegetables or vegetable mixtures other than potatoes, rice, or cereal-based products; and they must have a certain minimum nutrient level for each 100 calories.

What if the label says nothing more than a name, such as *mayonnaise?* For some items the law provides **standards of identity** and excuses manufacturers from the requirement of listing ingredients. Standards of identity exist for such foods as ice cream and mayonnaise—common foods that at one time were often prepared at home, so that the basic recipe was understood by almost everyone. Certain ingredients must be present in a specific percentage before the food may use the standard name. Any product like mayonnaise, for example, may use that name on the label only if it contains 65 percent by weight of vegetable oil, either vinegar or lemon juice, and egg yolk. The FDA does not have the authority to require that ingredients be listed for these foods, but it urges manufacturers to give the consumer more detailed information, and many manufacturers do so voluntarily.

TABLE B–2 Estimated Safe and Adequate Daily Dietary Intakes of Additional Selected Nutrients (United States)

Age (years)	Vitamins			Trace Elements[a]		
	Vitamin K (μg)	Biotin (μg)	Pantothenic acid (μg)	Copper (mg)	Manganese (mg)	Fluoride (mg)
0–0.5	12	35	2	0.5–0.7	0.5–0.7	0.1–0.5
0.5–1	10–20	50	3	0.7–1.0	0.7–1.0	0.2–1.0
1–3	15–30	65	3	1.0–1.5	1.0–1.5	0.5–1.5
4–6	20–40	85	3–4	1.5–2.0	1.5–2.0	1.0–2.5
7–10	30–60	120	4–5	2.0–2.5	2.0–3.0	1.5–2.5
11 +	50–100	100–200	4–7	2.0–3.0	2.5–5.0	1.5–2.5
Adults	70–140	100–200	4–7	2.0–3.0	2.5–5.0	1.5–4.0

Age (years)	Trace Elements[a]			Electrolytes		
	Chromium (mg)	Selenium (mg)	Molybdenum (mg)	Sodium (mg)	Potassium (mg)	Chloride (mg)
0–0.5	0.01–0.04	0.01–0.04	0.03–0.06	115–350	350–925	275–700
0.5–1	0.02–0.06	0.02–0.06	0.04–0.08	250–750	425–1,275	400–1,200
1–3	0.02–0.08	0.02–0.08	0.05–0.1	325–975	550–1,650	500–1,500
4–6	0.03–0.12	0.03–0.12	0.06–0.15	450–1,350	775–2,325	700–2,100
7–10	0.05–0.2	0.05–0.2	0.1–0.3	600–1,800	1,000–3,000	925–2,775
11 +	0.05–0.2	0.05–0.2	0.15–0.5	900–2,700	1,525–4,575	1,400–4,200
Adults	0.05–0.2	0.05–0.2	0.15–0.5	1,100–3,300	1,875–5,625	1,700–5,100

Because there is less information on which to base allowances, these figures are not given in the main table of the RDA and are provided here in the form of ranges of recommended intakes.

[a]Since the toxic levels for many trace elements may be only several times usual intakes, the upper levels for the trace elements given in this table should not habitually be exceeded.

TABLE B–3 Recommended Energy Intakes (United States) for Age Groups Based on Mean Heights and Weights

Age	Weight		Height		Energy Needs[a]	
(years)	(kg)	(lb)	(cm)	(in)	(cal)	(MJ)[b]
Infants						
0.0–0.5	6	13	60	24	kg × 115 (95–145)	kg × 0.48
0.5–1.0	9	20	71	28	kg × 105 (80–135)	kg × 0.44
Children						
1–3	13	29	90	35	1,300 (900–1,800)	5.5
4–6	20	44	112	44	1,700 (1,300–2,300)	7.1
7–10	28	62	132	52	2,400 (1,650–3,300)	10.1
Males						
11–14	45	99	157	62	2,700 (2,000–3,700)	11.3
15–18	66	145	176	69	2,800 (2,100–3,900)	11.8
19–22	70	154	177	70	2,900 (2,500–3,300)	12.2
23–50	70	154	178	70	2,700 (2,300–3,100)	11.3
51–75	70	154	178	70	2,400 (2,000–2,800)	10.1
76+	70	154	178	70	2,050 (1,650–2,450)	8.6
Females						
11–14	46	101	157	62	2,200 (1,500–3,000)	9.2
15–18	55	120	163	64	2,100 (1,200–3,000)	8.8
19–22	55	120	163	64	2,100 (1,700–2,500)	8.8
23–50	55	120	163	64	2,000 (1,600–2,400)	8.4
51–75	55	120	163	64	1,800 (1,400–2,200)	7.6
76+	55	120	163	64	1,600 (1,200–2,000)	6.7
Pregnant					+300	
Lactating					+500	

[a]The energy allowances for the young adults are for men and women doing light work. The allowances for the two older age groups represent mean energy needs over these age spans, allowing for a 2 percent decrease in basal (resting) metabolic rate per decade and a reduction in activity of 200 cal per day for men and women between 51 and 75 years, 500 cal for men over 75 years, and 400 cal for women over 75. The customary range of daily energy output, shown in parentheses, is based on a variation in energy needs of ± 400 cal at any one age, emphasizing the wide range of energy intakes appropriate for any group of people. Energy allowances for children through age 18 are based on median energy intakes of children these ages followed in longitudinal growth studies. The values in parentheses are tenth and ninetieth percentiles of energy intake, to indicate the range of energy consumption among individuals of these ages.
[b]MJ stands for megajoules (1 MJ = 1,000 kJ).

TABLE B–4 Recommended Nutrient Intakes for Canadians, 1984

Age	Sex	Weight (kg)	Protein (g/day)[a]	Fat-Soluble Vitamins		
				Vitamin A (RE/day)[b]	Vitamin D (μg/day)[c]	Vitamin E (mg/day)[d]
Months						
0–2	Both	4.5	11[f]	400	10	3
3–5	Both	7.0	14[f]	400	10	3
6–8	Both	8.5	17[f]	400	10	3
9–11	Both	9.5	18	400	10	3
Years						
1	Both	11	19	400	10	3
2–3	Both	14	22	400	5	4
4–6	Both	18	26	500	5	5
7–9	M	25	30	700	2.5	7
	F	25	30	700	2.5	6
10–12	M	34	38	800	2.5	8
	F	36	40	800	2.5	7
13–15	M	50	50	900	2.5	9
	F	48	42	800	2.5	7
16–18	M	62	55	1,000	2.5	10
	F	53	43	800	2.5	7
19–24	M	71	58	1,000	2.5	10
	F	58	43	800	2.5	7
25–49	M	74	61	1,000	2.5	9
	F	59	44	800	2.5	6
50–74	M	73	60	1,000	2.5	7
	F	63	47	800	2.5	6
75+	M	69	57	1,000	2.5	6
	F	64	47	800	2.5	5
Pregnancy (additional)						
1st Trimester			15	100	2.5	2
2nd Trimester			20	100	2.5	2
3rd Trimester			25	100	2.5	2
Lactation (additional)			20	400	2.5	3

[a]The primary units are expressed per kilogram of body weight. The figures shown here are examples.
[b]One retinol equivalent (RE) corresponds to the biological activity of 1 μg of retinol, 6 μg of β-carotene, or 12 μg of other carotenes.
[c]Expressed as cholecalciferol or ergocalciferol.
[d]Expressed as d-α-tocopherol equivalents, relative to which β- and γ-tocopherol and α-tocotrienol have activities of 0.5, 0.1, and 0.3 respectively.
[e]Expressed as total folate.
[f]Assumption that the protein is from breast milk or is of the same biological value as that of breast milk and that between 3 and 9 months adjustment for the quality of the protein is made.

Water-Soluble Vitamins			Minerals				
Vitamin C (mg/day)	Folacin (μg/day)[e]	Vitamin B$_{12}$ (μg/day)	Calcium (mg/day)	Magnesium (mg/day)	Iron (mg/day)	Iodine (μg/day)	Zinc (mg/day)
20	50	0.3	350	30	0.4[g]	25	2[h]
20	50	0.3	350	40	5	35	3
20	50	0.3	400	50	7	40	3
20	55	0.3	400	50	7	45	3
20	65	0.3	500	55	6	55	4
20	80	0.4	500	70	6	65	4
25	90	0.5	600	90	6	85	5
35	125	0.8	700	110	7	110	6
30	125	0.8	700	110	7	95	6
40	170	1.0	900	150	10	125	7
40	180	1.0	1,000	160	10	110	7
50	150	1.5	1,100	210	12	160	9
45	145	1.5	800	200	13	160	8
55	185	1.9	900	250	10	160	9
45	160	1.9	700	215	14	160	8
60	210	2.0	800	240	8	160	9
45	175	2.0	700	200	14	160	8
60	220	2.0	800	250	8	160	9
45	175	2.0	700	200	14[i]	160	8
60	220	2.0	800	250	8	160	9
45	190	2.0	800	210	7	160	8
60	205	2.0	800	230	8	160	9
45	190	2.0	800	220	7	160	8
0	305	1.0	500	15	6	25	0
20	305	1.0	500	20	6	25	1
20	305	1.0	500	25	6	25	2
30	120	0.5	500	80	0	50	6

[g]It is assumed that breast milk is the source of iron up to 2 months of age.

[h]Based on the assumption that breast milk is the source of zinc for the first 2 months.

[i]After the menopause the recommended intake is 7 mg/day.

Recommended intakes of energy and of certain nutrients are not listed in this table because of the nature of the variables upon which they are based. The figures for energy are provided in Table B–5. For nutrients not shown, the following amounts are recommended: thiamin, 0.4 mg/1,000 cal (0.48 mg/5,000 kJ); riboflavin, 0.5 mg/1,000 cal (0.6 mg/5,000 kJ); niacin, 7.2 NE/1,000 cal (8.6 NE/5,000 kJ); vitamin B$_6$, 15 μg, as pyridoxine, per gram of protein; phosphorus, same as calcium.

Recommended intakes during periods of growth are taken as appropriate for individuals representative of the mid-point in each age group.

All recommended intakes are designed to cover individual variations in essentially all of a healthy population subsisting upon a variety of common foods available in Canada.

SOURCE: *Recommended Nutrient Intakes for Canadians*, Health and Welfare Canada (Ottawa: Canadian Government Publishing Centre, 1984), Table X.I, pp. 179–180.

TABLE B–5 Average Energy Requirements (Canada)

| Age | Sex | Average Height (cm) | Average Weight (kg) | Requirements[a] | | | | | |
				cal/kg[b]	MJ/kg[b]	cal/day	MJ/day	cal/cm	MJ/cm
Months									
0–2	Both	55	4.5	120–100	0.50–0.42	500	2.0	9	0.04
3–5	Both	63	7.0	100–95	0.42–0.40	700	2.8	11	0.05
6–8	Both	69	8.5	95–97	0.40–0.41	800	3.4	11.5	0.05
9–11	Both	73	9.5	97–99	0.41	950	3.8	12.5	0.05
Years									
1	Both	82	11	101	0.42	1,100	4.8	13.5	0.06
2–3	Both	95	14	94	0.39	1,300	5.6	13.5	0.06
4–6	Both	107	18	100	0.42	1,800	7.6	17	0.07
7–9	M	126	25	88	0.37	2,200	9.2	17.5	0.07
	F	125	25	76	0.32	1,900	8.0	15	0.06
10–12	M	141	34	73	0.30	2,500	10.4	17.5	0.07
	F	143	36	61	0.25	2,200	9.2	15.5	0.06
13–15	M	159	50	57	0.24	2,800	12.0	17.5	0.07
	F	157	48	46	0.19	2,200	9.2	14	0.06
16–18	M	172	62	51	0.21	3,200	13.2	18.5	0.08
	F	160	53	40	0.17	2,100	8.8	13	0.05
19–24	M	175	71	42	0.18	3,000	12.4		
	F	160	58	36	0.15	2,100	8.8		
25–49	M	172	74	36	0.15	2,700	11.2		
	F	160	59	32	0.13	1,900	8.0		
50–74	M	170	73	31	0.13	2,300	9.6		
	F	158	63	29	0.12	1,800	7.6		
75+	M	168	69	29	0.12	2,000	8.4		
	F	155	64	23	0.10	1,500	6.0		

[a]Requirements can be expected to vary within a range of ± 30 percent, and are estimates based on expected patterns of activity.
[b]First and last figures are averages at the beginning and at the end of the 3-month period.

SOURCE: *Recommended Nutrient Intakes for Canadians*, 1984, Table II.I, pp. 22–23.

TABLE B–6 The U.S. RDA for Adults

Nutrients That Must Appear On the Label[b]	The U.S. RDA for Adults[a]	Nutrients That May Appear On the Label[b]	The U.S. RDA for Adults[a]
Protein (g), PER ≥ casein[c]	45	Vitamin D (IU)	400[e]
Protein (g), PER ≤ casein	65	Vitamin E (IU)	30[f]
Vitamin A (RE)	1000[d]	Vitamin B₆ (mg)	2.0
Vitamin C (ascorbic acid) (mg)	60	Folic acid (folacin) (mg)	0.4
Thiamin (vitamin B₁) (mg)	1.5	Vitamin B₁₂ (μg)	6
Riboflavin (vitamin B₂) (mg)	1.7	Phosphorus (g)	1.0
Niacin (mg)	20	Iodine (μg)	150
Calcium (g)	1.0	Magnesium (mg)	400
Iron (mg)	18	Zinc (mg)	15
		Copper (mg)	2
		Biotin (mg)	0.3
		Pantothenic acid (mg)	10

[a]Separate tables of U.S. RDA are published for infants, children, and pregnant and lactating women.

[b]whenever nutrition labeling is required.

[c]PER is an index of protein quality. Casein is milk protein.

[d]1000 RE was originally expressed as 5000 IU. 800 RE was originally expressed as 4000 IU.

[e]400 IU vitamin D is the same as 10 micrograms (μg).

[f]30 IU vitamin E is the same as 30 mg. 25 IU vitamin E is the same as 25 mg. The RDA for vitamin E has been lowered since 1968, when these tables were first published.

SOURCE: Adapted from *Food Technology* 28(7): 5, 1974.

Emergency Measures

When an emergency is at hand, fast, effective action can save a life, perhaps your own. On the other hand, attempts at help without knowledge of correct procedures can do more harm than no action at all. This appendix is inadequate to prepare you for administering emergency treatments, but is presented with the idea that it, alone, may some day be the only reference at hand in an emergency. The local Red Cross and hospitals offer first aid courses that can prepare you fully, so take one. Until then, here are techniques that can save a life until properly trained help arrives. In order of urgency—stop excessive bleeding, keep the person breathing, and treat for shock. In addition to these basics, there are tips specific to heart attack, burns, hypothermia (cold stress), poisonings, and emergency childbirth.

In a serious emergency, it is urgent that someone call for help at the earliest possible moment. If you are the only one available, give first aid first, then call. In most places in the United States, the emergency telephone number is 911. You may ask whoever answers to connect you with poison control, ambulance service, or whatever assisting organization you require.

THE MEDICINE CHEST

In order to offer emergency treatment, you must have access to supplies, or you must use makeshift substitutes for those that are not available. For example, freshly laundered clothing is an acceptable substitute for gauze used to cover wounds or burns. Each home medicine chest should be stocked with a variety of simple equipment, as listed in Table C–1. One of the simplest and most useful bandages is the "butterfly," made from strips of adhesive tape and used to close open wounds (see Figure C–1). Make a few of these in advance, and store them on the roll of adhesive tape. Also, a standard reference, such as the American Red Cross publication *First Aid and Personal Safety*, will help remind you of what to do in an emergency and should be kept close at hand.

Most accidents occur at home, but they occur on outings, too. Campers and hikers can carry a similar array of equipment, with the addition of a snake-bite kit that consists of a sharp instrument for lancing the bite (a shallow incision is made connecting the fang marks, just through the skin layers), a strap to tie around the limb between the bite and the heart to temporarily reduce blood flow to the bite (see later cautions on tourniquets), and a suction device to remove venom. Some people keep a medicine box in their car, so it goes wherever they go.

TABLE C–1 Standard Supplies for the Medicine Chest

Item	Purpose
Bandages and Dressings	
Rolled white gauze bandage, 2- and 3-inch widths	Wound wrap to hold sterile dressings or splints in place
Ready-to-apply sterile first aid dressings, individually packaged, various sizes	Padding to be applied directly to open wounds or burns
Triangular bandages, 36 × 36 inches	Diagonally folded sling for fractured or broken arm or shoulder; wrap to hold dressings in place; folded compress
Adherent dressing strips, 2- and 3-inch widths	Covering to be cut to size for simple wounds
Individually packaged adhesive bandages, various widths and shapes	Covering for minor cuts and scrapes
Medicines	
Aspirin or aspirin substitute	Pain reliever
Antiseptic cream or petroleum jelly	Sterile application for dressings, to prevent sticking to minor wounds
Liquid antiseptic	Cleanser for skin surfaces in cases of minor wounds
Calamine lotion	Agent for relieving itching from insect bites or exposure to skin irritants
Table salt packets	Treatment of shock with salted fluids
Syrup of ipecac	Emetic to induce vomiting in certain cases of poisoning
Activated charcoal	Adsorbent to bind certain types of poisons
Epsom salts	Laxative to speed passage of certain poisons through the digestive tract
Miscellaneous	
Adhesive tape	Fastening for bandages or dressings
Large safety pins	Fastening for bandages or slings
Tweezers	Splinter or insect stinger remover
Blunt-tipped scissors	Implement for severing lengths of bandage, adhesive tape, and the like
Thermometer(s)	Rectal or oral temperature taking
Hypoallergenic soap	Wound cleanser
Absorbent cotton, paper tissues	Absorbent dressing; wipe for cleansing wounds

SOURCE: Adapted from *Good Housekeepinig Family Health and Medical Guide* (New York: Hearst, 1980), p. 876; E. Kiester, Jr., ed., *Better Homes and Gardens New Family Medical Guide* (Des Moines: Meredith Corporation, 1982), p. 833.

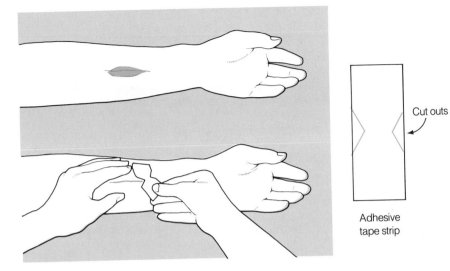

FIGURE C–1 The Butterfly Bandage
Strip

To close an open wound, make butterfly
strips from adhesive tape by cutting trian-
gles from each edge halfway along the
strip. Use one hand to close the wound,
and the other to apply the butterfly.

Cut outs

Adhesive
tape strip

TREATING WOUNDS AND CONTROLLING BLEEDING

Prompt treatment of wounds is necessary to prevent excessive bleeding and
infection. Everyone should know how to treat the five types of wounds:
abrasion, avulsion, incision, laceration, and **puncture** (see Miniglossary of
Wounds). Table C–2 shows how to treat each type. Wounds deeper than
the outer layers of skin are serious and should be evaluated by a health care
professional after first aid has been administered. Further, medical treatment
is required for any wound that has spurted blood, even if first aid has
controlled it. Medical treatment is also necessary for any wound that may
have involved muscles, tendons, ligaments, or nerves (indicated by paralysis
or numbness); any bite wound (animal or human); any heavily contaminated
wound; or any wound that contains soil or object fragments.

In order to determine the type and severity of the wound, look at it
carefully. If you can't see the wound because of clothing, cut or tear away
the clothing. The treatments proceed in the order of urgency for the protection of life. First, stop the blood flow from a wound that is bleeding
steadily until the person can receive professional emergency help. Figure
C–2 shows how to stop bleeding. Notice that the figure doesn't list a tourniquet for controlling bleeding; a tourniquet almost always kills the limb to
which it is applied and should be used rarely, if ever. In almost all cases,
bleeding can be controlled by direct pressure; just a few cases require the
addition of indirect pressure. Like the tourniquet, indirect pressure that
constricts an artery can damage the healthy tissue normally fed by that artery,
and should be used only in cases of severe hemorrhage where direct pressure
will not stop the flow. Elevate the injured part to encourage blood to drain
back into the body and to slow the blood flow to it.

BREATHING ASSISTANCE

Second in urgency to controlling beeding is restoring breathing. (A person
can live for a minute or two without breathing, but will bleed to death from
hemorrhage in just seconds.) People commonly choke on food at the table,

MINIGLOSSARY of Wounds

abrasion: a wound caused by rubbing
or scraping the skin, such as rug or rope
burns or skinned knees; typically, a thin
layer of skin is removed over an area of
flesh, leaving it open to infection.

avulsion: a lifting or removal of a flap of
skin and tissue, possibly involving torn
veins and arteries; often caused by
animal bites, motor vehicle and
machinery accidents, gunshots, or
explosions. This type of wound may
bleed excessively and later may become
infected.

incision: a straight-edged cut with
clean edges resulting from contact with
a sharp edge such as a knife or razor; if
deeper than the top skin layers, it may
bleed excessively and become infected
later on.

laceration: a cut that has jagged
edges, with bruised, torn tissue, possibly
involving veins and arteries; caused by
blows from heavy blunt objects.

puncture: a stab wound from a pointed
object, such as a nail or stick; the long,
narrow wound rarely bleeds excessively,
but is most likely to become infected,
possibly with anaerobic tetanus bacteria.
(See Chapter 15 for more about
infections.)

TABLE C–2 Treatment of Wounds

	Abrasion	Avulsion	Incision or Laceration	Puncture
Minor Wound Treatment	Wash with soap, water, and sterile gauze, wiping away from the center of the wound with a new surface at each wipe. Bathe the wound in rubbing alcohol, and cover with sterile gauze. Change gauze frequently.	Wash with soap and water. Place torn tissue in its original location, and bandage with butterfly strips and sterile gauze. Seek prompt medical help.	Wash out cut with soap and water. Use adhesive tape butterfly strips to close the wound, and cover with sterile gauze.	Wash the surface with soap and water, and remove the object (sliver, pin, or small nail) that has punctured the tissue. Seek prompt medical help.
Serious Wound Treatment	See a physician if the wound contains dirt that can't be washed away, is deeper than the top layers of skin, or is located where scarring would be objectionable.	Stop bleeding with pressure. Preserve any pieces of tissue removed from the body in moist sterile gauze, and return flaps to original positions. Do not attempt to return a dislocated organ (such as an eyeball or loop of intestine) to the body cavity; lightly cover it with moist, sterile gauze, and obtain immediate emergency care.	Stop the bleeding. Close the wound with butterfly strips. Cover with sterile gauze, and obtain emergency medical help.	If the wound is deep or large, do not attempt to remove the object (to do so could cause further injury or allow profuse bleeding). If necessary, cut the object free from its attachments so that the person and the object may be transported to an emergency facility.

and a person who is choking may need your help. First, ask this critical question: "Can you make any sound at all?" If the victim makes a sound, air is moving over the vocal cords, which means that some air can get into the lungs. In this case, the person might try bending over, coughing, and other self-help maneuvers before you intervene. Whatever you do, don't hit the victim on the back. If you do, the particle caught in the throat may become lodged in the air passage.

If the victim is unable to make a sound, you must act fast. To properly perform the techniques described here, a person should learn from a professional first aid instructor and practice on medical models. The objective of first aid is to clear the breathing passageway and to force air into and out of the lungs until spontaneous breathing resumes or professional emergency help arrives. It may take hours for help to arrive, but do not give up for at least four hours, even if the victim appears to be dead—the pulse may simply be weak, and recovery may be possible. (Figure 6–2 in Chapter 6 shows how to take a pulse.)

First, check inside the throat for tongue blockage or foreign matter, and clear the breathing passageway. Figure C–3 shows techniques for opening the airway and for cleaning out debris. After these measures, administer breathing assistance: kneel by the victim's head, tilt the chin up by pulling up on the back of the neck, pinch closed the nostrils, and blow into the mouth. (If the victim is a baby, cover both nose and mouth with your mouth, and blow small puffs of air.) Then listen closely for exhalation of air. If the air fails to enter the victim's lungs after a try or two, there may be an object lodged deep within the air passages. Quickly lift the person to standing or sitting on a chair, and perform the Heimlich maneuver as shown in Figure C–4 to remove lodged debris. Quickly return the person to the floor and

FIGURE C-2 Using Direct and Indirect Pressure to Control Bleeding

For direct pressure (A), use sterile gauze, if available, to cover the wound, and use your hand to apply pressure. Bleeding should stop or slow to oozing in under 30 minutes. For severe hemorrhage, indirect pressure (B) on an artery that feeds the damaged area can stop the flow. Select a place between the heart and the wound to apply indirect pressure. The points indicated here (C) are only a few of the possible pressure points. Like a tourniquet, indirect pressure robs healthy tissues fed by the artery, and may kill them; use indirect pressure only in severe hemorrhage when direct pressure fails to stem the flow of blood.

A. Direct pressure

B. Indirect pressure

C. Indirect pressure points

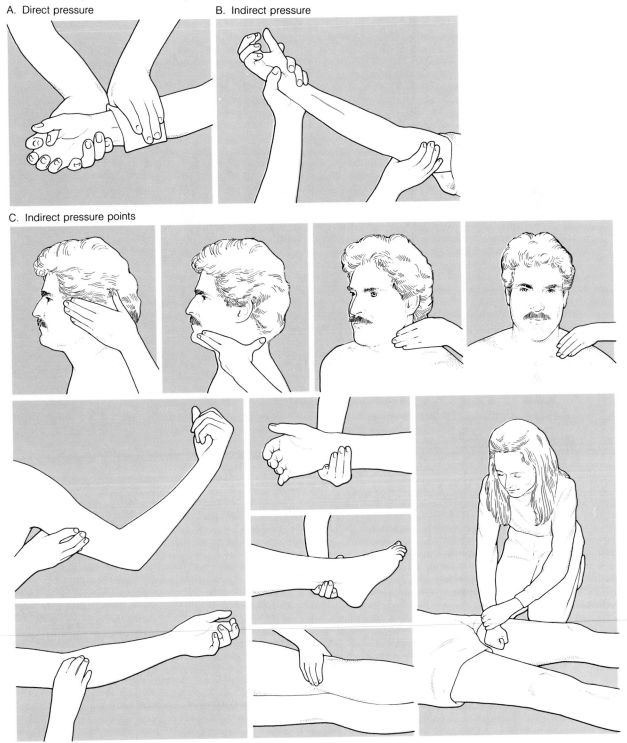

FIGURE C–3   Clearing the Airway

To clear debris from the mouth, turn the victim's head to the side, and use a finger to wipe out the debris. If the debris is lodged in the throat within finger's reach, try to catch an edge of the debris with a sweeping motion of a finger between the debris and the side of the throat, taking extreme care not to push the blockage further down toward the lungs. In children, use a small finger.

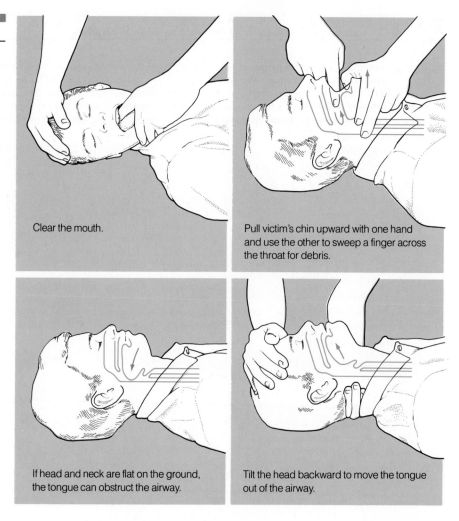

Clear the mouth.

Pull victim's chin upward with one hand and use the other to sweep a finger across the throat for debris.

If head and neck are flat on the ground, the tongue can obstruct the airway.

Tilt the head backward to move the tongue out of the airway.

FIGURE C–4   How to Perform the Heimlich Maneuver

Sit or stand the victim in front of you, and wrap you arms around the waist. Make a fist with one hand, and cover it with the other. Place the fist against the victim's abdomen, just below the rib cage. Use a sudden squeezing motion to thrust your fist into the victim's abdomen with a quick, upward motion. Repeat four times in rapid succession. The food or debris should be ejected by the force of the air escaping from the lungs.

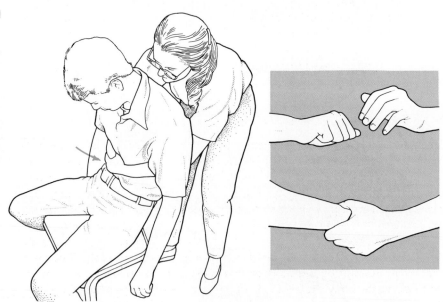

APPENDIX C ■■■ EMERGENCY MEASURES

begin again, clearing the mouth and throat, and start mouth-to-mouth breathing again. If the person is large or unconscious, you can perform the maneuver by allowing the victim to remain lying on his or her back. Kneel astride the thighs, and place both hands as shown in Figure C–4 below the rib cage; press quickly and firmly upward. Be sure to make contact with your fist *before* the thrust—don't punch, but press suddenly. If it is you who is choking, you can be your own rescuer by thrusting your fist into your own abdomen, or thrusting your body forward forcefully against a firmly placed object—the back of a chair, side of a table, or edge of a sink or stove.

You can tell whether someone who is unconscious is breathing by placing your face close to his or hers and listening and feeling for air coming out of the mouth or nose. If the chest is not moving, the person is not breathing, but chest movements can also be caused by muscle spasms that mimic breathing, and should not be trusted as the sole indicator. Normal breathing rate is about 17 breaths per minute.

Early signs of inadequate breathing are dizziness; headache; memory problems; pounding in the ears; rapid pulse; and cold, clammy skin. A minute later a light-skinned person may start to appear blue; the blueness can be seen in dark-skinned people in the fingernails, or in the edges of the inner membranes of the lips and eyelids. Further, pupils may dilate, breathing and pulse may be stopped or irregular, heartbeat may cease, and the person may lose consciousness. Appearance may differ among individuals; some appear bluish black or pale. A cherry red color indicates carbon monoxide suffocation. Death occurs in over 50 percent of people within five minutes after breathing stops; almost all others die within about ten minutes.

Drowning victims need breathing assistance. Before trying to move the victim completely out of the water, unless the water is so deep that you must do so, force air into the lungs with about ten breaths, using more pressure than normal to blow air past the water in the lungs. After the ten breaths have been delivered, move the victim out of the water, and undertake the breathing assistance as described above. The Heimlich maneuver has been recommended by some to reduce the amount of water in the lungs, but others consider it dangerous because it may cause vomiting, which can obstruct the lungs in an unconscious person. In any case, don't waste too much time trying to remove water while the lungs are starving for air—force air into them. It is normal for the victim to vomit water from the stomach in the recovery from drowning; turn the victim's head to the side to prevent choking.

TREATING FOR SHOCK

The condition called traumatic shock follows all injuries, including drownings. Its severity depends partly on the extent of physical injury and on the amount of blood lost, and partly on the victim's nervous system characteristics. Rough treatment, delayed treatment, emotional reactions, and pain worsen it. Every injury victim should be treated for shock as the third matter of business—bleeding first, then breathing, then treatment for shock.

Traumatic shock is not related to electric shock, diabetic shock, or others, but those medical conditions can certainly bring it on. Traumatic shock is a last-resort attempt by the body to save itself in the event of severe injury, to conserve the body's total blood supply by rerouting it from bleeding outer tissues to pools in the great vessels of the body. As circulation slows, vital

TABLE C–3 Treatment of Shock

1. Lay the victim flat to facilitate circulation. Elevate only those body parts that have been treated for bleeding. The feet may be raised slightly by resting them on a folded blanket or other object.
2. Loosen any constricting clothing, particularly collars, belts, and waistbands.
3. Regulate the victim's body temperature by covering with blankets and inserting padding such as spare clothing between the victim's body and the surface beneath.
4. If the victim is conscious and has no abdominal or head injuries, and if help is not likely to arrive within an hour, giving room-temperature fluids can help. Give small amounts—no more than half a glass—every 15 minutes, for as long as the victim accepts them. If salt is available, add a light sprinkle (not more than 1/8 tsp) to each half glass of fluid.

organs become starved for blood and for the oxygen that it carries—a condition as dangerous as breathing obstruction. People whose injuries would not have killed them have died of shock.

In shock, the victim's pulse becomes weak and rapid, and the skin becomes pale or mottled or bluish, cold, and clammy. Breathing becomes irregular, and the person feels weak. The pupils may dilate. The treatment for shock is relatively simple, and Table C–3 gives the details.

HEART ATTACK ASSISTANCE

The three first aid measures described above are basic to almost any injury or sudden illness, but there is much more to know about specific injuries, binding fractured bones, transporting victims, administering aid to a heart attack victim, and other specifics. It is worthwhile to note that heart attack and stroke victims are especially in need of help, even though their pain may be slight, and they may deny that a heart attack or stroke is occurring. Most heart attack victims die within an hour of the onset of symptoms, before professional help can be delivered. If you notice any of the symptoms of heart attack or stroke listed in Chapter 16, you should:

■ Call an emergency rescue service, and tell them to bring oxygen (or transport the victim to an emergency treatment facility).
■ Administer the breathing assistance described above when necessary, and treat for shock. Those trained in the chest compression technique called cardiopulmonary resuscitation (CPR) can do much more to prolong life after heart attack until professional help is available, but *the untrained should not attempt it.*

This appendix will cover four more emergencies where special help is needed: burns, hypothermia (cold stress), poisoning (including drug overdose), and emergency childbirth. There are many more, and you would be wise to seek out a first aid course to teach you what to do in case something unforeseen should befall you or someone near you.

TREATING BURNS

Burns are classified by the depth of the tissue injury. First-degree burns injure just the top layers of skin and appear as redness, with mild swelling and pain; they heal rapidly. A light sunburn and a mild scald are examples.

TABLE C–4 Standard Treatments for Burns

To treat first-degree burns:

- Submerge the burned part in cold water, or apply gauze soaked in cold water.
- Then, if exposure to soil is likely, layer dry gauze over the wet gauze to create a barrier to microbes.
- Never apply grease of any kind to any burn.

To treat second-degree burns:

- Treat as described above for first-degree burns, and seek medical treatment. Do not break blisters; remove tissue; or use antiseptic spray, cream, or any other product.
- Elevate burned part.

To treat third-degree burns:

- Elevate the burned part, especially the extremities.
- Cover the burn with many layers of sterile gauze.
- An ice pack with a dry surface may be applied to the burn, but do not apply water.
- Treat for shock, and arrange transportation to an emergency medical facility.
- Do not attempt to remove clothing or debris from the burn.

Second-degree burns involve deeper tissue damage and appear red or mottled, develop blisters, swell considerably, and are wet at the surface. A deep sunburn, flash burn from flammable fluid ignition, or contact with very hot liquid can cause second-degree burns. Third-degree burns involve deep tissue destruction and have a white or charred appearance; sometimes third-degree burns will appear to be second degree at first. Flame, ignited clothing, prolonged contact with hot fluids or objects, or electricity can all cause third-degree burns. Table C–4 shows the standard treatments for first-, second-, and third-degree burns.

TREATING HYPOTHERMIA

Hypothermia (literally, "low heat") is a condition marked by an abnormally low internal body temperature. It develops when body heat is lost to the environment faster than it can be replaced. As described in Chapter 14, a susceptible person in a cool room can develop hypothermia; the temperature of the surroundings does not have to be anywhere near freezing for the condition to occur. Susceptible people include older people who live alone, who do not shiver in response to cold, or who take certain medicines that interfere with their temperature-regulating mechanisms. Thousands of older people probably die of hypothermia each year; it affects about 10 percent of all persons over 65.

The signs of hypothermia include stiff muscles, with some trembling; shivering; puffy face; cold skin; problems with coordination; slowed breathing and heart rate; and pale or splotchy skin. As hypothermia progresses, the person may become confused and seem apathetic. If you suspect hypothermia, call an ambulance or rescue squad immediately; and while waiting for help, be careful not to do anything to make the victim's condition worse. Do *not* handle the person roughly (the heart is weak when the body is cold); do not attempt to rewarm the person with hot baths, electric blankets, or hot water bottles; and do not offer any food or drink. If the person is unconscious, do not raise the feet or legs, for the blood there is cooler than in other parts of the body and can further chill the body's core. Do wrap the person in available covering such as blankets, towels, pillows, scarves, or newspapers. Hypothermia is a dangerous, complicated medical problem, and the victim needs professional attention, so try to obtain help promptly.

TREATING POISONING

Any adverse effect on the body from a chemical substance is considered poisoning, from an overdose of drugs to chemical burns of the eyes. Poisonings pose difficult problems for those administering first aid, because they vary in symptoms and treatments according to the substance involved.

The most common household poisonings involve overdoses of aspirin or other over-the-counter pain relievers, eaten by children or taken by mistake by adults. In this case, if the victim is conscious, administer syrup of ipecac to induce vomiting, then give activated charcoal and transport the victim to an emergency facility. (Ipecac itself is a poison and some experts warn against its use. If you use it, follow label directions strictly.) This sequence is adequate for overdoses of most medications taken by mouth. If poisons are taken by injection, assistance in breathing may be required; it is always necessary to treat for shock and to seek immediate emergency assistance. Chapter 14 discussed ways of preventing poisonings. Table C–5 lists the

---

TABLE C–5 First Aid for Poisonings

If poisoning by mouth is suspected:
- If the victim is conscious, administer a glass of milk or water to dilute the poison while you get information.
- Try to identify the substance involved; read the labels of bottles, or ask the person.
- Call the nearest poison control center and ask how to treat the poisoning—what to administer, and when.
- Save any containers, as well as samples of any vomited material for inspection by emergency personnel.

If the poison was inhaled:
- Remove the person from the source of the gas to fresh air.
- Open all doors and windows.
- Treat skin and eyes as necessary, and call for an emergency rescue unit.
- Administer breathing assistance, if necessary.

If the poison is on the skin:
- Remove clothing that has been contaminated, and flood the affected skin for ten minutes with water. A shower works well for large areas. While flooding the skin, call the emergency rescue unit.
- After ten minutes, wash the affected area with soap and water.
- For rashes from poisonous plants, wash the affected area and all clothing with soap and water, dry the rash, and apply calamine lotion. Seek medical treatment if the reaction is severe.

If the poison is in the eye:
- Flood the eye with water (body temperature, if possible) for 15 minutes. Do this by having the victim lean over a water fountain or under a faucet or shower and allow a gentle flow to run through the affected eye, while blinking as much as possible. Direct the flow away from the nose. If no faucet is available, pour water from a cup or other object over the eye repeatedly for 15 minutes. After first aid has started, call an emergency rescue unit.

basic first aid steps for each type of poisoning, but there are hundreds of possible causes and treatments. An essential measure is to find out what chemical is involved, by reading the labels or by asking the person; then contact professionals at a poison control center for advice on how to proceed in each specific case. If the chemicals are illegally obtained drugs, do not try to protect the victim from legal action by not calling for help—the legalities are small when compared with loss of life.

EMERGENCY CHILDBIRTH

If you are in the presence of a woman who is delivering an infant without health care assistance, and you are truly beyond reach of medical help, she may want you to assist her. First, be absolutely certain that you are indeed outside of reach of medical assistance. If you can, summon whatever medical professional you are able to contact. While waiting for help to arrive, remember: childbirth is not like drowning or other dangerous medical emergencies. It is a normal body function, and women deliver babies every day around the world, with or without help. Your main function is to offer comfort to the woman, make sure the newborn is breathing, and clean up. Here's how:

■ Childbirth is messy. Spread clean sheets, towels or paper for the delivery.

■ Allow the woman to choose her own most comfortable position; provide props for her to lean on, if she desires them.

■ Once she is settled, encourage her to use a bedpan or other container for urinating or moving the bowels, rather than moving to a toilet. It is common for the woman to urinate or defecate during the delivery. If this happens, remove the soiled coverings or just cover them up with fresh ones.

■ Wash your hands with soap and water. Refrain from cleaning any part of the woman, especially around the vagina.

■ Expect the delivery to more or less follow the course described in Chapter 12. Do not interfere; do not pull or push on the infant; do not be upset if the woman yells out from her contractions. The condition is temporary and normal. Give encouragement.

■ Upon delivery, your first aid skills can come in handy. Make sure the newborn is breathing; clear away any obstruction blocking the airway. If the amniotic sac hasn't broken, break it gently, and uncover the baby's face. Use a clean cloth that doesn't leave particles to wipe the baby's face, but don't wipe the rest of the body.

■ Chances are it won't happen, but if the umbilical cord has wrapped around the baby's neck during delivery, ask the woman to stop pushing so that you can unwrap it. Slip the loop over the baby's head. Observe the baby for breathing after birth, and provide mouth-to-mouth assistance if no breathing has begun. Cover the infant's nose and mouth with your mouth.

■ Let the umbilical cord and the placenta be expelled naturally; put no tension on the cord. The cord contains blood that belongs to the baby and won't allow any back flow out of the baby's body, so you needn't cut it. Lightly wrap it up with the infant and placenta in a clean cloth for the health care professionals to deal with. If it will be a day or so before help arrives, wait until the cord stops pulsating to cut it (there's no hurry).

Tie a clean string or strip of gauze tightly around it 6 inches from the infant's body; place another tie an inch or so closer to the placenta, and cut between them with a clean knife.

■ Preserve the placenta for inspection by a health professional.

■ Place the baby near the mother; wipe the woman dry with clean cloth, and provide fluids or blankets if she requests them. Keep them both warm and dry. The baby may nurse and should be allowed to do so; nursing triggers contractions that shrink the woman's uterus and prevent excessive bleeding.

If you are convinced that the labor and delivery are not proceeding normally, make the woman as comfortable as possible, and transport her to the nearest emergency facility.

Chapter and Spotlight References

Chapter 1   Health Information and Behavior

1. N. B. Belloc and L. Breslow, Relationship of physical health status and health practices, *Preventive Medicine* 1 (1972): 409–421.

Spotlight 1   The Consumer and Health Quackery

1. U.S. Food and Drug Administration, *The Big Quack Attack: Medical Devices*, HHS publication no. (FDA) 80–4022, 1980.
2. D. Colburn, Quackery: Medical fraud is proliferating and the FDA can't seem to stop it, *Washington Post National Weekly Edition*, 8 July 1985, pp. 6–7.
3. A. H. Hayes, Jr., as cited by Colburn, 1985.

Chapter 2   Stress and Stress Management

1. The story of Dr. Selye's research into the nature of stress is told in (among others) H. Selye, *The Stress of Life* (New York: McGraw-Hill, 1956; rev. ed. 1976).
2. L. Sklar and H. Anisman, Stress and coping factors influence tumor growth, *Science* 205 (1979): 513–515.
3. P. W. Landfield, R. K. Baskin, and T. A. Pitler, Brain aging correlates: Retardation by hormonal-pharmacological treatments, *Science* 214 (1981): 581–584.
4. R. M. Sapolsky, L. C. Krey, and B. S. McEwen, The adrenocortical stress-response in the aged male rat: Impairment of recovery from stress, *Experimental Gerontology* 18 (1983): 55–64. A physical correlate of these alterations in function is a decline in the number of stress hormone receptors in specific sites; R. M. Sapolsky, L. C. Krey, and B. S. McEwen, Corticosterone receptors decline in a site-specific manner in the aged rat brain, *Brain Research* 289 (1983): 235–240.
5. H. Benson, *The Relaxation Response* (New York: Morrow, 1975).

Spotlight 2   Faith and Healing

1. N. Cousins, Anatomy of an illness (as perceived by the patient), *New England Journal of Medicine* 295 (1976): 1458–63. The sequel, which explores further the attitudes of physicians and patients and the importance of the patients' involvement in their own cure, is also stimulating reading: N. Cousins, What I learned from 3,000 doctors, *Saturday Review*, 18 February 1978, pp. 12–16.
2. O. Fennema, The placebo effect of foods, *Food Technology*, December 1984, pp. 37–67.
3. A.M. Gill, Pain and healing of peptic ulcer, *Lancet*, 8 March 1947, p. 291.
4. E. M. Widdowson, Mental contentment and physical growth, *Lancet* 1 (1951): 1316–1318.
5. Dr. Herbert Benson of the Beth Israel Hospital and Harvard Medical School, as quoted by B. Sullivan, Placebo effect: Medicine losing a valuable tool, *Miami Herald*, 8 April 1981, p. E1.
6. N. Chesanow, Is it time to take psychic healing seriously? *Family Health*, January 1979, pp. 22, 24, 26, 28.

Chapter 3   Emotional Health

1. From L. Raths, H. Merrill, and S. Sidney, *Values and Teaching* (Columbus, Ohio: Merrill, 1966), as cited in S. B. Simon, L. W. Howe, and H. Kirschenbaum, *Values Clarification, A Handbook of Practical Strategies for Teachers and Students*, rev. ed. (New York: Hart, 1978) p. 19.
2. H. Kirschenbaum, Current research in value clarification, in *Advanced Value Clarification* (La Jolla, Calif.: University Associates, 1977), as cited in Simon, Howe, and Kirschenbaum, p. 20.
3. D. E. Hamachek, *Encounters with the Self* (New York: Holt, Rinehart and Winston, 1971), pp. 248–251.
4. How your looks shape your life, *Parade*, 4 July 1982, pp. 11–12.

5. E. Erikson, *Childhood and Society* (New York: Norton, 1963).
6. A classic transactional analysis reference is E. Berne, *Games People Play: The Psychology of Human Relationships* (New York: Grove, 1964).
7. A. Maslow, *Toward a Psychology of Being* (Princeton, N.J.: Van Nostrand, 1968).
8. G. Sheehy, *Passages: Predictable Crises of Adult Life* (New York: Dutton, 1976).
9. J. Powell, *Why Am I Afraid to Tell You Who I Am?* (Chicago, Argus Communications, 1969).
10. A. C. Wassmer, *Making Contact* (New York: Dial, 1978), as cited in A. F. Grasha and D. S. Kirschenbaum, *Psychology of Adjustment and Competence* (Cambridge, Mass.: Whinthrop, 1980), p. 349.
11. R. N. Bolles, *What Color Is Your Parachute?: A Practical Manual for Job-Hunters and Career Changers* (Berkeley, Calif.: Ten Speed Press, 1987; comes out annually).
12. T. J. DeLong, Re-examining the career anchor model, *Journal of the American Dietetic Association* 81 (1981): 365.
13. H. Selye, as cited in Your job—Love it or leave it, *Executive Fitness Newsletter*, 30 December 1978, p. 1.
14. M. LaLonde, *A New Perspective on the Health of Canadians: A Working Document* (Ottawa: Information Canada, 1974), p. 61.
15. *Diagnostic and Statistical Manual of Mental Disorders*, 3rd ed. (Washington, D.C.: American Psychiatric Association, 1980), p. 8; often referred to as *DMS III*.
16. *Diagnostic and Statistical Manual*, 1980, p. 6.
17. A. Linne, A test for depression, *Family Health*, May 1981, pp. 10–11.
18. R. M. Hayden and G. J. Allen, Relationship between aerobic exercise, anxiety, and depression: Convergent validation by knowledgeable informants, *Journal of Sports Medicine* 24 (1984): 69–74.
19. J. H. Griest and coauthors, Running as treatment for depression, *Comprehensive Psychiatry* 20 (1979): 41–54.
20. D. Hales and R. Hales, Using the body to mend the mind, *American Health*, June

1985, first pp. 27–31 (issue contains two sets of pages 27–31).

21. D. J. Higdon, Pumping depression, *American Health*, April 1986, p. 26.

22. National Institute of Mental Health, Plain Talk about Feelings of Guilt (leaflet), DHEW publication no. (ADM) 79–580, 1979.

23. W. Barnhill, Psychiatry you can afford, *Family Health*, March 1981, p. 13.

Spotlight 3   Signals from Within

1. S.P. Dalvit, The effect of the menstrual cycle on patterns of food intake, *American Journal of Clinical Nutrition* 34 (1981): 1811–1815.

2. Treatment with a drug that raises serotonin neurotransmission reduces carbohydrate snack consumption. J. J. Wurtman, The involvement of brain serotonin in excessive carbohydrate snacking by obese carbohydrate cravers, *Journal of the American Dietetic Association* 84 (1984): 1004–1007.

3. E. B. Hook, Dietary cravings and aversions during pregnancy, *American Journal of Clinical Nutrition* 31 (1978): 1355–1362.

4. S. Begley and J. Carey, The clocks inside us, *Newsweek*, 1 December 1980, pp. 109–110.

5. Volunteers were most impaired in tests of reaction time when given alcohol in the morning. N. W. Lawrence, M. Herbert, and W. J. Jeffcoate, Circadian variation in effects of ethanol in man, *Pharmacology, Biochemistry and Behavior* 18 (Supplement 1, 1983): 555–558.

6. M. J. Thompson and D. W. Harsha, Our rhythms still follow the African sun, *Psychology Today*, January 1984, pp. 50–54.

7. D. Levitsky and E. Obarzanek, as cited in Exercising within several hours of eating can burn more kilocalories, *Journal of the American Dietetic Association* 83 (1983): 290.

8. D. Blazer and coauthors, Psychiatric disorders: A rural/urban comparison, *Archives of General Psychiatry* 42 (1985): 651–656.

9. The chapter "The Right Place" in E. O. Wilson's book *Biophilia* (Cambridge, Mass.: Harvard University Press, 1984), pp. 103–118, is especially illuminating on this subject. Studying the elements of natural habitats in this relation is B. Means, executive director, Coastal Plains Institute, Tallahassee, FL (personal communication, May 1985).

Chapter 4   Nutrition

1. Improved nutrition, *Public Health Reports Supplement*, September/October 1983, p. 132.

2. U.S. Department of Health and Human Services, Public Health Service, *Promoting Health, Preventing Disease: Objectives for the Nation* (Washington, D.C.: Government Printing Office, 1980), p. 73.

3. D.R. Gwatkin, How many die? A set of demographic estimates of the annual number of infant and child deaths in the world, *American Journal of Public Health* 70 (1980): 1268–1289.

4. D. Lonsdale and R. J. Shamberger, Red cell transketolase as an indicator of nutritional deficiency, *American Journal of Clinical Nutrition* 33 (1980): 205–211.

5. L.C. Pauling, *Vitamin C and the Common Cold* (San Francisco: W. H. Freeman, 1970).

6. H. Schaumberg and coauthors, Sensory neuropathy from pyridoxine abuse, *New England Journal of Medicine* 309 (1983): 445–448.

7. More B₆ toxicity reported, *Nutrition Forum*, November 1985, p. 84.

8. N. S. Scrimshaw, Functional consequences of iron deficiency in human populations, *Journal of Nutrition Science and Vitaminology* 30 (1984): 47–63.

Spotlight 4   Vitamin Supplements

1. R. L. Koretz and J. H. Meyer, Elemental diets: Facts and fantasies, *Gastroenterology* 78 (1980): 393–410.

2. L. Alhadeff, T. Gualtieri, and M. Lipton, Toxic effects of water-soluble vitamins, *Nutrition Reviews* 42 (1984): 33–40.

Chapter 5   Weight Control

1. G. Kolata, Obesity declared a disease (Research News), *Science* 227 (1985): 1019–1020.

2. T. B. Van Itallie, When the frame is part of the picture (Editorial), *American Journal of Public Health* 75 (1985): 1054–1055.

3. Consensus panel addresses obesity question, *Journal of the American Medical Association* 254 (1985): 1878.

4. T. B. Van Itallie and M. U. Yang, Current concepts in nutrition and diet and weight loss, *New England Journal of Medicine* 297 (1977): 1158–1161; Evaluation of 3 weight-reducing diets, *Nutrition and the MD*, March 1978. An experiment in which fasting caused increased weight loss but decreased fat loss compared with a low-calorie mixed diet was reported in M. F. Ball, J. J. Canary, and L. H. Kyle, Comparative effects of caloric restriction and total starvation on body composition in obesity, *Annals of Internal Medicine* 67 (1967): 60–67.

5. M. Simonton, An overview: Advances in research and treatment of obesity, *Food and Nutrition News*, March/April 1982.

6. The next three sections are adapted from Chapter 8, Energy balance and weight control, in *Understanding Nutrition*, 4th ed., by E. N. Whitney, E. M. N. Hamilton, and M. A. Boyle (St. Paul, Minn.: West, 1987).

Spotlight 5   Anorexia Nervosa and Bulimia

1. K. McCleary, Eating disorders: Daddy dearest, *American Health*, January/February 1986, p. 86.

2. M.A. Balaa and D. A. Drossman, *Anorexia Nervosa and Bulimia: The Eating Disorders*, *Disease a Month* (Chicago: Year Book Medical Publishers, June 1985), p. 38.

3. M. Baskind-Lodahl and J. Sirlin, The gorging-purging syndrome: Bulimarexia, *Psychology Today*, March 1977, pp. 50–52, 82, 85.

4. Balaa and Drossman, 1985, pp. 1–52.

5. H. G. Pope, Jr., J. I. Hudson, and D. Yurgelun-Todd, Anorexia nervosa and bulimia among 300 suburban women shoppers, *American Journal of Psychiatry* 141 (1984): 2, as cited by Balaa and Drossman, 1985.

Chapter 6   Fitness

1. R. S. Paffenbarger and coauthors, Physical activity, allcause mortality, and longevity of college alumni, *New England Journal of Medicine* 314 (1986): 605–613.

2. V. Gurley, A. Neuringer, and J. Massee, Dance and sports compared: Effects on psychological well-being, *Journal of Sports Medicine* 24 (1984): 58–68.

3. K. T. Francis and R. Carter, Psychological characteristics of joggers, *Journal of Sports Medicine* 22 (1982): 386–391; R. M. Hayden and G. J. Allen, Relationship between aerobic exercise, anxiety, and depression: Convergent validation by knowledgeable informants, *Journal of Sports Medicine* 24 (1984): 69–74.

4. Quantity and quality of exercise for developing and maintaining fitness in healthy adults, a position paper of The American College of Sports Medicine, *The Physician and Sportsmedicine* 6 (1978): 39–41.

5. N. E. Lane, D. A. Block, and H. H. Jones, Long distance running, bone density, and osteoarthritis, *Journal of the American Medical Association* 255 (1986): 1147–1151.

6. Quantity and quality of exercise, 1978.

7. S. Rainville and P. Vaccaro, Lipoprotein cholesterol levels, coronary artery disease and regular exercise: A review, *American Corrective Therapy Journal* 37 (1983): 161–165; B. Stamford, Improving coronary circulation, *The Physician and Sportsmedicine* 11 (1983): 163.

8. N. B. Belloc and L. Breslow, Relationship of physical health status and health practices, *Preventive Medicine* 1 (1972): 409–421.

9. K. Jung, Physical exercise therapy in juvenile diabetes mellitus, *Journal of Sports Medicine* 22 (1982): 23–31.

10. D. H.Garabrant and coauthors, Job activity and colon cancer risk, *American Journal of Epidemiology* 119 (1984): 1005–1014.

11. C. M.Tipton, Exercise, training, and hypertension, *Exercise and Sports Sciences Reviews* 12 (1984): 245–306.

12. J. G. Cannon and M. J. Kluger, Exercise enhances survival rate in mice infected with *Salmonella typhimurium*, *Proceedings of the Society for Experimental Biology and*

Medicine 175 (1984): 518–521; H. B. Simon, The immunology of exercise, *Journal of the American Medical Association* 252 (1984): 2735–2738; A. Viti and coauthors, Effect of exercise on plasma interferon levels, *Journal of Applied Physiology*, August 1985, pp. 426–428.

13. K. E.Powell and coauthors, Status of the 1990 objectives for physical fitness and exercise, *Public Health Reports*, 101 (1986): 15–19.

14. Some of the ideas presented here are from G. B. Dintiman and coauthors, *Discovering Lifetime Fitness* (St. Paul, Minn.: West, 1984).

15. C. A.Milesis, M. G. Fougeron, and H. Graham, Effect of active vs. passive recovery on cardiac time components, *Journal of Sports Medicine* 22 (1982): 147–153.

16. B. Anderson, *Stretching* (Bolinas, Calif.: Shelter, 1980). p. 12.

17. K. Hakkinen, M. Alen, and P. V. Komi, Neuromuscular, anaerobic, and aerobic performance characteristics of elite power athletes, *European Journal of Applied Physiology* 53 (1984): 97–105.

18. American College of Sports Medicine, Principles of exercise testing, in *Guidelines for Exercise Testing and Prescription* (Philadelphia: Lea & Febiger, 1986), pp. 34–35, 43.

19. C. E. Thompson and coauthors, Response of HDL cholesterol, apoprotein A-1, and LCAT to exercise withdrawal, *Atherosclerosis* 54 (1985): 65–73.

20. This discussion of food for the athlete is adapted from Controversy 7, Do athletes need a special diet? in *Nutrition: Concepts and Controversies*, 3rd ed., by E. M. N. Hamilton, E. N. Whitney, and F. S. Sizer (St. Paul, Minn.: West, 1985), pp. 178–185.

21. H. Haupt and G. D. Rovere, Anabolic steroids: A review of the literature, *American Journal of Sports Medicine* 12 (1984): 469–484; D. R. Lamb, Anabolic steroids in athletics: How well do they work and how dangerous are they? *American Journal of Sports Medicine* 12 (1984): 31–38; O. L. Webb, P. M. Laskarzewski, and C. J. Glueck, Severe depression of high-density lipoprotein cholesterol levels in weight lifters and body builders by self-administered exogenous testosterone and anabolic-androgenic steroids, *Metabolism* 33 (1984): 971–975; M. Alen and P. Rahkila, Reduced high-density lipoprotein-cholesterol in power athletes: use of male sex hormone derivatives, an atherogenic factor, *International Journal of Sports Medicine* 5 (1984): 341–342.

22. P. Astrand, Something old and something new . . . very new, *Nutrition Today*, June 1968, pp. 9–11.

23. G. R. Hagerman, Nutrition in part-time athletes, *Nutrition and the MD*, August 1981.

24. K. Keller and R. Schwarzkopf, Preexercise snacks may decrease exercise performance, *The Physician and Sportsmedicine* 12 (1984): 89–91.

25. J. Bergstrom and E. Hultman, Nutrition for maximal sports performance, *Journal of the American Medical Association* 221 (1972): 999.

26. F. T. O'Neil, M. T. Hynak-Hankinson, and J. Gorman, Research and application of current topics in sports nutrition, *Journal of the American Dietetic Association* 86 (1986): 1007–1015.

Spotlight 6   Sleep

1. J. Willis, On making it through the night, *FDA Consumer*, September 1979, pp. 4–7.

2. Willis, 1979.

3. P. Gunby, A drink a night keeps good slumber at bay (Medical News), *Journal of the American Medical Association* 246 (1981): 589.

4. Willis, 1979.

Chapter 7   Medicines, Other Drugs, and Drug Abuse

1. C. L. Thomas, ed., *Taber's Cyclopedic Medical Dictionary*, 14th ed. (Philadelphia: Davis, 1981), p. 431.

2. F. Taylor, Aspirin: America's favorite drug, *FDA Consumer*, December 1980/January 1981, pp. 12–16.

3. J. Henningfield, Addiction Research Center, National Institute of Drug Abuse, as cited by D. D. Edwards, Nicotine: A drug of choice? *Science News*, 18 January 1986, pp. 44–45.

4. Thomas, 1981, p. 32.

5. A. Smiley and coauthors, Effects of drugs on driving: Driving simulator tests of secobarbital, diazepam, marijuana, and alcohol, *Clinical and Behavioral Pharmacology Research Report*, DHHS publication no. (ADM) 85–1386, 1985.

6. G. T. Johnson, Marijuana: What are the risks? *Harvard Medical School Health Letter*, June 1980, pp. 1–3; D. Pine, Hungover driving, *Health*, May 1984, p. 12.

7. A. Hecht, Drugs and driving, *FDA Consumer*, September 1978, pp. 17–19.

8. M. S. Kramer, L. Naimark, and D. G. Leduc, Parental fever phobia and its correlates, *Pediatrics* 75 (1985): 1110–1113.

9. H. D. Jampel and coauthors, Fever and immunoregulation III: Hyperthermia augments the primary in vitro humoral immune response, *Journal of Experimental Medicine* 157 (1983): 1229–1238.

10. Many of the rules presented here are from U.S. Food and Drug Administration, *Selecting Your Own Medicine*, HHS publication no. (FDA) 76–3026, April 1980 (a leaflet available from the FDA Office of Public Affairs, 5600 Fishers Lane, Rockville, MD 20857).

11. Tidbits and morsels, *Nutrition and the MD*, January 1979, p. 6.

12. B. McPherrin, Mail order health fraud, *ACSH News and Views* September/October 1980, p. 10.

13. Ginseng abuse syndrome, *Nutrition and the MD*, September 1979, p. 4.

14. McPherrin, 1980.

15. R. O'Brien and S. Cohen, *The Encyclopedia of Drug Abuse* (New York: Facts on File, 1984), p. 1.

16. Thomas, 1981, p. 431.

17. G. M. Smith, Adolescent personality traits that predict young adult drug use, *Comprehensive Therapy* 12 (1986): 44–50.

18. Among many studies that show cocaine to be an effective reinforcer: T. G. Aigner and R. L. Balster, Choice behavior in rhesus monkeys: Cocaine vs. food, *Science* 201 (1978): 534–535.

19. N. Bejerot, *Addiction, an Artificially Induced Drive* (Springfield, Ill.: Charles C. Thomas, 1972), p. 5.

20. Bejerot, 1972, p. 19.

21. F. Bruno, Conclusions, remarks, perspectives and policy implications, in *Combatting Drug Abuse and Related Crime: Comparative Research on the Effectiveness of Socio-legal Preventive and Control Measures in Different Countries on the Interaction between Criminal Behavior and Drug Abuse* (Rome: Fratelli Palombi Editori, 1984), p. 160.

22. E. Hollister, Health effects of cannabis, *Pharmacological Reviews* 38, March 1986, pp. 1–20.

23. C. R. Creason and M. Goldman, Varying levels of marijuana use by adolescents and the amotivational syndrome, *Psychological Reports* 48 (1981): 447–454.

24. M. W. Fischman and C. R. Schuster, Cocaine selfadministration in humans, *Federation Proceedings* 41 (1982): 241–246.

25. From a self-administered questionnaire in a study of cocaine users by M. S. Gold, *800-Cocaine* (New York: Bantam, 1984), pp. 10–11. The book title is actually a national cocaine hotline number, 1–800-COCAINE.

26. Gold, 1984.

27. *The Case of the Frozen Addict*, a transcript of a "Nova" program, 18 February 1986, available from WGBH Transcripts, 125 Western Ave., Boston, MA 02134.

28. The list of symptoms of drug abuse comes from a letter to Ann Landers, *Tallahassee Democrat*, 14 January 1986.

Spotlight 7   Caffeine

1. G. A. Pincomb, W. R. Lovallo, and R. B. Passey, Effects of caffeine on vascular resistance, cardiac output and myocardial contractility in young men, *American Journal of Cardiology* 56 (1985): 119–122.

Chapter 8   Alcohol: Use and Abuse

1. W. J. Darby, The benefits of drink, *Human Nature*, November 1978, pp. 31–37.

2. K. Yano, G. G. Rhoads, and A. Kagan, Coffee, alcohol, and risk of coronary heart disease among Japanese men living in Hawaii, *New England Journal of Medicine* 297 (1977): 405–409.
3. Darby, 1978.
4. Tougher alcohol rules urged, *Tallahassee Democrat*, 18 February 1986.
5. D. Pine, hungover driving, *Health*, May 1984, p. 12.
6. *Facts on Alcoholism.*
7. G. Mirkin, The dynamics of drinking, *Health*, July/August 1981, pp. 44–45, 58.
8. C. S. Lieber and L. M. DeCarli, Animal models of ethanol dependence and liver injury in rats and baboons, *Federation Proceedings* 35 (1976): 1232–1236.
9. Getting pickled, *Scientific American*, April 1985, p. 76.
10. Alcohol-induced brain damage and its reversibility, *Nutrition Reviews* 38 (1980): 11–12; L. A. Cala and coauthors, Alcohol-related brain damage: Serial studies after abstinence and recommencement of drinking, *Australian Alcohol/Drug Review*, July 1984, pp. 127–140.
11. E. S. Pollack and coauthors, Prospective study of alcohol consumption and cancer, *New England Journal of Medicine* 310 (1984): 617.
12. Roe, 1984.
13. M. J. Eckardt and coauthors, Health hazards associated with alcohol consumption, *Journal of the American Medical Association* 246 (1981): 648–666.
14. E. Rubin, The "social" drinker (Questions and Answers), *Journal of the American Medical Association* 248 (1982): 2179.
15. E. S. Geller, in a study of 256 college students, as cited in S. Cunningham, Drunker by the pitcher, *Psychology Today*, March 1985, p. 80.
16. Some of the items in this list were adapted from *How to Be a Good Host: A Guide to Responsible Drinking*, a booklet available from the Bureau of Alcoholic Rehabilitation, P.O. Box 1147, Avon Park, FL 33825.
17. Adapted from the beauty of moderation, *Executive Fitness Newsletter*, 13 June 1981.
18. Adapted from U.S. Department of Health and Human Services, *Thinking about Drinking*, DHHS publication no. (ADM) 74–27, 1974.
19. One less for the road? *Time*, 20 May 1985, pp. 77–78.
20. Partly excerpted from *How to Be a Good Host*.

Spotlight 8   Alcoholism, the Disease

1. A. Silverstein and V. B. Silverstein, *Alcoholism* (Philadelphia: Lippincott, 1975), pp. 61–68.
2. P. Finn and P. A. O'Gorman, *Teaching about Alcohol* (Boston: Allyn and Bacon, 1981), p. 31.
3. M. J. Eckardt and coauthors, Health hazards associated with alcohol consumption, *Journal of the American Medical Association* 246 (1981): 648–666.
4. N. Bejerot, *Addiction: An Artificially Induced Drive* (Springfield, Ill.: Charles C. Thomas, 1972), p. 27.

Chapter 9   Smoking and Smokeless Tobacco

1. A redeeming quality in tobacco? *Health*, November/December 1981, p. 6.
2. R. Keeshan, Children and smoking, in *Smoking and Health*, proceedings of a conference commemorating the 20th anniversary of the first Surgeon General's Report on Smoking and Health, 11 January 1984, available from the American Council on Science and Health, 47 Maple St., Summit, NJ 07901.
3. *Tobacco Abuse*, a 1978 leaflet available from the Do It Now Foundation, Institute for Chemical Survival, P.O. Box 5115, Phoenix, AZ 85010.
4. These items are adapted from U.S. Department of Health and Human Services, *8 Reasons Young People Smoke*, HHS publication no. 200–75–0516, 1975.
5. Adapted from W. Pollin, Addiction is the key step in causation of all tobacco-related diseases (editorial), *World Smoking and Health*, Spring 1985, pp. 2–3.
6. O. F. Pomerleau and C. S. Pomerleau, Neuroregulators and the reinforcement of smoking: Toward a biobehavioral explanation, *Neuroscience and Biobehavioral Reviews* 8 (1984): 503–513.
7. W. Bennett, The nicotine fix, *Harvard Magazine*, July/August 1980, pp. 10–14; *Diagnostic and Statistical Manual of Mental Disorders*, 3rd ed. (Washington, D.C.: American Psychiatric Association, 1980), pp. 159–160.
8. C. B. Popescu, Cigarettes' secret ingredients, *ACSH News and Views*, January/February 1983, pp. 1–3.
9. D. Sogn, The effects of smoking, in *Inadvertent Modification of the Immune Response, the Effects of Foods, Drugs, and Environmental Contaminants: Proceedings of the Fourth FDA Science Symposium*, ed. I. M. Asher (Washington, D.C.: Government Printing Office, 1978), pp. 160–162.
10. J. Saltman, Emphysema: The growing problem of breathlessness, Public Affairs Pamphlet no. 326C, 3rd revised ed., 1983 (available from the American Lung Association, 381 Park Ave. South, New York, NY 10016.)
11. C. B. Popescu, Cigarettes and asbestos: A tale of two industries, *ACSH News and Views*, March/April 1983, pp. 1–3; Report: Smoking is riskier for workers than workplace exposure to hazardous substances, *Tallahassee Democrat*, 20 December 1985.
12. A. E. Reif, The causes of cancer, *American Scientist* 69 (1981): 437–447.
13. C. B. Popescu, Equal opportunity death? *ACSH News and Views*, November/December 1983, pp. 3, 14.
14. R. Cooper and B. E. Simmons, Cigarette smoking and ill health among black Americans, *New York State Journal of Medicine*, July 1985, pp. 344–349.
15. U. S. Department of Health and Human Services, Public Health Service, *Promoting Health, Preventing Disease: Objectives for the Nation* (Washington, D.C.: Government Printing Office, 1980), pp. 107–108.
16. J. W. Kikendall and coauthors, Effects of cigarette smoking on gastrointestinal physiology and non-neoplastic digestive disease, *Journal of Clinical Gastroenterology* 6 (1984): 65–78.
17. Drug effects can go up in smoke, *FDA Consumer*, March 1979 (reprint).
18. U. S. Department of Health and Human Services, 1980, pp. 107–108.
19. A. C. Higgins, Nutritional status and the outcome of pregnancy, *Journal of the Canadian Dietetic Association* 37 (1976): 17, abstracted in *Journal of the American Dietetic Association* 68 (1976): 580.
20. F. S. Anderson, I. Transbol, and C. Christiansen, Is cigarette smoking a promoter of the menopause? *Acta Medica Scandinavica* 212 (1982): 137–139.
21. D. J. Weeks, Do chronic cigarette smokers forget people's names? *British Medical Journal*, 22–29 December, 1979, p. 1627.
22. C. R. Soldatos and coauthors, Cigarette smoking associated with sleep difficulty, *Science* 207 (1980): 551–553.
23. Note what a cigarette packs in radiation (Correspondence), *New England Journal of Medicine* 307 (1982): 309–313.
24. H. J. Evans and coauthors, Sperm abnormalities and cigarette smoking, *Lancet*, 21 March 1981, pp. 627–629.
25. A. S. Ibrahim and A. S. Fatt-hi, Cigarette smoking and hearing loss, *World Smoking and Health*, Summer 1982, pp. 42–45.
26. A. I. Ismail, B. A. Burt, and S. A. Eklund, Epidemiologic patterns of smoking and periodontal disease in the United States, *World Smoking and Health*, Spring 1985, pp. 14–15.
27. Tobacco Institute: Cigarette fires human behavior problems, *Nation's Health*, October 1981.
28. "Unknown" risks of smoking, *Nation's Health*, July 1981.
29. Keeshan, 1984.
30. K. McCusker, E. McNabb, and R. Bone, Plasma nicotine levels in pipe smokers, *Journal of the American Medical Association* 248 (1982): 577–578; T. Pechacek and coauthors, Smoke exposure in pipe and cigar smokers: Serum thiocyanate levels, *Journal of the American Medical Association* 254 (1985): 3330–3332.
31. J. F. Bertram, M. E. Jones, and A. W. Rogers, Does structural recovery of bronchial epithelium follow the cessation of smoking? abstract cited in *Journal of Anatomy* 133 (1981): 479.
32. T. Hirayama, Passive smoking and lung cancer: Consistency of association, *Lancet*, 17 December 1983, pp. 1425–1426; D.

Trichopoulos and coauthors, Lung cancer and passive smoking, *International Journal of Cancer* 27 (1981): 1–4; L. Garfinkel, O. Auerbach, and L. Joubert, Involuntary smoking and lung cancer: A case-control study, *Journal of the National Cancer Institute* 75 (1975): 463–469.

33. K. A. Meister, Other people's cigarette smoke: The *real* whole story, *ACSH News and Views*, November/December 1981, p. 12.

34. *Risks for a Second-Hand Smoker*, a pamphlet prepared in consultation with former U.S. Surgeons General L. L. Terry, J. L. Steinfeld, and others by the Non-Smoker's Rights Association, 455 Spadina Ave., Suite 426A, Toronto, Ontario, M55 2G8, Canada.

35. G. N. Connolly and coauthors, The reemergence of smokeless tobacco, *New England Journal of Medicine* 314 (1986): 1020–1027.

36. A. G. Christen, The case against smokeless tobacco, Five facts for the health professional to consider, *Journal of the American Dental Association* 101 (1980): 464–469.

37. A. G. Christen, W. R. Armstrong, and R. K. McDaniel, Intraoral leukoplakia, abrasion, periodontal breakdown, and tooth loss in a snuff dipper, *Journal of the American Dental Association* 98 (1979): 584–586.

38. U.S. Department of Health and Human Services, 1980, pp. 107–108.

39. R. M. Carney and A. P. Goldberg, Weight gain after cessation of cigarette smoking: A possible role for adipose-tissue lipoprotein lipase, *New England Journal of Medicine* 310 (1984): 614–616.

40. Help wanted: No smokers need apply, *ACSH News and Views*, September/October 1982, p. 7.

Spotlight 9   Tobacco Advertising and Ethics

1. Is Liberty Worth Writing For? (advertisement).

2. Doctors Ought to Care (DOC) and Tobacco Products Liability Project (TPLP), Law Student Essay Competition (advertisement), *The Nation* 243, 13 December 1986, p. 688.

3. H. L. Sarokin, as cited in Three tobacco companies lose bid for mistrial, *Tallahassee Democrat*, 23 April 1988.

4. Sarokin, 1988.

5. Tobacco suit may be Pandora' box, *Tallahassee Democrat*, 18 January 1988.

6. DOC and TPLP, 1986.

7. DOC and TPLP, 1986.

Chapter 10   Intimacy, Pairing, and Commitment

1. I. Dierderen and L. Rorer, Do attitudes and background influence college students' sexual behavior? unpublished, presented at the American Psychological Association (1982), Washington, D.C.

2. B. Nicholson, Does kissing aid human bonding by semiochemical addiction? *British Journal of Dermatology* 3 (1984): 623–627.

3. H. Alzate, Vaginal eroticism and female orgasm: A current appraisal, *Journal of Sex and Marital Therapy*, Winter 1985, pp. 271–284.

4. L.R. Schover and J. LoPiccolo, Treatment effectiveness for dysfunctions of sexual desire, *Journal of Sex and Marital Therapy* 8 (1982): 179–197.

5. J.D. Chapman, Neuroendocrinologic developments in sexuality: Beta-endorphins in sexual desire phase disorders, *Journal of the American Osteopathic Association* 84 (1984): 368–371; J. D. Chapman, Sexual anhedonia: Disorders of sexual desire, *Journal of the American Osteopathic Association* 82 (Supplement, 1983): 709–714.

6. A. Hecht, Aphrodisiacs, *FDA Consumer*, December/January 1982–1983, p. 11.

7. W.H. Masters, V. E. Johnson, and R. C. Kolodny, *Human Sexuality*, 2nd ed. (Boston: Little, Brown, 1985), pp. 524–525.

8. M. Hughes and W. R. Gove, Living alone, social integration, and mental health, *American Journal of Sociology*, July 1981, pp. 48–74.

9. Hughes and Gove, 1981.

10. J. Bernard, *The Future of Marriage* (New Haven, Conn.: Yale University Press, 1982), pp. 3–53.

11. L. Cargan and M. Melko, *Singles: Myths and Realities* (Beverly Hills, Calif.: Sage, 1982), pp. 111–114.

12. W. G. Perry, Jr., *Forms of Intellectual and Ethical Development in the College Years: A Scheme* (New York: Holt, Rinehart and Winston, 1970).

13. C.R. Rogers, *Becoming Partners* (New York: Dell, 1972), pp. 199–202.

Spotlight 10   Gender and Power

1. R. LaRossa, A conflict approach to marriage: The problem of social order, *Conflict and Power in Marriage: Expecting the First Child* (Beverly Hills, Calif.: Sage, 1977), pp. 125–148.

2. L. Haas, Role-sharing couples: A study of egalitarian marriages, *Family Relations*, July 1980, pp. 289–296.

3. L.A. Peplau, Power in dating relationships, in J. Freeman, ed., *Women: A Feminist Perspective*, 2nd ed. (Palo Alto, Calif.: Mayfield, 1979), pp. 106–121.

4. T. L. Ruble, Sex stereotypes: Issues of change in the 1970s, *Sex Roles*, March 1983, pp. 397–402.

Chapter 11   Conception, Infertility, and Family Planning

1. J. M. Tanner, *Foetus into Man: Physical Growth from Conception to Maturity* (London: Open Books Publishing, 1978), pp. 36–51.

2. J. A. Collins and coauthors, Treatment-independent pregnancy among infertile couples, *New England Journal of Medicine* 309 (1983): 1201–1206.

3. F. F. Furstenberg, Jr., The social consequences of teenage parenthood, in *Adolescent Pregnancy and Childbearing: Findings from Research*, ed. C. S. Chilman, NIH publication no. 81–2077, 1980, pp. 267–308; National Technical Information Service, *Adolescent Pregnancy and Childbearing: Rates, Trends, and Research Findings from the CPR*, National Institute of Child Health and Human Development, 1984 (a paper available from NTIS, 5285 Port Royal Rd., Springfield, VA 22161).

4. The many sources for ratings of effectiveness do not agree exactly. The ratings listed here are taken from the carefully compiled Table 1.1 of R. A. Hatcher and coauthors, *Contraceptive Technology* (New York: Irvington, 1984), p. 3.

5. S. C. Hartz and coauthors, Factors associated with oral contraceptive use, *American Journal of Public Health* 70 (1980): 1105–1108.

6. The cancer steroid hormone study of the Centers for Disease Control and the National Institute of Child Health and Human Development: The reduction in risk of ovarian cancer associated with oral-contraceptive use, *New England Journal of Medicine* 316 (1987): 650–655.

7. J. Willis, Comparing contraceptives, *FDA Consumer*, May 1985, pp. 28–35.

8. D. W. Kaufman and coauthors, The effect of different intrauterine devices on the risk of pelvic inflammatory disease, *Journal of the American Medical Association* 250 (1983): 759–762.

9. A. J. Reingold, Toxic shock syndrome and the contraceptive sponge (Editorial), *Journal of the American Medical Association* 255 (1986): 242–243.

10. Hatcher and coauthors, 1984, p. 160.

11. J. D. Forrest and S. K. Henshaw, What U.S. women think and do about contraception, *Family Planning Perspectives* 15 (1983): 157–166.

12. Handy, 1982.

13. B. P. Sachs and coauthors, Reproductive mortality in the United States, *Journal of the American Medical Association* 247 (1982): 2789–2792.

14. S. K. Henshaw and coauthors, Abortion services in the United States, 1979 and 1980, *Family Planning Perspectives* 14 (1982): 5–15.

15. C. F. Westoff and coauthors, Abortions preventable by contraceptive practice, *Family Planning Perspectives* 13 (1981): 218–223.

Spotlight 11   Why People Don't Use Contraception

1. L. S. Zabin and coauthors, Adolescent sexual attitudes and behavior: Are they

consistent? *Family Planning Perspectives* 16 (1984): 181–185.

2. C. Lindemann, *Birth Control and Unmarried Young Women* (New York: Springer, 1975), as cited by M. Zelnik and J. F. Kantner, Sexual and contraceptive experience of young unmarried women in the United States, 1976 and 1971, in *Adolescent Pregnancy and Childbearing: Findings from Research*, ed. C. S. Chilman, NIH publication no. 81–2077, 1980, pp. 43–81.

3. G. Cvetkovich and B. Grote, Psychosocial development and social problems of teenage illegitimacy, in *Adolescent Pregnancy and Childbearing: Findings from Research*, ed. C. S. Chilman, NIH publication no. 81–2077, 1980, pp. 15–41.

4. M. Zelnik and J. F. Kantner, Sexual and contraceptive experience of young unmarried women in the United States, 1976 and 1971, in *Adolescent Pregnancy and Childbearing: Findings from Research*, ed. C. S. Chilman, NIH publication no. 81–2077, 1980, pp. 43–81.

5. Zabin and coauthors, 1984.

6. E. F. Jones and coauthors, Teenage pregnancy in developed countries: Determinants and policy implications, *Family Planning Perspectives* 17 (1985): 53–63.

7. G. P. Spanier, Sources of sex information and premarital sexual behavior, *Journal of Sex Research* 13 (1977): 73–88.

Chapter 12   Pregnancy, Childbirth, and Parenting

1. M. H. Kaufman, Ethanol-induced chromosomal abnormalities at conception, *Nature* 302 (1983): 258–260.

2. M. Wynn and A. Wynn, The influence of nutrition on the fertility of women, *Nutrition and Health* 1 (1982): 7–13.

3. M. Wynn and A. Wynn, Effect of nutrition on reproductive capability, *Nutrition and Health* 1 (1983): 165–178.

4. M. L. Doshi, Accuracy of consumer performed in-home tests for early pregnancy detection, *American Journal of Public Health* 76 (1986): 512–514.

5. J. M. Tanner, Growth before birth, in *Foetus into Man: Physical Growth from Conception to Maturity* (London: Open Books Publishing, 1978), p. 38.

6. G. M. Jonakait, M. C. Bohn, and I. B. Black, Maternal glucocorticoid hormones influence neurotransmitter phenotypic expression in embryos, *Science* 210 (1980): 551–553.

7. I. L. Ward and J. Weisz, Different effects of maternal stress on circulating levels of corticosterone, progesterone, and testosterone in male and female rat fetuses and their mothers, *Endocrinology* 114 (1984): 1635–1644.

8. E. Hackman and coauthors, Maternal birth weight and subsequent pregnancy outcome, *Journal of the American Medical Association* 250 (1983): 2016–2019.

9. U.S. Department of Health and Human Services, March of Dimes Birth Defects Foundation, *Working with the Pregnant Teenager: A Guide for Nutrition Educators* (Washington, D.C.: Government Printing Office, 1981), p. 3.

10. M. C. McCormick, S. Shapiro, and B. Starfield, High-risk young mothers: Infant mortality and morbidity in four areas of the United States, 1972–1978, *American Journal of Public Health* 74 (1983): 18–23.

11. J.-M. Delabar and coauthors, Beta amyloid gene duplication in Alzheimer's disease and karyotypically normal Down syndrome, *Science* 235 (1987): 1390–1392.

12. Z. A. Stein, A woman's age: Childbearing and child rearing, *American Journal of Epidemiology* 121 (March 1985): 327–343.

13. R. L. Naeye, Maternal age, obstetric complications, and the outcome of pregnancy, *Obstetrics and Gynecology* 61 (1983): 210–216.

14. D. S. Kriz, W. Dorchester, and R. K. Freeman, Advanced maternal age: The mature gravida, *American Journal of Obstetrics and Gynecology*, 1 May 1985, pp. 7–12.

15. National Institute of Child Health and Human Development, Little babies: Born too soon—Born too small, HHS publication no. (NIH) 77–1079, 1977.

16. *New York Trends and Approaches in the Delivery of Maternal and Child Care in Health Services*, sixth report of the WHO Expert Committee on Maternal and Child Health, as cited in *Journal of the American Dietetic Association* 71 (1977): 357; A. Petros-Barvazian and M. Behar, Low birth weight: What should be done to deal with this global problem? *WHO Chronicle* 32 (1978): 231–232.

17. I. J. Chasnoff and coauthors, Cocaine use in pregnancy, *New England Journal of Medicine* 313 (1985): 666–669; C. N. Chiang and C. C. Lee, *Prenatal Drug Exposure: Kinetics and Dynamics*, NIDA research monograph 60, 1985; T. M. Pinkert, *Current Research on the Consequences of Maternal Drug Abuse*, NIDA research monograph 59, 1985.

18. National Institute of Child Health and Human Development, Pregnancy and infant health, in *Smoking and Health: A Report of the Surgeon General*, HHS publication no. (PHS) 79–50066, 1979, pp. 8–1 through 8–93.

19. *Report of the Surgeon General*, 1979.

20. *Report of the Surgeon General*, 1979.

21. Food and Nutrition Board/Committee of the Mother and Preschool Child, *Alternative Dietary Practices and Nutritional Abuses in Pregnancy* (Washington, D.C.: National Academy Press, 1982), pp. 10–12.

22. D. N. Danforth, Cesarean section, *Journal of the American Medical Association* 253 (1985): 811–818.

23. A. S. Ragozin and coauthors, Effects of maternal age on parenting role, *Developmental Psychology* 18 (1982): 627–634.

24. C. M. Heinicke and coauthors, Pre-birth parent characteristics and family development in the first year of life, *Child Development* 54 (1983): 194–208.

25. H. R. Schaffer and P. E. Emerson, The development of social attachments in infancy, *Monographs of the Society for Research in Child Development* 29 (1964): 63–73.

26. T. R. Alley, Head shape and the perception of cuteness, *Developmental Psychology* 17 (1981): 650–654.

27. L. M. Baskett, Sibling status effects: Adult expectations, *Developmental Psychology* 21 (1985): 441–445.

Chapter 13   Mature Life, Aging, and Death

1. Summarized from G. Sheehy, *Pathfinders* (New York: Bantam, 1982).

2. F. H. Nuessel, The language of ageism, *Gerontologist* 22 (1982): 273–276.

3. S. M. Golant, *A Place to Grow Old: The Meaning of Environment in Old Age* (New York: Columbia University Press, 1984), pp. 137, 316.

4. Numbers show aging of America, *Tallahassee Democrat*, 17 February, 1985.

5. J. R. Bianchine, N. Gerber, and B. D. Andersen, Geriatric medicine, in *Current Concepts* (Kalamazoo, Mich.: Upjohn, 1981), pp. 6–8.

6. E. L. Schneider, *Cells and Aging*, NIH publication no. 74–1860, 1979.

7. E. L. Schneider and J. D. Reid, Jr., Life extension, *New England Journal of Medicine* 312 (1985): 1159–1168.

8. Schneider and Reid, 1985.

9. R. M. Sapolsky, L. C. Krey, and B. S. McEwen, The adrenocortical stress-response in the aged male rat: Impairment of recovery from stress, *Experimental Gerontology* 18 (1983): 55–64; R. M. Sapolsky, L. C. Krey, and B. S. McEwen, Corticosterone receptors decline in a site-specific manner in the aged rat brain, *Brain Research* 289 (1983): 235–240.

10. D. Blazer, Life events, mental health functioning and the use of health care services by the elderly, *American Journal of Public Health* 70 (1980): 1174–1179.

11. Benefits of estrogen replacement therapy outweigh risks, *Modern Medicine*, October 1986, p. 45.

12. R. S. Anderson, I. Transbol, and C. Christiansen, Is cigarette smoking a promoter of the menopause? *Acta Medica Scandinavica* 212 (1982): 137–139.

13. Live it up! *Health*, August 1985, p. 22.

14. Grow old—Gracefully, *Executive Fitness Newsletter*, 13 January 1979.

15. T. A. Salthouse, *Adult Cognition: An Experimental Psychology of Human Aging* (New York: Springer-Verlag, 1982), pp. 199–202.

16. Mental skills of the elderly; Lost and found, *Science News* 12 (1986): 244.

17. R. Kelly, Teaching a course on death and dying, in *Death and Dying Education*, ed.

R. O. Ulin (Washington, D.C.: National Education Association, 1977), pp. 45–48.

18. Kelly, 1977, p. 23.
19. Kelly, 1977, p. 23.
20. Kelly, 1977, p. 22.
21. *Hospice in America*, a brochure available from National Hospice Organization, Suite 307, 1901 North Fort Myer Dr., Arlington, VA 22209; S. V. Dobihal, Enabling a patient to die at home, *American Journal of Nursing*, August 1980, pp. 1448–1451.
22. S. T. Putnam and coauthors, Home as a place to die, *American Journal of Nursing*, August 1980, pp. 1451–1453.
23. Kelly, 1977, pp. 22–23.
24. Kelly, 1977, p. 23.
25. E. Kubler-Ross, *On Death and Dying* (look for the latest edition).
26. A. Worcester, *The Care of the Aged, The Dying and the Dead*, 2nd ed. (Springfield, Ill.: Charles C. Thomas, 1961), pp. 33–61.
27. Worcester, 1961.

Spotlight 13   Spiritual Health

1. L. S. Chapman, Developing a useful perspective on spiritual health: Love, joy, peace and fulfillment, *American Journal of Health Promotion*, Fall 1987, pp. 12–17.
2. J. B. Noss, *Man's Religions*, 6th ed. (New York: Macmillan, 1980), p. 2.
3. C. Darwin, a letter to two Dutch students from Utrecht, as cited by G. de Beer, *Charles Darwin: A Scientific Biography*, Natural History Library Edition (New York: Doubleday, 1965), p. 268.
4. L. Thomas, On the uncertainty of science, *Harvard Magazine*, September-October 1980, pp. 19–22.
5. A. Stevenson, as cited by H. A. Blackmun, Remarks at the commencement exercises of Mayo Medical School, *Mayo Clinic Proceedings* 55 (1980): 573–578.
6. L. P. Carroll and K. M. Dyckman, *Chaos or Creation: Spirituality in Mid-Life* (New York: Paulist Press, 1986), p. 142.
7. Carroll and Dyckman, p. 107.
8. Carroll and Dyckman, p. 117
9. Carroll and Dyckman, p. 142
10. E. Fox, *The Golden Key*, a leaflet (1931) from the Unity School of Christianity, Unity Village, Missouri 64065.
11. E. Fox, *The Sermon on the Mount* (New York: Harper and Row, 1938), p. 34.
12. N. V. Peale, *The Power of Positive Thinking*, (New York, Prentice-Hall, 1952), p. 109.

Chapter 14   Accident Prevention

1. Committee on Trauma Research, Commission on Life Sciences, National Research Council, and the Institute of Medicine, *Injury in America: A Continuing Public Health Problem* (Washington, D.C.: National Academy Press, 1985), p. 1.
2. American Red Cross, *Standard First Aid and Personal Safety*, 2nd ed. (Garden City, N.Y.: Doubleday, 1979), p. 219.
3. Adapted from American Red Cross, 1979, p. 157.
4. Newsfront, *Modern Medicine*, June 1986, p. 24.
5. A.V. Nero, Controlling indoor air pollution, *Scientific American* 258 (May 1988): 42–48
6. U.S. Department of Health and Human Services, Public Health Service, *Promoting Health, Preventing Disease: Objectives for the Nation* (Washington, D.C.: Government Printing Office, 1980), p. 39.
7. Adapted from American Red Cross, 1979, pp. 43–44.
8. American Red Cross, 1979, p. 224.

Chapter 15   Infectious Diseases

1. M.S. Insler and B. A. Gore, *Pseudomonas* keratitis and folliculitis from whirlpool exposure, *American Journal of Ophthalmology* 101 (1986): 41–43.
2. U.S. Department of Health and Human Services, Public Health Service, *Promoting Health, Preventing Disease: Objectives for the Nation* (Washington, D.C.: Government Printing Office, 1980), pp. 58–59.
3. S. Gilbert, Hospital-borne infections, *Science Digest* 93 (1985): 34.
4. H.D. Jampel and coauthors, Fever and immunoregulation: III. Hyperthermia augments the primary in vitro humoral immune response, *Journal of Experimental Medicine* 157 (1983): 1229–1238.
5. Don't share the air, *Science News* 129 (1986): 216.
6. J. G. Cannon and M. J. Kluger, Exercise enhances survival rate in mice infected with *Salmonella typhimurium*, *Proceedings of the Society for Experimental Biology and Medicine* 175 (1984): 518–521.
7. P.M. Layde, Pelvic inflammatory disease and the Dalkon shield (editorial), *Journal of the American Medical Association* 250 (1983): 796.
8. J.F. Rooney and coauthors, Acquisition of genital herpes from an asymptomatic sexual partner, *New England Journal of Medicine* 314 (1986): 1561–1564.
9. J.H. Nelson and coauthors, Dysplasia, carcinoma in situ, and early invasive cervical carcinoma, *CA—A Cancer Journal for Clinicians* 34 (1984): 306–327.
10. R.S. Ostrow and coauthors, Detection of papilloma virus DNA in human semen, *Science* 231 (1986): 731–733.
11. A. Hecht, AIDS progress report, *FDA Consumer*, February 1986, pp. 32–35.
12. E. M. Whelan, The AIDS epidemic: moving from complacency to action, *ACHS News & Views*, September/October 1986, pp. 1, 11–12.
13. C.A. Rosen, J. G. Sodroski, and W. A. Haseltine, The location of *cis*-acting regulatory sequences in the human T cell lymphotropic virus type III (HTLV-III/LAV) long terminal repeat, *Cell* 41 (1985): 813–823.
14. Newsfront, *Modern Medicine*, March 1987, p. 16.
15. Newsfront, *Modern Medicine*, September 1986, p. 15.
16. G. H. Friedland, B. R. Saltzman, and M. F. Rogers, Lack of transmission of HTLV-III/LAV infection to household contacts of patients with AIDS or AIDS-related complex with oral candidiasis, *New England Journal of Medicine* 314 (1986): 344–349.
17. D.N. Lawrence and coauthors, A model-based estimate of the average incubation and latency period for transfusion-associated AIDS, presented at the International Conference on Acquired Immunodeficiency Syndrome, Atlanta, April 14–17, 1985, as cited by C. B. Popescu, *Answers about AIDS: A report by the American Council on Science and Health*, January 1986 (a booklet available from ACSH, 1995 Broadway, New York, NY 10023).
18. J.M. Veasey, as quoted in Meeting highlights, *Modern Medicine*, September 1986, p. 26.
19. Committee on a National Strategy for AIDS, Institute of Medicine, National Academy of Sciences, *Confronting AIDS: Directions for Public Health, Health Care, and Research* (Washington, D.C.: National Academy Press, 1986).
20. M. A. Sande, Transmission of AIDS: The case against casual contagion, *The New England Journal of Medicine* 314 (1986): 380–382.

Spotlight 15   Allergy—Vandal of the Immune System

1. J. E. Vena and coauthors, Allergy related diseases and cancer: An inverse association, *American Journal of Epidemiology* 122 (1985): 66–74.

Chapter 16   Heart and Artery Disease

1. American Heart Association, *1986 Heart Facts* (Dallas: AHA, 1985), p. 1.
2. W. B. Kannel and coauthors, Risk factors and coronary disease, AHA Committee Report, *Circulation* 62 (1980): 449A-455A.
3. T. B. Jacobs, R. D. Bell, and J. D. Clements, Exercise, age and the development of myocardial vasculature, *Growth* 48 (1984): 148–157.
4. K. Przyklenk and A. C. Groom, Effects of exercise frequency, intensity, and duration on revascularization in the transition zone of infarcted rat hearts, *Canadian Journal of Physiology and Pharmacology* 63 (1985): 273–278.
5. C. M. Tipton, Exercise, training, and hypertension, *Exercise and Sports Sciences Reviews* 12 (1984): 245–306; R. S. Williams, R. A. McKinnis and F. R. Cobb, Effects of physical conditioning on left ventric-

ular ejection fraction in patients with coronary artery disease, *Circulation* 70 (July 1984): 69–75.

6. Committee on Reduction of Risk of Heart Attack and Stroke, American Heart Association, *Coronary Risk Handbook: Estimating Risk of Coronary Heart Disease in Daily Practice*, (Dallas: AHA, 1973).

7. Kannel and coauthors, 1980.

8. N. M. Kaplan, Non-drug treatment of hypertension, *Annals of Internal Medicine* 402 (1985): 359–373.

9. Institute of Food Technologists' Expert Panel on Food Safety and Nutrition, Dietary salt, *Food Technology*, January 1980, pp. 85–91; Joint National Committee on Detection, Evaluation, and Treatment of High Blood Pressure, *1980 Report*, NIH publication no. 81–1088, 1980).

10. D. A. McCarron, Low serum concentrations of ionized calcium in patients with hypertension, *New England Journal of Medicine* 307 (1982): 226–228.

11. O. H. Ford, S. F. Knutsen, and E. Arnesen, The Tromso heart study: Coffee consumption and serum lipid concentrations in men with hypercholesterolaemia: A randomised intervention study, *British Medical Journal* 290 (1985): 893–895.

12. S. Rainville and P. Vaccaro, Lipoprotein cholesterol levels, coronary artery disease and regular exercise: A review, *American Corrective Therapy Journal*, November/December 1983, pp. 161–165.

13. A. M. Fehily and coauthors, The effect of fatty fish on plasma lipid and lipoprotein concentrations, *American Journal of Clinical Nutrition* 38 (1983): 349–351; W. S. Harris and coauthors, in *Nutrition and Heart Disease* (London: Churchill Livingstone, 1983), as cited in Fish oils, serum lipids and platelet aggregation, *Nutrition and the MD*, January 1985.

14. D. Kromhout, E. B. Bosschieter, and C. D. Coulander, The inverse relation between fish consumption and 20-year mortality from coronary heart disease, *New England Journal of Medicine* 312 (1985): 1205–1209.

15. Try a little TLC, *Science 80*, January/February 1980, p. 15.

16. R. H. Rosenman and M. A. Chesney, The relationship of type A behavior pattern to coronary heart disease, *Activitas Nervosa Superior* (Prague) 22 (1980): 1–10.

17. B. J. Betz and C. B. Thomas, Individual temperament as a predictor of health or premature disease, *Johns Hopkins Medical Journal* 144 (1979): 81–89.

Spotlight 16   Diabetes

1. W. H. Herman, S. M. Teutsch, and L. S. Geiss, Closing the gap: The problem of diabetes mellitus in the United States, *Diabetes Care* 8 (1985): 391–406.

2. G. L. Burke, L. S. Webber, and S. R. Srinivasan, Fasting plasma glucose and insulin levels and their relationship to

cardiovascular risk factors in children: Bogalusa heart study, *Metabolism* 35 (1986): 441–446.

3. J. M. Couric, Diabetes is a controllable disease with a growth factor, *FDA Consumer*, November 1982, pp. 21–23.

Chapter 17   Cancer

1. U.S. Department of Health and Human Services, National Institutes of Health, *Cancer Prevention*, NIH publication no. 84-2671, 1984.

2. E. Whelan and F. Stare, Alcohol: How does it affect your body? *ACSH Media and Activity Update*, Spring 1981, pp. 8–9.

3. A.I. Holleb, ed., *The American Cancer Society Cancer Book* (Garden City, N.Y.: Doubleday, 1986).

4. J. C. Bailar and E. M. Smith, Progress against cancer? *New England Journal of Medicine* 314 (1986): 1226–1232.

5. L. Cunningham, *Malignant Melanoma of the Skin—An Increasingly Common Cancer* (pamphlet), American Council on Science and Health, 47 Maple St., Summit, NJ 07901, May 1986.

6. R. A. Lew and coauthors, Sun exposure habits in patients with cutaneous melanoma: A case control study, *Journal of Dermatologic Surgery and Oncology* 9 (1983): 981–986.

7. High-intensity tanning lamps, *FDA Consumer*, June 1985, p. 5.

8. A. E. Reif, The causes of cancer, *American Scientist*, July/August 1981, pp. 437–447.

9. N. A. Dreyer and E. Friedlander, Identifying the health risks from very low-dose sparsely ionizing radiation, *American Journal of Public Health* 72 (1982): 16–29; N. A. Dreyer and coauthors, The feasibility of epidemiologic investigations of the health effects of low-level ionizing radiation, *Final Report*, U.S. Nuclear Regulatory Commission publication NUREG/CR-1728, 1980, p. 33.

10. Inactivity may increase risk of colon cancer (Newsfront), *Modern Medicine*, February 1985, p. 33.

11. L. Temoshok, Biopsychosocial studies on cutaneous malignant melanoma: Psychosocial factors associated with prognostic indicators, progression, psychophysiology and tumor-host response, *Social Science and Medicine* 20 (1985): 833–840.

12. D. K. Wellisch and J. Yager, Is there a cancer-prone personality? *CA—A Cancer Journal for Clinicians* 33 (1983): 145–153.

13. P. L. Graves and coauthors, The Rorschach interaction scale as a potential predictor of cancer, *Psychosomatic Medicine* 48 (1986): 549–563.

14. J. H. Nelson and coauthors, Dysplasia, carcinoma in situ and early invasive cervical carcinoma, *CA—A Cancer Journal for Clinicians* 34 (1984): 306–327.

15. E. T. Fossel, J. M. Carr, and J. McDonagh, Detection of malignant tumors: Water-suppressed proton nuclear magnetic res-

onance spectroscopy of plasma, *New England Journal of Medicine* 315 (1986): 1369–1376.

16. B. Fisher, C. Redmond, and E. R. Fisher, Ten-year results of a randomized clinical trial comparing radical mastectomy and total mastectomy with or without radiation, *New England Journal of Medicine* 312 (1985): 674–681.

17. S. A. Rosenberg, Observations on the systemic administration of autologous lymphokine-activated killer cells and recombinant Interleukin-2 to patients with metastatic cancer, *New England Journal of Medicine* 313 (1985): 1485–1492.

18. O. C. Simonton, S. Matthews-Simonton, and T. F. Sparks, Psychological intervention in the treatment of cancer, *Psychosomatics* 21 (1980): 226–233.

Spotlight 17   Nutrition and Cancer

1. Council on Scientific Affairs, American Medical Association, Saccharin: Review of safety issues, *Journal of the American Medical Association* 254 (1985): 2622–2624.

2. P. Greenwald and coauthors, Feasibility studies of a low-fat diet to prevent or retard breast cancer, *American Journal of Clinical Nutrition* 45 (1987): 347–353.

3. E. L. Wynder, Dietary habits and cancer epidemiology, *Cancer* 43 (1979): 1955–1961, as cited by S. H. Brammer and R. L. DeFelice, Dietary advice in regard to risk for colon and breast cancer, *Preventive Medicine* 9 (1980): 544–549.

4. B. S. Reddy and coauthors, Nutrition and its relationship to cancer, *Advances in Cancer Research* 32 (1980): 238–245.

5. J. L. Werther, Food and cancer, *New York State Journal of Medicine*, August 1980, pp. 1401–1408.

Chapter 18   The Consumer and the Health Care System

1. Long-term care: Who pays? *NCL Bulletin*, May/June 1986, pp. 1, 6.

2. G. J. Church and coauthors, Sorry, your policy is canceled, *Time*, 24 March 1986, pp. 16–20, 23–26.

3. Equifax, an insurance benefit consulting firm, as cited by G. Akers, Containing the high cost of health care: New play-or-pay rules for health insurance, *Radcliffe Quarterly*, June 1985, pp. 31–32.

4. J. Creamer, The talking cure (Medical News), *American Health*, June 1985, p. 14.

5. Chiropractors: Healers or quacks? in *Health Quackery: Consumer Union's Report on False Health Claims, Worthless Remedies, and Unproved Therapies* (Mount Vernon, N.Y.: Consumer's Union, 1980), pp. 156–200.

Spotlight 18   Your Body—An Owner's Manual

1. T. Nordstrom, Steps to a healthy back, *Healthline*, May 1985, pp. 14–16.

2. J. Willis, Back pain: Ubiquitous, controversial, *FDA Consumer*, November 1983, pp. 5–7.

Chapter 19 Environmental Health

1. S. Begley, M. Miller, and M. Hager, The endless summer? *Newsweek*, 11 July 1988, pp. 18–20.
2. Begley, Miller, and Hager, 1988.
3. Threat to ozone layer looms unexpectedly large, *Tallahassee Democrat*, 2 February 1986; J. D. Bernal, *The Origin of Life* (Cleveland: World Publishing Company, 1967), pp. 100–109.
4. R. Crum, More on less ozone, *Harvard Magazine*, May/June 1987, pp. 4, 6.
5. D. Rigel, research physician from New York University Medical Center, reporting to an Energy and Commerce subcommittee hearing, March 1987, as cited in Associated Press, Action needed to save ozone, *Tallahassee Democrat*, 10 March 1987.
6. R. W. Shaw, Air pollution by particles, *Scientific American*, August 1987, pp. 96–103.
7. Three of the nation's leading doctors, testifying before a U.S. Senate subcommittee on environmental pollution, according to P. Shabecoff, Acid rain seen as posing risks for U.S. health, *New York Times*, 4 February 1987, p. A–12.
8. M. Weisskopf, Humans feel effect of fouled food chain,*Washington Post*, as cited by *Tallahassee Democrat*, 1 April 1986, pp. 1A–2A.
9. E. Magnuson and reporters, A problem that cannot be buried: The poisoning of America continues, *Time*, 14 October 1985, pp. 76–84.
10. Scientists alarmed by growing use of toxic chemicals, *Tallahassee Democrat*, 16 October 1985.
11. E. N. Whitney and E. M. N. Hamilton, *Understanding Nutrition*, 2nd ed. (St. Paul, Minn.: West, 1981), p. 511.
12. E. N. Whitney, E. M. N. Hamilton, and M. A. Boyle, *Understanding Nutrition*, 3rd ed. (St. Paul, Minn.: West, 1984), p. 441.
13. Getting the lead out, *Science News*, 24 October 1987, p. 269.
14. D. Faust and J. Brown, Moderately elevated blood lead levels: Effect on neuropsychological functioning in children, *Pediatrics* 80 (1987): 623–629.
15. E.M. N. Hamilton, E. N. Whitney, and F. S. Sizer, *Nutrition: Concepts and Controversies*, 3rd ed. (St. Paul, Minn.: West, 1985), p. 339; E. N. Whitney, E. M. N. Hamilton, and M. A. Boyle, *Understanding Nutrition*, 4th ed. (St. Paul, Minn.: West, 1981), pp. 464–465.
16. Getting the lead out, 1987.
17. The World Health Organization suggests not more than 3 mg/individual for adults; Evaluation of mercury, lead, cadmium and the food additives amaranth, diethylpyrocarbonate and octyl gallate, *WHO Food Additives Series No. 4*, World Health Organization, Geneva, as cited by D. G. Lindsay and J. C. Sherlock, Environmental contaminants, in *Adverse Effects of Foods*, by E. F. P. Jelliffe and D. B. Jelliffe (New York: Plenum Press, 1982), pp. 85–110.
18. *PCBs: Is the Cure Worth the Cost?*, a report (1985) by the American Council on Science and Health, 47 Maple St., Summit, NJ 07901.
19. *Dioxin in the Environment: Its Effect on Human Health*, a report (1984) by the American Council on Science and Health, 47 Maple St., Summit, NJ 07901.
20. Living, dangerously, with toxic wastes, *Time*, 14 October 1985, pp. 86–90; Magnuson and reporters, 1985.
21. Public Citizen, a consumer group founded by Ralph Nader in 1971, undated letter, 1986.
22. N. Maxwell, Chernobyl's message: Look again at containments in the United States, *Nucleus* (a quarterly reports from the Union of Concerned Scientists), pp. 3, 7.
23. Possible sites selected for nuclear-waste dump, *Tallahassee Democrat*, 17 January 1986.
24. M. W. Mikewell, The deforestation of Mount Lebanon, *The Geographical Review*, January 1969, pp. 1–28; J. J. Cloudsley-Thompson, Recent expansion of the Sahara, in Introduction to *Key Environments: Sahara Desert*, ed. J. J. Cloudsley-Thompson (Oxford, England: Pergamon Press, 1984), pp. 8–14.
25. Did you know? *Inform* (newsletter), 1986, 381 Park Ave. S, New York, NY 10016.
26. C. Uhl and G. Parker, Viewpoint: Our steak in the jungle, *BioScience* 36, November 1986, p. 642.
27. Uhl and Parker, 1986.
28. T. Peterson, Hunger and the environment, *Seeds*, October 1987, pp. 6–13.
29. U.S. Department of Agriculture Statistics, cited by J. D. Nations and D. I. Komer, Rainforests and the hamburger society, *Environment*, April 1983, pp. 12–20.
30. Nations and Komer, 1983.
31. Nations and Komer, 1983.
32. Nations and Komer, 1983.
33. L. Timberlake, *Only One Earth: Living for the Future* (New York: Sterling Publishing, 1987), as cited by Peterson, 1987.
34. R. T. Peterson, as cited by B. Yokel, president, Florida Audubon Society, in a letter to the members, 25 June 1986.
35. E.O. Wilson, *Biophilia: The Human Bond with Other Species* (Cambridge, Mass.: Harvard University Press, 1984) chapter titled The conservation ethic, pp. 119–140.
36. National Academy of Sciences, *Resources and Man* (1969 report), as cited by L. J. Gordon, Popullution: The 1981 APHA presidential address, *American Journal of Public Health* 72 (1982): 341–346.
37. B. Bull, Voodoo demography: What population problem? *The Amicus Journal*, Fall 1984, pp. 36–40.
38. L. J. Gordon, Popullution: The 1981 APHA presidential address, *American Journal of Public Health* 72 (1982): 341–346.
39. L. R. Brown and coauthors, *State of the World: A Worldwatch Institute Report on Progress toward a Sustainable Society* (New York: Norton, 1985), pp. 200–221.
40. *State of the World 1987: A Worldwatch Institute Report on Progress toward a Sustainable Society* (New York: Norton, 1987).

Spotlight 19 Personal Strategy— Voluntary Simplicity

1. The case for optimism, in *The Study of the Future: An Introduction to the Art and Science of Understanding and Shaping Tomorrow's World*, by E. Cornish and members and staff of the World Future Society (Washington, D.C.: World Future Society, 1977), pp. 34–37.
2. D. Elgin, *Voluntary Simplicity: Toward a Way of Life That Is Outwardly Simple, Inwardly Rich* (New York: Morrow, 1981), p. 25.
3. Elgin, 1981, pp. 32–34.
4. R. E. Pestle, T. A. Cornille, and K. Solomon, Lifestyle alternatives: Development and evaluation of an attitude scale, *Home Economics Research Journal*, December 1982, pp. 175–182.
5. Elgin, 1981, pp. 32–34.

Calorie Counter and Selected Nutrients in Foods

This appendix offers information on most of the foods people commonly eat. To present all the available data would require hundreds of pages, space not available here. Given limited space, we have chosen to present calories (because everyone wants to know them); the percentages of calories from protein, carbohydrate, and fat; fiber; cholesterol; and sodium contents of foods.

Keep a sense of perspective in using this table. Foods are not eaten singly, they are combined into diets—and diets may be beneficial or harmful. Foods, however, can pull diets in one direction or another, and the amounts eaten should be adjusted accordingly. For this reason, it can be useful to see what contributions individual foods make.

For a perspective on calories, remember that an average-sized adult man might require about 2,000 to 3,000 calories per day to maintain his weight; and a woman, about 1,200 to 2,200. With respect to the fat content of foods, remember (Chapter 4) that a widely accepted dietary goal is that no more than 30 percent of the day's calories should come from fat. Total dietary fiber for a day should perhaps add up to about 15 to 30 grams. Cholesterol recommendations probably need not be made for the general public, but people who are advised by their health care providers to restrict their cholesterol intakes may want to keep them below about 300 mg a day. As for sodium, current guidelines indicate that an intake of 2,000 to 3,000 mg a day might be desirable.

TABLE E–1 Food Composition

Key	Name	Measure	Energy (calories)	Protein/ Carbohydrate/ Fat (%)	Fiber (g)	Cholesterol (mg)	Sodium (mg)
	BEVERAGES						
	Alcoholic:						
	Beer:						
1	Regular (12 fl oz)	1½ cups	146	2/36/0*	0.5	0	19
1	Light (12 fl oz)	1½ cups	100[1]	3/18/0*	0.5	0	10
	Gin, rum, vodka, whiskey:						
1	90 proof	1½ fl oz	110	0/0/0*	0	0	.4
	Wine:						
1	Red	3½ fl oz	74	1/10/0*	0	0	6
1	White medium	3½ fl oz	70	1/5/0*	0	0	5
	Carbonated[3]:						
1	Cola beverage (12 fl oz)	1½ cups	151	1/100/0	0	0	14
1	Diet cola (12 fl oz)	1½ cups	2	40/60/0	0	0	21[4]
1	Ginger ale (12 fl oz)	1½ cups	124	1/100/0	0	0	25
1	Lemon-lime (12 fl oz)	1½ cups	149	0/100/0	0	0	41
	Coffee:[3]						
1	Brewed	1 cup	2[5]	8/90/2	t	0	5
	Fruit drinks,[6] noncarbonated:						
1	Fruit punch drink, canned	1 cup	118	0/99/1	0	0	56
1	Lemonade, prepared from frozen concentrate	1 cup	100	0/99/1	0.5	0	8
	Fruit and vegetable juices; see Fruit and Vegetable sections.						
	Tea:[3]						
1	Brewed	1 cup	2[5]	0/100/0	0	0	7
1	From instant, sweetened	1 cup	86	0/99/1	0	0	t
	DAIRY						
	Butter: see Fats and Oils						
	Cheese, natural:						
2	Blue	1 oz	100	24/3/73	0	21	39
2	Brie	1 oz	95	25/1/74	0	28	17
2	Camembert	1 oz	85	26/1/73	0	20	23
2	Cheddar, cut pieces	1 oz	114	25/1/74	0	30	17
	Cottage:						
2	Creamed, small curd	1 cup	215	50/11/39	0	31	85
2	Lowfat 2%	1 cup	205	63/17/20	0	19	91
2	Cream	1 oz	99	8/3/89	0	31	84
2	Gouda	1 oz	101	28/2/70	0	32	23
2	Monterey jack	1 oz	106	26/1/73	0	26	152
2	Mozzarella, made with part skim milk, low moisture	1 oz	80	40/5/55	0	15	150
2	Parmesan, grated	1 oz	129	37/3/60	0	22	528
2	Provolone	1 oz	100	29/2/69	0	20	248
2	Ricotta, made with whole milk	1 cup	428	26/7/67	0	124	207

*Alcohol contributes additional calories, bringing the total to 100%.

[1]Calories can vary from 78 to 131 for 12 fluid ounces.

[3]Sodium content varies depending on water source.

[4]Value for product sweetened with aspartame only; sodium is 32 mg if a blend of aspartame and sodium saccharin is used; 75 mg if just sodium saccharin is used.

[5]Calorie values are not available: this is a USDA estimate.

[6]Usually less than 10% fruit juice.

(For purposes of calculations, use "0" for t.)

Key: 1 = Bev 2 = Dairy 3 = Eggs 4 = Fat/Oil 5 = Fruit 6 = Bakery 7 = Grain 8 = Fish 9 = Meat 10 = Poultry 11 = Sausage 12 = Mixed Dishes 13 = Nuts/Seeds 14 = Sweets 15 = Veg/Leg 16 = Misc 22 = Soup/Sauce 25 = Fast Foods by Brand Name

TABLE E-1 Food Composition

Key	Name	Measure	Energy (calories)	Protein/ Carbohydrate/ Fat (%)	Fiber (g)	Cholesterol (mg)	Sodium (mg)
DAIRY (cont.)							
	Cheese, natural (cont.):						
2	Swiss	1 oz	107	30/4/66	0	26	74
	Pasteurized processed cheese products:						
2	American	1 oz	106	23/2/75	0	27	406
2	Swiss	1 oz	95	30/3/67	0	24	388
2	American cheese food	1 oz	93	24/9/67	0	18	337
2	American cheese spread	1 oz	82	24/12/64	0	16	381
	Cream, sweet:						
2	Half and half (cream and milk)	1 tbsp	20	8/14/78	0	6	6
2	Light, coffee or table	1 tbsp	30	5/8/87	0	10	6
2	Light whipping cream, liquid	1 tbsp	44	3/4/93	0	17	5
2	Heavy whipping cream, liquid	1 tbsp	51	2/3/95	0	20	6
2	Whipped cream, pressurized	1 tbsp	10	4/20/76	0	3	5
2	Cream, sour, cultured	1 tbsp	30	5/8/87	0	6	7
	Cream products-imitation and part dairy:						
	Coffee whitener:						
2	Frozen or liquid	1 tbsp	20	2/33/65	0	0	12
2	Powdered	1 tsp	11	0/39/61	0	0	4
2	Dessert topping, frozen	1 tbsp	15	0/29/71	0	0	1
2	Imitation sour cream	1 tbsp	29	4/12/84	0	0	14
	Milk, fluid:						
2	Whole milk	1 cup	150	21/30/49	0	33	120
2	2% Lowfat milk	1 cup	121	27/38/35	0	22	122
2	Skim milk	1 cup	86	39/56/5	0	4	126
2	Buttermilk	1 cup	99	33/47/20	0	9	257
	Milk, canned:						
2	Evaporated, whole	1 cup	340	20/29/51	0	74	267
2	Evaporated, skim	1 cup	200	39/59/2	0	10	293
	Milk, dried:						
2	Buttermilk	1 cup	464	36/51/13	0	83	621
2	Instant, nonfat	1 cup	244	40/58/2	0	12	373
	Milk beverages and powdered mixes:						
	Chocolate:						
2	Whole	1 cup	210	15/49/36	t	31	149
2	2% Fat	1 cup	180	18/57/25	t	17	151
2	Egg nog, commercial	1 cup	342	12/39/49	0	149	138

(For purposes of calculations, use "0" for t.)

Key: 1 = Bev 2 = Dairy 3 = Eggs 4 = Fat/Oil 5 = Fruit 6 = Bakery 7 = Grain 8 = Fish 9 = Meat 10 = Poultry 11 = Sausage 12 = Mixed Dishes 13 = Nuts/Seeds 14 = Sweets 15 = Veg/Leg 16 = Misc 22 = Soup/Sauce 25 = Fast Foods by Brand Name

TABLE E–1 Food Composition

Key	Name	Measure	Energy (calories)	Protein/ Carbohydrate/ Fat (%)	Fiber (g)	Cholesterol (mg)	Sodium (mg)
DAIRY (cont.)							
	Cream products (cont.):						
	Milk shakes:						
2	Chocolate (10 fl oz)	1¼ cups	360	11/63/26	0.5	37	273
2	Vanilla (10 fl oz)	1¼ cups	314	12/64/24	t	32	232
	Milk desserts, frozen:						
	Ice cream, regular (about 11% fat) vanilla:						
2	Hardened	1 cup	269	7/46/47	0	59	116
2	Soft Serve	1 cup	377	7/40/53	0	153	153
2	Ice cream, rich vanilla (about 16% fat), hardened	1 cup	349	6/44/50	0	88	108
	Ice milk, vanilla (about 4% fat):						
2	Hardened	1 cup	184	11/62/27	0	18	105
2	Soft serve (about 3% fat)	1 cup	223	14/68/18	0	13	163
2	Sherbet (2% fat)	1 cup	270	3/85/12	0	14	88
	Milk desserts, other:						
2	Custard, baked	1 cup	305	18/38/44	0	278	209
	Puddings, prepared from dry mix with whole milk:						
2	Chocolate, instant	1 cup	310	10/69/21	0.5	28	880
2	Rice	½ cup	155	10/67/23	t	15	140
2	Tapioca	½ cup	145	10/66/24	0	15	152
2	Vanilla, instant	½ cup	150	10/67/23	0	15	375
	Yogurt, lowfat:						
2	Fruit added[13]	1 cup	231	17/73/10	0.5	10	133
2	Plain	1 cup	144	33/45/22	0	14	159
2	Vanilla or coffee flavor	1 cup	193	23/64/13	0	11	150
2	Yogurt, made with nonfat milk	1 cup	127	42/55/3	0	4	173
2	Yogurt, made with whole milk	1 cup	138	23/30/47	0	29	104
EGGS							
3	Raw, large, whole, without shell	1 ea	79	32/3/65	0	274	69
	Cooked:						
3	Fried in butter	1 ea	95	27/2/71	0	278	162
3	Hard-cooked, shell removed	1 ea	79	32/3/65	0	274	69
3	Scrambled with milk and butter (also omelet)	1 ea	95	26/6/68	0	282	176

[13]Carbohydrate and calories vary widely—consult label if more precise values are needed.

(For purposes of calculations, use "0" for t.)

Key: 1 = Bev 2 = Dairy 3 = Eggs 4 = Fat/Oil 5 = Fruit 6 = Bakery 7 = Grain 8 = Fish 9 = Meat 10 = Poultry 11 = Sausage 12 = Mixed Dishes 13 = Nuts/Seeds 14 = Sweets 15 = Veg/Leg 16 = Misc 22 = Soup/Sauce 25 = Fast Foods by Brand Name

TABLE E–1 Food Composition

Key	Name	Measure	Energy (calories)	Protein/ Carbohydrate/ Fat (%)	Fiber (g)	Cholesterol (mg)	Sodium (mg)
FATS and OILS							
	Butter:						
4	Tablespoon	1 tbsp	100	t/0/99	0	31	116[14]
4	Pat (about 1 tsp)[15a]	1 ea	34	0/0/100	0	11	41[14]
4	Fats, cooking (vegetable shortening)	1 tbsp	115	0/0/100	0	0	0
	Margarine:						
4	Imitation (about 40% fat) soft	1 tbsp	50	0/0/100	0	0	136[14]
	Regular, hard (about 80% fat):						
4	Tablespoon	1 tbsp	100	t/t/99	0	0	133[14]
4	Pat[15a]	1 ea	36	0/0/100	0	0	47[14]
4	Regular, soft (about 80% fat)	1 tbsp	100	4/0/96	0	0	153[14]
	Spread (about 60% fat), hard:						
4	Tablespoon	1 tbsp	75	0/0/100	0	0	139[14]
4	Pat[15a]	1 ea	25	0/0/100	0	0	50[14]
4	Spread (about 60% fat) soft	1 tbsp	75	0/0/100	0	0	139[14]
	Oils:						
	Corn:						
4	Tablespoon	1 tbsp	125	0/0/100	0	0	0
	Olive:						
4	Tablespoon	1 tbsp	125	0/0/100	0	0	0
	Peanut:						
4	Tablespoon	1 tbsp	125	0/0/100	0	0	0
	Salad dressings/sandwich spreads:						
4	Blue cheese:	1 tbsp	75	4/5/91	t	3	164
	French:						
4	Regular	1 tbsp	85	0/5/95	t	0	188
4	Low calorie	1 tbsp	24	0/36/64	t	0	306
	Italian:						
4	Regular	1 tbsp	80	t/5/95	t	0	162
4	Low calorie	1 tbsp	5	0/26/74	t	0	136
	Mayonnaise:						
4	Regular	1 tbsp	100	1/2/97	0	8	80
4	Imitation	1 tbsp	35	0/23/77	0	4	75
4	Ranch style	1 tbsp	54	3/5/92	0	6	65
4	Salad dressing-mayo type	1 tbsp	58	1/24/75	0	4	105
4	Tartar sauce	1 tbsp	74	1/3/96	t	4	182
	Thousand Island:						
4	Regular	1 tbsp	60	1/15/84	t	4	110
4	Low calorie	1 tbsp	25	2/40/58	t	2	153
	Salad dressings, prepared from home recipe:						
4	Vinegar & oil	1 tbsp	70	0/0/100	0	0	0

[14]For salted butter or margarine; unsalted varieties contain 12 mg sodium per stick or ½ cup, 1.5 mg per tablespoon, or .5 mg per pat.
[15a]Pat is 1 in square, ⅓ in high; 90 per lb.

(For purposes of calculations, use "0" for t.)

Key: 1 = Bev 2 = Dairy 3 = Eggs 4 = Fat/Oil 5 = Fruit 6 = Bakery 7 = Grain 8 = Fish 9 = Meat 10 = Poultry 11 = Sausage 12 = Mixed Dishes 13 = Nuts/Seeds 14 = Sweets 15 = Veg/Leg 16 = Misc 22 = Soup/Sauce 25 = Fast Foods by Brand Name

TABLE E–1   Food Composition

Key	Name	Measure	Energy (calories)	Protein/ Carbohydrate/ Fat (%)	Fiber (g)	Cholesterol (mg)	Sodium (mg)
	FRUITS and FRUIT JUICES						
	Apples:						
	Raw, with peel:						
	2¾″ diam (about 3 per lb						
5	with cores)	1 ea	80	1/94/5	4.5	0	1
	3¼″ diam (about 2 per lb						
5	with cores)	1 ea	125	1/94/5	6.5	0	2
5	Dried, sulfured	10 ea	155	1/98/1	9.0	0	56[20]
5	Apple juice, bottled or canned[21]	1 cup	116	1/97/2	0.5	0	7
	Applesauce:						
5	Sweetened	1 cup	195	1/97/2	3.5	0	8
5	Unsweetened	1 cup	106	1/98/1	5.0	0	5
	Apricots:						
	Canned (fruit and liquid):						
5	Heavy syrup	1 cup	214	2/97/1	4.5	0	10
5	Juice pack	1 cup	119	5/95/0	4.5	0	9
	Dried:						
5	Dried halves	10 ea	83	6/92/2	3.5	0	3
	Avocado, raw, edible part only:						
5	Mashed, fresh, average	1 cup	370	4/17/79	6.5	0	24
	Bananas, raw, without peel:						
5	Whole, 8¾″ long (weighs 175g						
	with peel)	1 ea	105	4/92/4	3.5	0	1
5	Blackberries, raw	1 cup	74	5/89/6	9.5	0	0
	Blueberries:						
5	Raw	1 cup	82	4/90/6	5.0	0	9
	Frozen, sweetened:						
5	Cup	1 cup	185	2/97/1	7.0	0	3
	Cherries:						
5	Sour, red pitted, canned water pack	1 cup	90	8/90/2	2.5	0	17
5	Sweet, raw, without pits	10 ea	49	6/83/11	1.5	0	0
	Cranberry juices:						
5	Cranberry juice cocktail	1 cup	145	0/99/1	1.0	0	5
5	Cranberry sauce, canned, strained	¼ cup	105	1/98/1	0.5	0	20
	Dates:						
5	Whole, without pits	10 ea	228	3/96/1	7.0	0	2
5	Figs, dried	10 ea	477	4/92/4	24.0	0	21
	Fruit cocktail, canned, fruit and liquid						
5	Heavy syrup pack	1 cup	185	2/97/1	2.5	0	15
5	Juice pack	1 cup	115	4/96/0	2.5	0	10
	Grapefruit:						
	Raw 3¾ in diam, whole fruit weighs 1 lb 1 oz with refuse (peel, membrane, seeds):						
5	Pink/red, half fruit, edible part	1 half	37	7/91/2	1.5	0	0

[20]Unsulfured product contains less sodium.
[21]Also applies to pasteurized apple cider.

(For purposes of calculations, use "0" for t.)

Key: 1 = Bev 2 = Dairy 3 = Eggs 4 = Fat/Oil 5 = Fruit 6 = Bakery 7 = Grain 8 = Fish 9 = Meat 10 = Poultry 11 = Sausage 12 = Mixed Dishes 13 = Nuts/Seeds 14 = Sweets 15 = Veg/Leg 16 = Misc 22 = Soup/Sauce 25 = Fast Foods by Brand Name

TABLE E-1   Food Composition

Key	Name	Measure	Energy (calories)	Protein/ Carbohydrate/ Fat (%)	Fiber (g)	Cholesterol (mg)	Sodium (mg)
	FRUITS and FRUIT JUICES (cont.)						
	White, half fruit, edible						
5	part	1 half	39	7/91/2	1.5	0	0
5	Canned sections with liquid	1 cup	152	3/96/1	2.0	0	4
	Grapefruit juice:						
5	Raw	1 cup	96	5/93/2	0.5	0	2
	Canned:						
5	Unsweetened	1 cup	93	5/93/2	0.5	0	2
5	Sweetened	1 cup	115	5/94/1	0.5	0	5
	Frozen concentrate, unsweetened:						
5	Diluted with 3 cans water	1 cup	102	5/92/3	0.5	0	2
	Grapes, raw European type (adherent skin):						
5	Thompson seedless	10 ea	35	3/90/7	1.0	0	1
5	Tokay/Emperor, seeded types	10 ea	40	4/90/6	1.0	0	1
	Grape juice:						
5	Bottled or canned	1 cup	155	4/95/1	1.5	0	8
	Frozen concentrate, sweetened:						
5	Diluted with 3 cans water	1 cup	128	2/97/1	1.5	0	5
5	Kiwi fruit, raw, peeled (about 5 per lb with skin):	1 ea	46	6/89/5	1.5	0	4
5	Lemons, raw, without peel and seeds (about 4 per lb whole)	1 ea	17	9/84/7	1.5	0	1
	Lemon juice:						
	Fresh:						
5	Tablespoon	1 tbsp	4	0/100/0	t	0	.1
	Canned or bottled, unsweetened:						
5	Tablespoon	1 tbsp	5	0/100/0	t	0	3[33]
5	Mango, raw, edible part (weighs 300g with skin and seed)	1 ea	135	3/93/4	3.0	0	4
	Melons, raw, without rind and cavity contents:						
	Cantaloupe, 5 in diam (2⅓ lb whole, with refuse), orange						
5	flesh:	½ ea	94	9/85/6	2.5	0	24
5	Honeydew, 6½ in diam (5¼ lb whole with refuse) slice = 1/10 melon	1 pce	45	5/94/2	1.5	0	13
5	Nectarines, raw, without pits, 2½ in diam	1 ea	67	7/86/7	3.0	0	0
	Oranges, raw:						
5	Whole without peel and seeds 2⅝ in diam (weighs about 180 g with peel and seeds)	1 ea	60	7/90/3	3.0	0	t
	Orange juice:						
5	Fresh, all varieties:	1 cup	111	6/90/4	0.5	0	2

[33]Sodium benzoate is added as a preservative.

(For purposes of calculations, use "0" for t.)

Key: 1 = Bev 2 = Dairy 3 = Eggs 4 = Fat/Oil 5 = Fruit 6 = Bakery 7 = Grain 8 = Fish 9 = Meat 10 = Poultry 11 = Sausage 12 = Mixed Dishes 13 = Nuts/Seeds 14 = Sweets 15 = Veg/Leg 16 = Misc 22 = Soup/Sauce 25 = Fast Foods by Brand Name

TABLE E–1 Food Composition

Key	Name	Measure	Energy (calories)	Protein/ Carbohydrate/ Fat (%)	Fiber (g)	Cholesterol (mg)	Sodium (mg)
	FRUITS and FRUIT JUICES (cont.)						
5	Canned, unsweetened	1 cup	105	6/91/3	0.5	0	5
	Frozen concentrate:						
5	Diluted with 3 parts water by volume	1 cup	110	5/94/1	1.0	0	2
	Peaches:						
	Raw:						
5	Whole, 2½ in diam, peeled, pitted (about 4 per lb with peels and pits)	1 ea	37	6/94/0	2.0	0	0
	Canned, fruit and liquid:						
	Heavy syrup pack						
5	Half	1 ea	60	2/98/0	1.5	0	5
	Juice pack						
5	Half	1 ea	34	5/95/0	1.5	0	3
	Dried:						
5	Uncooked	10 ea	311	5/92/3	10.5	0	9
	Frozen, sliced, sweetened:						
5	Cup, thawed measure	1 cup	235	3/96/1	5.5	0	16
	Pears:						
	Raw, with skin, cored:						
5	Bartlett, 2½ in diam (about 2½ per lb, whole)	1 ea	98	2/92/6	5.0[36]	0	1
5	Bosc, 2½ in diam (about 3 per lb, whole)	1 ea	85	3/92/5	4.0[36]	0	t
5	D'Anjou, 3 in diam (about ½ lb, whole)	1 ea	120	2/93/5	6.0[36]	0	t
	Canned, fruit and liquid:						
	Heavy syrup pack:						
5	Half	1 ea	59	1/98/1	1.5[36]	0	4
	Juice pack:						
5	Half	1 ea	38	3/97/0	1.5[36]	0	3
5	Dried halves	10 ea	459	3/95/2	19.0	0	10
	Pineapple:						
5	Raw chunks, diced	1 cup	76	3/90/7	3.0	0	2
	Canned, fruit and liquid:						
	Heavy syrup pack:						
5	Slices	1 ea	45	2/98/0	0.5	0	1
	Juice pack:						
5	Slices	1 ea	35	2/98/0	0.5	0	1
5	Pineapple juice, canned, unsweetened	1 cup	140	3/96/1	1.0	0	3

[35]Dietary fiber data varies 2.4 to 3.4 grams per 100 grams for fresh pears; 1.6 to 2.6 grams per 100 grams for canned pears.

(For purposes of calculations, use "0" for t.)

Key: 1 = Bev 2 = Dairy 3 = Eggs 4 = Fat/Oil 5 = Fruit 6 = Bakery 7 = Grain 8 = Fish 9 = Meat 10 = Poultry 11 = Sausage 12 = Mixed Dishes 13 = Nuts/Seeds 14 = Sweets 15 = Veg/Leg 16 = Misc 22 = Soup/Sauce 25 = Fast Foods by Brand Name

TABLE E–1 Food Composition

Key	Name	Measure	Energy (calories)	Protein/ Carbohydrate/ Fat (%)	Fiber (g)	Cholesterol (mg)	Sodium (mg)
	FRUITS and FRUIT JUICES (cont.)						
	Plums, without pits:						
	Raw:						
5	Medium 2⅛ in diam	1 ea	36	5/86/9	1.5	0	t
	Canned, purple, with liquid:						
	Heavy syrup pack:						
5	Plums	3 ea	98	2/97/1	2.0	0	21
	Juice pack:						
5	Cup	1 cup	146	3/97/0	5.5	0	3
5	Plums	3 ea	55	3/97/0	2.0	0	1
	Prunes, dried, pitted:						
5	Uncooked (10 prunes with pits weigh 97 g):	10 ea	201	4/94/2	13.5[40]	0	3
5	Prune juice-bottled or canned	1 cup	181	3/97/0	3.0	0	10
	Raisins, seedless:						
5	One packet, ½ oz	1 ea	41	4/96/0	1.0	0	2
	Raspberries:						
5	Raw	1 cup	60	7/84/9	9.0	0	0
	Frozen, sweetened:						
5	Cup, thawed measure	1 cup	255	3/96/1	13.5	0	3
	Strawberries:						
5	Raw, whole, capped	1 cup	45	7/82/11	3.5	0	2
	Frozen, sliced, sweetened:						
5	Cup, thawed measure	1 cup	245	2/97/1	5.5	0	8
	Tangerines, without peel and seeds:						
5	Raw (2⅜ in diam)	1 ea	37	5/91/4	1.5	0	1
	Watermelon, raw, without rind and seeds						
5	Piece, 1 in thick by 10 in diam (weighs 2 lb with refuse)	1 pce	152	7/82/11	2.5	0	10
5	Diced	1 cup	50	7/82/11	1.0	0	3
	BAKED GOODS: BREADS, CAKES, COOKIES, CRACKERS, PIES, PANCAKES, TORTILLAS						
6	Bagel, plain, enriched, 3½ in diam	1 ea	200	15/77/8	0.5	0	245
	Biscuits:						
6	From mix	1 ea	94	9/60/31	0.5	t	265
	Breads:						
	Cracked wheat bread (¼ cracked wheat flour, ¾ enr wheat flour):						
6	Slice (18 per loaf)	1 pce	65	14/75/11	1.5	0	106
	French/Vienna bread, enriched:						
6	Vienna, slice 4¾ × 4 × ½ in	1 pce	70	14/73/13	0.5	0	145
	French toast: see Mixed dishes, key 12						
	Italian bread, enriched:						
6	Slice 4½ × 3¼ × ¾ in	1 pce	83	13/84/3	0.5	0	176

[40]Dietary fiber data can vary to a lower value of approx 8.1 grams for 10 prunes.

(For purposes of calculations, use "0" for t.)

Key: 1 = Bev 2 = Dairy 3 = Eggs 4 = Fat/Oil 5 = Fruit 6 = Bakery 7 = Grain 8 = Fish 9 = Meat 10 = Poultry 11 = Sausage 12 = Mixed Dishes 13 = Nuts/Seeds 14 = Sweets 15 = Veg/Leg 16 = Misc 22 = Soup/Sauce 25 = Fast Foods by Brand Name

TABLE E–1 Food Composition

Key	Name	Measure	Energy (calories)	Protein/ Carbohydrate/ Fat (%)	Fiber (g)	Cholesterol (mg)	Sodium (mg)
	BAKED GOODS (cont.)						
	Breads (cont.):						
	Mixed grain bread, enriched:						
6	Slice (18 per loaf)	1 pce	65	12/75/13	1.0	0	106
	Oatmeal bread, enriched:						
6	Slice(18 per loaf)	1 pce	65	13/72/15	1.0	0	124
6	Pita pocket bread, enr, 6½ in round	1 ea	165	15/80/5	0.5	0	339
	Pumpernickel break (⅔ rye flour, ⅓ enr wheat flour):						
6	Slice, 5 × 4 × ⅜ in	1 pce	80	14/74/12	1.5	0	277
	Raisin bread, enriched:						
6	Slice (18 per loaf)	1 pce	68	11/76/13	0.5	0	92
	Rye bread, light (⅓ rye flour, ⅔ enr wheat flour):						
6	Slice, 4¾ × 3¾ × ⁷⁄₁₆ in	1 pce	65	13/74/13	1.5	0	175
	Wheat bread[45] (blend of enr wheat flour and whole wheat flour):						
6	Slice (18 per loaf)	1 pce	65	14/72/14	1.5	0	135
	White bread, enriched:						
6	Slice (18 per loaf)	1 pce	65	13/74/13	0.5	0	129
	Whole wheat bread:						
6	Slice (16 per loaf)	1 pce	70	16/69/15	3.0	0	180
	Bread stuffing, prepared from mix:						
6	Dry type	¼ cup	125	7/39/54	0.5	0	314
6	Moist type, with egg	¼ cup	105	8/38/54	0.5	17	256
	Cakes[46], prepared from mixes:						
6	Boston cream pie, ⅛ cake	1 pce	260	4/68/28	0.5	20	225
	Coffee cake:						
6	Piece, ⅙ cake	1 pce	230	8/65/27	0.5	47	310
	Devil's food with chocolate frosting:						
6	Piece, ¹⁄₁₆ of cake	1 pce	235	5/66/29	0.5	37	181
6	Cupcake, 2½ in diam	1 ea	120	5/64/31	t	19	92
	Gingerbread:						
6	Piece, ⅑ of cake	1 pce	174	5/73/22	0.5	1	192
	Yellow, with chocolate frosting, 2 layer:						
6	Piece, ¹⁄₁₆ of cake	1 pce	235	5/66/29	0.5	36	157
	Cakes from home recipes with enriched flour:						
	Carrot cake, cream cheese frosting:						
6	Piece, ¹⁄₁₆ of 9 × 13 in sheet cake 2¼ × 3¼ in	1 pce	385	4/48/48	0.5	74	279
	Fruitcake, dark, 7½ in diam tube-2¼ in high:						
6	Piece, ¹⁄₃₂ of cake, ⅔ in arc	1 pce	165	5/58/37	1.0	20	67

[45] A blend of white and whole wheat flour—no official ratio specified.

[46] Excepting angel food cake, cakes were made from mixes containing vegetable shortening, and frostings were made with margarine. All mixes use enriched flour.

(For purposes of calculations, use "0" for t.)

Key: 1 = Bev 2 = Dairy 3 = Eggs 4 = Fat/Oil 5 = Fruit 6 = Bakery 7 = Grain 8 = Fish 9 = Meat 10 = Poultry 11 = Sausage 12 = Mixed Dishes 13 = Nuts/Seeds 14 = Sweets 15 = Veg/Leg 16 = Misc 22 = Soup/Sauce 25 = Fast Foods by Brand Name

TABLE E–1 Food Composition

Key	Name	Measure	Energy (calories)	Protein/ Carbohydrate/ Fat (%)	Fiber (g)	Cholesterol (mg)	Sodium (mg)
	BAKED GOODS (cont.)						
	Cakes (cont.):						
	Sheet cake, plain, unckd white frosting:						
6	Piece, 1/9 of cake	1 pce	445	4/68/28	0.5	70	275
	Pound cake:						
6	Piece, 1/17 of loaf	1 pce	120	7/53/40	t	32	97
	Cakes, commercial:						
	Snack cakes:						
6	Chocolate w/creme filling, 2 small cakes per package	1 ea	105	4/63/33	t	15	105
6	Sponge cake w/creme filling, 2 small cakes per package	1 ea	155	2/69/29	t	7	155
	White cake with white frosting, 2 layer cake, 8 or 9 in:						
6	Piece, 1/16 of cake	1 pce	260	5/64/31	0.5	3	176
	Yellow cake with chocolate frosting, 2 layer cake:						
6	Piece, 1/16 of cake	1 pce	245	4/59/37	0.5	38	192
	Cheesecake:						
6	Piece, 1/12 of cake	1 pce	278	7/37/56	0.5	170	204
	Cookies made with enriched flour:						
	Brownies with nuts:						
6	Commercial with frosting, 1½ × 1¾ × 7/8 in	1 ea	100	4/59/37	t	14	59
6	Home recipe, 1¾ × 1¾ × 7/8 in	1 ea	95	5/41/54	t	18	51
	Chocolate chip cookies:						
6	Commercial, 2¼ in diam	4 ea	180	5/56/39	t	5	140
6	Home recipe, 2⅓ in diam	4 ea	185	4/50/46	1.0	18	82
6	From refrigerated dough, 2¼ in diam	4 ea	225	4/54/42	t	22	173
6	Fig bars	4 ea	210	4/80/16	1.0	27	180
6	Oatmeal raisins cookies, 2⅝ in diam	4 ea	245	5/59/36	t	2	148
6	Peanut butter cookie, home recipe, 2⅝ in diam	4 ea	245	6/44/50	1.0	22	142
6	Sandwich-type cookies, all	4 ea	195	4/59/37	t	0	189
	Shortbread cookies:						
6	Commercial, small	4 ea	155	5/50/45	t	27	123
6	Sugar cookies from refrigerated dough, 2½ in diam	4 ea	235	3/52/45	t	29	261
6	Vanilla wafers	10 ea	185	4/62/34	t	25	150
6	Corn chips	1 oz	155	5/42/53	0.5	0	233
	Crackers:						
6	Cheese crackers	10 ea	50	7/44/49	t	6	112
6	Cheese crackers with peanut butter	4 ea	150	11/47/42	t	4	338
6	Graham crackers	2 ea	60	7/71/22	1.5	0	86
6	Melba toast, plain	1 pce	20	18/70/12	t	0	44
6	Rye wafers, whole grain	2 ea	55	8/75/17	1.5	0	115
6	Saltine crackers	4 ea	50	8/72/20	t	4	165
6	Snack-type crackers, Ritz	3 ea	45	5/47/48	t	0	90
6	Wheat cracker, thin	4 ea	35	11/55/34	0.5	0	69

(For purposes of calculations, use "0" for t.)

Key: 1 = Bev 2 = Dairy 3 = Eggs 4 = Fat/Oil 5 = Fruit 6 = Bakery 7 = Grain 8 = Fish 9 = Meat 10 = Poultry 11 = Sausage 12 = Mixed Dishes 13 = Nuts/Seeds 14 = Sweets 15 = Veg/Leg 16 = Misc 22 = Soup/Sauce 25 = Fast Foods by Brand Name

TABLE E-1 Food Composition

Key	Name	Measure	Energy (calories)	Protein/ Carbohydrate/ Fat (%)	Fiber (g)	Cholesterol (mg)	Sodium (mg)
	BAKED GOODS (cont.)						
	Crackers (cont.):						
6	Whole wheat wafers	2 ea	35	11/53/36	0.5	0	59
6	Croissant, 4½×4×1¾ in	1 ea	235	8/46/46	0.5	13	452
	Danish pastry:						
6	Round piece, plain, 4¼ in diam, 1 in high	1 ea	220	7/46/47	0.5	49	218
6	Round piece with fruit	1 pce	235	6/46/48	0.5	56	233
	Doughnuts:						
6	Cake type, plain, 3¼ in diam	1 ea	210	5/45/50	0.5	20	192
6	Yeast-leavened, glazed, 3¾ in diam	1 ea	235	7/44/49	0.5	21	222
	English muffin:						
6	Plain, enriched	1 ea	140	14/79/7	1.5	0	378
	Muffins, 2½ in diam, 1½ in high:						
	From commercial mix:						
6	Blueberry	1 ea	140	7/62/31	1.5	45	225
6	Bran	1 ea	140	8/67/25	2.0	28	385
6	Cornmeal	1 ea	145	8/57/35	1.5	42	291
	Pancakes, 4 in diam:						
6	Buckwheat, from mix; egg and milk added	1 ea	55	36/48/16	1.5	20	125
6	Plain, from mix; egg, milk, oil added	1 ea	60	14/55/31	0.5	16	160
	Pies, 9 in diam; pie crust made with veg shortening, enriched flour:						
	Apple pie[55]:						
6	Piece, ⅙ of pie	1 pce	405	4/58/38	3.0	0	476
	Banana cream pie[56]:						
6	⅙ of pie	1 pce	320	8/57/35	1.5	15	422
	Cherry pie[55]:						
6	Piece, ⅙ of pie	1 pce	410	4/58/38	2.5	0	480
	Chocolate cream pie[57]:						
6	Piece, ⅙ of pie	1 pce	311	9/54/37	0.5	15	428
	Custard pie:						
6	Piece, ⅙ of pie	1 pce	293	11/46/43	0.5	148	333
	Lemon meringue pie[55]:						
6	Piece, ⅙ of pie	1 pce	355	5/59/36	1.0	137	395
	Peach pie[55]:						
6	Piece, ⅙ of pie	1 pce	405	3/59/38	3.0	0	423
	Pecan pie[55]:						
6	Piece, ⅙ of pie	1 pce	583	4/61/35	1.5	137	304
	Pumpkin pie[55]:						
6	Piece, ⅙ of pie	1 pce	375	9/54/37	2.5	109	325
	Pies, fried, commercial:						
6	Apple	1 ea	255	3/49/48	1.5	14	326
6	Cherry	1 ea	250	3/49/48	1.5	13	371
	Pretzels, made with enriched flour:						
6	Thin sticks, 2¼ in long	10 ea	10	10/82/8	t	0	48

[55]Recipes updated for latest USDA values for fruits/nuts/fruit juice.
[56]Recipe based on pie crust, cooked vanilla pudding, 2 bananas.
[57]Based on values for pie crust, cooked chocolate pudding with meringue.

(For purposes of calculations, use "0" for t.)

Key: 1 = Bev 2 = Dairy 3 = Eggs 4 = Fat/Oil 5 = Fruit 6 = Bakery 7 = Grain 8 = Fish 9 = Meat 10 = Poultry 11 = Sausage 12 = Mixed Dishes 13 = Nuts/Seeds 14 = Sweets 15 = Veg/Leg 16 = Misc 22 = Soup/Sauce 25 = Fast Foods by Brand Name

TABLE E–1 Food Composition

Key	Name	Measure	Energy (calories)	Protein/ Carbohydrate/ Fat (%)	Fiber (g)	Cholesterol (mg)	Sodium (mg)
	BAKED GOODS (cont.)						
	Pretzels (cont.):						
6	Thin twists, 3¼ × 2¼ × ¼ in	10 ea	240	10/82/8	1.5	0	966
	Rolls and buns, enriched:						
	Commercial:						
6	Hotdog bun	1 ea	115	12/71/17	1.0	0	241
6	Hamburger bun	1 ea	129	12/71/17	1.0	0	271
6	Hard roll, white, 3¾ in diam, 2 in high	1 ea	155	13/76/11	1.0	0	313
6	Submarine roll or hoagie, 11½ × 3 × 2½ in	1 ea	400	12/80/8	2.0	0	683
6	Toaster pastry, fortified	1 ea	210	4/71/25	0.5	0	248
	Tortillas:						
6	Corn, enriched, 6 in diam	1 ea	65	12/75/13	1.0	0	1
6	Flour, 8 in diam	1 ea	105	9/69/22	1.0	0	134
6	Taco shell	1 ea	48	7/56/37	0.5	0	50
	Waffles, 7 in diam:						
6	From home recipe	1 ea	245	11/42/47	1.5	102	445
6	From mix, egg/milk added	1 ea	205	13/52/35	1.5	59	515
	GRAIN PRODUCTS: CEREALS, FLOUR, GRAINS, PASTA and NOODLES, POPCORN						
	Barley, pearled:						
7	Cooked	1 cup	196	9/88/3	4.5	0	2
	Breakfast cereals, hot, cooked:						
	Corn grits (hominy) cooked:						
7	White, instant, prepared from packet	1 ea	80	10/88/2	0.5	0	343
	Cream of Wheat®, cooked:						
7	Regular, quick, instant	1 cup	140	11/85/4	0.5	0	5[64,65]
7	Mix 'n eat, plain, packet	1 ea	100	12/84/4	0.5	0	241
7	Malt-O-Meal® cereal, cooked	1 cup	122	12/86/2	0.5	0	2[65]
	Oatmeal or rolled oats, cooked:						
7	Regular, quick, instant, non-fortified	1 cup	145	16/69/15	9.0	0	1[65]
	Instant, fortified:						
7	Plain, from packet	¾ cup	104	17/69/14	7.0	0	285[60]
7	Flavored, from packet	¾ cup	160	12/77/11	6.5	0	254[60]
7	Whole wheat cereal, cooked	1 cup	110	15/79/6	5.5	0	3
	Breakfast cereals, ready to eat:						
7	All-Bran®	⅓ cup	70	15/81/4	8.5	0	320
7	Cheerios®	1 cup	89	15/71/14	1.0	0	246
7	Corn Flakes, Kellogg's®	1¼ cup	110	9/91/0	0.5	0	351
7	40% Bran Flakes, Kellogg's®	1 cup	125	13/83/4	5.5	0	363
7	Grape Nuts®	½ cup	202	20/79/1	3.5	0	394
7	Nature Valley® Granola	1 cup	503	9/57/34	7.5	0	232
7	Product 19®	1 cup	126	10/88/2	0.5	0	378
7	Raisin Bran, Kellogg's®	1 cup	211	9/85/6	6.0	0	386
7	Rice Krispies, Kellogg's®	1 cup	112	7/91/2	t	0	340
7	Puffed Rice	1 cup	56	6/92/2	t	0	t
7	Shredded Wheat	¾ cup	115	11/83/6	4.0	0	3

[60]Salt added.

[64]For regular and instant cereal. For quick cereal, sodium is 142 mg.

[65]Cooked without salt. If salt added as directed, sodium content is 390 mg for Cream of Wheat, 324 mg for Malt-O-Meal, 374 mg for oatmeal.

(For purposes of calculations, use "0" for t.)

Key: 1 = Bev 2 = Dairy 3 = Eggs 4 = Fat/Oil 5 = Fruit 6 = Bakery 7 = Grain 8 = Fish 9 = Meat 10 = Poultry 11 = Sausage 12 = Mixed Dishes 13 = Nuts/Seeds 14 = Sweets 15 = Veg/Leg 16 = Misc 22 = Soup/Sauce 25 = Fast Foods by Brand Name

TABLE E–1   Food Composition

Key	Name	Measure	Energy (calories)	Protein/ Carbohydrate/ Fat (%)	Fiber (g)	Cholesterol (mg)	Sodium (mg)
	GRAIN PRODUCTS (cont.)						
	Breakfast cereals (cont.):						
7	Special K®	1½ cup	125	20/79/1	0.5	0	298
7	Sugar Frosted Flakes®	1 cup	133	5/94/1	0.5	0	284
7	Total®	1 cup	116	11/84/5	2.5	0	409
7	Wheaties®	1 cup	101	10/86/4	3.5	0	363
	Bulgar:						
7	Cooked	1 cup	246	17/79/4	7.0	0	3
	Cornmeal:						
7	Degermed, enriched, cooked	1 cup	120	9/87/4	1.0	0	1
	Macaroni, cooked:						
7	Tender stage, cold	1 cup	115	13/84/3	1.0	0	1
7	Tender stage, hot	1 cup	155	13/83/4	1.0	0	1
	Noodles:						
7	Egg noodles, cooked	1 cup	200	14/77/9	t	50	3
7	Chow mein, dry	1 cup	220	10/46/44	t	5	450
	Popcorn:						
7	Air popped, plain	1 cup	30	13/76/11	1.5	0	1
7	Popped in veg oil/salted	1 cup	55	7/43/50	1.5	0	86
7	Sugar syrup coated	1 cup	135	6/88/6	0.5	0	1
	Rice:						
7	Brown rice, cooked	1 cup	232	8/87/5	4.0	0	0
	White, enriched, all types:						
7	Cooked without salt	1 cup	223	7/92/1	1.0	0	0
7	Instant, prepared without salt	1 cup	180	8/91/1	0.5	0	0[66]
	White, parboiled/converted rice:						
7	Cooked, hot	1 cup	186	8/91/1	0.5	0	9
7	Wild rice, cooked	½ cup	92	16/82/2	2.5	0	2
	Spaghetti, cooked:						
7	Tender stage, hot	1 cup	155	13/84/3	1.0	0	1
7	Wheat bran	½ cup	38	18/70/12	8.0	0	3
	Wheat germ:						
7	Toasted	1 cup	431		3.0	0	2
7	Whole grain wheat, cooked	⅓ cup	28	13/81/6	1.0	0	2
	FISH and SHELLFISH						
	Clams:						
8	Canned, drained	3 oz	85	60/9/31	t	54	102
	Cod:						
8	Baked with butter	3½ oz	114	63/0/37	0	60	224
8	Batter fried	3½ oz	199	39/15/46	0	55	100
8	Poached, no added fat	3½ oz	94	89/0/11	0	60	110
8	Crab meat, canned	1 cup	135	75/3/22	0	135	1350
8	Fish sticks	2 ea	140	36/24/40	t	52	106
	Flounder/sole, baked with lemon juice:						
8	With margarine	3 oz	120	54/0/46	0	55	151
8	Without added fat	3 oz	80	88/0/12	0	57	101

[66]If prepared with salt as directed, sodium would equal 608 mg.

(For purposes of calculations, use "0" for t.)

Key: 1 = Bev 2 = Dairy 3 = Eggs 4 = Fat/Oil 5 = Fruit 6 = Bakery 7 = Grain 8 = Fish 9 = Meat 10 = Poultry 11 = Sausage 12 = Mixed Dishes 13 = Nuts/Seeds 14 = Sweets 15 = Veg/Leg 16 = Misc 22 = Soup/Sauce 25 = Fast Foods by Brand Name

TABLE E–1   Food Composition

Key	Name	Measure	Energy (calories)	Protein/ Carbohydrate/ Fat (%)	Fiber (g)	Cholesterol (mg)	Sodium (mg)
	FISH and SHELLFISH (cont.)						
8	Haddock, breaded/fried[67]	3 oz	175	38/16/46	t	75	123
	Halibut, broiled with butter and						
8	lemon juice	3 oz	140	60/0/40	0	62	103
8	Ocean perch, breaded/fried	3 oz	185	33/15/52	t	66	138
	Oysters:						
	Raw:						
8	Eastern	1 cup	160	54/22/24	0	120	175
8	Pacific	1 cup	160	52/20/28	0	120	185
	Cooked:						
8	Eastern, breaded, fried	1 ea	90	24/24/52	0	35	70
8	Western, simmered	3½ oz	135	46/24/30	0	77	165
	Salmon:						
8	Canned pink, solids and liquid	3 oz	120	60/0/40	0	34	443
8	Broiled or baked	3 oz	140	65/0/35	0	60	55
8	Smoked	3 oz	150	50/0/50	0	51	1700
8	Atlantic sardines canned, drained	3 oz	175	49/0/51	0	85	425
8	Scallops, breaded, from frozen	6 ea	195	32/21/47	t	70	298
	Shrimp:						
8	Cooked, boiled	3½ oz	109	88/0/12	0	147	180
8	Canned, drained	3 oz	100	87/4/9	0	128	1955
8	Fried, 7 medium[69]	3 oz	200	32/22/46	t	168	384
8	Trout, broiled with butter and lemon juice	3 oz	175	50/1/49	0	71	122
	Tuna, canned, drained solids:						
8	Oil pack	3 oz	165	60/0/40	0	55	303
8	Water pack	3 oz	135	93/0/7	0	48	468
	MEAT and MEAT PRODUCTS						
	Beef, cooked:[70]						
	Braised, simmered, pot roasted:						
	Relatively fat, like chuck blade:						
	Lean and fat, piece						
9	2½ × 2½ × ¾ in	3 oz	325	27/0/73	0	87	51
9	Lean only	2.2 oz	170		0	66	44
	Relatively lean, like round:						
9	Lean and fat, piece						
	4⅛ × 2¼ × ¾ in	3 oz	220	48/0/52	0	81	43
9	Lean only	2.8 oz	175	58/0/42	0	75	40
	Ground beef, broiled, patty 3 × ⅝ in:						
9	Lean	3 oz	230	37/0/63	0	74	65
9	Regular	3 oz	245	53/0/47	0	76	70
9	Liver, fried	3 oz	185	51/15/34	0	410	90
	Roast, oven cooked, no added liquid:						
	Relatively fat, rib:						
9	Lean and fat, piece 4⅛ × 2¼ × ½ in	3 oz	315	25/0/75	0	72	54

[67]Dipped in egg, milk and breadcrumbs; fried in vegetable shortening.
[69]Dipped in egg, breadcrumbs, and flour; fried in vegetable shortening.
[70]Outer layer of fat removed to about ½ in of the lean. Deposits of fat within the cut remain.

(For purposes of calculations, use "0" for t.)

Key: 1 = Bev 2 = Dairy 3 = Eggs 4 = Fat/Oil 5 = Fruit 6 = Bakery 7 = Grain 8 = Fish 9 = Meat 10 = Poultry 11 = Sausage 12 = Mixed Dishes 13 = Nuts/Seeds 14 = Sweets 15 = Veg/Leg 16 = Misc 22 = Soup/Sauce 25 = Fast Foods by Brand Name

TABLE E–1   Food Composition

Key	Name	Measure	Energy (calories)	Protein/ Carbohydrate/ Fat (%)	Fiber (g)	Cholesterol (mg)	Sodium (mg)
	MEAT and MEAT PRODUCTS (cont.)						
	Beef (cont.):						
9	Lean only	2.2 oz	150	46/0/54	0	49	45
	Relatively lean, round:						
9	Lean and fat, piece						
	2½ × 2½ × ¾ in	3 oz	205	46/0/54	0	62	50
9	Lean only	2.6 oz	135	66/0/34	0	52	46
	Steak, broiled, sirloin:						
9	Lean and fat, piece 2½ × 2½ × ¾ in	3 oz	240	41/0/59	0	77	53
9	Lean only	2.5 oz	150	62/0/38	0	64	48
9	Beef, canned, corned	3 oz	185	49/0/51	0	80	802
9	Beef, dried, chipped	2.5 oz	145	73/0/27	0	46	3053
	Lamb, cooked:						
	Chops (3 per lb with bone):						
	Arm chop, braised:						
9	Lean and fat	2.2 oz	220	37/0/63	0	77	46
9	Lean only	1.7 oz	135	52/0/48	0	59	36
	Loin chop, broiled:						
9	Lean and fat	2.8 oz	235	38/0/62	0	78	62
9	Lean only	2.3 oz	140	58/0/42	0	60	54
	Leg, roasted:						
9	Lean and fat, piece						
	4⅛ × 2¼ × ½ in	3 oz	205	43/0/57	0	78	57
9	Lean only	3 oz	163	60/0/40	0	76	58
	Pork, cured, cooked (see also Sausages):						
9	Bacon, medium slices	3 pce	109	78/0/22	0	16	303
9	Canadian-style bacon	2 pce	86	55/3/42	0	27	719
	Ham, roasted:						
9	Lean and fat, 2 pieces						
	4⅛ × 2¼ × ¼ in	3 oz	207	36/0/64	0	53	1009
9	Lean only	3 oz	133	67/0/33	0	47	1128
9	Ham, canned, roasted	3 oz	140	52/1/47	0	35	908
	Pork, fresh, cooked:						
	Chops, loin (cut 3 per lb with bone):						
	Broiled:						
9	Lean and fat	3.1 oz	275	36/0/64	0	84	61
9	Lean only	1 ea	166	58/0/42	0	71	56
	Pan fried:						
9	Lean and fat	1 ea	334	25/0/75	0	92	64
9	Lean only	1 ea	178	44/0/56	0	71	57
	Leg, roasted:						
9	Lean and fat, piece						
	2½ × 2½ × ¾ in	3 oz	250	34/0/66	0	79	50
9	Lean only	3 oz	187	53/0/47	0	80	54

(For purposes of calculations, use "0" for t.)

Key: 1 = Bev 2 = Dairy 3 = Eggs 4 = Fat/Oil 5 = Fruit 6 = Bakery 7 = Grain 8 = Fish 9 = Meat 10 = Poultry 11 = Sausage 12 = Mixed Dishes 13 = Nuts/Seeds 14 = Sweets 15 = Veg/Leg 16 = Misc 22 = Soup/Sauce 25 = Fast Foods by Brand Name

TABLE E-1 Food Composition

Key	Name	Measure	Energy (calories)	Protein/ Carbohydrate/ Fat (%)	Fiber (g)	Cholesterol (mg)	Sodium (mg)
	MEAT and MEAT PRODUCTS (cont.)						
	Pork (cont.):						
	Rib, roasted:						
9	Lean and fat, piece						
	2½ × 2½ × ¾ in	3 oz	270	32/0/68	0	69	37
9	Lean only	2½ oz	175	48/0/52	0	56	33
	Shoulder, braised:						
9	Lean and fat, 3 pieces,						
	2½ × 2½ × ¼ in	3 pce	295	31/0/69	0	93	75
9	Lean only	2.4 oz	165	55/0/45	0	76	68
	Veal, medium fat, cooked:						
	Veal cutlet, braised or broiled,						
9	4⅛ × 2¼ × ½ in	3 oz	185	52/0/48	0	109	56
	POULTRY and POULTRY PRODUCTS						
	Chicken, cooked:						
	Fried batter dipped:						
10	Breast (5.6 oz with bones)	1 ea	364	39/14/47	t	119	385
10	Drumstick (3.4 oz with bones)	1 ea	193	33/15/54	t	62	194
10	Thigh	1 ea	238	32/13/55	t	80	248
10	Wing	1 ea	159	25/14/61	t	39	157
	Fried, flour coated:						
10	Breast (4.2 oz with bones)	1 ea	218	60/3/37	t	88	74
10	Drumstick (2.6 oz with bones)	1 ea	120	45/3/52	t	44	44
10	Thigh	1 ea	162	42/5/53	t	60	55
10	Wing	1 ea	103	33/3/64	t	26	25
	Roasted:						
10	Dark meat	1 cup	286	56/0/44	0	130	130
10	Light meat	1 cup	242	75/0/25	0	118	108
10	Breast, without skin	½ ea	142	80/0/20	0	73	64
10	Drumstick	1 ea	76	69/0/31	0	41	42
10	Thigh	1 ea	153	42/0/58	0	58	52
10	Chicken meat, stewed, all types	1 cup	248	64/0/36	0	116	98
10	Chicken liver, simmered	1 ea	30	54/19/27	0	126	10
	Turkey, roasted, meat only:						
10	Dark meat	3 oz	159	64/0/36	0	72	67
10	Light meat	3 oz	133	81/0/19	0	59	54
	Poultry food products (see also Sausages):						
10	Canned, boneless chicken	5 oz	235	55/0/45	0	88	714
10	Gravy and turkey, frozen package	5 oz	95	36/28/36	0.5	26	787
10	Turkey loaf breast meat	2 pce	46	86/0/14	0	17	608
	SAUSAGES and LUNCHMEATS						
	Bologna:						
11	Beef and pork	1 pce	89	15/4/81	0	16	289
11	Turkey	2 pce	113	28/2/70	0	56	498
	Brown and serve sausage links,						
11	cooked	1 ea	50	15/1/84	0	9	105
	Frankfurter (see also Chicken Frankfurter):						
11	Beef and pork	1 ea	145	14/3/83	0	23	504

(For purposes of calculations, use "0" for t.)

Key: 1 = Bev 2 = Dairy 3 = Eggs 4 = Fat/Oil 5 = Fruit 6 = Bakery 7 = Grain 8 = Fish 9 = Meat 10 = Poultry 11 = Sausage
12 = Mixed Dishes 13 = Nuts/Seeds 14 = Sweets 15 = Veg/Leg 16 = Misc 22 = Soup/Sauce 25 = Fast Foods by Brand Name

TABLE E–1 Food Composition

Key	Name	Measure	Energy (calories)	Protein/ Carbohydrate/ Fat (%)	Fiber (g)	Cholesterol (mg)	Sodium (mg)
	SAUSAGES and LUNCHMEATS (cont.)						
	Frankfurter (cont.):						
11	Turkey	1 ea	102	25/3/72	0	44	550
	Ham:						
11	Ham luncheon meat, canned						
	3 × 2 × ½ in	1 pce	70	15/2/83	0	13	271
11	Ham lunchmeat, regular	2 pce	103	40/7/53	0	32	746
11	Ham lunchmeat, extra lean	2 pce	75	62/3/35	0	27	810
11	Turkey ham	2 pce	75	61/1/38	0	32	565
11	Pork sausage link, cooked[75]	1 ea	50	22/1/77	0	11	168
	Salami:						
11	Pork and beef	2 pce	145	23/3/74	0	37	607
11	Turkey	2 pce	111	34/1/65	0	46	535
11	Dry, beef and pork	2 pce	85	22/2/76	0	16	372
11	Sandwich spread, pork and beef	1 tbsp	35	13/20/67	0	6	152
11	Vienna sausage, canned	1 ea	45	15/3/82	0	8	152
	MIXED DISHES						
12	Beef and vegetable stew, homemade	1 cup	220	29/27/44	3.5	71	292
12	Beef pot pie, homemade[76]	1 pce	515	16/31/53	1.0	42	596
12	Chicken and noodles, home recipe	1 cup	365	25/29/46	1.0	103	600
12	Chicken chow mein, canned	1 cup	95	26/66/8	5.0	8	725
12	Chicken pot pie, home recipe[76]	1 pce	545	17/31/52	1.5	56	594
12	Chili con carne with beans, canned	1 cup	339	22/37/41	5.0	28	1354
12	Chop suey with beef and pork	1 cup	300	34/17/49	2.5	68	1053
12	Cole slaw[78]	1 cup	84	6/64/30	2.5	10[145]	28
12	French toast, home recipe[143]	1 pce	156	16/40/44	1.0	140	257
	Macaroni and cheese:						
12	Canned[79]	1 cup	230	16/45/39	1.5	24	730
12	Home recipe[49]	1 cup	430	16/37/47	1.0	44	1086
12	Quiche lorraine[76], ⅛ of 8 in quiche	1 pce	600	9/19/72	0.5	285	653
	Spaghetti (enriched) in tomato sauce:						
	With cheese:						
12	Canned	1 cup	190	12/79/9	2.5	3	955
12	Home recipe	1 cup	260	14/56/30	2.5	8	955
	With meatballs:						
12	Canned	1 cup	260	19/46/35	3.0	23	1220
12	Home recipe	1 cup	330	22/36/42	3.0	89	1009
	Burrito[80]:						
12	Beef and bean	1 ea	390	21/40/39	5.0	52	516
12	Bean	1 ea	322	16/57/27	8.0	15	1030
	Cheeseburger:						
12	Regular	1 ea	300	20/36/44	1.5	44	672
12	4 oz patty	1 ea	524	21/28/51	2.5	104	1224

[49]Made with margarine.
[75]One patty (8 per pound) of bulk sausage is equivalent to 2 links.
[76]Crust made with vegetable shortening and enriched flour.
[78]Recipe: 41% cabbage, 12% celery, 12% table cream, 12% sugar, 7% green pepper, 6% lemon juice, 4% onion, 3% pimiento, 3% vinegar, 2% salt, dry mustard, and white pepper.
[79]Made with corn oil.
[80]Made with a 10½ inch diameter flour tortilla.
[143]Recipe: 35% whole milk, 32% white bread, 29% egg and cooked in 4% margarine.

(For purposes of calculations, use "0" for t.)

Key: 1 = Bev 2 = Dairy 3 = Eggs 4 = Fat/Oil 5 = Fruit 6 = Bakery 7 = Grain 8 = Fish 9 = Meat 10 = Poultry 11 = Sausage 12 = Mixed Dishes 13 = Nuts/Seeds 14 = Sweets 15 = Veg/Leg 16 = Misc 22 = Soup/Sauce 25 = Fast Foods by Brand Name

TABLE E–1 Food Composition

Key	Name	Measure	Energy (calories)	Protein/ Carbohydrate/ Fat (%)	Fiber (g)	Cholesterol (mg)	Sodium (mg)
	MIXED DISHES (cont.)						
12	Chicken patty sandwich	1 ea	436	23/31/46	1.5	68	2732
12	Corn dog	1 ea	330	12/33/55	t	37	1252
12	Enchilada	1 ea	235	25/30/45	2.0	19	1332
12	English muffin with egg, cheese, bacon	1 ea	360	20/35/45	1.5	213	832
	Fish sandwich:						
12	Regular with cheese	1 ea	420	15/37/48	1.5	56	667
12	Large without cheese	1 ea	470	15/35/50	1.5	90	621
	Hamburger with bun:						
12	Regular	1 ea	245	27/18/55	1.5	32	463
12	4 oz patty	1 ea	445	23/34/43	1.5	71	763
12	Hotdog/frankfurter and bun	1 ea	260	13/33/54	1.0	23	745
12	Cheese pizza, ⅛ of 15 in round[76]	1 pce	290	20/53/27	2.0	56	699
12	Roast beef sandwich	1 ea	345	26/39/35	1.5	55	757
12	Beef taco	1 ea	195	18/31/51	1.0	21	456
12	Potato salad with mayonnaise and egg[81]	1 cup	358	8/35/57	3.5	170	1323
12	Tuna salad[83]	1 cup	375	35/20/45	2.5	80	877
	NUTS, SEEDS, and PRODUCTS						
	Almonds:						
	Whole, dried:						
13	Ounce	1 oz	167	13/13/74	3.0[85]	0	3[86]
13	Almond butter	1 tbsp	101	9/12/79	1.5	0	2[87]
13	Brazil nuts, dry (about 7)	1 oz	186	8/7/85	2.5	0	0
	Cashew nuts:						
	Dry roasted, salted:						
13	Ounce	1 oz	163	10/21/69	1.5	0	181[88]
	Oil roasted, salted:						
13	Ounce	1 oz	163	10/19/71	1.5	0	177[89]
	Coconut:						
	Raw:						
13	Shredded/grated[91]	1 cup	283	4/16/80	11.0	0	16
	Dried, shredded/grated:						
13	Unsweetened	1 cup	515	4/13/83	19.0	0	29
13	Sweetened	1 cup	466	2/37/61	19.0	0	244
	Filberts (hazelnuts), chopped:						
13	Ounce	1 oz	179	8/9/83	2.0	0	1
	Macadamia nuts, oil roasted, salted:						
13	Ounce	1 oz	204	4/7/89	1.0	0	74[92]
	Mixed nuts, salted:						
13	Dry roasted	1 cup	814	11/16/73	11.0	0	91[93]
13	Roasted in oil	1 cup	876	10/13/77	11.0	0	926[93]

[76]Crust made with vegetable shortening and enriched flour.

[81]Recipe: 62% potatoes, 12% egg, 8% mayonnaise, 7% celery, 6% sweet pickle relish, 2% onion, 1% each for green pepper, pimiento, salt, and dry mustard.

[83]Made with drained chunk light tuna, celery, onion, pickle relish, and mayonnaise-type salad dressing.

[85]Values reported for dietary fiber in almonds vary from 7.0 to 14.3 per 100 grams.

[86]Salted almonds contain 1108 mg sodium per cup, 221 mg sodium per ounce.

[87]Salted almond butter contains 72 mg sodium per tablespoon.

[88]Dry roasted cashews without salt contain 21 mg of sodium per cup or 4 mg per ounce.

[89]Oil roasted cashews without salt contain 22 mg sodium per cup or 5 mg per ounce.

[91]1 cup packed = 130 grams

[92]Macadamia nuts without salt contain 9 mg sodium per cup or 2 mg per ounce.

[93]Mixed nuts without salt contain about 15 mg sodium per cup.

(For purposes of calculations, use "0" for t.)

Key: 1 = Bev 2 = Dairy 3 = Eggs 4 = Fat/Oil 5 = Fruit 6 = Bakery 7 = Grain 8 = Fish 9 = Meat 10 = Poultry 11 = Sausage
12 = Mixed Dishes 13 = Nuts/Seeds 14 = Sweets 15 = Veg/Leg 16 = Misc 22 = Soup/Sauce 25 = Fast Foods by Brand Name

TABLE E–1 Food Composition

Key	Name	Measure	Energy (calories)	Protein/ Carbohydrate/ Fat (%)	Fiber (g)	Cholesterol (mg)	Sodium (mg)
	NUTS, SEEDS and PRODUCTS (cont.)						
	Peanuts:						
	Oil roasted, salted:						
13	Ounce	1 oz	165	17/12/71	2.0	0	123[94]
	Dried, unsalted:						
13	Ounce	1 oz	161	17/11/72	2.5	0	5
13	Peanut butter	1 tbsp	95	18/10/72	1.0	0	75[95]
	Pecans, halved, dried:						
13	Ounce	1 oz	190	4/10/86	1.5[96]	0	3[97]
13	Pine nuts/pinyon, dried	1 oz	161	7/11/82	1.5	0	20
13	Pistachio nuts, dried, shelled	1 oz	164	13/16/71	1.5	0	2[98]
13	Pumpkin kernels, dried, unsalted	1 oz	154	17/12/71	1.5	0	5[99]
13	Sesame seeds, hulled, dry	¼ cup	221	17/6/77	6.0	0	15
	Sunflower seed kernels:						
13	Dry	¼ cup	205	15/12/73	2.0	0	1
13	Oil roasted	¼ cup	208	13/9/78	2.0	0	205[100]
	Black walnuts, chopped:						
13	Ounce	1 oz	172	15/7/78	2.5	0	0
	English walnuts, chopped:						
13	Ounce	1 oz	182	8/11/81	2.0	0	3
	SWEETENERS and SWEETS (see also Dairy (milk desserts) and Baked Goods):						
14	Caramel, plain or chocolate	1 oz	115	3/74/23	t	1	64
	Chocolate (see also Syrups and Miscellaneous):						
	Milk chocolate:						
14	Plain	1 oz	145	5/42/53	0.5	6	23
14	With almonds	1 oz	150	7/36/57	1.0	5	23
14	With peanuts	1 oz	155	12/24/64	1.5	3	19
14	With rice cereal	1 oz	140	6/50/44	1.0	6	46
14	Sweet dark chocolate	1 oz	150	3/40/57	1.0	0	5
	Fondant candy, uncoated (mints, candy corn, other)						
14	candy corn, other)	1 oz	105	0/100/0	0	0	57
14	Fudge, chocolate	1 oz	115	2/75/23	t	1	54
14	Hard candy, all flavors	1 oz	109	0/100/0	0	0	7
14	Marshmallows	4 ea	90	3/97/0	0	0	25
14	Gelatin salad/dessert	½ cup	70	10/90/0	t	0	55
	Honey:						
14	Tablespoon	1 tbsp	65	0/100/0	0	0	1
	Jam or preserves:						
14	Tablespoon	1 tbsp	54	1/99/0	t	0	2
	Jellies:						
14	Tablespoon	1 tbsp	49	0/100/0	0	0	4
14	Popsicle, 3 oz when fluid	1 ea	70	0/100/0	0	0	11
	Sugars:						
14	Brown sugar	1 tbsp	51	0/100/0	0	0	6

[94]Peanuts without salt contain 22 mg sodium per cup or 4 mg per ounce.
[95]Peanut butter without added salt contains 3 mg sodium per tablespoon.
[96]Dietary fiber data calculated/derived from data on other nuts.
[97]Salted pecans contain 816 mg sodium per cup and 214 mg per ounce.
[98]Salted pistachios contain approx 221 mg sodium per ounce.
[99]Salted pumpkin/squash kernels contain approx 163 mg sodium per ounce.
[100]Unsalted sunflower seeds contain 1 mg sodium per ¼ cup.

(For purposes of calculations, use ''0'' for t.)

Key: 1 = Bev 2 = Dairy 3 = Eggs 4 = Fat/Oil 5 = Fruit 6 = Bakery 7 = Grain 8 = Fish 9 = Meat 10 = Poultry 11 = Sausage 12 = Mixed Dishes 13 = Nuts/Seeds 14 = Sweets 15 = Veg/Leg 16 = Misc 22 = Soup/Sauce 25 = Fast Foods by Brand Name

TABLE E–1 Food Composition

Key	Name	Measure	Energy (calories)	Protein/ Carbohydrate/ Fat (%)	Fiber (g)	Cholesterol (mg)	Sodium (mg)
	SWEETENERS and SWEETS (cont.)						
	Sugars (cont.):						
	White sugar, granulated						
14	Tablespoon	1 tbsp	45	0/100/0	0	0	t
	White sugar, powdered, sifted	1 tbsp	24	0/100/0	0	0	t
	Syrups:						
	Chocolate:						
14	Thin type	2 tbsp	85	5/90/5	1.0	0	36
14	Fudge type	2 tbsp	125	6/61/33	1.0	0	42
14	Molasses, blackstrap	2 tbsp	85	0/100/0	0	0	38
	Pancake table syrup (corn and						
14	maple)	¼ cup	244	0/100/0	0	0	38
	VEGETABLES and LEGUMES						
15	Alfalfa seeds, sprouted	1 cup	10	44/41/15	1.0	0	2
15	Artichoke, cooked globe (300 g with						
	refuse)	1 ea	53	18/79/3	4.0	0	79
	Asparagus, green, cooked:						
	From raw:						
15	Cuts and tips	½ cup	22	33/57/10	1.5	0	4
15	Spears, ½ in diam at base	4 spears	15	34/56/10	1.0	0	2
	From frozen:						
15	Cuts and tips	1 cup	50	33/56/11	3.0	0	7
15	Spears, ½ in diam at base	4 spears	17	33/54/13	1.0	0	2
15	Canned, spears, ½ in diam at base	4 spears	11	35/42/23	1.5	0	278[101]
15	Bamboo shoots, canned, drained slices	1 cup	25	30/55/15	3.5	0	9
	Beans (see also Great northern beans, Kidney beans, Navy beans, Pinto beans, Refried beans, Soybeans):						
15	Black beans, cooked	1 cup	225	26/71/3	15.5	0	1
	Lima beans:						
	Thin-seeded (baby), cooked						
15	from frozen	½ cup	94	25/72/3	5.0	0	26
	Snap bean/green beans, cuts and french style:						
15	Cooked from raw	1 cup	44	18/75/7	3.0	0	4
15	Cooked from frozen	1 cup	36	17/79/4	3.5	0	17
15	Canned, drained	1 cup	26	20/77/3	2.0	0	340[104]
	Navy beans, canned:						
	Pork and beans with						
15	tomato sauce	1 cup	311	20/61/19	18.5	10	1181
	Pork and beans with sweet						
15	sauce	1 cup	383	16/56/28	18.0	8	969
15	Beans with frankfurters	1 cup	365	21/35/44	17.5	30	1374
	Bean sprouts (mung):						
15	Raw	1 cup	32	32/63/5	1.5	0	6
	Beets:						
	Cooked from fresh:						
15	Sliced or diced	½ cup	26	14/86/0	2.0	0	42
	Canned:						
15	Sliced or diced	½ cup	27	11/86/3	2.0	0	233[106]
15	Pickled slices	½ cup	74	5/94/1	2.5	0	301

[101]Special dietary pack contains 3 mg sodium.
[104]Dietary pack contains 3 mg sodium.
[106]Dietary pack contains 39 mg sodium.

(For purposes of calculations, use "0" for t.)

Key: 1 = Bev 2 = Dairy 3 = Eggs 4 = Fat/Oil 5 = Fruit 6 = Bakery 7 = Grain 8 = Fish 9 = Meat 10 = Poultry 11 = Sausage 12 = Mixed Dishes 13 = Nuts/Seeds 14 = Sweets 15 = Veg/Leg 16 = Misc 22 = Soup/Sauce 25 = Fast Foods by Brand Name

TABLE E–1　Food Composition

Key	Name	Measure	Energy (calories)	Protein/ Carbohydrate/ Fat (%)	Fiber (g)	Cholesterol (mg)	Sodium (mg)
	VEGETABLES and LEGUMES (cont.)						
	Blackeyed peas, cooked:						
15	From fresh, drained	1 cup	179	29/65/6	7.0	0	7
15	From frozen, drained	1 cup	224	25/71/4	7.5	0	9
	Broccoli:						
	Raw:						
15	Chopped	1 cup	24	33/58/9	3.5	0	24
15	Spears	1 spear	42	33/59/8	5.5	0	41
	Cooked from raw:						
15	Spears	1 spear	53	32/61/7	7.5	0	20
15	Chopped	1 cup	46	32/62/6	6.5	0	16
	Cooked from frozen:						
15	Spears	1 spear	8	36/64/0	1.0	0	7
15	Chopped	1 cup	51	36/61/3	6.0	0	44
	Brussels sprouts:						
15	Cooked from raw	1 cup	60	28/64/8	5.5	0	17
15	Cooked from frozen	1 cup	65	28/65/7	5.0	0	36
	Cabbage, common varieties:						
15	Raw, shredded or chopped	1 cup	16	16/79/5	1.5	0	12
15	Cooked, drained	1 cup	32	15/76/9	4.0	0	29
	Chinese cabbage:						
15	Bok choy or pak-choi, cooked, drained	1 cup	20	41/48/11	3.5	0	57
	Carrots:						
	Raw:						
15	Whole, 7½ × 1⅛ in	1 carrot	31	8/89/3	2.0	0	25
	Cooked, sliced, drained:						
15	Cooked from raw	½ cup	35	9/89/2	3.0	0	52
15	Cooked from frozen	½ cup	26	13/87/0	2.5	0	43
15	Canned, sliced, drained	½ cup	17	18/74/8	2.0	0	176[108]
15	Carrot juice	¾ cup	73	9/88/3	2.5	0	54
	Cauliflower:						
15	Raw, flowerets	½ cup	12	29/71/0	1.5	0	7
	Cooked, drained, flowerets:						
15	From raw	½ cup	15	28/67/5	1.5	0	4
15	From frozen	1 cup	34	27/65/8	4.0	0	33
	Celery, pascal-type, raw:						
15	Large outer stalk, 8 × 1½ in (at root end)	1 stalk	6	18/82/0	1.0	0	35
	Chickpeas (see Garbanzo)						
	Collards, cooked, drained:						
15	From raw	1 cup	20	27/65/8	4.0	0	27
15	From frozen	1 cup	61	27/65/8	5.0	0	85
	Corn:						
	Cooked, drained:						
15	From raw, on cob, 5 in long	1 ear	83	11/80/9	3.5	0	13
15	From frozen, on cob, 3½ in long	1 ear	59	12/82/6	3.0	0	3
15	Kernels, cooked from frozen	½ cup	67	13/87/0	4.0	0	4

[108]Dietary pack contains 31 mg sodium.

(For purposes of calculations, use "0" for t.)

Key: 1 = Bev 2 = Dairy 3 = Eggs 4 = Fat/Oil 5 = Fruit 6 = Bakery 7 = Grain 8 = Fish 9 = Meat 10 = Poultry 11 = Sausage 12 = Mixed Dishes 13 = Nuts/Seeds 14 = Sweets 15 = Veg/Leg 16 = Misc 22 = Soup/Sauce 25 = Fast Foods by Brand Name

TABLE E–1   Food Composition

Key	Name	Measure	Energy (calories)	Protein/ Carbohydrate/ Fat (%)	Fiber (g)	Cholesterol (mg)	Sodium (mg)
	VEGETABLES and LEGUMES (cont.)						
	Corn (cont.):						
	Canned:						
15	Cream style	½ cup	93	8/88/4	6.5	0	365[110]
15	Whole kernel, vacuum pack	1 cup	166	11/84/5	10.0	0	572[111]
	Cowpeas (see Blackeyed peas)						
15	Cucumber with peel, ⅛ in thick, 2⅛ in diam	6 slices	4	20/80/0	0.5	0	1
15	Eggplant, cooked	1 cup	45	10/83/7	6.0	0	5
15	Garbanzo beans (chickpeas), cooked	1 cup	270	22/65/13	8.5	0	11
15	Great northern beans, cooked	1 cup	210	26/70/4	12.5	0	13
15	Escarole/curly endive, chopped	1 cup	8	14/39/47	1.0	0	11
15	Kidney beans, canned	1 cup	230	25/72/3	20.0	0	968
15	Lentils, cooked from dry	1 cup	215	28/68/4	10.0	0	26
	Lettuce:						
	Butterhead/Boston types:						
15	Leaves, 2 inner or outer	2 leaves	2	40/60/0	0.5	0	t
	Iceberg/crisphead:						
15	Wedge, ¼ of head	1 wedge	18	29/57/14	2.5	0	12
15	Chopped or shredded	1 cup	7	30/59/11	1.0	0	5
	Romaine:						
15	Chopped	1 cup	9	37/54/9	1.0	0	4
	Mushrooms:						
15	Raw, sliced	½ cup	9	28/63/9	1.0	0	1
15	Cooked from raw, pieces	½ cup	21	26/61/13	2.0	0	2
15	Canned, drained	½ cup	19	26/67/7	2.0	0	332
	Mustard greens:						
15	Cooked from raw	1 cup	21	47/43/10	3.0	0	22
15	Cooked from frozen	1 cup	28	38/52/10	4.0	0	38
15	Navy beans, cooked from dry	1 cup	225	26/70/4	16.5	0	13
	Okra, cooked:						
15	From fresh pods	8 pods	27	20/77/3	3.0	0	4
15	From frozen slices	½ cup	34	19/74/7	3.0	0	3
	Onions:						
	Raw:						
15	Chopped	1 cup	54	13/81/6	2.5	0	3
15	Sliced	1 cup	39	13/81/6	2.0	0	2
15	Cooked, drained, chopped	½ cup	30	10/84/6	1.5	0	8
15	Dehydrated flakes	¼ cup	45	9/91/0	1.5	0	3
15	Onions, spring, chopped, bulb and top	½ cup	13	24/76/0	1.5	0	2
15	Onion rings, breaded, prepared from frozen	2 rings	80	5/40/55	t	0	75
	Parsley:						
	Raw:						
15	Chopped	½ cup	10	25/75/0	2.0	0	12
15	Freeze dried	¼ cup	4	40/60/0	0.5	0	5
	Peas (see also Blackeyed peas):						
15	Edible pods, cooked	1 cup	67	30/65/5	5.0	0	6
	Green:						
15	Canned, drained	½ cup	59	25/71/4	5.5	0	186[113]
15	Cooked from frozen	½ cup	63	26/71/3	7.5	0	70

[110]Dietary pack contains 4 mg sodium per ½ cup.
[111]Dietary pack contains 6 mg sodium per cup.
[113]Dietary pack contains 1.7 mg sodium.

(For purposes of calculations, use "0" for t.)

Key: 1 = Bev 2 = Dairy 3 = Eggs 4 = Fat/Oil 5 = Fruit 6 = Bakery 7 = Grain 8 = Fish 9 = Meat 10 = Poultry 11 = Sausage 12 = Mixed Dishes 13 = Nuts/Seeds 14 = Sweets 15 = Veg/Leg 16 = Misc 22 = Soup/Sauce 25 = Fast Foods by Brand Name

TABLE E–1 Food Composition

Key	Name	Measure	Energy (calories)	Protein/ Carbohydrate/ Fat (%)	Fiber (g)	Cholesterol (mg)	Sodium (mg)
	VEGETABLES and LEGUMES (cont.)						
	Peas (cont.):						
15	Split, green, cooked from dry	1 cup	230	27/71/2	10.0	0	26
	Peppers, hot:						
	Hot green chili:						
15	Canned	½ cup	17	12/88/0	1.0	0	10
15	Raw	1 pepper	18	17/83/0	1.0	0	3
15	Jalapenos, chopped, canned	½ cup	17	11/70/19	2.5	0	995
	Peppers, sweet, green:						
15	Whole pod (90 g with refuse), raw	1 pod	18	12/75/13	1.5	0	2
15	Pinto beans, cooked from dry	1 cup	265	23/74/3	19.0	0	3
	Potatoes						
	Baked in oven, 4¾ × 2⅓ in diam:						
15	With skin	1 potato	220	8/91/1	4.5	0	16
15	Flesh only	1 potato	145	8/91/1	4.0	0	8
	Boiled, about 2½ in diam:						
15	Peeled before boiling	1 ea	116	8/91/1	1.5	0	7
	French-fried, strips 2 to 3½ in long, frozen:						
15	Oven heated	10 strips	111	6/59/35	1.5	0	15
15	Fried in veg oil	10 strips	158	5/49/46	1.5	0	108
15	Hashed brown, from frozen	1 cup	340	6/49/45	1.5	0	53
	Mashed:						
15	Home recipe with milk and margarine	1 cup	222	7/59/34	1.0	4[123]	619
15	Prepared from flakes; water, milk, butter, salt added	1 cup	237	6/51/43	1.0	4[123]	697
	Potato products, prepared:						
	Au gratin:						
15	From dry mix	1 cup	228	9/53/38	4.0	12	1076
15	From home recipe[119]	1 cup	322	15/34/51	4.5	56[120]	1064
	Potato salad (see Mixed foods)						
	Scalloped:						
15	From dry mix	1 cup	228	9/52/39	4.5	27	835
15	Home recipe[124]	1 cup	210	13/49/38	4.5	29[125]	821
15	Potato chips	14 chips	148	5/37/58	0.5	0	133[126]
15	Red radishes	10 radishes	7	14/76/10	1.0	0	11
15	Refried beans, canned	1 cup	295	24/67/9	22.0	0	1228
15	Sauerkraut, canned with liquid	1 cup	44	16/79/5	4.5	0	1561
	Soybean products:						
15	Miso	3 tbsp	88	23/53/24	1.0[128]	0	1534
15	Tofu, piece 2½ × 2¾ × 1 in	1 pce	86	40/12/48	2.0[128]	0	8
	Spinach:						
15	Raw, chopped	1 cup	12	40/49/11	2.5	0	44

[119]Recipe: 55% potatoes; 30% whole milk; 9% cheddar cheese; 3% butter; 2% flour; 1% salt.

[120]For butter; if margarine is used, cholesterol = 37 mg.

[123]For margarine; if butter is used, cholesterol = 25 mg for 29 total mg.

[124]Recipe: 59% potatoes; 36% whole milk; 2% butter; 2% flour; 1% salt.

[125]For butter; if margarine is used cholesterol = 15 mg.

[126]If no salt is added, sodium = 2 mg.

[128]Estimate based on cooked soybeans.

(For purposes of calculations, use "0" for t.)

Key: 1 = Bev 2 = Dairy 3 = Eggs 4 = Fat/Oil 5 = Fruit 6 = Bakery 7 = Grain 8 = Fish 9 = Meat 10 = Poultry 11 = Sausage 12 = Mixed Dishes 13 = Nuts/Seeds 14 = Sweets 15 = Veg/Leg 16 = Misc 22 = Soup/Sauce 25 = Fast Foods by Brand Name

TABLE E–1 Food Composition

Key	Name	Measure	Energy (calories)	Protein/ Carbohydrate/ Fat (%)	Fiber (g)	Cholesterol (mg)	Sodium (mg)
	VEGETABLES and LEGUMES (cont.)						
	Spinach (cont.):						
	Cooked, drained:						
15	From raw	1 cup	41	40/51/9	6.0	0	126
15	From frozen (leaf)	1 cup	53	35/60/5	6.5	0	163
15	Canned, drained solids	1 cup	50	38/46/16	7.5	0	683[129]
	Squash, summer varieties, cooked slices:						
15	Crookneck	1 cup	36	16/78/6	3.0	0	2
15	Zucchini	1 cup	29	13/87/0	3.0	0	5
	Squash, winter varieties, cooked:						
15	Acorn, baked, mashed	1 cup	83	7/91/2	6.0	0	6
15	Butternut, baked cubes	1 cup	83	7/91/2	5.0	0	7
	Sweet potatoes:						
	Cooked, 5 × 2 in diam:						
15	Baked in skin, peeled	1 potato	118	7/92/1	3.0	0	12
15	Boiled without skin	1 potato	160	5/93/2	4.0	0	20
15	Candied, 2½ × 2 in	1 pce	144	2/78/20	2.0	0[131]	74
	Canned:						
15	Solid pack, mashed	1 cup	258	8/91/1	6.5	0	191
	Tomatoes:						
	Raw:						
15	Whole, 2⅗ in diam	1 tomato	24	16/75/9	2.0	0	10
15	Cooked from raw	1 cup	60	15/76/9	5.5	0	25
15	Canned, solids and liquid	1 cup	47	16/74/10	2.0	0	390[134]
15	Tomato juice, canned	1 cup	42	15/83/2	1.5	0	881[135]
	Tomato products, canned:						
15	Paste	1 cup	220	15/77/8	6.0	0	170[136]
15	Puree	1 cup	102	14/84/2	4.0	0	49[137]
15	Sauce	1 cup	74	15/81/4	3.0	0	1481[138]
	Turnip greens, cooked:						
15	From raw (leaves and stems)	1 cup	29	19/73/8	4.0	0	41
15	From frozen (chopped)	½ cup	24	37/54/9	2.5	0	12
15	Vegetable juice cocktail, canned	1 cup	46	12/85/3	1.5	0	883
	Vegetables, mixed:						
15	Canned, drained	1 cup	77	21/75/4	6.5	0	243
15	Frozen, cooked, drained	1 cup	107	18/80/2	7.5	0	64
	Water chestnuts, canned:						
15	Slices	½ cup	35	6/94/0	0.5	0	6
	MISCELLANEOUS						
16	Basil, ground	1 tbsp	11	18/70/12	1.0	0	2
	Catsup:						
16	Tablespoon	1 tbsp	18	7/93/0	t	0	156
16	Celery seed	1 tsp	8	17/37/46	0.5	0	4
16	Chili powder	1 tsp	8	12/54/34	0.5	0	26

[129]Dietary pack contains 58 mg sodium.

[131]For recipe using margarine; if butter is used cholesterol = 8 mg.

[134]Dietary Pack contains 31 mg sodium.

[135]If no salt is added, sodium content is 24 mg.

[136]If salt is added, sodium content is 2070 mg.

[137]If salt is added, sodium content is 998 mg.

[138]With salt added.

(For purposes of calculations, use "0" for t.)

Key: 1 = Bev 2 = Dairy 3 = Eggs 4 = Fat/Oil 5 = Fruit 6 = Bakery 7 = Grain 8 = Fish 9 = Meat 10 = Poultry 11 = Sausage 12 = Mixed Dishes 13 = Nuts/Seeds 14 = Sweets 15 = Veg/Leg 16 = Misc 22 = Soup/Sauce 25 = Fast Foods by Brand Name

TABLE E–1 Food Composition

Key	Name	Measure	Energy (calories)	Protein/ Carbohydrate/ Fat (%)	Fiber (g)	Cholesterol (mg)	Sodium (mg)
	MISCELLANEOUS (cont.)						
	Chocolate:						
16	Baking	1 oz	145	8/17/75	2.0	0	1
	Semi-sweet, milk, and dark chocolates (see Sweets and Sweeteners)						
16	Cinnamon	1 tsp	5	0/100/0	0.5	0	1
16	Curry powder	1 tsp	5	10/58/32	0.5	0	1
	Garlic:						
16	Cloves	4 cloves	18	17/83/0	t	0	2
16	Powder	1 tsp	9	20/80/0	t	0	1
16	Gelatin, dry, plain	1 envelope	25	100/0/0	1.0	0	6
16	Ginger root, raw, sliced	5 slices	8	11/89/0	t	0	1
	Mustard, prepared, packet (1 packet=1						
16	tsp)	1 tsp	4	21/32/47	t	0	63
16	Miso (see Vegetables, soybean products)						
	Olives:						
16	Green	10 olives	45	3/3/94	1.5	0	936
16	Ripe, pitted[140]	10 olives	50	3/22/75	1.5	0	410
16	Onion powder	1 tsp	5	10/90/0	t	0	1
16	Oregano, ground	1 tsp	5	12/61/27	t	0	t
16	Paprika	1 tsp	6	13/57/30	0.5	0	1
16	Pepper, black	1 tsp	5	12/88/0	0.5	0	1
	Pickles:						
16	Dill, medium, 3¾ × 1¼ in diam	1 pickle	5	24/66/10	1.0	0	928
16	Fresh pack, slices, 1½ in diam × ¼ in thick	4 slices	20	5/95/0	0.5	0	201
16	Sweet, small, about 2½ × ¾ in diam	1 pickle	20	0/100/0	t	0	107
16	Pickle relish, sweet	1 tbsp	20	0/100/0	0.5	0	107
	Popcorn (see Grains)						
16	Salt	1 tsp	0	0/0/0	0	0	2132
16	Vinegar, cider	1 tbsp	2	0/100/0	0	0	t
	SOUPS, SAUCES, and GRAVIES						
	Soups, canned, condensed:						
	Prepared with equal volume of whole milk:						
22	Clam chowder, New England	1 cup	163	23/41/36	2.5	22	992
22	Cream of chicken	1 cup	191	16/31/53	t	27	1046
22	Cream of mushroom	1 cup	205	12/29/59	0.5	20	1076
22	Tomato	1 cup	160	14/54/32	0.5	17	932
	Prepared with equal volume of water:						
22	Bean with bacon	1 cup	173	18/52/30	2.5	3	952
22	Beef broth, bouillon, consomme	1 cup	16	56/21/23	0	1	782
22	Beef noodle	1 cup	84	23/43/34	t	3	952
22	Chicken noodle	1 cup	75	21/49/30	t	7	1106
22	Chicken rice	1 cup	60	23/48/29	1.0	7	815
22	Clam chowder, Manhattan	1 cup	78	19/57/24	1.0	2	1808
22	Cream of chicken	1 cup	115	11/32/57	0.5	10	986
22	Cream of mushroom	1 cup	130	6/30/64	1.5	2	1032
22	Minestrone	1 cup	80	20/53/27	1.0	2	911
22	Split pea with ham	1 cup	189	21/58/21	0.5	0	1008

[140]This is the most recent tested data from the California Olive industry, October 1986.

(For purposes of calculations, use "0" for t.)

Key: 1 = Bev 2 = Dairy 3 = Eggs 4 = Fat/Oil 5 = Fruit 6 = Bakery 7 = Grain 8 = Fish 9 = Meat 10 = Poultry 11 = Sausage 12 = Mixed Dishes 13 = Nuts/Seeds 14 = Sweets 15 = Veg/Leg 16 = Misc 22 = Soup/Sauce 25 = Fast Foods by Brand Name

TABLE E–1 Food Composition

Key	Name	Measure	Energy (calories)	Protein/ Carbohydrate/ Fat (%)	Fiber (g)	Cholesterol (mg)	Sodium (mg)
	SOUPS, SAUCES, and GRAVIES (cont.)						
	Soups (cont.):						
22	Tomato	1 cup	86	9/72/19	0.5	0	872
22	Vegetable beef	1 cup	79	28/51/21	1.0	5	956
22	Vegetarian vegetable	1 cup	70	11/66/23	1.0	0	823
	Soups, dehydrated:						
	Unprepared, dry products:						
22	Bouillon	1 packet	15	24/24/52	0	1	1019
22	Onion	1 packet	20	14/70/16	t	t	627
	Prepared with water:						
22	Chicken noodle	¾ cup	40	19/59/22	t	2	957
22	Onion	¾ cup	20	15/69/16	t	0	635
22	Tomato vegetable	¾ cup	41	14/71/15	0.5	0	856
	Sauces:						
	From dry mixes:						
22	Cheese sauce, prepared with milk	1 cup	305	20/30/50	t	53	1565
22	Hollandaise, prepared with water	1 cup	240	8/22/70	—	52	1564
22	White sauce, prepared with milk	1 cup	240	16/35/49	0.5	34	797
	Ready to serve:						
22	Barbeque sauce	1 tbsp	10	7/58/35	t	0	128
22	Soy sauce	1 tbsp	11	48/52/0	0	0	1029
	Gravies:						
	Canned:						
22	Beef	1 cup	124	27/35/38	0.5	7	117
22	Chicken	1 cup	189	9/27/64	t	5	1375
22	Mushroom	1 cup	120	10/44/46	0.5	0	1357
	FAST FOODS BY BRAND NAME						
	McDONALD'S[142]						
25	Chicken McNuggets®	—	323	24/17/59	—	73	512
25	Hamburger	—	263	19/43/38	—	29	506
25	Cheeseburger	—	328	19/36/45	—	41	743
25	Quarter Pounder®	—	427	23/27/50	—	81	718
25	Quarter Pounder® w/Cheese	—	525	23/23/54	—	107	1220
25	Big Mac®	—	570	17/28/55	—	83	979
25	Filet-O-Fish®	—	435	14/33/53	—	45	799
25	Mc D.L.T.®	—	680	18/23/59	—	101	1030
25	French fries, regular	—	220	5/48/47	—	9	109
25	Biscuit w/sausage, egg	—	585	14/25/61	—	285	1301
25	Egg McMuffin®	—	340	22/36/42	—	259	885
25	Hot cakes w/butter, syrup	—	500	6/75/19	—	47	1070
25	English muffin w/butter	—	186	11/63/26	—	15	310
25	Hash brown potatoes	—	125	5/45/50	—	7	325
25	Chocolate shake	—	383	10/69/21	—	30	300
25	Hot fudge sundae	—	357	8/65/27	—	27	170
25	Apple pie	—	253	3/46/51	—	12	398
25	McDonaldland® Cookies	—	308	5/64/31	—	10	358

[142]*Source:* McDonald's Corp, Oak Brook, Illinois. Nutrient analyses by Hazelton Laboratory of America (formerly Raltech Scientific Services Inc), Madison, Wisconsin.

(For purposes of calculations, use "0" for t.)

Key: 1 = Bev 2 = Dairy 3 = Eggs 4 = Fat/Oil 5 = Fruit 6 = Bakery 7 = Grain 8 = Fish 9 = Meat 10 = Poultry 11 = Sausage 12 = Mixed Dishes 13 = Nuts/Seeds 14 = Sweets 15 = Veg/Leg 16 = Misc 22 = Soup/Sauce 25 = Fast Foods by Brand Name

TABLE E–1 Food Composition

Key	Name	Measure	Energy (calories)	Protein/ Carbohydrate/ Fat (%)	Fiber (g)	Cholesterol (mg)	Sodium (mg)
	FAST FOODS (cont.)						
	WENDY'S[143]						
25	Single hamburger, multigrain bun	—	340	30/24/46	—	67	290
25	Bacon cheeseburger, white bun	—	460	25/20/55	—	65	860
25	Chicken sandwich, multigrain bun	—	320	32/40/28	—	59	500
25	Chili, 8 oz	—	260	32/40/28	—	30	1070
25	French fries, regular	—	280	5/50/45	—	15	95
25	Taco salad	—	390	23/36/41	—	40	1100
25	Frosty dairy dessert	—	400	8/60/32	—	50	220
25	Hot stuffed baked potatoes	—	250	10/83/7	—	t	60
25	Ham & cheese omelet	—	250	29/10/61	—	450	405
25	Breakfast sandwich	—	370	18/36/46	—	200	770
25	French toast, 2 slices	—	400	11/46/43	—	115	850
25	Home fries	—	360	4/41/55	—	20	745
	COCA-COLA[144]						
25	Coca-Cola classic®	—	144	0/100/0	—	—	—
25	Coca-Cola®	—	154	0/100/0	—	—	—
25	Cherry Coke®	—	154	0/100/0	—	—	—
25	Diet Coke®**	—	1	0/100/0	—	—	—
25	Sprite®	—	142	0/100/0	—	—	—
25	Mr. Pibb®	—	142	0/100/0	—	—	—
25	Mello Yello®	—	172	0/100/0	—	—	—
25	Ramblin' Root Beer®	—	158	0/100/0	—	—	—
25	Fanta® Orange	—	164	0/100/0	—	—	—
25	Fanta® Grape	—	168	0/100/0	—	—	—
25	Fanta® Root Beer	—	158	0/100/0	—	—	—
25	Fanta® Ginger Ale	—	126	0/100/0	—	—	—
25	Hi-C® Orange***	—	152	0/100/0	—	—	—
25	Hi-C® Lemon***	—	142	0/100/0	—	—	—
25	Hi-C® Punch***	—	154	0/100/0	—	—	—
25	Hi-C® Grape***	—	164	0/100/0	—	—	—
25	Tab®**	—	1	0/100/0	—	—	—
25	Diet Sprite®**	—	3	0/100/0	—	—	—
25	Minute Maid® Orange	—	160	0/100/0	—	—	—
	ARBY'S[145]						
25	Roast beef, regular	—	350	25/36/39	—	39	590
25	Beef 'n Cheddar®	—	490	20/42/38	—	51	1520
25	Chicken breast sandwich	—	592	19/39/42	—	57	1340
25	French fries	—	211	4/62/34	—	6	30
25	Bac'n Cheddar Deluxe	—	561	20/26/54	—	78	1385

[143]*Source:* Wendy's International Inc, Dublin, Ohio. Nutrient analyses: entree items, Hazelton Laboratory of America (formerly Raltech Scientific Services Inc), Madison, Wisconsin; other items, US Department of Agriculture Handbook #8.

[144]*Source:* The Coca-Cola Co, Atlanta, Georgia.
Nutritive value of fountain products, 12-oz servings without ice. **Sweetened with an aspartame-saccharin blend. Bottled and canned versions of Diet Coke and Diet Sprite are sweetened with 100% NutraSweet, a registered trademark of The NutraSweet Co for aspartame. ***Hi-C soft drinks do not contain fruit juice and are not the same as Hi-C fruit-juice-containing drinks produced by Coca-Cola Foods, a division of The Coca-Cola Co. *Source:* The Coca-Cola Co, Atlanta, Georgia.

[145]*Source:* Arby's Inc, Atlanta, Georgia. Nutritional analyses by Arby's Laboratory and other independent testing laboratories.

Key: 1 = Bev 2 = Dairy 3 = Eggs 4 = Fat/Oil 5 = Fruit 6 = Bakery 7 = Grain 8 = Fish 9 = Meat 10 = Poultry 11 = Sausage 12 = Mixed Dishes 13 = Nuts/Seeds 14 = Sweets 15 = Veg/Leg 16 = Misc 22 = Soup/Sauce 25 = Fast Foods by Brand Name

TABLE E–1 Food Composition

Key	Name	Measure	Energy (calories)	Protein/ Carbohydrate/ Fat (%)	Fiber (g)	Cholesterol (mg)	Sodium (mg)
	FAST FOODS (cont.)						
	ARBY'S (cont.):						
25	Hot Ham 'n Cheese	—	353	30/37/33	—	50	1655
25	Turkey Deluxe	—	375	25/34/41	—	39	850
25	Baked potato	—	290	11/88/1	—	0	12
25	Taco	—	619	15/46/39	—	145	1065
25	Vanilla shake	—	295	11/59/30	—	30	245
25	Chocolate shake	—	384	9/65/26	—	32	300
25	Jamocha shake	—	424	8/71/21	—	31	280
25	Roasted chicken breast	—	254	71/3/26	—	200	930
25	Roasted chicken leg	—	319	53/1/46	—	214	995
25	Chicken salad sandwich	—	386	19/34/47	—	30	630
	BURGER KING[146]						
25	Whopper Sandwich®	—	640	17/26/57	—	94	842
25	Whopper® w/cheese	—	723	17/24/59	—	117	1126
25	Double Beef Whopper®	—	850	21/24/55	—	—	1080
25	Double Beef Whopper® w/cheese	—	950	21/23/56	—	—	1535
25	Hamburger	—	275	21/41/38	—	37	509
25	Cheeseburger	—	317	21/37/42	—	48	651
25	French fries, regular	—	227	5/43/52	—	14	160
25	Onion rings, regular	—	274	6/41/53	—	0	665
25	Apple pie	—	305	4/60/36	—	4	412
25	Chocolate shake, medium	—	320	10/57/33	—	—	202
25	Vanilla shake, medium	—	321	11/61/28	—	—	205
25	Whaler® Fish Sandwich	—	488	15/36/49	—	84	592
25	Whaler® w/Cheese	—	530	16/34/50	—	95	734
25	Ham and cheese sandwich	—	471	20/37/43	—	70	1534
25	Chicken sandwich	—	688	15/33/52	—	82	1423
25	Chicken Tenders®	—	204	38/19/43	—	47	636
25	Scrambled egg platter w/bacon	—	536	14/25/61	—	378	975
	DAIRY QUEEN[147]						
25	Cone, regular	—	240	10/64/26	—	15	80
25	Dipped cone, regular	—	340	7/50/43	—	20	100
25	Sundae, regular	—	310	6/71/23	—	20	120
25	Shake, regular	—	710	8/68/24	—	50	260
25	Malt, regular	—	760	7/72/21	—	50	260
25	Float	—	410	5/80/15	—	20	85
25	Banana split	—	540	7/75/18	—	30	150
25	Parfait	—	430	8/74/18	—	30	140
25	Peanut Buster Parfait	—	740	9/50/41	—	30	250
25	Double Delight	—	490	7/56/37	—	25	150
25	Hot Fudge Brownie Delight	—	600	6/57/37	—	20	225
25	Strawberry shortcake	—	540	7/75/18	—	25	215
25	Freeze	—	500	7/71/22	—	30	180
25	Mr. Misty®, regular	—	250	0/100/0	—	0	10
25	Mr. Misty® Kiss	—	70	0/100/0	—	0	10
25	Mr. Misty® Freeze	—	500	7/72/21	—	30	140
25	Mr. Misty® Float	—	390	5/78/17	—	20	95
25	Buster Bar	—	460	9/35/56	—	10	175

[146]*Source*: Burger King Corp Inc. Nutritional analyses by Hazelton Laboratory of America (formerly Raltech Scientific Services Inc), Madison, Wisconsin, and Campbell Laboratories, Camden, New Jersey.

[147]*Source*: International Dairy Queen Inc, Minneapolis, Minnesota. Nutrient analyses by Hazelton Laboratory of America (formerly Raltech Scientific Services Inc), Madison Wisconsin.

Key: 1 = Bev 2 = Dairy 3 = Eggs 4 = Fat/Oil 5 = Fruit 6 = Bakery 7 = Grain 8 = Fish 9 = Meat 10 = Poultry 11 = Sausage 12 = Mixed Dishes 13 = Nuts/Seeds 14 = Sweets 15 = Veg/Leg 16 = Misc 22 = Soup/Sauce 25 = Fast Foods by Brand Name

TABLE E–1 Food Composition

Key	Name	Measure	Energy (calories)	Protein/ Carbohydrate/ Fat (%)	Fiber (g)	Cholesterol (mg)	Sodium (mg)
	FAST FOODS (cont.)						
	DIARY QUEEN (cont.):						
25	Dilly Bar	—	210	6/39/55	—	10	50
25	DQ Sandwich	—	140	8/67/25	—	5	40
25	Single hamburger	—	360	23/37/40	—	45	630
25	Single w/cheese	—	410	24/32/44	—	50	790
25	Hot dog	—	280	16/31/53	—	45	830
25	Hot dog w/chili	—	320	16/28/56	—	55	985
25	Hot dog w/cheese	—	330	18/25/57	—	55	990
25	Fish filet sandwich	—	400	20/41/39	—	50	875
25	Chicken sandwich	—	670	17/28/55	—	75	870
25	French fries, small	—	200	4/51/45	—	10	115
25	Onion rings	—	280	5/44/51	—	15	140
	JACK IN THE BOX[148]						
25	Hamburger	—	276	18/43/39	—	29	521
25	Cheeseburger	—	323	20/39/41	—	42	749
25	Jumbo Jack®	—	485	21/31/48	—	64	905
25	Jumbo Jack® w/Cheese	—	630	20/29/51	—	110	1665
25	Moby Jack®	—	444	14/35/51	—	47	820
25	Regular taco	—	191	16/33/51	—	21	406
25	Club pita	—	284	31/43/26	—	43	953
25	Chicken Supreme	—	601	20/26/54	—	60	1582
25	Sausage Crescent	—	584	15/19/66	—	187	1012
25	Scrambled eggs breakfast	—	719	14/31/55	—	260	1110
25	Chicken strips dinner	—	689	23/38/39	—	100	1213
25	Sirloin steak dinner	—	699	22/43/35	—	75	969
25	Cheese nachos	—	571	11/34/55	—	37	1154
25	Taco salad	—	377	33/10/57	—	102	1436
25	French fries, regular	—	221	4/48/48	—	8	164
25	Onion rings	—	382	5/41/54	—	27	407
25	Hash brown potatoes	—	68	6/44/50	—	0	15
25	Vanilla shake	—	320	12/71/17	—	25	230
25	Strawberry shake	—	320	12/68/20	—	25	240
25	Chocolate shake	—	330	14/67/19	—	25	270
25	Apple turnover	—	410	4/44/52	—	15	350
	KENTUCKY FRIED CHICKEN[149]						
	Original Recipe®						
25	Center Breast*	—	257	40/12/48	—	93	532
25	Drumstick*	—	147	37/9/54	—	81	269
25	Thigh*	—	278	26/12/62	—	122	517
	Extra Crispy®						
25	Center Breast*	—	353	31/16/53	—	93	842
25	Drumstick*	—	173	29/14/57	—	65	346
25	Thigh*	—	371	21/15/64	—	121	766
25	Kentucky Nuggets (one)	—	46	25/19/56	—	12	140
	Kentucky Nugget Sauce (oz)						
25	Barbeque	—	35	3/82/15	—	1	450
25	Sweet and Sour	—	58	1/90/9	—	1	148
25	Kentucky Fries	—	268	7/50/43	—	2	89
25	Mashed potatoes	—	59	13/78/9	—	1	228

[148]*Source:* Jack in the Box Restaurants, Foodmaker, Inc, San Diego, California. Nutrient analyses by Hazelton Laboratory of America (formerly Raltech Scientific Services Inc), Madison, Wisconsin.

[149]*Source:* Kentucky Fried Chicken Corp. Nutrient analyses by Hazelton Laboratory of America (formerly Raltech Scientific Services Inc), Madison, Wisconsin.

*edible portion

Key: 1 = Bev 2 = Dairy 3 = Eggs 4 = Fat/Oil 5 = Fruit 6 = Bakery 7 = Grain 8 = Fish 9 = Meat 10 = Poultry 11 = Sausage 12 = Mixed Dishes 13 = Nuts/Seeds 14 = Sweets 15 = Veg/Leg 16 = Misc 22 = Soup/Sauce 25 = Fast Foods by Brand Name

TABLE E–1   Food Composition

Key	Name	Measure	Energy (calories)	Protein/Carbohydrate/Fat (%)	Fiber (g)	Cholesterol (mg)	Sodium (mg)
	FAST FOODS (cont.)						
	KENTUCKY FRIED CHICKEN (cont.):						
25	Chicken gravy	—	59	13/30/57	—	2	398
25	Buttermilk biscuit	—	269	8/47/45	—	1	521
25	Potato salad	—	141	5/36/59	—	11	396
25	Baked beans	—	105	20/70/10	—	1	387
25	Corn on the cob	—	176	11/73/16	—	1	21
25	Cole slaw	—	103	5/45/50	—	4	171
	LONG JOHN SILVER'S[150]						
25	3 Pc Fish & Fryes	—	853	20/30/50	—	106	2025
25	Fish & More	—	978	14/33/53	—	88	2124
25	3 Pc Fish Dinner	—	1180	16/31/53	—	119	2797
25	4 Pc Chicken Planks Dinner	—	1037	16/32/52	—	25	2433
25	6 Pc Chicken Nuggets Dinner	—	699	13/30/57	—	25	853
25	Fish & Chicken	—	935	16/31/53	—	56	2076
25	Seafood platter	—	976	12/35/53	—	95	2161
25	Clam dinner	—	955	8/40/52	—	27	1543
25	Batter fried shrimp dinner	—	711	9/34/57	—	127	1297
25	Oyster dinner	—	789	8/40/52	—	55	763
25	2 Pc Kitchen-Breaded Fish Dinner	—	818	13/37/50	—	76	1526
25	Fish sandwich platter	—	835	15/40/45	—	75	1402
25	Seafood salad	—	426	18/20/62	—	113	1086
25	Hush puppies	—	145	8/49/43	—	1	405

[150]*Source:* Long John Silver's Inc, Lexington, Kentucky. Nutrient analyses by Department of Nutrition and Food Science, University of Kentucky.

Key: 1 = Bev 2 = Dairy 3 = Eggs 4 = Fat/Oil 5 = Fruit 6 = Bakery 7 = Grain 8 = Fish 9 = Meat 10 = Poultry 11 = Sausage 12 = Mixed Dishes 13 = Nuts/Seeds 14 = Sweets 15 = Veg/Leg 16 = Misc 22 = Soup/Sauce 25 = Fast Foods by Brand Name

Index

Numbers in boldface type refer to glossary entries. Numbers followed by an italic *n* refer to footnotes. Letters A, B, C, D, E refer to appendixes.

■ A

Medicines, 127, 130–136, **150**. *See also* Drugs; *specific entries, for example:* Antibiotics; Interleukin 2
Meditation, 34, **36**
Megadoses of nutrients, 76, **82**, 246
Melanomas, 343, **358**. *See also* Skin cancer
Menopause, 264, 265, **276**
Menstrual cycle, 194, **212**. *See also* Premenstrual syndrome
Menstruation, 194, **212**
Mental confusion, 266–267
Mental disorders, 53–55, **62**
Mental retardation, 310–311. *See also* Brain damage
Mentor, 49, **62**
Mercy killing, **276**
Metabolism
   aerobic, 110 112, **121**
   anaerobic, 110–112, **121**
   basal, 90, 101
   of carbohydrates, and diabetes, 340–341
   and exercise, 96
Metastasizing of cancer cells, 344, **358**
Microbes (microorganisms), 299, **317**
Middle age, health monitoring during, 368. *See also* Adulthood; Aging process
Midwives, 257, **258**
Milk products, 78, 79, 80, E
Mind-altering (psychoactive) drugs, 129–130, 137, **150**. *See also specific entries, for example:* Alcohol, Marijuana; Tranquilizers
Minerals, 67, 73–78, **82**. *See also* Orthomolecular psychiatrists
   calcium, 74, 76
   as electrolytes, 78, **82,** 120
   iron, 75, 77–78
   sodium, 75, 78, 79, **83,** 120
   trace, 75, 77, **83**
   in water, 396, **416**
Mineral supplements, 85
Minilalaparotomy, 228, **232**
Minimum Daily Requirements, **B**
Minipill (oral contraceptive), 222, **232**
Minor tranquilizers, **131**
Miracle cures, 7, 39
Miscarriage (spontaneous abortion), **231,** 240
Misconceptions in adulthood, 261
MOC (maximum oxygen consumption), **122**
Moderate drinkers, 156, **168**
Moderation in alcohol use, 156–159, **168–169**
Modified radical mastectomy, **358**. *See also* Mastectomy
Molds, 303, **317**
Molybdenum, 75
Mongolism (Down's syndrome), 243–244, 245

Monogamous marriage, **212**
Monogamous relationships, 209, **212**. *See also* Marriage
Monogamy, sexual, 209, **212**
Morning sickness, 241
Mortality. *See* Death; Life expectancy
Motherhood. *See* Childbirth; Pregnancy; Surrogate motherhood
Motivation, 8–10, **16**
Motives, 8, **16**
Motorcycle accidents, 284
Mucus, 177, **189**
Multiple sclerosis, **300**
Mumps, **300**, 305, 307
Muscle endurance, 107, 112, **122**
Muscle fibers, 110, **121**
Muscle relaxants, **131**
Muscle relaxation, progressive, 33–34, 36
Muscles
   abdominal, 282
   atrophy of, 110, **121**
   cancer of, 343
   as connective tissue, 114
   in fitness, **113,** 113–114, 119
   heart, 108
   hypertrophy of, 110, **122**
   involuntary (smooth), 107, **122**
   nutrition for, 117–120
   voluntary (striated), 107, **122**
Muscle stimulators in weight loss, 93
Muscle strength, 107, 112
Mutation of genes, 344, **358**
Myelomas, 343, **358**
Myocardial infarction (heart attack), 325–326, **338**
Myoclonic jerk, 123, **124**

■ N

NA (Narcotics Anonymous), 61, 165
Naprapaths, 378
Narcotics, **131,** 140–141, **150**
Narcotics Anonymous (NA), 61, 165
National Council Against Health Fraud, 7n
"Natural" (on labels), 7, 85
Natural childbirth, 258
Natural rhythms, 63–65
Naturopaths, 378
Needs, hierarchy of (Maslow), 48, 209, 277
Nervous system, 25–26, 92, 349
Neurotransmitters, 63, **64**
News about health, 6–7
Niacin, 73, 74
Nickel, 75
Nicotine, 175, 181, **189**
Nicotine-containing gum, 187
Nipple stimulation, 197
Nitrites, 361–362, **362**
Nitrosamines, 361–362, **362**

Nocturnal emissions, 301, **212**
Noise pollution, 408, **416**
Nonassertive behavior, 50–52, **62**
Nonconformists, 52, **62**
Non-Smoker's Rights Association, 182n
Norepinephrine (noradrenaline), 27, **35–36**
Norms, sexual, 194, 196
Nosocomial infections, 305, **317**
N.P. (nurse practitioner), 7, 374–375, **375**
Nuclear families, **255**. *See also* Children; Parenting
Nuclear power plants, 405–407
Nurse practitioners (N.P.s, R.N.P.s), 7, 374–375, **375**
Nursing homes, **373**
Nutrient deficiences
   mineral, 78, 85
   vitamin, 84–85
Nutrients, 67, **82,** B, E. *See also specific entries, for example:* Carbohydrates; Minerals; Vitamins
   overdoses and megadoses of, 76, **82,** 246
   during pregnancy, 242–243
Nutrient standards, B
Nutrient supplements, 84–85
Nutrition, 67–85, A. *See also* Diet *entries;* Food *entries*
   and alcohol, 68
   and cancer, 360–363
   and fitness, 116–121
   for muscles, 117–120
   and oral contraceptives, 223
   over-, 67, **82**
   before pregnancy, 238
   during pregnancy, 242–243
   under-, 67, **83**
Nutritional guidelines, **B**
Nutritionists, 378
Nutrition strategies, 78–82

■ O

OA (Overeaters Anonymous), 61, 97
Obesity, 69, 87, 101, 264
Occupational Safety and Health Administration (OSHA), 293n, A
Occupations and fitness, 109
Old age, health monitoring during, 369. *See also* Aging process
Oncogenes, 344, 348, **358**
One-day surgery centers, **373**
Open marriage, **212**
Opiates, 140–141
Opportunists (pathogenic), 299, **317**
Oral behavior as defense mechanism, **33**
Oral cancer, 183, **188,** 345, **358**
Oral contraceptives, 180, 221–224, **232**
"Organic" (on labels), 7, 85
Orgasm, 193–194, 200, 201, **212**. *See also* Sexual intercourse

Prepayment system for health care, 373, **379**

Prescription drugs, 130–131, 135–136, **150**. *See also* Medicines; *specific entries, for example:* Antibiotics; Digitalis; Fertility drugs in pregnancy, 245

Primary sex characteristics, 194, **212**

Private (proprietary) hospitals, **373**

Problem drinkers, 156, **169**

Prodrome of diseases, **305**

Progesterone, 194, **195**
synthetic (progestin), 222, **232**. *See also* Oral contraceptives

Progressive muscle relaxation, 33–34, **36**

Progressive overload principle, **122**

Projection as defense mechanism, **33**

Promoters in cancer, 343, **358**

Proof as alcohol percentage, 155, **169**

Proprietary (private) hospitals, 373

Prostaglandins, 127, **150**, 325

Protein, 67, 71–72, **82**, 91, 118, B, E *See also* Lipoproteins
percentages in foods, E

Protein-energy malnutrition (PEM), 72, **83**

Psychiatrists, **60**

Psychoactive (mind-altering) drugs, 129–130, 137, **150**. *See also specific entries, for example:* Alcohol; Marijuana; Tranquilizers

Psychoanalysis, **60**

Psychoanalysts as therapists, **60**

Psychological dependence on drugs, 129, **150**. *See also* Drugs, dependence on

Psychological problems
of aging process, 265

Psychologists are therapists, **60**

Psychosocial stressors, 21, 22

Psychotherapy, 61, **62**

Puberty, 194

Pubic lice, 310, 311

Public health centers, 366, 372

Pulse (heart rate), 110, 114

Puncture wounds, C

Pyridoxine, 74

■ Q

Quackery, 18, **19**, 46, 133, 324, 356, 376. *See also* Fraud

■ R

Radiation. *See also* X-rays
in cancer detection, 352
as cancer risk, 345–347
in cancer treatment, 355
in homes, 291–293
during pregnancy, 245, 247
ultraviolet, 346, 394

Radical mastectomy, 354, **358**

Radioactive waste, 405–406

Radioactivity, defined, 405, **416**

Radon, 292, **295**

Rainforest Action Network, 411*n*

Rainforests, loss of, 408–411

Rape prevention, 289–291

Rapid-eye movement (REM) sleep, **124**

Ratchet effect (yoyo effect) of dieting, 96, **101**

Rationalization as defense mechanism, **33**

R.D. (registered dietitian), 85, **375**, 376

RDA (Recommended Dietary Allowances), 91, **B**

Recommended Dietary Allowance (RDA), 91, **B**

Recommended Nutrient Intakes for Canadians, (RNI), **B**

Recovery in stress response, 21–24, **36**

Recreational drug use, 137, **150**

Registered dietitians (R.D.s), 85, **375**, 376

Registered nurses (R.N.s), **375**

Registration of health care providers, 376, **379**

Regression as defense mechanism, **33**

Relationships
commitment in, 208–211, **211**
power in, 213–214

Relaxation response, 33–35, **36**. *See also* Stress response

Relaxation techniques, 35, 335–336

REM (rapid-eye-movement) sleep, **124**

Repression as defense mechanism, **33**

Reproductive systems, female and male, 193–195

Resentment as emotional problem, 58–59

Reservoirs (of infection), 303, **317**

Resistance in stress response, 21–24, **36**

Resolution phase of sexual response cycle, 200, 201, **212**

Resting heart rate (pulse), 110, 114

Reye's syndrome, 132*n*

Rhythm method of contraception, 226, **232**

Riboflavin, 74

Risk
in contraception, 219–228
infectious diseases, 299–303
in pregnancy, 243–245

Risk factors
for cancer. *See* Cancer, risk factors for
for cardiovascular disease, **338**

R.N. (registered nurse), **375**

RNI (Recommended Nutrient Intakes for Canadians), **B**

R.N.P. (nurse practitioner), 7, 374–375, **375**

Rogers, Carl, 208–209

Role confusion, 47

Roles, gender, 194, **211**

Roughage (fiber), 69, **83**

Rubella (German measles), 246, **256**, 307

■ S

Saccharin, 247, 360

Safety of drugs, 130–136, **150**

Salt, 75, 78, 79, **83,** 120

Sarcomas, 343, **358**

Scrotum, 193, 194, **195**

Seattle, Chief, 412

Sebum, 302, **303**

Secondary sex characteristics, 194, **212**

Second-hand smoking, 181–182, 345

Sedatives, **131**, 140–141, 144

Selective forgetting, 33

Selenium, 75

Self
in relation to others, 49–53
in relation to society, 52–53

Self-actualization in hierarchy of needs, 48, **62**

Self-care in health, 132, 367–369, 381–386

Self-concept, 44–49. *See also* Gender identity

Self-doubt and shame, 47

Self-esteem, 44–46

Self-help groups, 61, A
for alcoholism, 165
for cancer patients, 357
in weight loss, 97

Self-hypnosis, 34, **36**

Self-image in self-esteem, 44–45

Self-talk, 59
positive, 45, **62**, 116, 356–357

Semen, 193, **195**. *See also* Artificial insemination; Sperm *entries*

Senility, 266–267, **276**

Sensuousness, 196, **212**

Septic abortion, **231**

Serotonin, 63, **64,** 124

Sets of exercise, 114, **122**

Sewage, 396–399

Sex. *see also* Gender *entries;* Love
biological, 193–196
defined, **212**

Sex characteristics, primary and secondary, 194, **212**

Sex education, 233–234

Sex glands (gonads), 193–196, **211**. *See also* Ovaries; Testes (testicles)

Sex organs
external (genitals), 193–196, **211**
internal, examining, 383, 385

Sex play, 197–198, **212**

Sexual abuse of children, 251, **255**

Sexual activity, 196–203. *See also* Sexual intercourse
and acquired immune deficiency syndrome, 315–316
and aging process, 264
and gender roles, 194, 196
masturbation as, 196
during pregnancy, 241
problems and strategies in, 201–203

Acknowledgments

Inside Back Cover. Reprinted courtesy of the Metropolitan Life Insurance Company.

Inside Back Cover. Reprinted courtesy of the Metropolitan Life Insurance Company.

Page 5, Life Choice Inventory. From "The Longevity Game©," by Northwestern Mutual Life Insurance Company, Milwaukee, Wisconsin. Copyright © 1978. Used with permission.

Page 10, Fig. 1–2. Based partly on *Slim Chance in a Fat World*, by R.B. Stuart and B. Davis (Champaign, Ill: Research Press, 1972), Figure 2, p. 76; and partly on *Self-Control-Power to the Person*, by M.J. Mahoney and C.E. Thoreson (Monterey, Calif.: Brooks/Cole Publishing, 1974), Chapter 1, pp. 3–19.

Page 22, Table 2–2. Reprinted with permission from "The Social Readjustment Rating Scale," by T.H. Holmes ad R.H. Rahe. In *Journal of Psychosomatic Research, 2*, 213–218. Copyright © 1979, Pergamon Journals, Ltd.

Page 45, Life Choice Inventory. Adapted from *Encounters with the Self*, by Don E. Hamachek. Copyright © 1971 by Holt, Rinehart and Winston, Inc. Reprinted by permission of Holt, Rinehart and Winston, Inc.

Page 79, Table 4–5. Reprinted with permission of the Dairy Council of California.

Page 80, Life Choice Inventory. Developed by Liberty Life Insurance Company, Greenville, S.C. and Roger Sargent, University of South Carolina. Used with permission of Liberty Life Insurance Company.

Page 109, Life Choice Inventory. Reprinted by permission of Russell Pate, University of South Carolina.

Page 119, Fig. 6–5. Adapted from "Something Old Something New . . .Very New," by P. Astrand. In *Nutrition Today*, June 1968, pp. 9–11.

Page 132, Fig. 7–3. Adapted from Self-medication and Self-care: An Update, in *Self-Medication: The New Era, A Symposium*, 31 March 1980. (Washington D.C.: The Proprietary Association, 1980), p. 5.

Page 139, box material. Adapted from *Managing the "Drugs" in Your Life*, by S. J. Levy. Copyright © 1983 by McGraw-Hill. All rights reserved.

Pages 148, Life Choice Inventory. Adapted from *Managing the "Drugs" in Your Life*, by S. J. Levy. Copyright © 1983 by McGraw-Hill. All rights reserved.

Page 171, box material. From "How Do You Score on Drink Quiz?" *Chicago Tribune*, October 26, 1975. Copyright © 1975, Chicago Tribune Company. All rights reserved. Used with permission.

Page 179, Table 9–1. Adapted from *Smoking or Health: It's Your Choice*, a report by the American Council on Science and Health, January 1984. Used with permission.

Page 199, Table 10–1. Adapted from "Come Ons and Put Offs: Unmarried Students' Strategies for Having and Avoiding Sexual Intercourse," by N. B. McCormick. In *Psychology of Women Quarterly*, 1979, 4, 192–211. Copyright © Human Science Press, New York. Reprinted with permission of the publisher.

Page 220, Life Choice Inventory. Adapted from "Choosing a Contraceptive: Effectiveness, Safety, and Important Personal Considerations," by R. A. Hatcher. In *Contraceptive Technology 1986–87* (New York: Irvington Publishers, 1987), pp. 1–18. Used with permission of the author.

Page 244, Table 12–1. Adapted from "Nonnutritional Factors Affecting Fetal Growth," by R. G. Newcombe. In *American Journal of Clinical Nutrition*, April

Credits for Chapter-Opening Art and Photos

Chapter 4 Garry Gay, The Image Bank.

Chapter 5 Printed by permission of the Estate of Norman Rockwell. Copyright © 1953.

Chapter 6 Al Satterwhite, The Image Bank.

Chapter 7 "Swans reflecting Elephants" (detail) by Salvador Dali, 1937. Geneva Collection Cavalieri Holding. Giraudon/Art Resource. © Demart Pro Arte/ARS N.Y., 1989.

Chapter 8 Hans Wolf, The Image Bank.

Chapter 9 "Nighthawks" by Edward Hopper, 1942, oil on canvas, 76.2 × 144 cm, Friends of American Art Collection, 1942.51 © 1988 The Art Institute of Chicago. All Rights Reserved.

Chapter 10 "The Luncheon of the Boating Party" (detail) by Pierre Auguste Renoir, 1881. The Phillips Collections, Washington, D.C.

Chapter 11 Michel Tcherevkoff, The Image Bank.

Chapter 12 Cliff Feulner, The Image Bank.

Chapter 13 © Barry Root. Represented by Jacqueline Dedell.

Chapter 14 Printed by permission of the Estate of Norman Rockwell. Copyright © 1919.

Chapter 15 "Slip Slidin' Away" by Edward McCain. © Edward McCain.

Chapter 16 "The Candy Store." (detail). 1969. Oil and Synthetic polymer on canvas. 47 3/4 × 68 3/4 inches. Collection of Whitney Museum of American Art. Purchase, with funds from the Friends of the Whitney Museum of Art. 69.21.

Chapter 17 Jules, Zalon. The Image Bank.

Chapter 18 Original painting by Marvin Mattelson.

Chapter 19 Reprinted with permission of the artist. All rights reserved. Copyright 1986 by Gene Boyer.

Photo Credits

Chapter 1 3 Jodi Buren, Sygma; 11 D. Degnan, H. Armstrong Roberts; 17 David J. Farr, Imagesmythe, Inc.;

Chapter 2 23 Jeff Persons, Stock, Boston; 34 (*top*) Peter Menzel; 34 (*bottom*) Bill Stanton, International Stock Photography; 37 Kay Chernush, The Image Bank;

Chapter 3 42 (*top left*) Co. Rentmeester, The Image Bank; 42 (*bottom left*) P. Eising, The Image Bank; 42 (*right*) Tom McHugh, Photo Researchers, Inc; 50 Cary Wolinsky, Stock, Boston; 53 Charles Gupton, Stock, Boston; 54 Flip Chalfant, The Image Bank; 56 Peter Southwick, Stock, Boston; 58 (*left*) Eric Meola, The Image Bank; 58 (*right*) Alan Becker, The Image Bank; 59 Peter Menzel; 63 David McMurtrey;

Chapter 4 68 Mark A. Mittelman, Taurus Photos; 69 Ray Stanyard; 77 Courtesy of Gjon Mill; 81 Peter Menzel; 84 Bonnie Reuch, The Image Bank;

Chapter 5 99 Anne Gardon, Taurus Photos; 102 George S. Zimbel, Monkmeyer;

Chapter 6 111 (*top*) John Blaustein, Woodfin Camp & Associates; 111 (*Bottom*) Peter Menzel; 112 A. Tannenbaum, Sygma; 116 Arthur Grace, Stock, Boston; 123 Peter Russell Clemens, International Stock Photography;

Chapter 7 133 Michael Heron, Monkmeyer; 135 Ray Ellis/Science Source, Photo Researchers, Inc.; 142 M. Salas, The Image Bank; 148 Peter Menzel; 152 Sam Abell, Woodfin Camp & Associates: